CURRENT TRENDS IN SPHINGOLIPIDOSES AND ALLIED DISORDERS

ADVANCES IN EXPERIMENTAL MEDICINE AND BIOLOGY

CURRENT TRENDS IN SPHINGOLIPIDOSES AND ALLIED DISORDERS

Edited by

Bruno W. Volk

Isaac Albert Research Institute of the Kingsbrook Jewish Medical Center
and
Downstate Medical Center
State University of New York

and

Larry Schneck

Neuroscience Center of the Kingsbrook Jewish Medical Center
Downstate Medical Center
State University of New York
and
Birth Defects Center of the Isaac Albert Research Institute

PLENUM PRESS • NEW YORK AND LONDON

Library of Congress Cataloging in Publication Data

Symposium on the Current Trends in Sphingolipidoses and Allied Disorders, 5th,
    Downstate Medical Center, 1975. Current trends in sphingolipidoses and allied
    disorders.

    (Advances in experimental medicine and biology; v. 68)
    The symposium was held "under the auspices of the Isaac Albert Research In-
stitute of the Kingsbrook Jewish Medical Center, the Department of Pathology,
Downstate Medical Center, State University of New York, Brooklyn, New York,
and the National Tay-Sachs and Allied Diseases Association, Inc., New York."
    Includes bibliographical references and index.
    1. Sphingolipidoses–Congresses. 2. Lipid metabolism disorders–Congresses. I.
Volk, Bruno W. II. Schneck, Larry. III. Title. IV. Series [DNLM: 1. Lipid meta-
bolism, Inborn errors–Congresses. 2. Sphingolipidosis–Congresses. W1 AD559 v.
68 1975/WD202.L5 I64c 1975]
RC632.S67S94 1975   616.3'99   76-2586
ISBN 978-1-4684-7737-5   ISBN 978-1-4684-7735-1 (eBook)
DOI 10.1007/ 978-1-4684-7735-1

Proceedings of the Symposium on the Current Trends in Sphingolipidoses and
Allied Disorders held at the Downstate Medical Center, State University of New
York, Brooklyn, N. Y., October 20-21, 1975

© 1976 Plenum Press, New York
Softcover reprint of the hardcover 1st edition 1976
A Division of Plenum Publishing Corporation
227 West 17th Street, New York, N. Y. 10011

United Kingdom edition published by Plenum Press London
A Division of Plenum Publishing Company, Ltd.
Davis House (4th Floor), 8 Scrubs Lane, Harlesden, London, NW10 6SE, England

Preface

The present volume contains the scientific contributions to
the Fifth International Symposium on "Current Trends in Sphingolipidoses and Allied Disorders" under the auspices of the Isaac
Albert Research Institute of the Kingsbrook Jewish Medical Center,
the Department of Pathology, Downstate Medical Center, State University of New York, Brooklyn, New York, and the National Tay-Sachs
and Allied Diseases Association, Inc., New York.

A review of the four previous Symposia shows the increase in
scope of the scientific exploration in this rapidly expanding field.
The first meeting, held in 1958, was devoted to the discussion almost entirely of Tay-Sachs disease. The majority of the work
emanated from local laboratories. The participants at the present
Symposium came from many other domestic and foreign research in-
stitutions. The scope of the papers presented at these meetings
and the interest shown in the Symposium demonstrates the significance attached by the scientific community to the problems of these
hereditary diseases. The reasons for this are apparent, when one
considers the contributions during recent years to our basic knowledge by lipid and enzyme chemistry, genetics, and neuropathology.
Partly because of the hereditary nature of these diseases any new
discovery in this field has general meaning and permits cautious
generalization well beyond its clinical significance.

The complexity of the brain lipids has presented the biochem-
ist with a continuous challenge as to the development of adequate
methods for their analysis and characterization and inspired electron microscopists to investigate the fine structure of the affected tissues. Many of the authors who explored the mucopolysaccharidoses and leucodystrophies as well as the sphingolipidoses
have given recognition to the investigative efforts held in common
by the otherwise diverse disease processes.

The multiphasic approach to the study of these disorders has
resulted in a considerable cross-fertilization within related
fields and also has lead to the discoveries of new diseases. Up

to this date many enzyme deficiencies underlying most of these genetic afflictions have been elucidated.

Since the last Symposium held in 1971, the problems of prevention and possible therapy of these diseases have been given considerable attention. Laboratory screening procedures which are designed to detect carriers of these various disorders have been made available and the prospective identification of heterozygotes has become a powerful adjunct in genetic counseling.

A unique feature of this Symposium was the constant awareness of the clinical implications of the fundamental studies presented. This was due not only to the participation of clinicians and the presentation of papers by them, but also to the existence at Kingsbrook Jewish Medical Center of a clinical unit which is devoted exclusively to the care and study of patients with inborn errors of lipid metabolism.

Because of the lack of time the following papers could not be presented at the Symposium. However, the Editors feel that because of their quality and informational content they deserve to be included in the book: Kamoshita et al., Collins et al., Dubois et al., and Hösli.

The Editors are indebted to Mrs. Renee Brenner, Mrs. Sarah Ginsberg, and Mrs. Ethel Ginsburg, secretaries at the Isaac Albert Research Institute, as well as to Miss Raie Sones, Administrative Assistant, State University of New York, Downstate Medical Center. Moreover, the contributions of Mr. Herbert A. Fischler, Chief Medical Photographer, in the technical management of the Symposium are gratefully acknowledged.

The Editors hope that the collection of the scientific papers heard at these meetings will convey to the readers a comprehensive survey of this complicated subject and may stimulate still other workers to apply their scientific skills to this area of investigation.

Finally, they would like to thank the staff of Plenum Publishing Corporation for their excellent preparation and for the prompt publication of these proceedings.

B.W.V.
L.S.
Brooklyn, New York

October, 1975

Contents

SIMPLE ULTRA-MICROTECHNIQUES FOR GENETIC COMPLEMENTATION

ANALYSIS AND EARLY PRENATAL DIAGNOSIS OF SPHINGOLIPIDOSES

P. HÖSLI

Dept. Molecular Biology

Institut Pasteur, 25 rue du Dr. Roux, Paris, France

There are two good reasons for introducing simple ultra-micro enzyme assays into clinical work : one is the frequent sparsity of the materials available for diagnostic procedures ; the other is the restricted availability and the high costs of natural substrates. Microchemical methods of limited sensitivity have been successfully introduced into practical clinical work by Mattenheimer (10). Ultra-microchemistry, which has been defined as the measurement of substrates or of enzyme activites in volumes of less than 10 μl, has, on the other hand, not been widely employed by clinicians ; this is probably due to the fact that the only practical ultra-micro-technique, Lowry's enzymatic cycling method (9), is too involved to be used in the daily routine.

The purpose of the present paper is to make available to practitioners simple microtechniques which have been developed since 1963. These techniques, which are based on the design of the *Plastic Film Dish* and the development of the *Parafilm Micro Cuvette*, respectively, allow the observation, selection and isolation of specific cells with the phase microscope and the quantitative measurement of enzyme activities in single isolated cells.

ULTRA-MICROTECHNIQUES

The *Plastic Film Dish (PFD)* : Cell Cultivation on Plastic Films (2,3,7)

The *PFD*, which we made commercially available from TECNOMARA (3), consists of a tripartite reusable metal holder and a disposable plastic film. After the rapid mounting of the plastic film,

the *PFD* is comparable to a Petri-dish with a very thin, transparent
and absolutely flat, non-toxic surface on which the cells grow.
The bottom of the *PFD* is so thin that the cells on it can be
observed with high-power phase objectives on an inverted microscope.
This allows the morphological typing of cells (e.g. fibroblast-
like versus epithelial-like) in prenatal diagnosis, or the selection of single heteropolykaryons for genetic complementation
analysis, by marking the plastic film around the selected cell.

Subsequently the cell culture in the *PFD* is washed, shock-
frozen in liquid nitrogen and lyophilized in conventional ways.
Plastic film leaflets carrying either a counted number of morphologically typed amniotic cells (prenatal diagnosis) or a marked
heteropolykaryon (complementation analysis) are then cut out of
the *PFD*-bottom. This is done by hand, with a scalpel under the
stereo-microscope.

The *Parafilm Micro Cuvette (PMC)* : Quantitative Enzyme Activity
Assays at the Single Cell Level (1,2,3,4,6,7)

The obvious and simple principle of the *PMC*-technique
consists of enforcing an optimal signal to noise ratio which
allows one to quantify small amounts of product with commercially
available instruments. The noise, i.e., the blank, in an enzyme
reaction is almost invariably due to the amount of substrate
employed in the enzyme reaction. If one tries to assay the enzyme
activity of a single cell by incubating it for 12 minutes in 1 ml
of substrate one finds, for example, a signal to noise ratio of
1:10,000 ; by decreasing the incubation volume to 0.1 µl one
ameliorates the ratio 10,000 times ; by prolonging the incubation
time to 10 hours one finally improves the signal to noise ratio
about 500,000 times. The *PMC*-technique permits the incubation,
in a simple way, of very small volumes of enzyme reaction mixtures
for many hours. Immediately before use, the disposable *PMC's* are
pressed on a teflon mold into parafilm strips. At present this
is done by hand, but a simple instrument for preparing the disposable *PMC's* automatically, will soon become commercially available.
With a constriction pipette the *PMC's* are filled with 0.3 µl of a
fluorogenic or radioactive substrate and each of them is loaded
with a plastic film leaflet carrying the lyophilized cells isolated
from the *PFD*. Strips with 10 *PMC's* are covered with a second parafilm strip and cold-sealed with a teflon rod. This seal is completely water-vapor tight ; the small incubation volumes are therefore
perfectly protected against evaporation and resist long-term
incubation at 37°C either in a dry atmosphere or submerged in a
water-bath. Various hydrolases release methylumbelliferone from
the appropriate artificial substrates while most dehydrogenases
will reduce NAD(P). Both free methylumbelliferone and NAD(P)H
become strongly fluorescent in alkaline solution providing a
sensitive procedure for the assay of many enzymes. The enzyme

reaction in the *PMC* is stopped by diluting the 0.3 µl reaction mixture with 0.5 ml of alkaline buffer, the strongly fluorescent
products being measured with a conventional spectrophotofluorimeter
(Perkin Elmer, MPF-4).

If radioactive substrates have been used the whole content of
the *PMC's*, after incubation, is pushed onto chromatographic paper
and the substrate and product are separated by conventional
chromatography or high-voltage electrophoresis. The radioactive
product is measured with a liquid scintillation counter. Fig.1
illustrates the outcome of an α-galactosidase assay of isolated
human fibroblasts, making use of an artificial fluorogenic substrate. Each point corresponds to the mean of 10 independent cell
isolations. This is important as the single cells have been
isolated from asynchronously growing cell cultures and therefore
display strong cell cycle dependent variations in enzyme activities.
If one looks, however, at the mean of 10 independent cell isolations,
there is a very strict quantitative relationship between the numbers
of cells incubated, i.e. 1,2,4,8,16 cells, and the enzyme activities
found ; this in spite of the fact that the α-galactosidase has a
low activity. The few enzyme molecules of one single fibroblast,
which in the *PMC* are exposed to a relatively large surface, are
protected against surface denaturation by adding 0.05% w/v purified
BSA to the enzyme reaction mixture. It is also necessary to study
very carefully the stability of enzymes which require long incubation
times ; for example, as shown in Fig.2, α-galactosidase is unstable
at 37°C, but stable for at least 10 hours at 25°C.

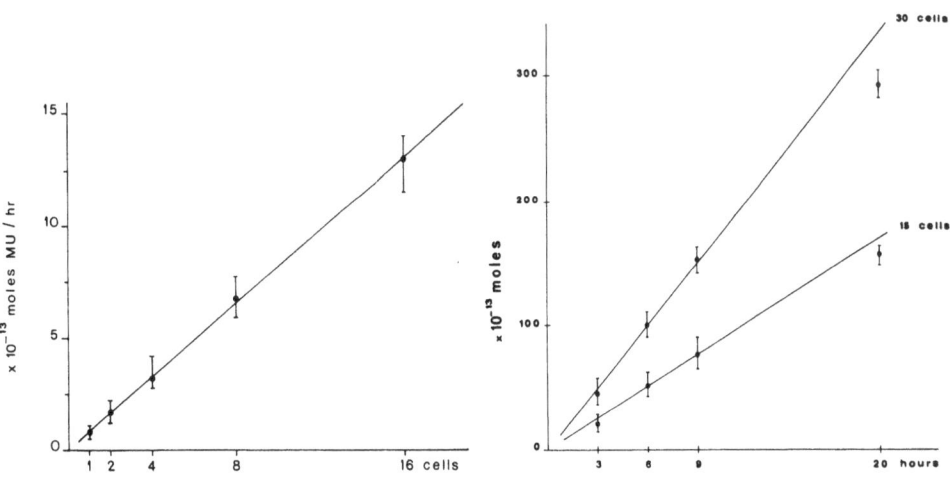

Fig.1 and Fig.2. α-galactosidase assay with 4-methylumbelliferyl-
α-D-galactopyranoside 8 mM, pH 4.8, at 25°C ; Fig.1 incubation for
12 hours ; in both graphs the means and ranges of 10 independent
cell isolations are indicated.

Micro-Isoenzyme Electrophoresis

Two techniques for routinely carrying out micro-isoenzyme electrophoresis have been developed :
Method A : The plastic film leaflets with the lyophilized cells are preincubated for 1/2 hour in cold buffer in a PMC. The enzymes leak out of the lyophilized cells and into the buffer ; 0.25 µl aliquots of this enzyme-loaded buffer are applied to Phoroslide cellulose acetate strips (Millipore corp.) and isoenzyme electrophoresis is done in a conventional way (cf. Fig.6).
Method B : The plastic film leaflet with the lyophilized cells is directly put on top of the Phoroslide strip (cells toward the gel). The electric field extracts and separates the isoenzyme fractions in one step without any loss of material (cf. Fig.8). Three points concerning the microtechniques should be especially stressed :
1°) The PMC-technique allows, in principle, the assay of any enzyme. If natural substrates are desirable one can either employ radioactive compounds or couple the enzyme reaction to a NAD or NADP dependent system.
2°) Enzyme activities are expressed per cell ; gene dosage measurements, which are important for the separation of homo- and heterozygotes, are much more accurate than with the current macro methods which express enzyme activities in terms of the total cell protein content.
3°) These ultra-microtechniques do not involve micromanipulation ; they are simple, easy to learn and demand little special equipment.

THE "HETEROPOLYKARYONTEST" : SYSTEMATIC COMPLEMENTATION ANALYSIS IN MAN (5,8)

The principle of genetic complementation analysis consists of bringing two different mutant genomes, with the same phenotypic defect, such as an enzyme deficiency, into one common cytoplasm. If the two mutants complement we have to assume that they are genetically different. Somatic cell hybrids have been used for genetic complementation analysis in man. These were produced by virus-assisted cell fusion and isolated by chemical selection. The use of hybrids has, however, several disadvantages. First, viable hybrid cell clones have to develop. Second, only a very few selective systems are available. Third, chromosomes are lost during the establishment of hybrid clones making the continuous monitoring of the karyotype necessary. Fourth, the establishment and selection of hybrid cell clones will always be time consuming and costly. All these difficulties could be overcome by applying the present microtechniques which permit one to visually select and isolate single heteropolykaryons and to routinely measure the enzyme activities of the isolated heteropolykaryons. To develop the "heteropolykaryontest" we chose two diploid human β-galactosidase deficient cell strains, i.e. GM1-gangliosidosis-cells and I-cells

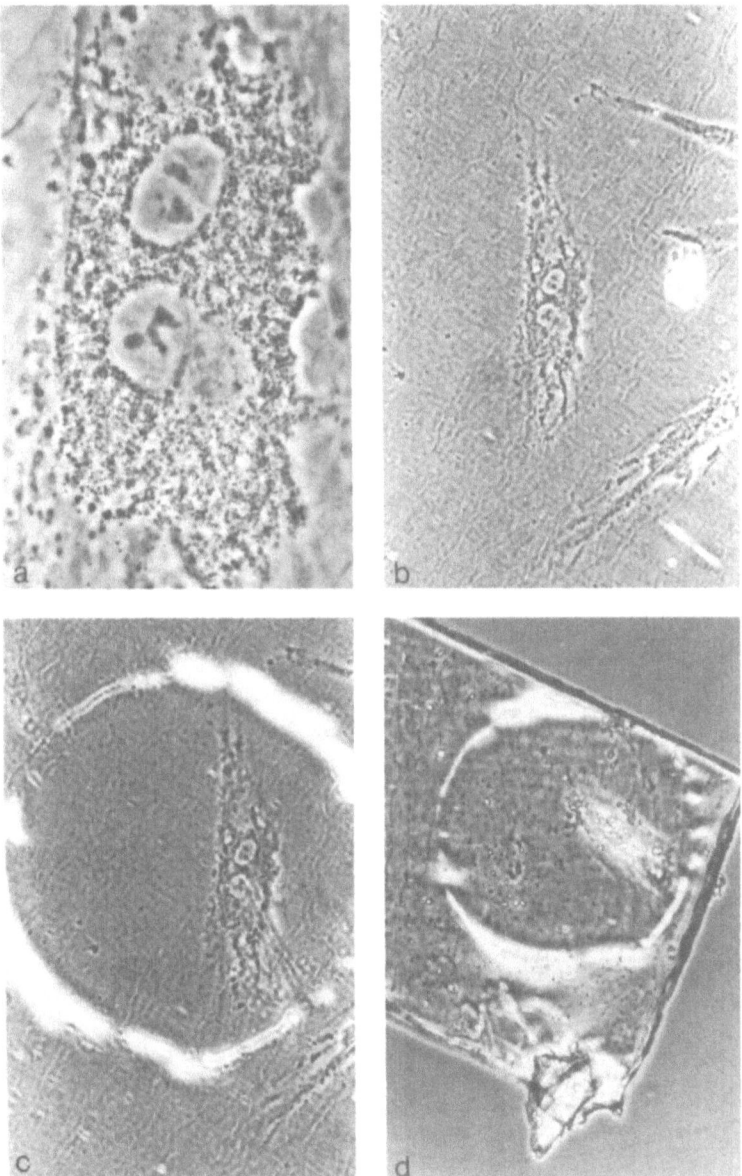

Fig.3a. I-cell-homobikaryon, phase contrast
Fig.3b and 3c. Same cell, before and after marking
Fig.3d. Same cell, lyophilized and isolated from the PFD-bottom

which, having single and multiple lysosomal enzyme deficiencies, respectively, should be genetically different and therefore display intergenic complementation. The two mutant cell strains were fused with inactivated Sendai-virus in a 1:1 ratio and seeded onto the bottom of a *PFD*. Three days later bikaryons were visually selected and marked on the *PFD*-bottom (Fig.3) ; after lyophilization the marked bikaryons were isolated from the *PFD*-bottom and transferred into *PMC's* to monitor the appearance of β-galactosidase activities. We expected that half of the bikaryons should be heterobikaryons and therefore display intergenic complementation. This expectation was confirmed by the appearance of β-galactosidase activities in half of the bikaryons while all mononuclear non-fused parental cells stayed β-galactosidase deficient (Fig.4). In practice, instead of bikaryons, we isolate polykaryons with 10 nuclei which guarantees the presence of both parental mutant nuclei in each of the poly-karyons. In principle, it is therefore possible to detect genetic complementation with one single heteropolykaryon.

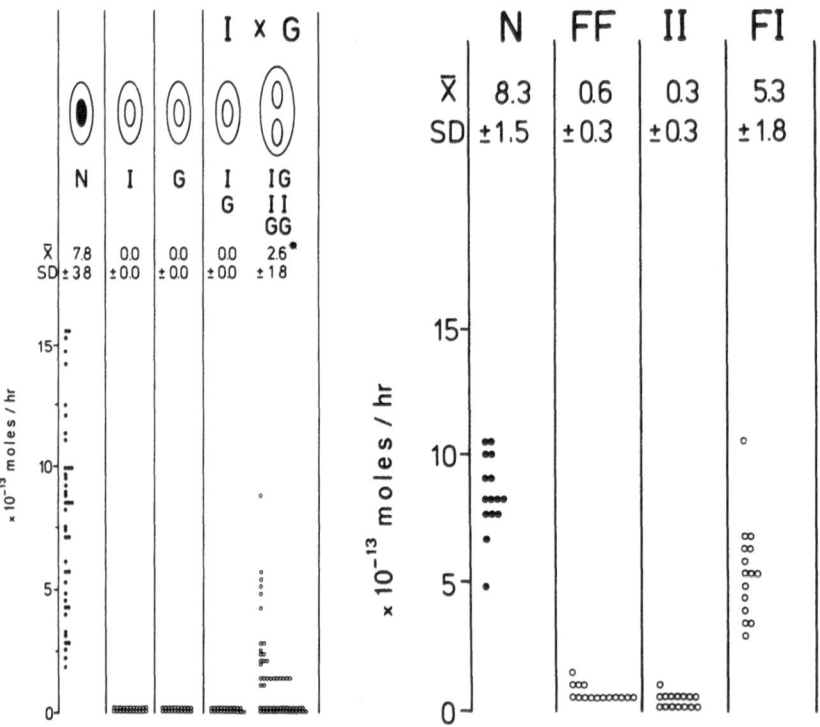

Fig.4. Cross between I-cells and GM1-cells ; single cells monitored for β-galactosidase activities.

Fig.5. Cross between I-cells and Fabry-cells ; polykaryons monitored for α-galactosidase activities.

To demonstrate the reliability of the "heteropolykaryontest"
we performed crosses between I-cells, which are deficient for
β-galactosidase, α-galactosidase, α-mannosidase, etc... and
Landing-cells (deficient for β-galactosidase), Fabry-cells (deficient for α-galactosidase) and mannosidosis (deficient for α-mannosidase), respectively. As expected, we find in all three cases three
days after the cell fusion signs of intergenic complementation
at the single heteropolykaryon level (Fig.5).
    Practically, genetic complementation analysis is employed
1) to detect genetic heterogeneity ; 2) to classify human hereditary disease ; 3) to predict the nature of the protein molecule
involved.

Demonstration of Genetic Heterogeneity

    Different I-cell strains have been crossed in all possible
permutations and the isolated heteropolykaryons were monitored for
the appearance of β-galactosidase activity. In repeat experiments
interallelic complementation could clearly be demonstrated, indicating that the 5 unrelated I-cell mutants belong to the same
cistron and that the primary cause of I-cell disease is probably
a defect in a processing gene (11) which codes for a homopolymeric
protein.

Classification of Human Hereditary Disease

    The cells of 7 unrelated cases of Landing's disease were
crossed. By monitoring the heteropolykaryons for the appearance
of β-galactosidase activity we found 3 different non-overlapping
classes of mutants : complementation was detected between the
classes, but not within them, indicating that the complementation
was most probably intergenic. If these results can be confirmed
with more patient material we have to infer that in man at least
3 cistrons code for β-galactosidase. This genetic classification
corresponds to Pinsky's biochemical classification (12).

Genetic Prediction of the Nature of the Protein Molecule Involved

    Two Sandhoff-cell strains were crossed with three Tay-Sachs-
cell strains and monitored by micro enzyme electrophoresis for
hexosaminidase A and B (using the previously described micro-
electrophoretic method A).
(Fig.6 : on the left are the control extracts,
        on the right extracts of 10 pooled heteropolykaryons)
In all Tay-Sachs x Sandhoff crosses, but only in these, a hexosaminidase – A faction becomes clearly visible, indicating intergenic complementation and thus the heteropolymeric nature of the
hexosaminidase A (8).

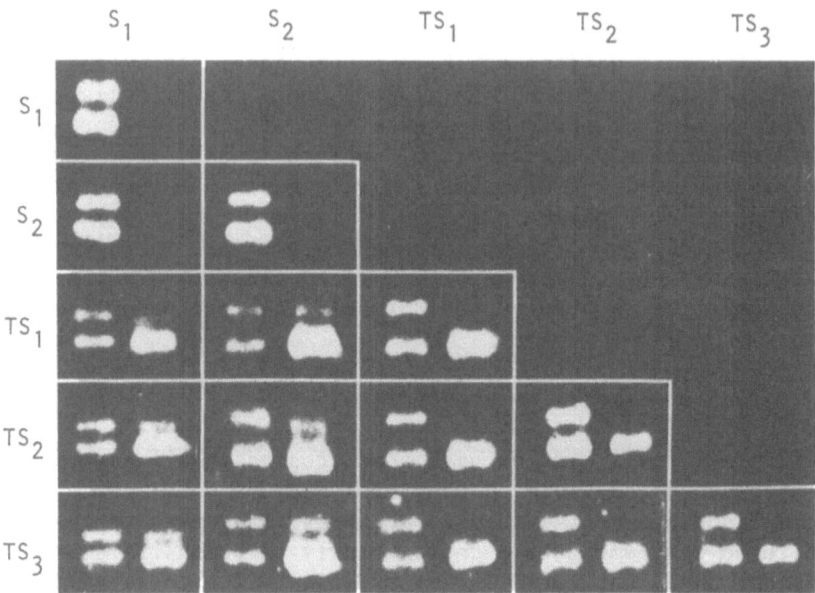

Fig.6. Tay-Sachs-cells crossed with Sandhoff-cells, monitored for
hexosaminidase A and B ; control extracts on the left, polykaryon
extracts on the right.

RAPID PRENATAL DIAGNOSIS IN EARLY PREGNACY WITH
AMNIOTIC FLUID CELLS (1,4,6,7,8)

Early prenatal diagnosis is important not only for psychologi-
cal reasons (fetal movements) but because the risk of a selective
abortion increases with the length of the pregnancy. With the described microtechniques prenatal diagnosis by amniocentesis can
be regularly achieved before the 17th week of the pregnancy (7,8).

With methylumbelliferyl coupled fluorogenic substrates we
can diagnose the different types of GM1-gangliosidoses, GM2-
gangliosidoses, Gaucher's disease and Fabry's disease at the
single cell level ; in addition, we are developing the specific
enzyme assays for the single sphingolipidoses by employing radioactive natural substrates.

In practice one uses, of course, all the amniotic cell
material available.

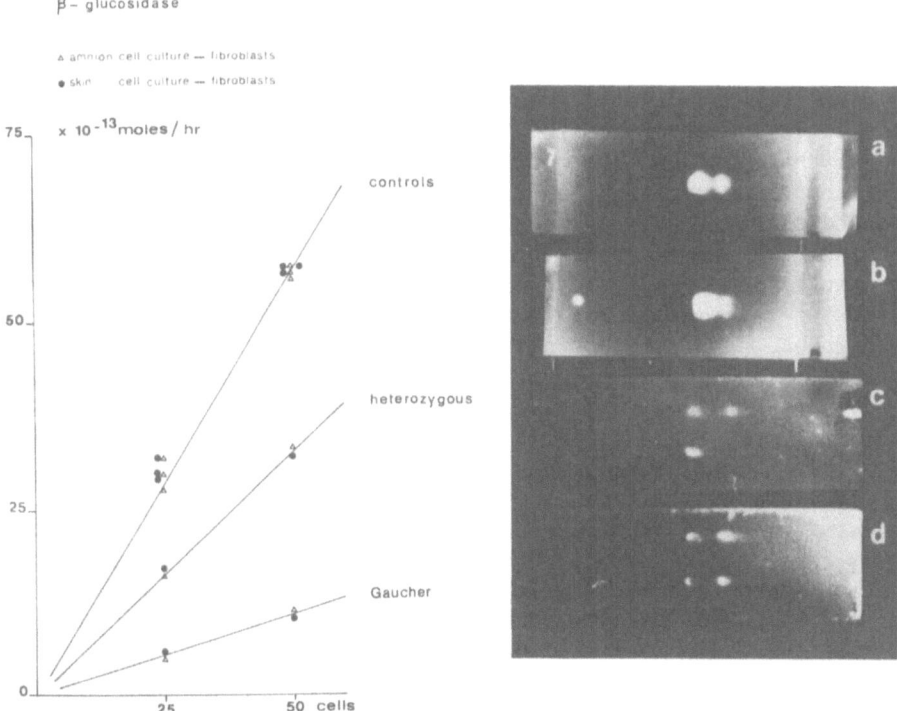

Fig.7 and Fig.8. Prenatal diagnosis of pregnancies at risk for
sphingolipidoses.
Fig.8. Micro-enzyme electrophoresis of hexosaminidases :
Fig.8a. Control, 200 cells ; Fig.8b. Prenatal diagnosis, Tay-Sachs-
heterozygote, 200 cells.
Fig.8c. Normal and Tay-Sachs control, 50 cells ; Fig.8d. Prenatal
diagnosis, normal fetus, 50 cells.

Fig.7 and Fig.8 give examples of early prenatal diagnoses
carried out with the present microtechniques in pregnancies at
risk for sphingolipidoses. Fig.7 demonstrates that hetero- and
homozygotes can be easily separated (due to the expression of
the enzyme activities per cell) and that cells of one morphological
type display identical enzyme activities, whether isolated from
the amniotic fluid or from fetal or adult skin.

PROSPECTS FOR PRENATAL SCREENING OF GENETIC
DEFECTS WITH UNSPECIFIC BIOCHEMICAL MARKERS

To avoid the tragic birth of index cases one should be daring enough to look for ways to eventually screen all pregnancies for a very large number of possible fetal genetic defects.

For that purpose, one would have to be able to isolate fetal cells from the maternal blood and to screen these cells with fully automated ultra-microassays for unspecific biochemical markers which would indicate inborn errors of metabolism, as well as chromosomal aberrations. Some years ago, we proposed alkaline phosphatase as a promising candidate for such a marker. In the meantime, we learned how to induce alkaline phosphatase reproducibly in lysosomal mutants and there is now a real possibility to use this induction to diagnose any lysosomal disease at the single cell level.

Whilst studying I-cells it became obvious that there is a kind of coordinate regulation of the activities of the acid lysosomal hydrolases and of alkaline phosphatase. All non-deficient lysosomal enzymes, as well as alkaline phosphatase, show higher than normal activities. As the alkaline phosphatase activity is extremely low in normal fibroblasts its dramatic increase upon induction is particularly useful as a diagnostic tool. We therefore concentrated on this enzyme and experimented with the following working hypothesis.

The lysosomal acid hydrolases and the alkaline phosphatase cooperate in the intracellular digestion of various polymers ; their activities are regulated in a coordinate fashion. The stimulus for the coordinate induction of these enzyme activities is the retention of any kind of polymer in the cell. This stimulus is short and weak under physiological conditions where polymers are rapidly degraded ; it is long-lasting and strong whenever a polymer is retained due to the lack of a necessary catabolic enzyme. Feeding a sphingomyelinase deficient Niemann-Pick-cell with sphingomyelin will induce within a few hours a large increase in the alkaline phosphatase activity. An α-glucosidase deficient Pompe-cell on the other hand, will not be stimulated by feeding with spingomyelin (Fig. 9). Conversely, the Pompe-cell, but not so the Niemann-Pick-cell, will react on feeding glycogen.

Challenged with a cocktail containing various polymers, the normal cell will show a weak increase of the alkaline phosphatase activity which returns to its original low value after washing out the cocktail ; a lysosomal mutant, however, will store the polymers that it cannot digest and will therefore react with a long-lasting increase of the alkaline phosphatase activity (Fig.10).

The function of the alkaline phosphatase is unfortunately unknown ; its universal occurence seems to indicate,however, that it is important. Therefore, it made sense to screen various aberrations for a rise in alkaline phosphatase activity.

To our great satisfaction cystic fibrosis, the most frequent inborn error in Caucasian populations (which at present cannot be

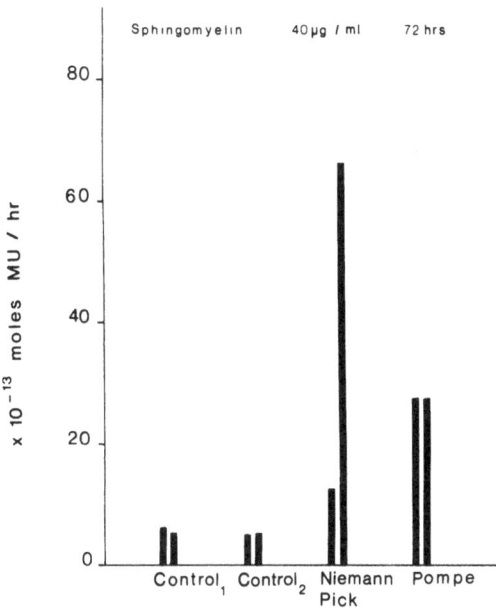

Fig.9. Alkaline phosphatase activities (20 fibroblasts) before
and after induction with 40 μg sphingomyelin/ml medium.

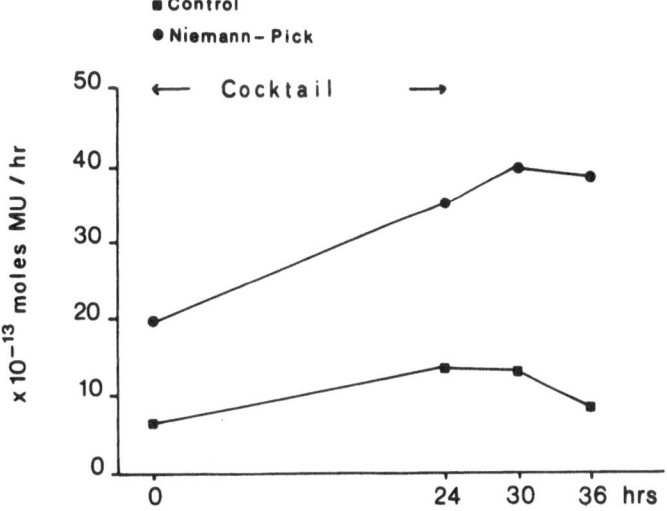

Fig.10. Alkaline phosphatase activities in normal and Niemann-Pick-
cells (20 fibroblasts), induced with a cocktail containing 40 μg
sphingomyelin, 40 μg glycogen and 40 μg cystine per ml of medium.

diagnosed prenatally) shows an impressive rise in alkaline phosphatase activity.

Even more exciting is the observation that chromosomal aberrations, i.e. the trisomies 13,18,21,XXY and the monosomy XO show increases in the alkaline phosphatase activities. It will obviously be very important to learn how to control the alkaline phosphatase induction in cystic fibrosis and in the various trisomies.

We believe that it soon will become possible to isolate, in early pregnancy, fetal cells from the maternal blood ; these fetal cells will be challenged in vitro with a cocktail containing the various polymers ; genetically defective cells (with either an inborn error or a chromosomal aberration) will react with a rise in alkaline phosphatase activity ; in these suspect cases amniocentesis will be performed to confirm the suspected genetic defect on amniotic fluid cells.

REFERENCES

1. de Bruyn, C.H.M.M., Oei, T.L. and Hösli, P., Quantitative radio-chemical enzyme assays in single cells : purine phosphoribosyl transferase activities in cultured fibroblasts, submitted.

2. Hösli, P., Zellkultur und Zellgenetik, Anat. Anz. 120, 583 (1967)

3. Hösli, P., Tissue Cultivation on Plastic Films, Zürich, Tecnomara (1972)

4. Hösli, P., Microtechniques for rapid prenatal diagnosis of inborn errors of metabolism in early pergnancy,Prenat.Diagn. Newsletter (Canada), 1, 10 (1972).

5. Hösli, P., Microtechniques for the detection of intergenic and interallelic complementation in man, Bull. Europ. Soc. Hum. Gen. p.32 (1972)

6. Hösli, P., de Bruyn, C.H.M.M. and Oei, T.L., Development of a micro HG-PRT activity assay : premiminary complementation studies with Lesch-Nyhan cell strains. In "Purine Metabolism in Man" (O. Sperling, A. de Vries, J.B. Wijngaarden Eds.), New York, Plenum Press, 1974, p.11.

7. Hösli, P., Microtechniques for rapid prenatal diagnosis in early pregnancy. In "Birth Defects"(A. Motulsky and W. Lenz, Eds.), Amsterdam, Excerpta Medica, 1974, p.226.

8. Hösli, P., Microbiochemical analysis of hereditary errors of metabolism. In "Proc. Third Int. Congr. of the Int. Ass. for the Scient. Study of Mental Deficiency"(D.A.A. Primrose Ed.) Warsaw, Polish Medical Publishers, 1974, p.394

9. Lowry, O.H. and Passoneau, J.V.A., A flexible system of enzymatic analysis, New York,Academic Press (1972)

10. Mattenheimer, H., Micromethods for the Clinical and Biochemical Laboratory, Ann Harbor Science Publishers, Inc. (1970)

11. Paigen, K., Swank, R.T., Tomino, S. and Ganschow, R.E., The Molecular genetics of mammalian glucuronidase, J. Cell. Physiol., 85, 379 (1975)

12. Pinsky, L. Miller, J., Shanfield, B., Watters, G. and Wolfe, L.S., GM1 gangliosidosis in skin fibroblast culture : enzymatic differences between types 1 and 2 and observations on a third variant, Am. J. Hum. Genet., 26, 563 (1974).

STORAGE AND EXCRETION OF OLIGOSACCHARIDES AND GLYCOPEPTIDES IN THE GANGLIOSIDOSES

Leonhard S. Wolfe and N. M. K. Ng Ying Kin

Donner Laboratory of Experimental Neurochemistry
Montreal Neurological Institute, McGill University
Montreal, Quebec, H3A 2B4 Canada

G_{M1}-Gangliosidosis

Electron microscopical studies of visceral tissues from the infantile form of G_{M1}-gangliosidosis (Type I or generalized gangliosidosis) show extensive cytoplasmic vacuolation of parenchymal cells, histiocytes, fibrocytes and lymphocytes (9,23-25, 29,33,36,44). Indeed, in the liver, the majority of the hepatocytes are packed with membrane-limited vacuoles filled with highly water-soluble, α-amylase-resistant, PAS-positive material. Similar morphological features are also seen in an affected fetus at 17 weeks of gestation with in addition intense vacuolation of the syncytiotrophoblasts of the placenta (16,28). Vacuolation of hepatocytes is much less marked in the Type II late infantile or juvenile form of G_{M1}-gangliosidosis (9,11,27). It was recognized early in the descriptions of this disease that the material stored in the vacuoles was unlikely to be G_{M1}-ganglioside since the ultrastructural features were quite different from the neuronal membranous cytoplasmic bodies characteristic of ganglioside storage. Earlier chemical studies of not too rigorous a nature established that the liver from Type I G_{M1}-gangliosidosis contained excessive amounts of polysaccharides rich in galactose and N-acetylglucosamine and fractions containing some mannose were also recognized (5,32-34,44). Various rather non-specific names have been given to these materials in the literature: undersulfated keratan sulfate, keratan sulfate-like polysaccharides, sialomucopolysaccharide, glucosaminogalactan, glycosaminoglycans. The predominant idea in the past was that the principal component of the visceral accumulations was derived from cartilage keratan sulfate (4,5,32,34,39). The major part of the glycosaminoglycan

chain of keratan sulfate consists of alternating galactose $\beta1\rightarrow4$
N-acetylglucosamine $\beta1\rightarrow3$ disaccharide units variably sulfated and
joined probably through a short mannose-containing sequence to
N-acetylgalactosamine linked O-glycosidically to a serine or threo-
nine unit of the protein moiety. The almost complete lack of
activity of β-galactosidase isozymes in the Type I disease could
account not only for the glycolipid accumulations in neurones but
the inability to degrade completely keratan sulfates and be related
possibly to the skeletal abnormalities seen clinically. In addition
the urine of Type I G_{M1}-gangliosidosis patients contained large
amounts of unsulfated polysaccharides which were not precipitated
by cetyl pyridinium chloride and earlier studies as far as they
went suggested these compounds were keratan-like (5,26). However,
the major fractions were of low molecular weight of 3000-4000.
Similar fractions were found in large excess after being labelled
with ^{14}C-galactose, from a fibroblast cell line of a patient (4).
No increase in any of the uronic acid-containing glycosaminoglycans
has been found in the urine or tissues of G_{M1}-gangliosidosis
patients.

Over the past two years we have re-examined by much more
rigorous chemical methods the structures of the water-soluble oligosaccharides and glycopeptides obtained from the liver and urine from
a number of cases of G_{M1}-gangliosidosis Type I. Space does not
permit a detailed account of these studies which have been for the
most part published (19,20,45,46). Several homogeneous fractions
from both liver and urine of structurally related compounds have
been isolated and purified and their complete structures determined
utilizing enzymatic and physicochemical methods and permethylation
analyses coupled with gas chromatography-mass spectrometry identification of the partially methylated alditol and 2-deoxy-2-N-
methylacetamido hexitol acetates. Proton magnetic resonance
spectroscopy at 100 and 220 MHz was particularly valuable for the
determination of anomeric configurations. It was clear that all
the fractions we had studied which had molecular weights below 3000
were oligosaccharides or small glycopeptides with a branched chain
structure, galactose at the non-reducing termini and a trimannosyl-
N-acetylglucosamine core of quite dissimilar structure to the
keratan sulfates. Structures similar to partially degraded keratan
sulfates may exist as has been reported recently (39,42), but we
have not characterized such material. This report therefore will
briefly summarize our results on the oligosaccharide storage and
excretion, present further observations on the structure of the
glycopeptides and discuss the origin of these compounds.

We found that a convenient method for isolation of the non-
ganglioside low molecular weight oligosaccharides and glycopeptides
from G_{M1}-gangliosidosis liver was homogenization in 10 volumes of
chloroform-methanol (2:1) followed by extraction again with

chloroform-methanol-water (1:2:0.3). After centrifuging, the upper
phase material was removed, the lower phase re-extracted with water,
the upper phases combined, evaporated to dryness and the gangliosides removed by repeated extraction with dry chloroform-methanol
(2:1). The oligosaccharide-containing materials were precipitated
with four volumes of ethanol and separated into fractions on Bio-
Gel P-10 columns (46). It is important to mention that extraction
with 20 volumes of chloroform-methanol as conventionally done in
the delipidation of tissues did not extract nearly as much oligosaccharide material. The delipidated residue was digested twice
for 24 hours at 65° with papain under standard conditions, centrifuged and the supernatant dialysed extensively at 0°. The dialysate
was then fractionated on Bio-Gel into glycopeptide and oligosaccharide fractions as described above. The non-dialysable fraction
after papain digestion was found to be a complex mixture of higher
molecular weight compounds with less than 30% hexose composition
and we did not further examine this fraction. The compounds in the
urine were cleanly isolated by dialysis, ethanol precipitation and
Bio-Gel chromatography. Table 1 summarizes the yields of oligosaccharide and glycopeptide fractions found in one of our cases.
Similar results were obtained for 3 other Type I cases. The con-
sistency in composition and relative amounts of fractions 3-5 from
the liver of all our cases was particularly striking. Variability
in amount and composition was only seen in fractions 1 and 2.
Fractions 3-5 from both the chloroform-methanol-water and the dialysed papain-digested residue accounted for 70 percent of the total
extractable oligosaccharides and glycopeptides. It is worth noting
that the urine dialysate contained negligible quantities of fraction
1 and 2.

The fraction 4 oligosaccharide was found to have the structure
shown in Figure 1. The oligosaccharide in fraction 5 was found to
have identical structure to fraction 4 except it lacked the Gal
β1→4 GlcNAc disaccharide linked β1→4 to the monosubstituted mannose
residues. The anomeric absorptions determined from the proton
magnetic resonance spectra for the glycopeptide and oligosaccharide fractions are listed in Table 2. In fractions 3, 4 and 5 the
galactosyl residues are clearly β-linked, there are two types of
β-linked N-acetylglucosamine and three mannose anomeric protons
indicate three different environments and it is not possible to
unequivocally assign these to α or β configurations by PMR evidence
alone (see 46).

Recently we have extended our chemical studies of the glycopeptide fractions particularly fraction 3 (see Table 1 and ref. 46).
We wished to know if the trimannosyl core was linked through a
single N-acetylglucosamine to a peptide through asparagine or by a
chitobiosyl unit (GlcNAc β1→4 GlcNAc). The GlcNAc-Asparagine bonds
of the fraction 3 glycopeptide was cleaved by treatment with 2.5 M
NaOH for 3 hours at 90° (13) or 1 M NaOH-1 M NaBH$_4$ for 6 hours at

Table 1.   Glycopeptide and oligosaccharide fractions isolated from liver and urine of G_{M1}-gangliosidosis, Type I by BioGel P-6 chromatography

		Fractions			
	1 (void volume)	2	3	4	5
M.W.	>4,500	3000	2200	1800	1400
Liver					
C-M-H_2O extraction mg/100 g liver	134	64	128	169	70
Residue, papain digested, dialysate mg/100 g liver	107	50	154	203	90
Urine					
Dialysate mg/100 ml	0	5	75	165	137
Lowry protein %	10-20	9	<5	0	0
Sugars present	Gal GlcNAc GalNAc little Man	Gal GlcNAc Man	Gal GlcNAc Man	Gal GlcNAc Man	Gal GlcNAc Man
Composition	Mixture	glycopeptide	glycopeptide	decasaccharide	octasaccharide

Details of the Bio-Gel fractionation patterns are given in Ref. 46.

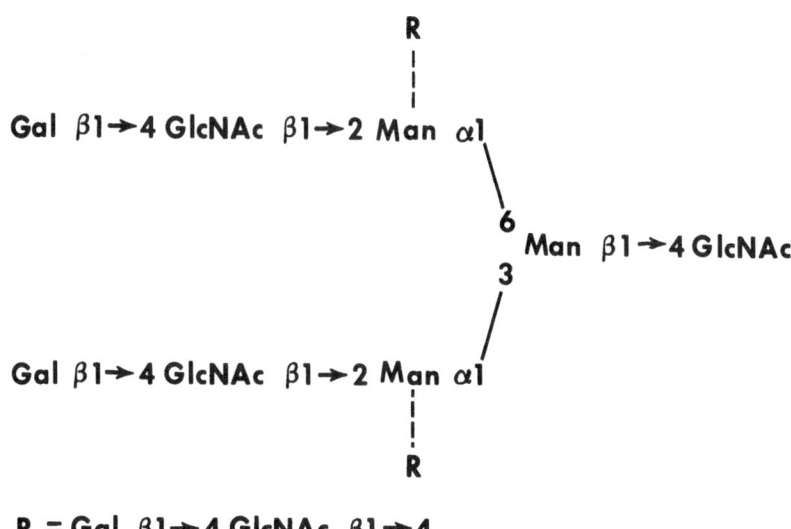

Figure 1. Structure of the major oligosaccharide accumulating
           in the liver of G_{M1}-gangliosidosis patients.

Table 2. Anomeric absorptions in ppm of various oligosaccharide
          fractions from G_{M1}-gangliosidosis liver dissolved in D_2O

Sugar residues		Fractions			
		1	3	4	5
Gal (terminal) β		4.96*	4.96*	4.96*	4.96*
GlcNAc (non-reducing) β		5.06†	5.06†	5.06†	5.06†
GlcNAc (reducing)		none	5.68 (very weak)	5.68	5.68
Trimannosyl Core	1.	5.23	5.23	5.23	5.23
	2.	none	5.39	5.39	5.39
	3.	5.63	5.61	5.61	5.61

External standard, tetramethylsilane. Spectra measured with a
Varian HA-100 spectrometer. See ref. 20, 46 for detailed spectra.

* doublet J=7Hz
† broad signal

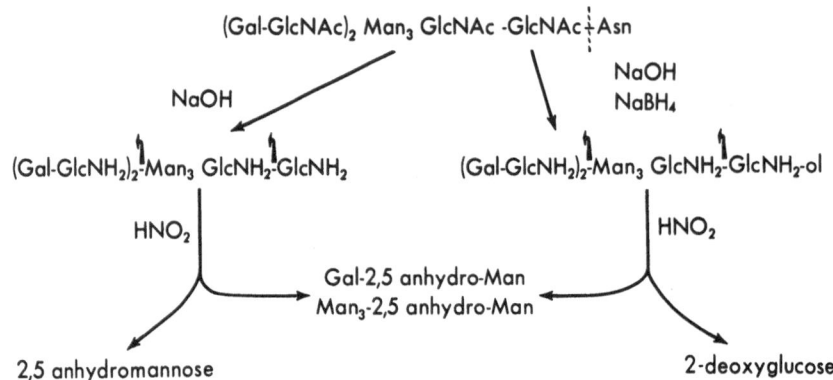

Figure 2. Outline of the scheme for base hydrolysis and
nitrous acid degradation of fraction 3 glycopeptides from G_{M1}-gangliosidosis liver and the
products identified by gas chromatography and
mass spectrometry.

100° (see 2). The resultant oligosaccharides with glucosamine or
glucosaminitol at the reducing termini were desalted and purified
on Sephadex G-10 and then subjected to nitrous acid degradation
(13) as outlined in Figure 2. In the case of alkaline hydrolysis
followed by nitrous acid deamination, 2,5 anhydromannose was
identified by gas chromatography-mass spectrometry of the tri-
methylsilyl ether derivative of the alditol on a 3% OV-1 column.
The alditol acetate was identified on a 3% ECNSS-M column. This
free 2,5 anhydromannose must have originated from a chitobiosyl
unit since glucosaminidic linkages are known to undergo nitrous
acid degradation. Further confirmation of this was obtained by
subjecting the product of reductive alkaline hydrolysis of the
fraction 3 glycopeptide to nitrous acid deamination. In this
case free 2-deoxyglucose was identified. It is well known that
the major product of nitrous acid deamination of glucosaminitol is
2-deoxyglucose (10). The other products were Gal-2,5 anhydroman
and Man_3-2,5 anhydroman which after $NaBH_4$ reduction followed by
acid hydrolysis (1 N HCl, 10 hours, 100°) yielded galactose,
mannose and 2,5 anhydromannitol identified by gas chromatography
as the acetates or alditol acetates. These results indicate that
the reducing terminus of the fraction 3 glycopeptide contains a
chitobiosyl unit. This is most probably linked to asparagine
since after strong alkaline hydrolysis aspartic acid was found by
thin layer chromatography on cellulose.

G_{M2}-Gangliosidosis

Accumulation of N-acetylglucosamine-containing oligosaccharides or glycopeptides in liver or brain or their excretion in the urine was not found in Tay Sachs disease cases (β-N-acetylhexosaminidase deficiency of component A) (18). However, in Sandhoff's disease (G_{M2}-gangliosidosis, variant O) in which there is a deficiency of both the A and B components of β-N-acetylhexosaminidase (see 24,25) greatly increased amounts of two highly water-soluble oligosaccharide fractions were found in the liver (18). N-acetylglucosamine was present at both the non-reducing and reducing termini and proton magnetic resonance and permethylation studies showed a trimannosyl core structure identical to that found in G_{M1}-gangliosidosis oligosaccharides. The oligosaccharide structure is shown in Figure 3.

Recently we had the opportunity to analyse the dialysable fraction from the urine of another case of Sandhoff's disease (19). Two oligosaccharide fractions not present in Tay Sachs disease urine or normal subjects were found (Figure 4). Permethylation and PMR studies showed that these fractions contained oligosaccharides of similar structure to those found in the liver (Figure 3). It is interesting that glycopeptides were not found in liver or urine of Sandhoff disease patients. Strecker and Montreuil (31) have reported

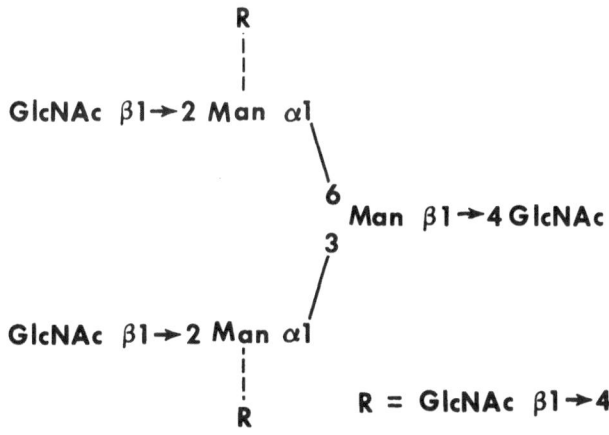

Figure 3. Structure of the major heptasaccharide accumulating in the liver of Sandhoff disease. A hexasaccharide lacking the $\beta 1 \to 4$ linked GlcNAc at the non-reducing terminal was also isolated.

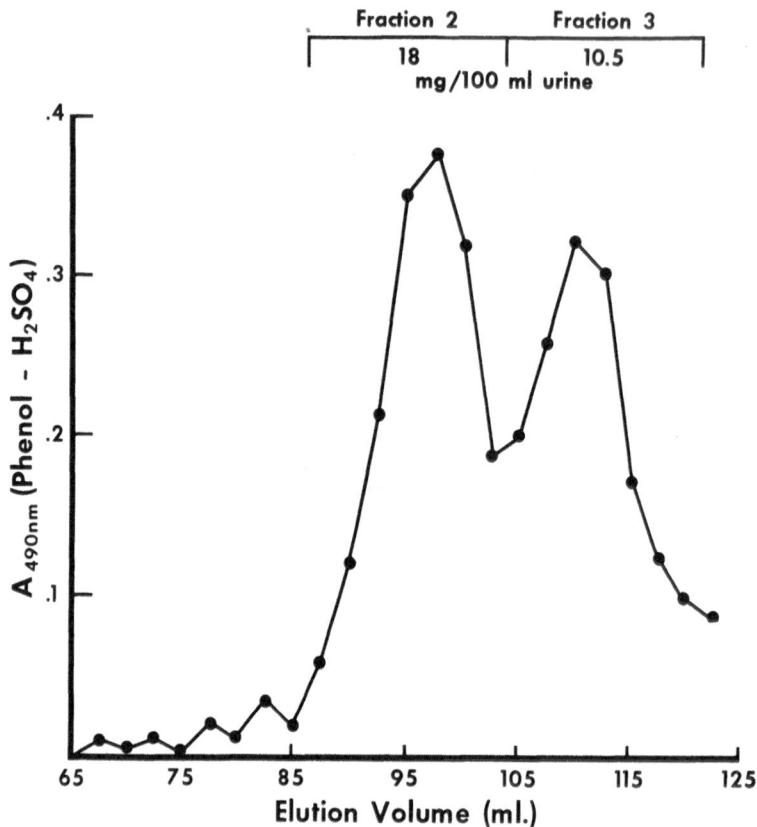

<u>Figure 4.</u>   Elution profile on Sephadex G-25 of dialysable
            oligosaccharides from the urine of a patient
            with Sandhoff's disease.

oligosaccharides in the urine of Sandhoff's disease which only
contained mannose and N-acetylglucosamine but no detailed structures were given. Excretion of uronic acid-containing glycosaminoglycans was not increased (1,31). The report of glycosaminoglycan storage and defective catabolism in cultured fibroblasts
from Sandhoff's disease (6) is curious and not readily explained
particularly since no increase of these compounds has been
observed in other tissues.

Discussion

The glycolipid, oligosaccharide and glycopeptide substances
accumulating in neuronal and visceral tissues identified so far in
G_{M1}- and G_{M2}-gangliosidosis are summarized in Table 3. The
question whether or not some glycopeptides derived from keratan
sulfate are stored and excreted is still not satisfactorily resolved.

Table 3

Compounds Accumulating in Tissues or Excreted in The Gangliosidoses

G$_{M1}$-gangliosidosis		G$_{M2}$-gangliosidosis	
Type I	Type II	Tay-Sachs	Sandhoff
G$_{M1}$-ganglioside Asialo G$_{M1}$-ganglioside (Gal-GlcNAc)$_2$ Man$_3$ GlcNAc$_2$-Asn-peptide (Gal-GlcNAc)$_{2\ or\ 3}$ Man$_3$ GlcNAc Desulfated Glycopeptides from KS		G$_{M2}$-ganglioside Asialo-G$_{M2}$-ganglioside	G$_{M2}$-ganglioside Asialo-G$_{M2}$-ganglioside Globoside GlcNAc$_{2\ or\ 3}$ Man$_3$ GlcNAc

The "keratosulfate-like" glycopeptide reported by Tsay and Dawson (39,40,42) of molecular weight approximately 1800 was not identified in our papain-digested dialysates of delipidated liver. Furthermore, the structure reported is not in accord with the core structure proposed for cartilage keratan sulfate by Hirano and Meyer (12). The presence of N-acetylgalactosamine and 3-linked galactose was detected in our studies but only in the void volume fractions of the Bio-Gel P-6 columns which represented a minor amount of the total hexose-containing materials from the liver (46 and Table 1). However this is unsatisfactory evidence for the presence of a keratan type structure since some glycopeptides from blood group glycoproteins contain similar sugars and linkages (15, 17). Calatroni (3) has also isolated N-acetylgalactosamine-containing glycopeptides from G$_{M1}$-gangliosidosis Type I liver but only from non-dialysable fractions obtained after papain digestion. In the dialysate only trace amounts of galactosamine were present, the major part being oligosaccharides which contained only galactose, mannose and N-acetylglucosamine.

We have suggested (20,45,46) that a possible origin of the glycopeptides and oligosaccharides is from erythrocyte MN-active glycoproteins (Glycophorin) since the carbohydrate sequences described by Winzler (38,43) and the Kornfelds (see 8) are almost identical except for the absence of sialic acid and fucose to those found in G$_{M1}$-gangliosidosis. Recent precise carbohydrate sequence studies of glycopeptides derived from immunoglobulins (IgE, IgM and IgG) have also revealed that they contain similar structures to the fraction 5 oligosaccharide isolated in G$_{M1}$-gangliosidosis except for the presence of sialic acid, fucose and chitobiosyl residue (2,8,35,37). The fraction 3 glycopeptides, however, we have shown do contain a chitobiosyl unit (Figure 2). Thus defective catabolism of immunoglobulin carbohydrate sequences may also contribute to the stored and excreted compounds in the gangliosidoses. The occurrence

of free oligosaccharides together with glycopeptides containing
a chitobiosyl unit linked to asparagine strongly suggests that an
endo-β-N-acetylglucosaminidase is present in human liver. The
existence of such a glycoprotein endo-glucosaminidase has recently
been reported in the rat and pig (21). In Sandhoff's disease
there is storage and excretion of only oligosaccharides and no
glycopeptide was identified (18). Possibly this is related to a
stereospecificity of endo-glucosaminidases which might be more
active on glycopeptide substrates lacking non-reducing galactose
termini.

A scheme for the catabolism of erythrocyte and immunoglobulin
glycoproteins is shown in Figure 5. Absence of β-galactosidase or
β-N-acetylglucosaminidase activity in G_{M1}-gangliosidosis and
Sandhoff's disease respectively, we propose, would result in the
failure to catabolise common intermediate glycopeptides. It is
pertinent to note here that in mannosidosis, an α-mannosidase
deficiency disease, a Man α1→3 Man β1→4 GlcNAc trisaccharide is
excreted in the urine (22). In addition, several mannose-containing
oligosaccharides almost certainly derived from the inner mannosyl

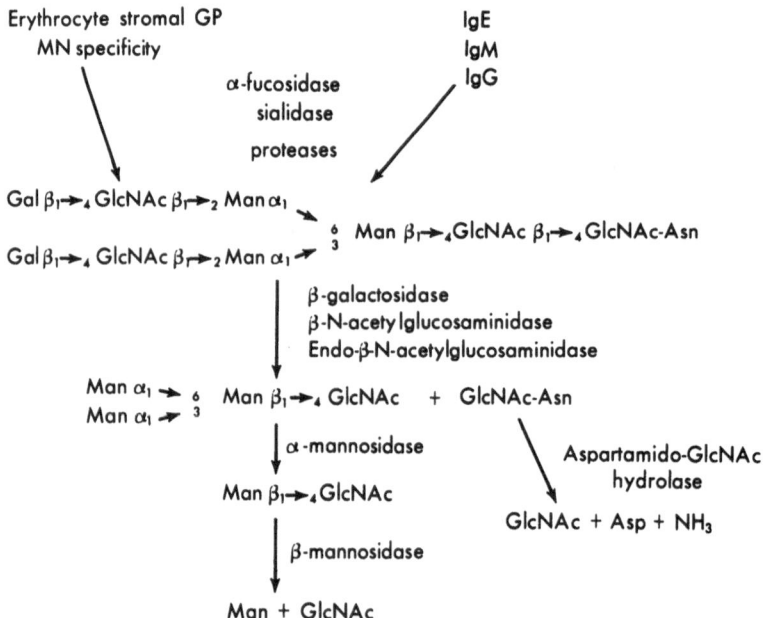

Figure 5. Suggested pathway for the catabolism of
           erythrocyte and immunoglobulin glycoproteins.

core of various glycoproteins have been reported to accumulate in liver, spleen, brain and cultured fibroblasts (see 22 and 41) in this disease.

It is well known that cells can take up glycoproteins readily by pinocytosis. The pinocytotic vesicles can fuse to form vacuoles which become secondary lysosomes (phagosomes) which normally would contain the enzymes for complete degradation of glycoproteins. In the absence of β-galactosidase or β-N-acetylglucosaminidase activity, the glycopeptides and oligosaccharides derived from incomplete glycoprotein metabolism would accumulate initially in vacuoles of the tissues responsible for the major part of their turnover (liver, spleen). Saturation of storage capacity in the parenchymal cells of these tissues could lead to overflow into the circulation followed by re-uptake by many other tissues and account for the widespread visceral vacuolation seen pathologically. The low molecular weight of the undegradable compounds would also permit glomerular filtration and appearance in the urine. The exceedingly small amounts of the carbohydrate compounds present in brain in contrast to the large ganglioside storage indicates a barrier of entry into the brain. Indeed, the small accumulation in the brain could well be accounted for by uptake into the vascular endothelial cells.

In infants with G_{M1}-gangliosidosis Type I up to 1 g of the glycopeptides and oligosaccharides are excreted each day. Calculations based on immunoglobulin and erythrocyte turnover time in infants, total blood immunoglobulin and stromal glycoprotein carbohydrate content indicate that the major part of the oligosaccharide excretion could be derived from these sources alone. The large amounts of these oligosaccharides and glycopeptides excreted in the urine of G_{M1}-gangliosidosis Type I patients could provide a ready source of presently unavailable key acceptor molecules for investigations on the specificity of and products formed in glycosyl transferase reactions. Furthermore, recent evidence implicates the participation of polyisoprenol derivatives as lipid intermediates in oligosaccharide transfer to protein (7,14,30). The synthesis of oligosaccharide-lipid intermediates using the pure urinary oligosaccharides from G_{M1}-gangliosidosis as precursor in studies of these transfer reactions is of considerable interest. Thus, detailed biochemical studies of the storage materials in inherited disorders of glycosphingolipid and glycoprotein catabolism can have important implications in the solution of other problems in biochemical research.

This research was supported by a Grant MT-1345 to L.S.W. from the Medical Research Council of Canada.

REFERENCES

1. Applegarth, D. A. and Bozoian, G. Mucopolysaccharide storage
    in Organs of a Patient with Sandhoff's Disease. Clin. Chim.
    Acta, 39, 269, 1972.

2. Baenzinger, J., Kornfeld, S. and Kochwa, S. Structure of the
    Carbohydrate Units of IgE. J. Biol. Chem., 249, 1889, 1897,
    1974.

3. Calatroni, A. Fractionation and Characterization of Glyco-
    peptides and Oligosaccharides from the Liver of a Patient with
    G_{M1}-Gangliosidosis Type I. Ital. J. Biochem., 23, 329, 1974.

4. Callahan, J. W., Pinsky, L. and Wolfe, L. S. G_{M1}-Gangliosidosis
    Type II: Studies on a Fibroblast Cell Strain. Biochem. Med.,
    4, 295, 1970.

5. Callahan, J. W. and Wolfe, L. S. Isolation and Characterization
    of Keratan Sulfates from the Liver of a Patient with G_{M1}-
    Gangliosidosis Type I. Biochim. Biophys. Acta, 215, 527, 1970.

6. Cantz, M. and Kresse, H. Sandhoff Disease: Defective Glycos-
    aminoglycan Catabolism in Cultured Fibroblasts. Eur. J.
    Biochem., 47, 581, 1974.

7. Chen, W. W., Lennarz, W. J., Tarentino, A. L. and Maley, F. A.
    Lipid-linked Oligosaccharide Intermediate in Glycoprotein
    Synthesis in Oviduct. J. Biol. Chem., 250, 7006, 1975.

8. Cook, G. M. W. and Stoddart, R. W. Surface Carbohydrates of
    the Eukaryotic Cell. Academic Press, London, pp. 140-154,
    1973.

9. Derry, D. M., Fawcett, J. S., Andermann, F. and Wolfe, L. S.
    Late Infantile Systemic Lipidosis. Neurology, 18, 340, 1968.

10. Foster, A. B. Deamination of D-glucosamine, D-glucosaminic
    acid and D-glucosaminol. Chem. and Ind. (London), 627, 1955.

11. Gonatas, N. K. and Gonatas, J. Ultrastructural and Biochemical
    Observations on a Case of Systemic Late Infantile Lipidosis.
    J. Neuropath. Exp. Neurol., 24, 318, 1965.

12. Hirano, S. and Meyer, K. Enzymatic Degradation of Corneal and
    Cartilaginous Keratosulfates. Biochem. Biophys. Res. Comm.,
    44, 1371, 1971.

13. Isemura, S., and Schmid, K. Studies on the Carbohydrate Moiety of α_1-Acid Glycoprotein (Orosomucoid) by Using Alkaline Hydrolysis and Deamination by Nitrous Acid. Biochem. J., 124, 591, 1971.

14. Lennarz, W. J. Lipid Linked Sugars in Glycoprotein Synthesis. Science, 188, 986, 1975.

15. Lloyd, K. O., Kabat, E. A. and Licerio, E. Immunochemical Studies on Blood Groups XXXVIII. Biochemistry, 7, 2976, 1968.

16. Lowden, J. A., Cutz, E., Conen, P. E., Rudd, N. and Doran, T. A. Prenatal Diagnosis of G_{M1}-Gangliosidosis. New Engl. J. Med., 288, 225, 1973.

17. Montgomery, R. Glycoproteins. In, The Carbohydrates IIB, Ed. Pigman, W. and Horton, D. Academic Press, New York, 627-709, 1970.

18. Ng Ying Kin, N. M. K. and Wolfe, L. S. Oligosaccharides accumulating in the Liver from a Patient with G_{M2}-Gangliosidosis Variant O. Biochem. Biophys. Res. Comm., 59, 837, 1974.

19. Ng Ying Kin, N. M. K. and Wolfe, L. S. The Structures of Oligosaccharides and Glycopeptides in the Urine of G_{M1} and G_{M2}-Gangliosidosis. Fed. Proc., 34, 634, 1975.

20. Ng Ying Kin, N. M. K., and Wolfe, L. S. Characterization of Oligosaccharides and Glycopeptides Excreted in the Urine of G_{M1}-Gangliosidosis Patients. Biochem. Biophys. Res. Comm., 66, 123, 1975.

21. Nishigaki, M., Muramatsu, T. and Kobata, A. Endoglycosidases acting on Carbohydrate Moieties of Glycoproteins. Biochem. Biophys. Res. Comm., 59, 638, 1974.

22. Nordén, N. E., Lundblad, A., Svensson, S., Okermann, P. and Autio, S. A Mannose-containing Trisaccharide Isolated from Urines of Three Patients with Mannosidosis. J. Biol. Chem., 248, 6210, 1973.

23. O'Brien, J. S. Generalized Gangliosidosis. J. Pediatrics, 75, 167, 1969.

24. O'Brien J. S. Ganglioside Storage Diseases. Adv. Human Gen., 3, 39, 1972.

25. O'Brien, J. S., Okada, S. and Ho, M. W. Ganglioside Storage
     Diseases. Fed. Proc., 30, 956, 1971.

26. Orii, T., Minami, R., Sukegawa, K., Sato, S., et al. A New
     Type of Mucolipidosis with β-galactosidase Deficiency and
     Glycopeptiduria. Tohoku J. Exp. Med., 107, 303, 1972.

27. Patel, V., Goebel, H. H., Watanabe, I. and Zeman, W. Studies
     on G_{M1}-Gangliosidosis, Type II. Acta Neuropath., 30, 155,
     1974.

28. Percy, A. K., McCormick, U. M., Kaback, M. M. and Herndon,
     R. M. Ultrastructure Manifestations of G_{M1} and G_{M2}
     Gangliosidosis in Fetal Tissues. Arch. Neurol., 28, 417, 1973.

29. Petrelli, M. and Blair, J. D. The Liver in G_{M1}-Gangliosidoses
     Types 1 and 2. Archiv. Path., 99, 111, 1975.

30. Pless, D. D. and Lennarz, W. J. A Lipid-Linked Oligosaccharide
     in Glycoprotein Synthesis. J. Biol. Chem., 250, 7014, 1975.

31. Strecker, G. and Montreuil, J. Description d'une oligosac-
     charidosurie accompagnant une gangliosidose G_{M2} à deficit
     total en N-acetylhexosaminidases. Clin. Chim. Acta, 33, 395,
     1971.

32. Suzuki, K. Cerebral G_{M1}-Gangliosidosis: Chemical Pathology of
     Visceral Organs. Science, 159, 1471, 1968.

33. Suzuki, K., Suzuki, K. and Chen, G. C. Morphological, histo-
     chemical and biochemical studies on a case of systemic Late
     Infantile Lipidosis (Generalized Gangliosidosis). J.
     Neuropath. Exp. Neurol., 27, 15, 1968.

34. Suzuki, K., Suzuki, K., Kamoshita, S. Chemical pathology of
     G_{M1}-Gangliosidosis. J. Neuropath. Exp. Neurol., 28, 25, 1969.

35. Tai, T., Ito, S., Yamashita, K., Muramatsu, T. and Kobata, A.
     Asparagine-linked Oligosaccharide Chains of IgG: A Revised
     Structure. Biochem. Biophys. Res. Comm., 65, 968, 1975.

36. Takebayashi, S., Bassewitz, D. B. von, and Themann, H.
     Ultrastructural Alterations of the Kidney in Generalized
     Gangliosidosis G_{M1}. Vidch. Arch. Zellpath., 5, 301, 1970.

37. Tarentino, A. L., Plummer, T. H. and Maley, F. A. The core
     oligosaccharide of IgM. Fed. Proc., 34, 591, 1975.

38. Thomas, D. B. and Winzler, R. J. Structure of Glycoproteins of Human Erythrocytes. Biochem. J., 124, 55, 1971.

39. Tsay, G. C. and Dawson, G. Structure of the "Keratosulfate-like" Material in Liver from a Patient with G_{M1}-Gangliosidosis. Biochem. Biophys. Res. Comm., 52, 759, 1973.

40. Tsay, G. C. and Dawson, G. Glycopeptide Storage in Fibroblasts from Patients with Inborn Errors of Glycoprotein and Glyco-sphingolipid Catabolism. Biochem. Biophys. Res. Comm., 63, 807, 1975.

41. Tsay, G. C., Dawson, G. and Matalon, R. Glycopeptide Storage in Skin Fibroblasts Cultures from a Patient with α-Mannosidase Deficiency. J. Clin. Investig., 56, 711, 1975.

42. Tsay, G. C., Dawson, G. and Yu-Teh-Li. Structures of the Glyco-peptide Storage Material in G_{M1}-Gangliosidosis. Biochim. Biophys. Acta, 385, 305, 1975.

43. Winzler, R. J. The Glycoproteins of Plasma Membranes. In, Glycoproteins. Ed. A. Gottschalk, Elsevier, Amsterdam, 1268-1293, 1972.

44. Wolfe, L. S., Callahan, J., Fawcett, J. S., Andermann, F. and Scriver, C. R. G_{M1}-gangliosidosis without chondrodystrophy or visceromegaly. Neurology, 20, 23, 1970.

45. Wolfe, L. S., Clarke, J. T. R. and Senior, R. G. Biochemical Studies of G_{M1}-Gangliosidosis and Ceramide Trihexosidosis. In, Sphingolipids, Sphingolipidoses and Allied Disorders, Ed. B. W. Volk, Plenum, New York, 373-384, 1972.

46. Wolfe, L. S., Senior, R. G. and Ng Ying Kin, N. M. K. The Structures of Oligosaccharides Accumulating in the Liver of G_{M1}-Gangliosidosis, Type I. J. Biol. Chem., 249, 1828, 1974.

GLYCOPROTEIN CATABOLISM IN BRAIN TISSUE IN THE LYSOSOMAL ENZYME

DEFICIENCY DISEASES

Eric G. Brunngraber, Leonard G. Davis, Javaid I. Javaid,
  and Bruno Berra
Missouri Institute of Psychiatry, School of Medicine,
University of Missouri-Columbia, 5400 Arsenal Street,
St. Louis, Mo. 63139; Illinois State Psychiatric
Institute, 1601 W. Taylor Street, Chicago, Ill. 60612;
and Istituto Di Chimica Biologica Dell'Universita Di
Milano, Facolta di Medicina, Via Saldini 50, Milano,Italy

Glyocoproteins of brain tissue contain two major classes of
heteropolysaccharide side chain, both of which are attached to the
polypeptide chain of the protein moiety by means of an alkali-stable
beta-aspartylglycosamine linkage (1). These carbohydrate-rich
structures are readily liberated as soluble glycopeptides upon
treatment of the denatured glycoproteins with proteolytic enzymes
such as papain or pronase. The acidic sialoglycopeptides thus
released account for approximately 65% of the glycoprotein-carbohydrate in brain tissue. These substances contain N-acetylneuraminic
acid, galactose, mannose, N-acetylglucosamine, and fucose; some of
these heteropolysaccharide polymers also contain sulfate-ester
groups. A hypothetical structure for these glycopeptides is depicted
(Fig. 1).

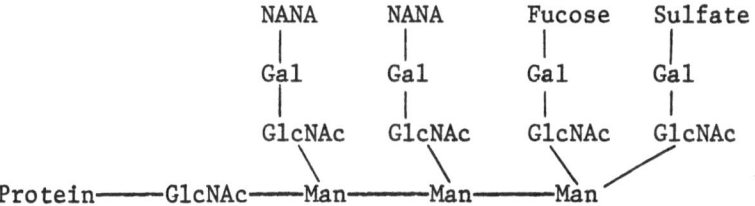

Fig.1. Hypothetical structure for non-dialyzable acidic sialoglycopeptides from brain, based on that propsed for oligosaccharides
associated with fetuin (2). NANA = N-acetylneuraminic acid; Gal =
galactose; GlcNAc = N-acetylglucosamine; Man = mannose.

The polymer consists of internally located mannose residues joined to the N-acetylglucosamine residue that is linked to the peptide chain. The mannose residues also serve as branch points for the more external side branches consisting of --N-acetylglu-cosamine--galactose--NANA (or fucose, sulfate). Sulfate and fucose groups are depicted as attached to galactose. However, it is equally likely that these substances may be linked to N-acetylglucos-amine residues. It does not appear to be likely that a single heteropolysaccharide of this type would contain more than one sulfate or fucose residue per oligosaccharide molecule (1).

Approximately 25% of the glycoprotein-carbohydrate of brain tissue is associated with mannose-rich oligosaccharide polymers that have the capability of binding to the lectin, Concanavalin A (3,4). These oligosaccharides, recovered as mannose-rich glyco-peptides after the action of papain on defatted brain tissue resi-dues, contain six moles of mannose and two moles of N-acetylgluco-samine per glycopeptide molecule.

The lysosome is most probably the subcellular organelle that accomplishes the degradation of a major part of the glycoprotein molecule. Aronson and De Duve (5) found that the isolated rat liver lysosome was capable of cleaving approximately one half of the peptide bonds of the glycoprotein substrate, fetuin. Most of the terminal sialic acid groups were quickly cleaved in this in vitro system, but the release of galactose and N-acetylglucosamine proceeded more slowly and did not exceed 50% of the theoretical yield. Enzymatic release of mannose could not be detected and it was assumed that the branch points in the heteropolysaccharide structures were relatively resistant to attack. Although little is known regarding the sequence of degradative steps that serve to dismantle the glycoprotein structure, in vivo, it is clear that the lysosome contains all of the enzymes required for the task. It appears likely that the degradation of the oligosaccharide poly-mers attached to glycoproteins proceeds by sequential cleavage of the sugar residues located at the exposed non-reducing termini of the various chains of which the polymer is composed. Thus, a sequential attack by neuraminidase, beta-galactosidase, beta-N-ace-tylglucosaminidase, and alpha mannosidase will cleave the hypo-thetical oligosaccharide depicted in Fig. 1. When a specific glyco-sidase activity is deficient, as in GM2 or GM1 gangliosidosis, it is expected that glycopeptides that contain the sugar residue at the non-reducing termini that serves as the appropriate substrate for the missing enzyme will accumulate. The failure of the enzyme to cleave the terminal sugar will, in addition, prevent the cleavage of the more internally located sugars by the appropriate glycosidases. Thus, in GM1-gangliosidosis, the exposed galactose residues are not cleaved due to the absent or defective beta-galactosidase. This will prevent the action of beta-hexosaminidase and alpha-

mannosidase, enzymes known to be present at normal or above normal
levels in this disease. Consequently, the tissue will accumulate
bound mannose and N-acetylglucosamine, as well as galactose, in
the form of partially degraded oligosaccharide chains. In this
analysis, it is assumed that the deficient beta-galactosidase
responsible for the cleavage of terminal galactose in GM1 is also
responsible for the degradation of the prosthetic groups of glycoproteins. This appears to be the case (6).

The absence of beta-galactosidase in GM1-gangliosidosis and
beta-hexosaminidase in GM2-gangliosidosis would be expected to
affect the degradation of the acidic sialo-oligosaccharides which
contain galactose and N-acetylglucosamine in their external
branches. The mannose-rich oligosaccharide chains, which contain
mannose residues in their terminal non-reducing positions (3,4)
are presumably catabolized in a normal manner, at least up to the
stage at which all external mannose groups had been removed. Consequently, a major proportion of the accumulated oligosaccharides
in GM1- and GM2-gangliosidosis consists of breakdown products
derived from the acidic sialo-oligosaccharide polymers.

Degradation of glycoproteins, in vivo, requires the combined
action of proteases and glycosidases. One possible sequence consists of a pathway in which the heteropolysaccharide chains are
attacked by glycosidases prior to substantial cleavage of the peptide chains. In this case, glycoproteins with incompletely degraded heteropolysaccharide side chains would accumulate, if the
required glycosidase is deficient. A second possibility is a
process whereby glycoprotein degradation proceeds by the simultaneous action of lysosomal proteases and glycosidases. Alternatively,
a considerable portion of the peptide chain may be cleaved prior
to cleavage of the oligosaccharide units. In either case, glycopeptides with partially degraded oligosaccharide chains would
accumulate. Tingey (7) has provided evidence that this may be the
case in GM2-gangliosidosis. Defatted brain tissue was extracted
with boiling water and the hexosamine content of the extract was
estimated. The amount of water soluble bound-hexosamine extracted
from the brain tissue was approximately five times that extracted
from control brains. Approximately half of the accumulated protein-
bound hexosamine could be extracted in this way. It appears
probable that the accumulated product existed in the form of glycopeptides of a wide variety of molecular sizes. Glycopeptides
produced by the action of proteases and glycosidases may become
sufficiently small so that beta-aspartyl-N-acetylglucosaminidase
is enabled to split the bond between asparagine and the heteropolysaccharide chain. The size and structure of the oligosaccharide
unit appears to be less important for the action of this enzyme,
than the peptide portion of the molecule. For the enzyme to act,
the asparagine unit must not be linked to another amino acid (8).

In aspartylglycosaminuria, a genetically linked disease in which
the activity of this enzyme is defective, a number of aspartyl
oligosaccharides accumulate in brain and other tissues (9), and
are excreted in excess in the urine (10). Thus, one would expect
that oligosaccharides as well as glycopeptides would accumulate
in GM1- and GM2-gangliosidosis.

Since oligosaccharides have not been observed to accumulate
in brain tissue in these cases, it appears that the activity of
the beta-aspartyl-N-acetylglucosaminidase may not be significant
in GM1- or GM2-gangliosidosis. The accumulated product appears to
bear a negative charge (11); it is not extracted from brain tissue
by aqueous chloroform-methanol. On the other hand, oligosaccharides
derived from glycoproteins have been shown to accumulate in the
liver of patients with GM1-gangliosidosis (12-15); glycopeptides
also accumulate (16-20). It is of interest that the oligosaccharides, which are very soluble in water, are partially extracted from liver tissue by means of aqueous chloroform-methanol, and
can subsequently be partitioned into an upper aqueous phase where
they contaminate the ganglioside preparation (12-15,18,19). Since
this has not been observed in brain tissue, the accumulated material presumably exists in the form of glycopeptides the peptide
moiety of which increases its polarity and insolubility in organic
solvents. Oligosaccharides have been observed to accumulate in
the liver in Sandhoff's variant of GM2-gangliosidosis. The heptasaccharide which accumulates has a trimannosyl core and contains
N-acetylglucosamine at non-reducing termini (21).

While accumulated oligosaccharides have not been definitely
observed in brain tissue in either GM1 or GM2 gangliosidosis,
oligosaccharides have been shown to accumulate in brain tissue in
fucosidosis (22) and mannosidosis (23,24). Glycopeptides that
contain fucose--alpha(1→6)N-acetylglucosamine linkages and oligosaccharides containing fucose-galactose-N-acetylglucosamine sequences were reported to accumulate in the brain in fucosidosis
(22). The fucose residue blocks the degradation of the chain of
which it forms the terminal portion: the entire chain therfore
accumulates in the absence of alpha-fucosidase, as predicted earlier (25). In mannosidosis, mannose-rich oligosaccharides containing approximately 5 mannose residues and 1 N-acetylglucosamine
residue were readily extracted from brain gray matter with water.
Thus it appears that the beta-aspartyl-N-acetylglucosaminidase
was active in brain tissue in these diseases.

Use of Concanavalin A to separate glycopeptides: In the studies
to be discussed in the following sections, defatted brain tissue
was treated with papain to convert all of the glycoprotein mater-
ial--intact glycoproteins and partially degraded glycoprotein der-
ivatives--into glycopeptides. Glycosaminoglycans and nucleic

acids, which are also solubilized by the proteolytic enzymes, were removed by precipitation with cetylpyridinium chloride (26). Subjection of the glycopeptide preparation to prolonged dialysis provides a non-dialyzable glycopeptide preparation that consists primarily of the acidic sialoglycopeptides. The dialyzable glycopeptides include the mannose-rich material. However, a large precentage of the dialyzable N-acetylneuraminic acid is associated with acidic sialoglycopeptides that predominate in the non-dialyzable preparation. In addition, both dialyzable and non-dialyzable glycopeptide preparations contain several minor glycopeptide components that appear to differ from the major glycopeptide classes insofar as their carbohydrate composition and molecular size is concerned.

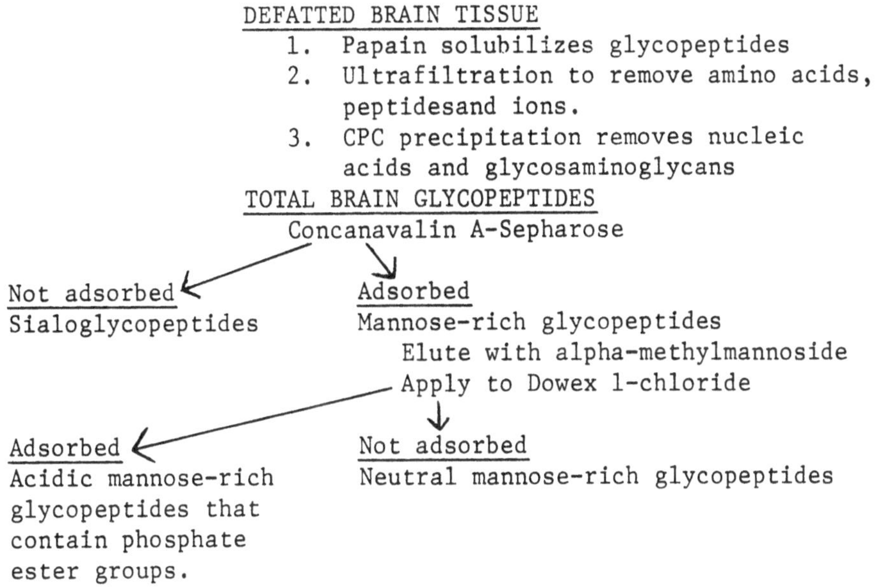

DEFATTED BRAIN TISSUE
    1. Papain solubilizes glycopeptides
    2. Ultrafiltration to remove amino acids,
       peptidesand ions.
    3. CPC precipitation removes nucleic
       acids and glycosaminoglycans
TOTAL BRAIN GLYCOPEPTIDES
    Concanavalin A-Sepharose

Not adsorbed   Adsorbed
Sialoglycopeptides   Mannose-rich glycopeptides
                  Elute with alpha-methylmannoside
             Apply to Dowex 1-chloride

Adsorbed   Not adsorbed
Acidic mannose-rich   Neutral mannose-rich glycopeptides
glycopeptides that
contain phosphate
ester groups.

Figure 2. Flow chart for separation of sialoglycopeptides, mannose-rich, neutral glycopeptides, and phosphorylated mannose-rich glycopeptides.

More recently, affinity chromatography has been employed to separate glycopeptide fractions (Fig. 2). After treatment of the defatted tissue residue with papain, the solubilized glycopeptides were subjected to ultrafiltration to remove amino acids, small peptides and ions. Nucleic acids and glycosaminoglycans were removed by precipitation with cetylpyridinium chloride as before, and the total glycopeptide preparation was applied to columns of concanavalin A-Sepharose. Acidic sialoglycopeptides, as well as most of the minor glycopeptide fractions, were not adsorbed to the lectin. The mannose-rich glycopeptides were adsorbed to the concanavalin A and subsequently were eluted with alpha-methylman-

noside (3,4). After removal of alpha-methylmannoside by ultrafiltration, it was possible to separate the mannose-rich glycopeptide
fraction into neutral and acidic forms by utilization of Dowex 1-
chloride anion exchange chromatography. The acidic mannose-rich
glycopeptides appear to be similar to the neutral fraction in carbohydrate composition and molecular size, except that they contain
phosphate ester groups that are attached to one of the carbohydrate
residues (probably mannose) of the oligosaccharide chains. The
existance of carbohydrate-bound phosphate ester groups has been
confirmed by NMR studies and the isolation of monosaccharide-phos-
phate esters after partial acid hydrolysis (27) as well as by
isolation of the parent phosphoglycoproteins from rat brain tissue
by means of affinity chromatography on concanavalin A-Sepharose.

Dialyzable glycopeptide preparations that had been previously
isolated from various pathological tissues (28-31) were applied
to concanavalin A-Sepharose columns. No evidence for the accumulation of glycopeptide-carbohydrate had previously been noted for
Krabbe's disease (31) and this served as an appropriate control
for the present comparisons. Approximately half of the dialyzable
glycopeptide preparation was found to bind to concanavalin A-Sepharose (Table I). On the other hand, only 16 and 25% of the dial-

TABLE I

	Total dialyzable glycopeptide (umoles hexose/ gram (fresh))	% that binds to concana- valin A	Mannose-rich glycopeptides (umoles hexose/ gram (fresh))
GM1-gangliosidosis	2.99	16	0.48
GM2-gangliosidosis	2.18	25	0.55
Nieman-Pick Disease	1.44	23	0.33
Krabbe's Disease	0.65	50	0.32

yable glycopeptide-hexose obtained from brain tissue of cases with
GM1 and GM2 gangliosidosis (variant B) was retained by the lectin.
The stored materials in these diseases do not bind to concanavalin A and presumably do not contain the terminal mannose linkages
that permit interaction with the lectin. As noted above, the
stored material in GM1 and GM2 gangliosidosis are breakdown products derived from the sialoglycopeptides and presumably contain
terminal galactose and N-acetylglucosamine residues. Having lost
terminal NANA groups (GM1 gangliosidosis) and terminal NANA plus
galactose (GM2 gangliosidosis), the partly degraded materials
have been rendered dialyzable.

In the case of Nieman-Pick disease, it had been found that the acidic sialoglycopeptides showed a two-fold elevation. A large proportion of these materials appeared in the dialyzable glycopeptide preparation and consequently the percentage of the dialyzable glycopeptide-hexose that bound to concanavalin A was only 23%. The concentration of the mannose-rich glycopeptides was not elevated.

Normal and diseased brain tissue samples were processed according to the procedure of Fig. 2. The concentration of mannose-rich glycopeptides in samples of cerebral gray matter from Tay-Sachs disease was not different from that found in the newborn normal gray matter (Table II): Krabbe's disease showed a small elevation. The significance of this is uncertain since the Krabbe brain sample was that of a 20 month old child. The percentage of mannose-rich glycopeptides that contain phosphate ester groups was approximately the same in the three cases studied.

TABLE II

	Mannose-Rich Glycopeptides ugr/gram fresh gray matter	% that contain PO_4 ester groups
Newborn control	0.122	36%
Tay-Sachs Disease	0.119	34%
Krabbe's Disease	0.174	31%

Although an analysis of three specimens is insufficient to draw firm conclusions, preliminary experiments suggest a possible marked age-dependence of the concentration of acidic and neutral mannose-rich glycopeptides in brain tissue (Table III). The concentration of the phosphorylated glycopeptides was highest in the newborn but reached adult levels by 15 years of age. The neutral mannose-rich glycopeptides were present at highest levels at 15 years of age, but showed a marked decrease by 62 years of age.

TABLE III

Age	Total Con A Binding Glycopeptides	Neutral Con A binding Glycopeptides	Acidic Con A binding Glycopeptides
	ugr hexose/g fresh wt		
New Born	122	73	42
15-year old	283	253	15
62-year old	50	31	13

GM2-Gangliosidosis: The concentration and composition of the non-
dialyzable acidic sialoglycopeptides in cerebral gray matter from
Tay-Sachs Disease (GM2-gangliosidosis, Variant B) was similar to
that of the normal controls (11). However, the concentration of
the dialyzable glycopeptide-carbohydrate was elevated (11,29).
Dialyzable glycopeptide-galactose was not appreciably affected by
the disease while dialyzable glycopeptide-mannose and -N-acetyl-
glucosamine showed four and three fold elevations respectively (29).
(Table IV). As noted above, the concentration of concanavalin A-
binding, mannose-rich glycopeptides was not appreciably increased in
this disease; therefore the accumulated mannose and N-acetylglucosamine was associated with glycopeptides that do not contain
mannoside structures capable of interacting with the lectin. The
accumulated degradation product is presumably derived from sialoglycopeptides that had been partially degraded by the action of
neuraminidase and beta-galactosidase to provide a glycopeptide
that was enriched in both N-acetylglucosamine and mannose. Similar
findings were observed in a case of Sandhoff's disease (GM2-ganglio-
sidosis, Variant 0) (29).

     Suzuki, et. al. (32) noted an increase in the hexosamine content
of fatted tissue residues obtained from the gray matter of a case
of GM2-gangliosidosis, Variant 0; marked elevation of the hexosamine content of an aqueous extract from cerebral gray matter was
also noted. Only a moderate increase in protein-bound hexosamine
was noted in the B-variant. No increase in glycoprotein content
was noted in a case of juvenile GM2-gangliosidoses (33). This
variant of the disease was qualitatively similar to, but quantitatively milder than Tay-Sachs disease. Bogoch (34) has reported
an elevation of glycoprotein content in Tay-Sachs disease. Balint
and Kyriadides (35) reported an increase in glycoprotein-hexosamine
content of the red blood cell in Tay-Sachs disease; the content
of N-acetylneuraminic acid was normal (36). Thus red blood cells
appear to reflect the situation in the brain: elevation of hexosamine but normal NANA levels.

GM1-Gangliosidosis: The accumulated material of glycoprotein origin
in GM1-gangliosidosis was derived from the acidic sialoglycopeptides (28,37). Terminal NANA residues are cleaved, thereby exposing
galactose groups. Degradation of the chain cannot continue and
glycopeptides or oligosaccharides with terminal galactose residues
accumulate. A part of this material is dialyzable, and galactose,
mannose, and N-acetylglucosamine in the dialyzable glycopeptide
preparation was found to be elevated (Table IV). A part of the
accumulated material remains in the non-dialyzable fraction, account-
ing for the elevation of these sugars in this preparation.
Patel, et. al. (38) studied the brain tissue of a six year old
boy afflicted with GM1-gangliosidosis of type II. Although there

TABLE IV

GLYCOPEPTIDE-CARBOHYDRATE CONTENT OF CEREBRAL GRAY MATTER

	NANA	Fucose	HexNAc	Man	Gal
	umoles/g fresh				
Non-Dialyzable	Glycopeptides				
Control, 3 yrs.	0.64	0.54	1.50	0.69	1.00
Control, 8 yrs.	0.72	0.55	1.94	1.13	1.04
GM2-gangliosidosis, B variant	0.77	0.49	1.81	0.98	1.20
GM2-gangliosidosis, O variant	0.54	0.51	2.02	0.79	0.96
GM1-gangliosidosis, Type I	0.75	0.52	2.69	1.43	1.90
GM1-gangliosidosis, Type I	0.69	0.40	1.56	1.43	1.68
Krabbe's Disease	0.89	0.41	1.81	1.08	1.13
Niemann-Pick Disease	1.53	0.90	2.80	1.63	1.70
MLD, juvenile	0.44	0.50	1.92	2.14	
Dialyzable	Glycopeptides				
Control, 3 yrs.	0.11	0.26	0.60	0.72	0.32
Control, 8 yrs.	0.21	0.22	1.03	0.56	0.43
GM2-gangliosidosis, B variant	0.24	0.37	1.93	2.97	0.52
GM2-gangliosidosis, O variant	0.15	0.45	2.69	2.82	0.58
GM1-gangliosidosis, Type I	0.10	0.15	1.36	1.07	0.88
GM1-gangliosidosis, Type I	0.37	0.23	1.67	1.87	1.12
Krabbe's Disease	0.10	0.14	0.58	0.44	0.21
Niemann-Pick Disease	0.28	0.30	1.25	1.02	0.42
MLD, juvenile	0.11	0.37	0.89	1.03	

Age at death: GM2-gangliosidosis, B variant (20 mos); GM2-gang-
liosidosis, O-variant (15 mos); GM1-gangliosidosis, Type I (15
mos); GM1-gangliosidosis, Type I (7 mos); Krabbe's Disease (20
mos); Niemann Pick Disease (15 mos); MLD (onset 8 yrs, death
20 yrs).

was no evidence of glycoprotein accumulation in the liver, brain
tissue showed a 2.5 fold elevation in glycoprotein-galactose content. Accumulation of oligosaccharides in liver tissue (39) has
been discussed above. Wolf et. al. (40) found a decrease in
sialoglycopeptide levels in the brain tissue of a case of gangliosidosis of type II, but no values were given for the dialyzable
glycopeptides derived from this tissue. A marked increase in the
urinary excretion of undersulfated keratan sulfate was noted.

Niemann-Pick and Gaucher's Diseases: The primary lesions in Niemann-
Pick and Gauchers diseases are respectively a deficiency of
sphingomyelinase and glucosylcerebroside beta-glucosidase activity.
Neither of these enzymes are involved in glycoprotein degradation.
Nevertheless, accumulation of glycoprotein or glycoprotein degrad-

ation products have been reported to occur in these diseases.
Elevation of protein-bound hexosamine in Niemann-Pick disease was
noted by Norman et. al. (41), Tingey (7), and Svennerholm (42).
Brunngraber, et. al. (30) found that the increased concentation
of protein-bound hexosamine was due to the elevation of both
glycosaminoglycans and the acidic sialoglycopeptides derived from
brain glycoproteins (Table IV). The dialyzable, mannose-rich
glycopeptides, on the other hand, were present in normal concentration. Svennerholm (42-44) reported an elevation of protein-
bound hexosamine in brain tissue in Gaucher's Disease. Kanfer,
et. al. (45) extracted a Gaucher spleen with chloroform-methanol
and treated the protein residue with papain and pronase. A two-
fold accumulation of hexosamine, fucose, hexose, and NANA in glycopeptides that remained unprecipitated with cetylpyridinium chloride
was noted.

    Niemann-Pick and Gaucher's disease may represent conditions
in which a primary brain lesion affects the degradation of a multi-
macromolecular complex, the degradation or transport of which is
inhibited as a consequence of the failure of the cell to degrade
one of its components. For example, turnover of plasma membranes
may involve the sequential degradation of a variety of macromolecular components. Failure to degrade one of the components of the
system may inhibit the degradation of the entire complex, or block
its transport to degradative sites. In Niemann-Pick disease, failure
to degrade sphingomyelin results in the accumulation of gangliosides, glycoproteins, glycosaminoglycans and cholesterol as well
as sphingomyelin; all of these components are prominent plasma
membrane constituents.

Krabbe's Disease: No remarkable changes were noted in the concentration of glycosaminoglycans and glycopeptides derived from brain
gray matter glycoproteins from a 20 month old child afflicted with
Krabbe's Disease (31). Tingey and Edgar (46) had found no elevation
in protein-bound hexosamine in Krabbe's Disease, although they
noted an elevation in white matter. It has been reported (47)
that the missing enzyme activity in this disease is that of the
cerebroside beta-galactosidase; activities against lactosylceramide
and asialoganglioside GM1 were normal. Since the beta-galactosidase that removes the terminal galactose residue from asialoganglioside GM1 appears to be capable of cleaving the terminal galactose
residues of desialidated glycoproteins (asialofetuin), the failure
to find an accumulation of degradation products derived from glycoproteins was not unexpected.

Metachromatic Leukodystrophy: Numerous reports have indicated that
the concentration of protein-bound hexosamine in white matter from
some, if not all, forms of metachromatic leukodystrophy is increased
(7,46,48-56). These chemical findings were supported by a number

of histochemical investigations (55,57-60). The primary metachromatic storage product, the sulfatides, were removed from tissue
slices by the use of organic solvents. A periodic acid-Schiff
positive granular material remained in the tissue after the extraction. This positive PAS reaction is often attributed to the accumulation of glycosaminoglycans. However, glycosaminoglycans generally show a considerably weaker reaction with the periodic acid-
Schiff reagents than that produced by the carbohydrate residues
associated with glycoproteins. Since brain glycoproteins contain
heteropolysaccharide chains with sulfate ester groups (1), it
appears that the accumulated material may be derived from these
substances as well as sulfated glycosaminoglycans. Accumulation
of both glycosaminoglycans and glycoprotein degradation products
may be substantial in the multiple sulfatase deficiency forms of
metachromatic leukodystrophy (61). Eto, _et. al._ (62) have suggested
that sulfatase B, deficient in the multiple sulfatase deficiency
forms of the disease, may be the enzyme responsible for the cleavage of sulfate ester groups from glycopeptides and glycoproteins.

A juvenile form of metachromatic leukodystrophy, with onset
at 8 years of age and death at 20 years, was found to lack arylsulfatase A activity, although arylsulfatase B levels showed no
significant deviation from normal control values (63). The sulfatide level in white matter was elevated by two fold. Glycosaminoglycan levels were normal, but the hexosamine and hexose content
of the non-dialyzable acidic sialoglycopeptide preparation presented
a 55 to 100% elevation compared to the normal control values obtained for 8 and 72 year old white matter (Table V). There was no
significant change in the concentration of dialyzable glycopeptide
hexose and hexosamine in white matter, and no remarkable changes
were noted in gray matter (Table IV).

TABLE V

Glycopeptide-Carbohydrate Content of Cerebral White Matter

	NANA	Fucose	HexNAc	Hex
		umoles/g fresh		
Non-dialyzable Glycopeptides				
Control, 8 yr old	0.46	0.24	1.10	1.30
Control, 72 yr old	0.40	0.17	0.80	1.12
MLD, juvenile	0.39	0.34	1.71	2.17
GM2-gangliosidosis, variant B	0.65	0.38	2.36	1.79
GM1-gangliosidosis, Type I.	0.83	0.55	2.04	4.08
Dialyzable Glycopeptides				
Control, 8 yr old	0.18	0.17	1.08	0.81
Control, 72 yr old	0.09	0.16	0.54	0.76
MLD, juvenile	0.07	0.37	0.85	1.16
GM2-gangliosidosis, variant B	0.18	0.34	1.72	1.51
GM1-gangliosidosis, Type I.	0.37	0.23	1.67	2.99

The Neuronal Ceroid-Lipofuscinoses (64): Late infantile amaurotic
idiocy (Jansky-Bielschowski type) and the juvenile form of amaurotic idiocy (Batten-Vogt-Spielmeyer type) have generally shown a
reduction in the glycoprotein-carbohydrate content of gray matter
(65-67) with normal levels in white matter. Landolt (68) presented
an atypical case (Spielmeyer-Vogt) in which a small decrease in
glycoprotein-NANA was observed in gray matter with no significant
change in white matter. The case was that of a 21 year old female
with onset at 6 years of age. Adelman et. al. (69) recently
reported a case with clinical features that resembled those of
Batten Disease or the late infantile amaurotic idiocy of Jansky-
Bielschowski type. The gray matter of this case presented a 77%
increase in glycoprotein-NANA concentration. An increase in the
concentration of the non-dialyzable sialoglycopeptide derived from
gray matter glycoproteins led the authors to suggest a possible
defect in glycoprotein catabolism. Landolt (68) had also described
a case of the Batten or Bielschowski type in which glycoprotein
NANA was increased in both gray and white matter. The foregoing
suggests a possible aberration of glycoprotein catabolism in some
forms of the neuronal ceroid-lipofuscinoses.

Acknowledgement: This work was supported in part by NATO Research
Grant No. 951.

1.   E. G. Brunngraber, H. Hof, J. Susz, B. D. Brown, A. Aro,
      and I. Chang. Glycopeptides from rat brain glycoproteins.
      Biochim. Biophys. Acta, 304, 781, 1973.

2.   R. G. Spiro. Glycoproteins. Ann. Rev. Biochem., 39, 599, 1970.

3.   J. I. Javaid, H. Hof, and E. G. Brunngraber. Preparation
      and properties of concanavalin A-binding glycopeptides
      derived from rat brain glycoproteins. Biochim. Biophys. Acta,
      404, 74, 1975.

4.   H. I. Hof, J. P. Susz, J. I. Javaid, and E. G. Brunngraber.
      Concanavalin A-binding-glycopeptides from rat brain glyco-
      proteins. Neurobiology, in press.

5.   N. N. Aronson, Jr., and C. de Duve. Digestive activity of ly-
      sosomes. J. Biol. Chem., 243, 4564, 1968.

6.   A. G. W. Norden, L. L. Tennant, and J. S. O'Brien. GM1 gang-
      lioside beta-galactosidase A. J. Biol. Chem., 249, 7969,1974.

7.   A. Tingey. The results of glycolipid analysis in certain
      types of lipidoses and leucodystrophy. J. Neurochem., 3,
      230, 1959.

8.   H. Kohno, I. Yamashina. Purification and properties of 4-L-
     aspartylglycosylamine amindohydrolase from hog kidney.
     Biochim. Biophys. Acta, 258, 600, 1972.

9.   J. Palo, H. Savolainen. Biochemical diagnosis of aspartylgly-
     cosaminuria. Ann. Clin. Res., 5, 156, 1973.

10. R. J. Pollitt, and K. M. Pretty. The glycoasparagines in
     urine of a patient with aspartylglycosaminuria. Biochem. J.,
     141, 141, 1974.

11. E. G. Brunngraber, L. A. Witting, C. Haberland, and B. Brown.
     Glycoproteins in Tay-Sachs Disease: Isolation and carbohy-
     drate composition of glycopeptides. Brain Res., 38, 151, 1972.

12. K. Suzuki. Cerebral GM1-gangliosidosis: Chemical pathology
     of visceral organs. Science, 159, 1471, 1968.

13. K. Suzuki, K. Suzuki, S. Kamoshita. Clinical pathology of
     GM2-gangliosidosis. J. Neuropathol. Exp. Neurol., 28, 25,
     1968.

14. Y. Suzuki, A. C. Crocker, K. Suzuki. GM1-gangliosidosis.
     Arch. Neurol. (Chic.), 24, 58, 1971.

15. L. S. Wolfe, R. G. Senior, and N. M. K. Ng Ying Kin. The
     structures of oligosaccharides accumulating in the liver of
     GM1-gangliosidosis, Type 1. J. Biol. Chem., 249, 1828, 1974.

16. G. C. Tsay, G. Dawson, Y-T. Li. Sturcture of the glycopeptide
     storage material in GM1 gangliosidosis. Sequence determina-
     tion with specific endo- and exoglycosidases. Biochim. Biophys.
     Acta, 385, 305, 1975.

17. A. Calatroni. Fractionation and characterization of glyco-
     peptides and oligosaccharides from the liver of a patient with
     GM1-gangliosidosis, Type 1. Ital J. Biochem., 23, 329, 1974.

18. L. S. Wolfe, J. T. R. Clarke, R. G. Senior. Biochemical
     studies on GM1-gangliosidosis. Adv. in Exptl. Med. and Biol.,
     19, 373, 1971.

19. J. W. Callahan, L. S. Wolfe. Isolation and characterization
     of keratan sulfates from the liver of a patient with GM1
     gangliosidosis, Type I. Biochim. Biophys. Acta, 215, 527, 1970.

20. G. C. Tsay, G. Dawson. Structure of the "keratan-sulfate-like"
     material in liver from a patient with GM1-gangliosidosis
     (beta-D-galactosidase deficiency). Biochem. Biophys. Res.Communs,

52, 759, 1973.

21. N. M. K. Ng Ying Kin, L. S. Wolfe. Oligosaccharides accumula-
     ting in the liver from a patient with GM2-gangliosidosis
     Variant o (Sandhoff-Jatzekewitz Disease). Biochem. Biophys.
     Res. Communs. 59, 837, 1974.

22. G. C. Tsay and G. Dawson. Glycopeptide storage in fibroblasts
     from patients with inborn errors of glycoprotein and glycoli-
     pid catabolism. Biochem. Biophys. Res. Communs., 63, 807, 1975.

23. P. A. Ockerman. Mannosidosis: Isolation of oligosaccharide
     storage material from brain. J. Pediat., 75, 360, 1969.

24. N. E. Norden, A. Lundblad, P. A. Ockerman, R. D. Jolly. Mann-
     osidosis in angus cattle. Partial characterization of two
     mannose containing oligosaccharides. FEBS Lett., 35, 209, 1973.

25. E. G. Brunngraber. Neuropathology of glycopeptides derived
     from brain glycoproteins. Adv. Exptl Med. and Biol., 25,
     255, 1972.

26. E. G. Brunngraber, B. D. Brown, and H. Hof. Determination of
     gangliosides glycoproteins, and glycosaminoglycans in brain
     tissue. Clin. Chim. Acta, 32, 159, 1971.

27. L. G. Davis, J. Javaid, and E. G. Brunngraber. To be published

28. B. Berra, S. DiPalma, and E. G. Brunngraber. Altered levels
     of tissue gangliosides and glycoproteins in the infantile
     form of GM1-gangliosidosis. Clin. Chim. Acta, 57, 301, 1974.

29. E. G. Brunngraber, B. D. Brown, and A. Aro. Glycoproteins
     in brain tissue of the O-variant of GM2 gangliosidosis. J.
     Neurochem., 22, 125, 1974.

30. E. G. Brunngraber, B. Berra, and V. Zambotti. Altered levels
     of tissue glycoproteins, gangliosides, glycosaminoglycans
     and lipids in Niemann-Pick's Disease. Clin. Chim, Acta, 48,
     173, 1973.

31. B. Berra, E. G. Brunngraber, V. Aguilar, A. Aro, and V.
     Zambotti. Gangliosides, glycoproteins, and glycosaminoglycans
     in Krabbe's Disease. Clin. Chim. Acta, 47, 325, 1973.

32. Y. Suzuki, J. C. Jacob, K. Suzuki, K. N. Kutty, and K. Suzuki.
     GM2 gangliosidosis with total hexosaminidase deficiency.
     Neurology, 21, 313, 1971.

33. K. Suzuki, K. Suzuki, I. Radin, N. Ishii. Juvenile GM2
     gangliosidosis. Clinical variant of Tay-Sachs Disease or a
     New Disease. Neurology, 20, 190, 1970.

34. S. Bogoch. Brain glycoproteins and intercellular recognition.
     Tay-Sachs Disease and intracellular recognition. Adv. Exptl.
     Med. and Biol., 19, 127, 1972.

35. J. A. Balint and E. C. Kyriadides. Studies on red cell stromal
     proteins in Tay-Sachs Disease. J. Clin. Invest., 47, 1858, 1972.

36. M. Pourfar and S. Levy. Clin. Chem., 17, 332, 1971.

37. E. G. Brunngraber, B. Berra, and V. Zambotti. Brain glyco-
     proteins in GM1-gangliosidosis: Isolation and carbohydrate
     composition of glycopeptides. FEBS Lett., 34, 350, 1973.

38. V. Patel, H. H. Goebel, I. Watanabe, W. Zeman. Studies on
     GM1-gangliosidosis, Type II. Acta Neuropathol., 30, 155, 1974.

39. T. Yutaka, S. Okada, K. Mimaki, T. Sugita, H. Yabuuchi.
     Enzymatic study of GM1 gangliosidosis. Clin. Chim. Acta, 59,
     283, 1975.

40. L. S. Wolfe, J. Callahan, J. S. Fawcett, G. Andermann, C. R.
     Scriver. GM1 gangliosidosis without chondrodystrophy or
     visceromegaly. Neurology, 20, 23, 1970.

41. R. M. Norman, A. H. Tingey, M. C. Fowler. Niemann-Pick Disease,
     Proceedings of the Fifth Internatl. Congr. on Neuropathol.,
     Zürich, 1965, Amsterdam, Excerta Medical Foundation, 1966,
     p. 143.

42. L. Svennerholm. Lipidoses, Metab. Physiol. Significance
     Lipids, Proc., Cambridge, Engl. 553, 1963.

43. L. Svennerholm. The metabolism of gangliosides in cerebral
     lipidoses. In: Inborn Disorders of Sphingolipid Metabolism,
     S. M. Aronson and B. W. Volk, eds., Pergamon Press, Oxford,
     1967, p. 169.

44. L. Svennerholm and P. Sourander. Combined histological and
     chemical investigations on brain autopsy material in lipidoses.
     Proceedings of the Fifth Internatl. Congr. on Neuropathol.,
     Zürich, 1965, Amsterdam, Excerta Medical Foundation, 1966,
     p. 342.

45. J. N. Kanfer, M. Stein, C. Spielvogel. Recent observations
     on Gaucher's Disease. Adv. Exp. Med. Biol., 19, 225, 1972.

46. A. H. Tingey, and G. W. F. Edgar. A contribution to the chemistry of the leukodystrophies. J. Neurochem., 10, 817, 1963.

47. Y. Suzuki and K. Suzuki. Glycosphingolipid beta-galactosidases. II. Electrofocusing characterization of the enzymes in human globoid cell leukodystrophy (Krabbe's Disease). J. Biol. Chem. 249, 2105, 1974.

48. J. N. Cumings. Chemistry of disease of the central nervous system, Metabolism, Clin. and Exptl., 9, 219, 1960.

49. L. Svennerholm. Some aspects of the biochemical changes in leukodystrophy. In: Brain Lipids, Lipoproteins, Leukodystrophies, J. Folch-Pi and H. Bauer, eds., Elsevier, Amsterdam, 1963, p. 104.

50. B. Hagberg, P. Sourander, L. Svennerholm, and H. Voss. Late infantile metachromatic leukodystrophy of the genetic type. Acta Paediat., (Uppsala), 49, 135, 1960.

51. G. W. F. Edgar. Anatomo-chemical research in demyelinating conditions and inborn errors in metabolism. Proc. of the Fifth Internal. Congr. on Neuropathol., Zürich, 1965, Amsterdam, Excerpta Medical Foundation, 1966, p. 328.

52. P. L. Masters, W. B. MacDonald, M. M. P.Ryan, and J. N. Cumings. Arch. Disease Childhood, 39, 345, 1964.

53. H. Yabuuchi, S. Okada, M. Honda, and J. Hanai. Pathological and biochemical study of metachromatic leukodystrophy. Med. J. Osaka Univ., 18, 361, 1968.

54. E. de Vries, L. van Bogaert, and G. W. F. Edgar. New observations on familial idiocy with spongy degeneration of nerve centers. Rev. Neurol., 98, 271, 1958.

55. H. Urich. Histochemical observations on metachromatic leukodystrophy. Intern. Kongr. Neuropathol., Proc. 4th; Munich, 1961, p. 42.

56. J. N. Cumings and M. Kremer. Biochemical aspects of neurological disorders. F. A. Davis, Pub., Philadelphia, 1965.

57. H. Hollaender. Histochemical demonstration of mucopolysaccharides in sulfatide granules formed during the intracellular storate of cerebroside sulfate esters in metachromatic leukodystrophy. J. Neurochem., 12, 335, 1965.

58. R. M. Norman, H. Urich, and A. H. Tingey. Metachromatic leukoencephalopathy: a form of lipidosis. Brain, 83, 369, 1960.

59. A. Resibois-Gregoire. Electron microscopic studies of metachromatic leukodystrophy. II. Compound Nature of the Inclusions. Acta Neuropathol. (Berlin) 9, 244, 1967.

60. P. Sourander. Histopathological studies in sulfatide lipidosis (metachromatic leukodystrophy). Acta Pathol. Microbiol., Scand. Suppl., 154, 83, 1962.

61. H. W. Moser, M. Sugita, M. D. Harrison, M. William. Liver glycolipids, steroid sulfates, and steroid sulfatases in a form of metachromatic leukodystrophy associated with multiple forms of sulfate deficiency. Adv. Exp. Med. Biol., 19, 429, 1972.

62. Y. Eto, S. Rampini, U. Wiesmann, and N. N. Herschkowitz. Enzymatic studies of sulfatases in tissues of the normal human and in metachromatic leukodystrophy with multiple sulfatase deficiencies: arylasulfatases A, B, and C, cerebroside sulfatase, psychosine sulfatase and steroid sulfatases. J. Neurochem., 23, 1161, 1974.

63. C. Haberland, E. G. Brunngraber, L. Witting, and A. Daniels. Juvenile metachromatic leukodystophy. Case report with clinical, histopatholgical, ultrastructural, and biochemical observations. Acta Neuropathol. (Berlin), 26, 93, 1973.

64. W. Zeman and A. N. Siakotos. The neuronal ceroid-lipofuscinoses. In: Lysosomes and Storage Diseases, H. G. Hers and F. Van Hoof, eds., Academic Press, New York, 1973, p. 519.

65. P. F. Borri and G. J. M. Hooghwinkel. Comparative studies of glycolipids, and carbohydrate moieties in brain and visceral organs in amaurotic idiocy and gargoylism. Pathol. Eur., 3, 416, 1968.

66. G. W. F. Edgar and L. V. van Bogaert. Anatomo-chemical study of the white matter in late infantile amaurotic idiocy. In: Inborn Disorders of Sphingolipid Metabolism. S. M. Aronson and B. W. Volk, eds., Pergamon Press, Oxford, 1967, p. 75.

67. C. Haberland, E. G. Brunngraber, L. A. Witting, and H. Hof. Late infantile amaurotic idiocy (LIAI). Neurology, 22, 305, 1972.

68. R. Landolt. Biochemical studies on two cases of neuronal
     lipid storage diseases. Pathol. Eur., 3, 440, 1968.

69. L. S. Adelman, E. Young, N. H. Bass. Abnormal accumulation
     of sialoglycoprotein in a case of late infantile amaurotic
     idiocy. Neurology, 24, 1045, 1974.

COMPONENT FORMS OF ACID HYDROLASES IN SUBCELLULAR GRANULES FROM

HUMAN LEUCOCYTES

R.B. Ellis and A.D. Patrick

MRC Clinical Genetics Unit and Department of
Chemical Pathology, Institute of Child Health
London, WC1N 1EH, England

During the last decade, the basic enzyme defects of many
lysosomal storage disorders have been elucidated and this has led
to the development of relatively simple laboratory tests for their
precise diagnosis. The routine application of such tests has
revealed that variant forms of these disorders usually exist and
that these variants are often characterised by relative deficiencies of the component activities of a multi-component enzyme. A
fuller understanding of the clinical, genetic, and biochemical
differences between such variants will require detailed investigations into the physicochemical and biological characteristics
of the component forms of the enzymes associated with each disorder.
For many types of cell there is considerable evidence of heterogeneity of hydrolase-containing particles, and it is possible that
this reflects some differentiation of their digestive functions.
In the case of a multi-component hydrolase, this differentiation
might be manifested further in the variable distribution of these
components in the different particles. Knowledge of such variable
distribution might then help to explain the biological functions
of the enzyme components. This report is concerned with the
resolution and subcellular localisation of the component forms of
N-acetyl-β-D-glucosaminidase, the lysosomal hydrolase associated
with Tay-Sachs disease and its variants.

EXPERIMENTAL

Preparation of subcellular fractions of human leucocytes

Fresh heparinised blood (20 ml) from a normal adult was mixed
with 2 vols. of dextran (3% w/v) in 0.9% NaCl and left at room
temperature for 25 min. The supernatant was removed and centrifuged

at 600g for 5 min (MSE Mistral 6L) at 4° (all subsequent procedures
were carried out at this temperature). The leucocyte pellet was
subjected to hypotonic lysis (1) and recentrifuged at 600g for
5 min. After careful removal of erythrocyte ghosts, the pellet was
washed with 0.25 M sucrose (2 ml) and finally resuspended in sucrose
solution (2 ml). The cells were then disrupted at 20kHz for 12 sec
using a 50W ultrasonic disintegrator (Ultrasonics Ltd., Shipley,
Yorks.). Under these conditions, there was only a slight release
of acid hydrolases into solution. After removal of the nuclear
fraction by centrifugation (MSE Mistral 6L) at 600g for 10 min, an
aliquot of the post-nuclear supernatant fraction (0.4 ml) was
layered on a sucrose density gradient (consisting of seven 0.3 ml
layers of approximately equal density increment from 1.15 to 1.30;
allowed to diffuse for 3 h at 4°) and centrifuged at 115,000g for
2 h (MSE Superspeed 50 with 3 x 3 ml swing-out rotor, r_{av} 7.1 cm).
About 25 fractions (0.1 ml) were collected using an MSE tube-
piercer. They were quickly frozen in a methanol-solid CO_2 bath
and stored at $- 20^o$.

Preparation of subcellular fractions of purified human granulocytes and lymphocytes

The leucocyte-rich supernatant obtained after sedimentation of
whole blood in dextran, as described above, was carefully layered
on Lymphoprep (8 ml; Nyegaard & Co., Oslo, Norway) and centrifuged
at 400g for 40 min at 20°. Granulocytes were present in the sedimented pellet. After removal of contaminant erythrocytes by
hypotonic lysis the granulocytes were sonicated as described for
the mixed leucocyte preparation. Lymphocytes, which were concentrated at the Lymphoprep-sample interface were collected by pipette,
diluted with an equal volume of isotonic saline, and centrifuged
at 600g for 10 min. The pellet was suspended in saline (2 ml),
layered onto a further 8 ml of Lymphoprep, and centrifuged at 400g
for 40 min at 20°. The interfacial layer was again collected and
centrifuged at 600g for 10 min. The pellet was suspended in
0.25 M sucrose (0.4 ml) and sonicated as described for leucocyte
preparations. Subcellular fractionation of purified granulocyte and
lymphocyte post-nuclear supernatants was carried out exactly as
described for mixed leucocytes.

Enzyme Assays

The appropriate 4-methylumbelliferyl glycosides were used in
the determination of the activities of N-acetyl-β-D-glucosaminidase
(2) and β-D-galactosidase (3).

For the assay of acid phosphatase, disodium β-glycerophosphate
(10 μmol; adjusted to pH 5.0) was incubated with the enzyme at 37°
in sodium acetate buffer, pH 5.0 (4.0 μmol) in a total volume of

60 μl. The reaction was stopped by the addition of 20% w/v trichloroacetic acid (60 μl) and inorganic phosphate was determined in the supernatant by the method of Fiske and SubbaRow (4).

Alkaline phosphatase was assayed at 37° in a mixture containing disodium p-nitrophenylphosphate (0.9 μmol), glycine-NaOH buffer, pH 10.5 (6.0 μmol), $MgCl_2$(0.06 μmol), and enzyme in a final volume of 120 μl. The reaction was stopped by the addition of 20 mmol/l NaOH (1.0 ml) and the absorbance measured at 405 nm.

Protein was measured according to the method of Lowry et al (5).

Chromatographic Resolution of N-acetyl-β-D-glucosaminidase components

DEAE-cellulose microcolumn chromatography coupled with auto-mated assay of enzyme activity in the column effluent was carried out by slight modifications to the method previously described (6). The concentration of substrate, 4-methylumbelliferyl-2-acetamido-2-deoxy-β-D-glucopyranoside, was reduced to 0.33 mg/ml of buffer (54 mmol/l citric acid - 92 mmol/l Na_2HPO_4, pH 4.5, and albumin was added (0.1 mg/ml). A second 4-way valve was added to the line between the gradient-maker bottle and the pump tube leading to the column inlet, and this was used for sample loading. The method used to form the salt gradient was altered: instead of pumping KCl into an open mixer at half the rate at which liquid was withdrawn, the gradient-maker bottle was closed and connected directly to a reservoir of KCl. In this arrangement, the volume of liquid (10 ml) in the mixer remained constant. Nominal flow rates (ml/min) were as follows: a) through column, 0.32; b) air, 0.23; c) buffer-substrate, 0.16; d) stop solution, 0.25 mol/l glycine-NaOH, pH 10.4, 0.42; and e) pull-through flow-cell, 0.8. It took 8 min. for a specimen to pass through the 37^oC incubation coil.

Subcellular fractions were thawed, frozen again in a methanol-solid CO_2 bath and thawed. Aliquots (20 μl) of each fraction were diluted with 10 mmol/l sodium phosphate, pH 6.0 (500 μl) just before chromatography. Samples were loaded for 1.0 min. A 300 mmol/l KCl solution in 10 mmol/l sodium phosphate, pH6.0, was connected to the gradient maker 3.5 min after the start of sample loading. The fluorimeter sensitivity setting was not changed during the assay of all fractions from one sucrose density gradient analysis.

RESULTS AND DISCUSSION

In the classical studies of de Duve and colleagues it was shown that acid phosphatase of rat liver sediments differently from mito-chondrial marker enzymes and possesses structure-linked latency. The finding that other acid hydrolases shared this property and sedimented at the same density as acid phosphatase led to the development of the lysosome concept (7,8).

A more detailed examination of the distribution of acid hydrolase activities in particulate fractions of rabbit heterophil
leucocytes separated by isopycnic centrifugation or by zonal sedimentation revealed a complex pattern for each enzyme, with up to
three partially resolved peaks (9,10). These biochemical findings,
and their correlation with morphological studies, clearly indicated
the occurrence of more than one type of cytoplasmic granule. In
order of decreasing density, these have been described as primary
(or azurophil) granules, containing a large proportion of the acid
hydrolase activities of the cells and the myeloperoxidase;
secondary (or specific) granules, containing most of the alkaline
phosphatase but very little acid hydrolase activity; tertiary
granules, containing the remainder of the acid hydrolase activity;
and, finally, very low density material containing all of a thiol-
dependent acid p-nitrophenyl phosphatase. The primary and
secondary granules have been well-characterised but there is some
controversy about the origin of the tertiary granules (11).

The subcellular distribution of acid hydrolases in human polymorphonuclear leucocytes was found to be similar to that described
for rabbit but alkaline phosphatase was associated with particles
of much lower density (12,13). These findings have been confirmed
in the present work; Fig. 1 shows the distributions of acid hydrolases and of alkaline phosphatase obtained by isopycnic centrifugation
of human leucocytes. The patterns for a purified granulocyte preparation were similar. Three partially resolved peaks of activity
for acid β-glycerophosphatase and also β-D-galactosidase were
observed at modal densities of 1.22, 1.19 and 1.15. Morphological
studies were not made, and so it is difficult to correlate these
fractions with those characterised in rabbit granulocytes (9,10).
The fraction with a modal density of 1.22 presumably included
azurophil granules because it also contained the bulk of the myeloperoxidase activity (not shown in Fig. 1). Kane and Peters (14),
in an analysis of subcellular particles from human granulocytes,
recognized that certain hydrolases showed a broad distribution and
could not be readily assigned to either the specific or azurophil
granules. They suggested that the observed distribution indicated
the presence of a third type of hydrolase-containing granule corresponding to the tertiary granule described by Baggiolini et al (9,10).
A similar result was found in the present study for N-acetyl-β-D-
glucosaminidase; there was a single, complex peak with maximum activity
at density 1.20-1.21 but significant activity was also found throughout the range 1.23 to 1.15.

In all the studies of the distribution of acid hydrolases in
subcellular fractions discussed above, only the total activity of
each enzyme was assayed. But it is well known that most, if not all,
of these hydrolases occur in multi-component forms. A study of the
distribution of the components of one acid hydrolase, N-acetyl-β-D-
glucosaminidase, was therefore undertaken to determine whether or not

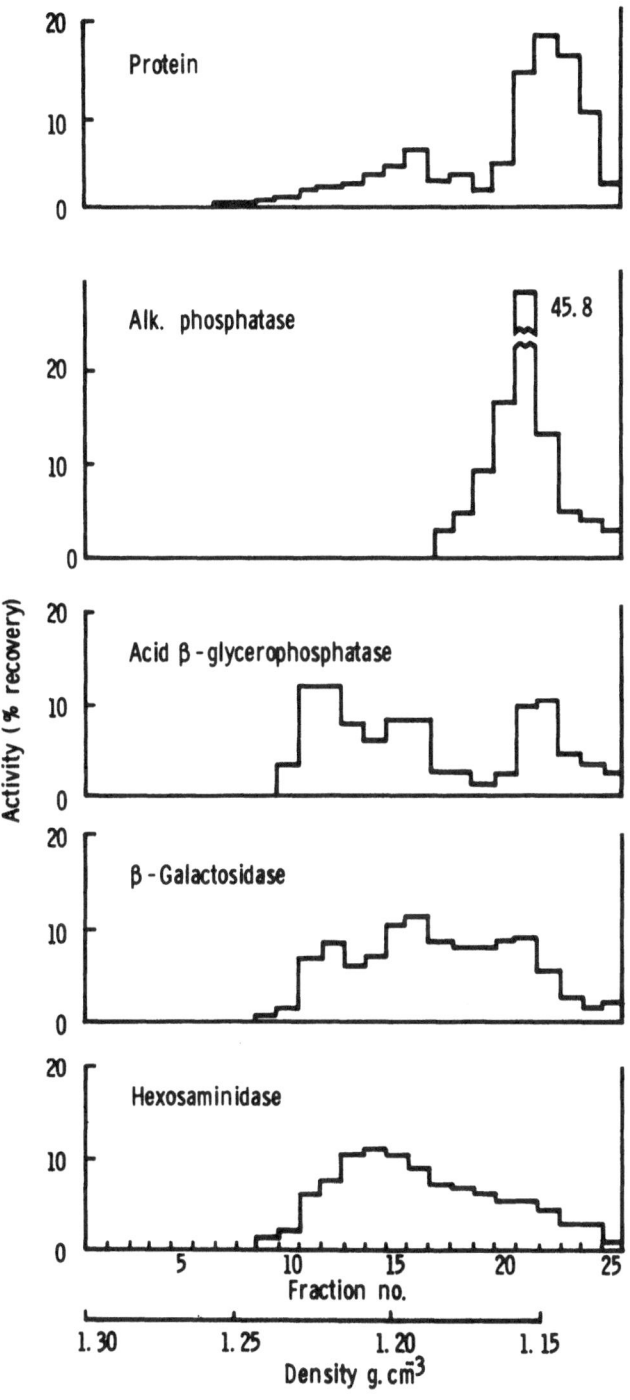

Fig.1. Distribution of enzymic activities after isopycnic
centrifugation of a 600xg supernatant of sonicated human leucocytes.

the complex profile of total activity could be explained as the
aggregate of simpler distributions of the different component forms.
These studies were made possible by the development of a sensitive
method of chromatography of acid hydrolases on microcolumns of DEAE-
cellulose coupled with continuous automated assay of enzyme activity
in the column effluent (6).

The elution profile of N-acetyl-β-D-glucosaminidase activity
from a control homogenate of human grey matter is shown in the top
trace of Fig. 2. Resolution into four components is clearly seen
and these have been defined as B, I_1, I_2, and A in order of elution
(15,16). The elution profile from a leucocyte homogenate is shown
in the trace below that of grey matter in Fig. 2. The B, I_1, and
A components are present as distinct peaks but the I_2 component is
indicated only by a change of slope. Though the shape of the A
peak of grey matter is symmetrical, that of leucocytes is skewed
towards the leading edge. This has been consistently observed in
many experiments.

The asymmetry of the leucocyte A peak was an indication of the
probable occurrence of more than one constituent and this was clearly
demonstrated by chromatography of the subcellular fractions obtained
by isopycnic centrifugation (Fig. 2, traces 10-26; the numbers refer
to the fractions and correspond to those used in the studies of total
activities recorded in Fig. 1).

The peak maximum of component A of low density fractions (nos.
17-26) occurred at the same position in the elution profile as that
of the total leucocyte preparation, whereas the denser fractions
(nos. 10-15) gave a peak maximum about 3 min earlier. Fraction 16
gave an A peak with a complex shape similar to that seen for the
whole homogenate. A minor peak, corresponding in its position of
elution to the major component of serum, was most prominent in
fractions 17 and 18 and was presumably also present in fraction 16;
it was not apparent in denser fractions. In contrast, a component
with a peak maximum at about 40 min was confined to the denser
fractions (nos. 12 to 14). N-acetyl-β-D-glucosaminidase component A
of human leucocytes is therefore shown to be composed of at least
three forms and these different forms appear to be preferentially
associated with particulate fractions of different density. This
provides evidence in support of the original hypothesis that the
complex pattern of the distribution of glucosaminidase activity in
density gradient fractions can be regarded as the sum of simpler
distributions of different component forms.

Baggiolini et al (9) have drawn attention to the importance of
using a single cell type in studies of the distribution of enzymes
in subcellular particles but the leucocyte preparations used in the
studies described above contained both granulocytes and lymphocytes.

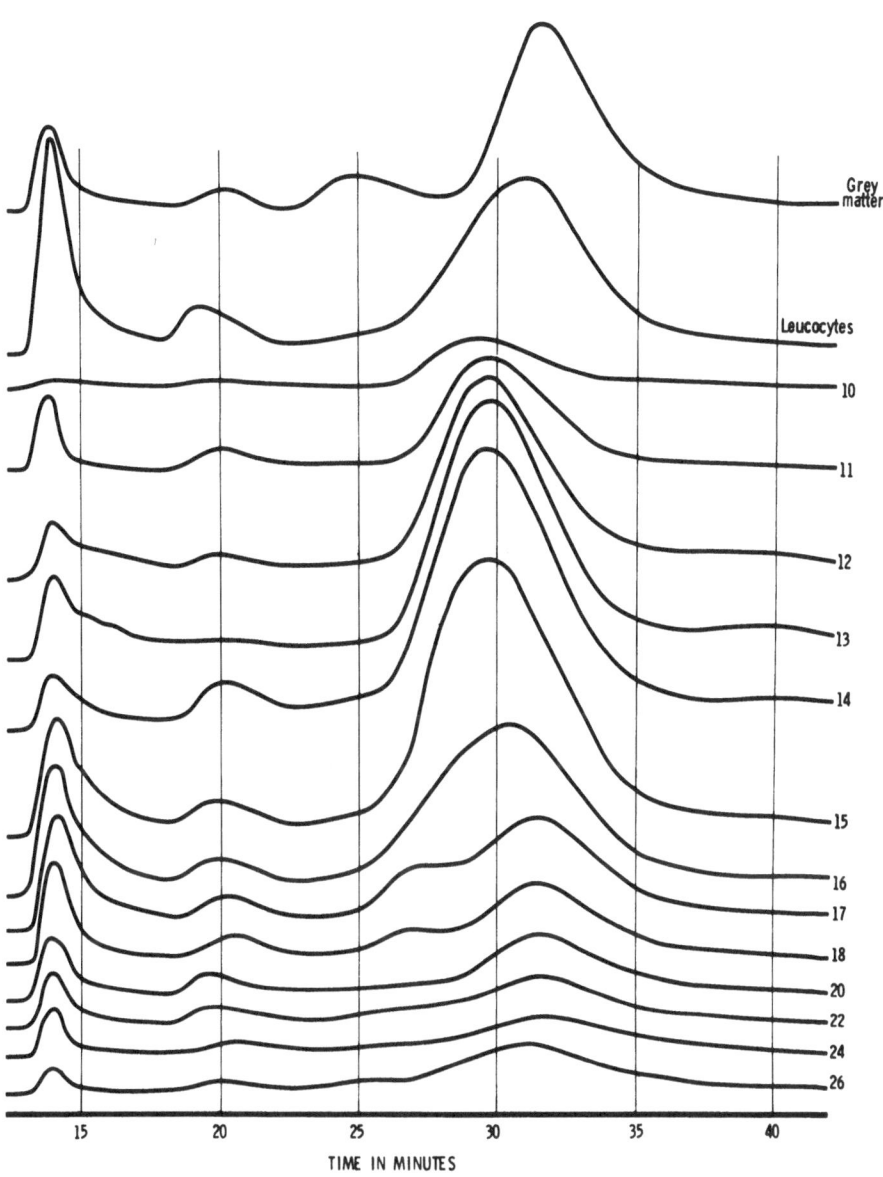

Fig.2. DEAE-cellulose chromatography of hexosaminidase in
fractions obtained by isopycnic centrifugation of a 600xg
supernatant of sonicated human leucocytes. Fraction numbers
correspond to those given in Fig.1.

It was therefore not possible to know if the different types of
particle were all present in one type of cell. An attempt was made
to gain additional information by studying the elution profiles of
glucosaminidase from purified lymphocytes (97% mononuclear cells)
and granulocytes (99% polymorphonuclear cells). These profiles are
given in Fig. 3 together with those of the mixed leucocyte preparation
and of control serum. It can be seen that the profile for the
purified granulocytes (Fig. 3c) is closely similar to that of the
mixed leucocytes (Fig. 3a), the principal difference being the
relatively greater proportion of component B in mixed leucocytes.
However, the pattern found for the glucosaminidase of purified
lymphocytes (Fig. 3b) was clearly different from that of mixed
leucocytes (Fig. 3a), though it resembled that of the least dense
leucocyte subcellular fractions (Fig. 2, curve 26) and of grey
matter (Fig. 2).

It should be noted that the elution profiles shown in any
figure were obtained within a few hours of all other profiles
recorded in the same figure and that the positions of peak maxima
were highly reproducible. However, the profiles in different
figures were obtained at quite different times, using different
sets of pump tubes on the Autoanalyser, and they cannot therefore
be directly compared.

Subcellular fractionation of the purified granulocyte and
lymphocyte preparations was carried out by isopycnic centrifugation
on a sucrose density gradient under the conditions used for mixed
leucocytes. The glucosaminidase profiles of granulocyte fractions
(Fig. 4) corresponded closely to those found for the equivalent
fractions of mixed leucocytes; the denser fractions again had an A
component which was eluted earlier than that of the lighter fractions,
and the minor A component in fractions of intermediate density was
also seen. Thus the three different forms of glucosaminidase A
appear to be present in subcellular particles of different density
in a single type of cell.

Glucosaminidase components in lymphocyte granules had a much
simpler distribution; only one form of component A was seen in all
fractions (Fig. 5). It corresponded in its position of elution to
that of the lighter fractions from granulocytes. Component B was
found to be relatively increased in lymphocytes. This finding
could be relevant to the detection of carriers of Tay-Sachs disease
since a high lymphocyte count would be expected to lower the ratio
of component A to component B.

Agglutination artefacts can be a serious problem in studies of
subcellular components. In an attempt to prevent or minimize their
formation, the procedures developed by Baggiolini et al (9,10) were
adopted. In particular, postnuclear supernatants were always applied

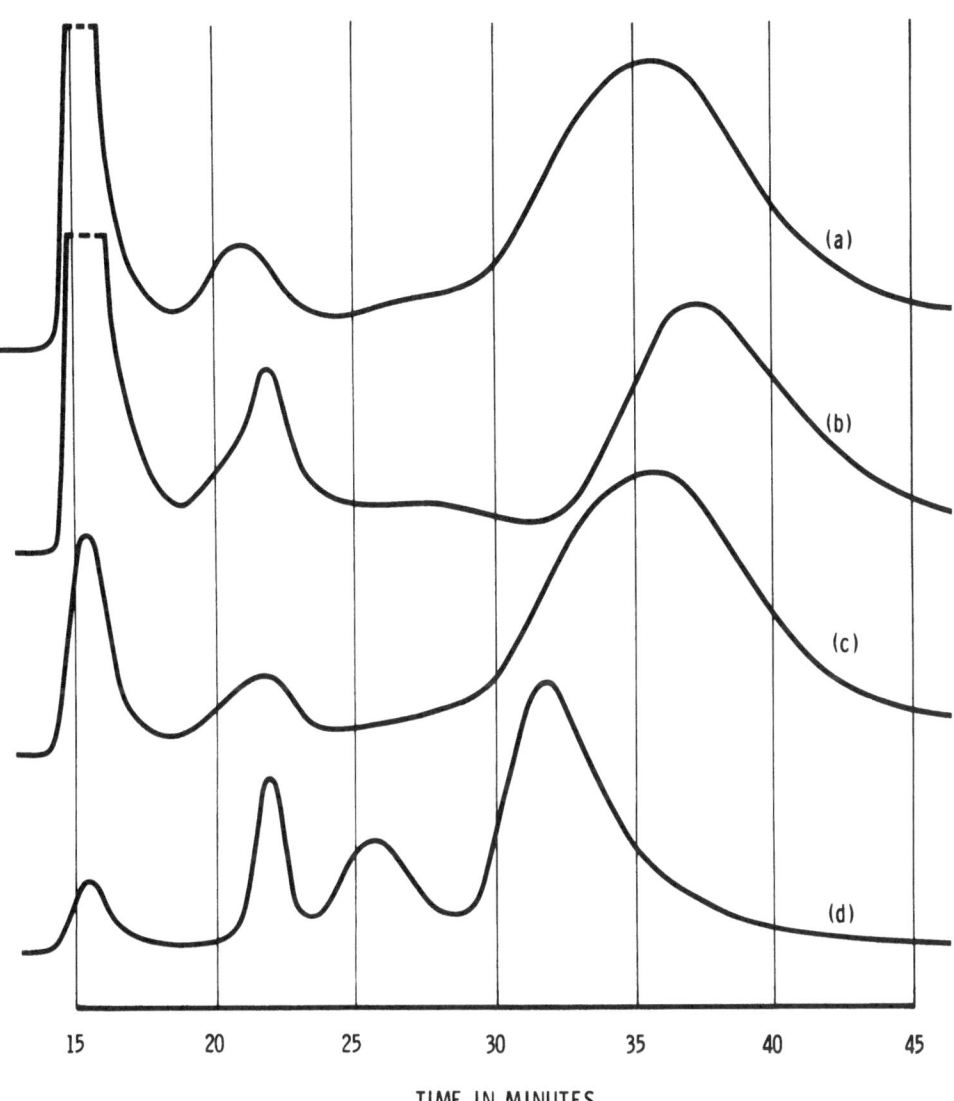

TIME IN MINUTES

Fig.3. DEAE-cellulose chromatography of hexosaminidase in
a) leucocytes; b) lymphocytes; c) granulocytes; and d) serum.

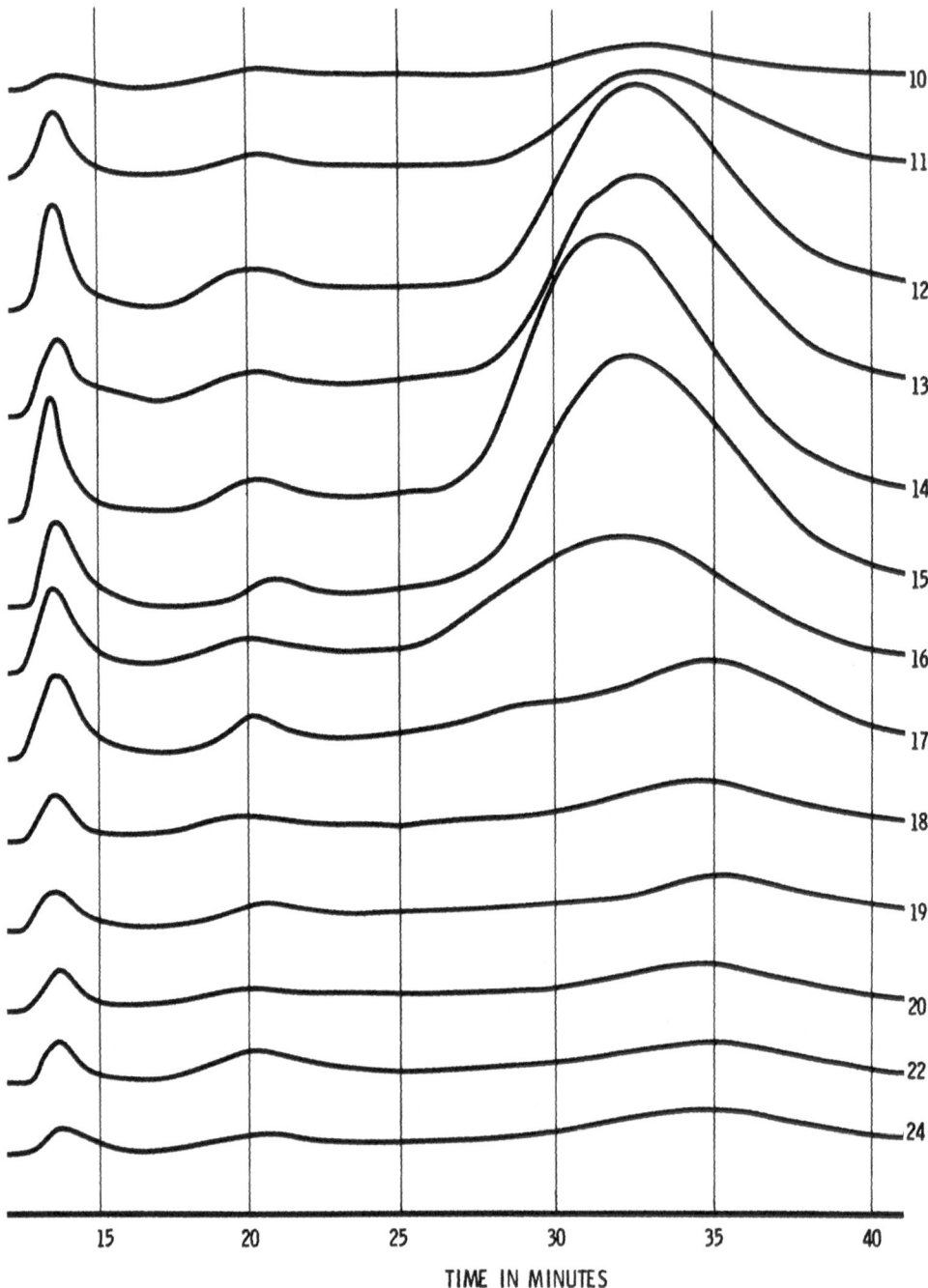

Fig.4. DEAE-cellulose chromatography of hexosaminidase in
fractions obtained by isopycnic centrifugation of a 600xg
supernatant of sonicated human granulocytes.

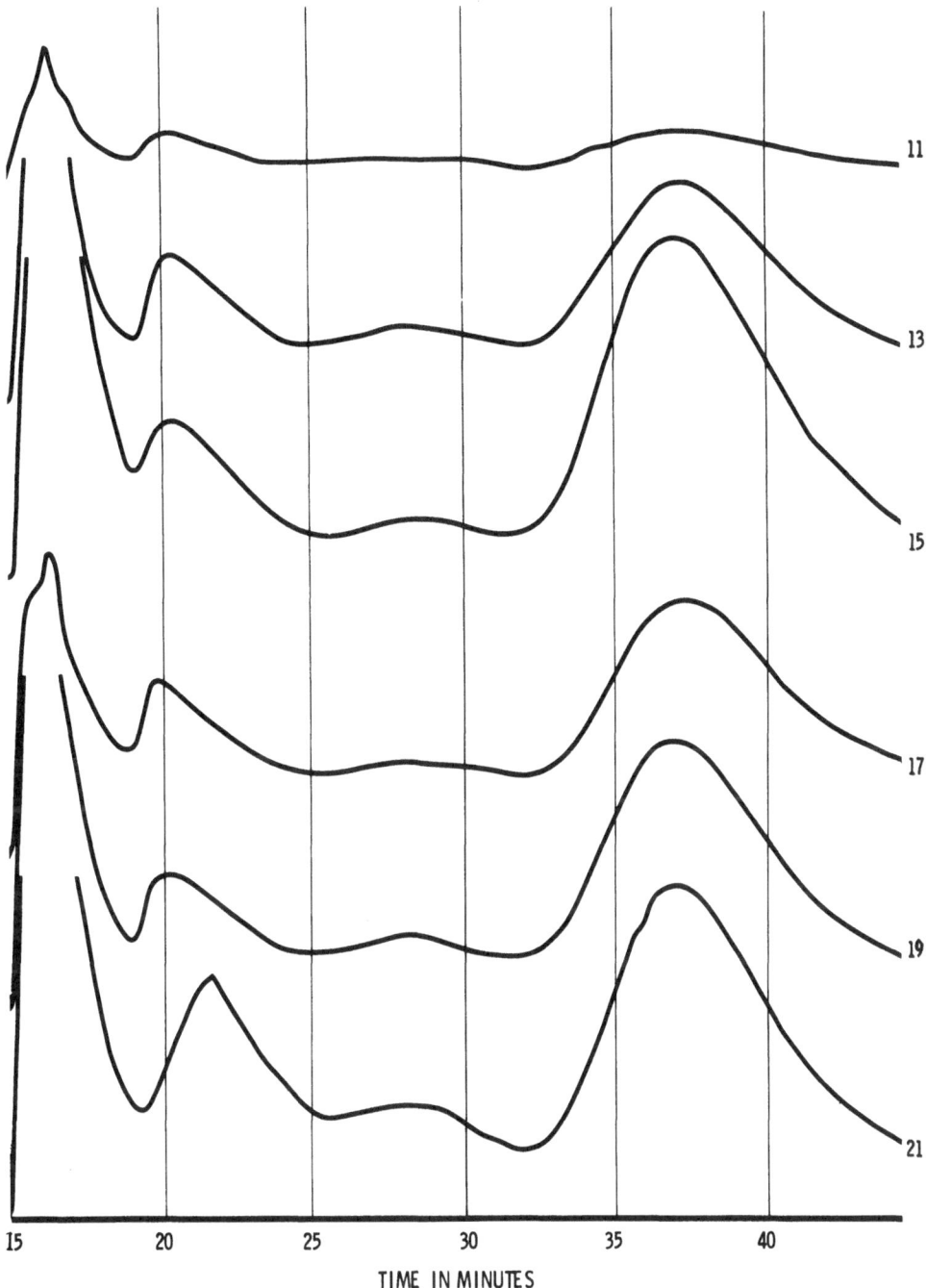

TIME IN MINUTES

Fig.5. DEAE-cellulose chromatography of hexosaminidase in
fractions obtained by isopycnic centrifugation of a 600xg
supernatant of sonicated human lymphocytes.

directly to the density gradient, thus avoiding agglutination
resulting from resuspension of centrifuged pellets. The restriction
of alkaline phosphatase activity to a sharp, non-sedimenting band
suggests that agglutination was insignificant in our fractionation.

A great deal of effort and ingenuity has gone into devising
optimum conditions for the separation of the different classes of
postnuclear cytoplasmic granules (17). But the fractions obtained
have been analysed, in almost all cases, only for the total
activities of their enzyme contents, though it has been widely
recognized that many of these enzymes are present in multi-component
forms. The results reported in this paper suggest that more meaning-
ful distinctions between density fractions will result from a study
of the distributions of each component form, rather than that of
total enzymic activities. This concept has also been recognized by
Dewald et al (18) who used polyacrylamide gel electrophoresis to
separate the different forms of neutral proteases in subcellular
fractions of human and rabbit polymorphonuclear leucocytes.

The different component forms of an acid hydrolase may represent
different proteins with separate functions, and there is evidence
for this from studies of the variant types of lysosomal storage disorders. For example, globoside storage in visceral organs is found
only in cases of the Sandhoff variant of Tay-Sachs disease and these
are the only cases reported to lack glucosaminidase component B (19).
In addition, Hayase and Kritchevsky (20) showed that hexosaminidase
A of human aorta and serum could be separated into several bands by
polyacrylamide gel electrofocusing, and Bach and Suzuki (21) have
recently reported on the heterogeneity of human hepatic hexosaminidase
A activity towards natural glycosphingolipid substrates. This is
relevant to the findings we report and suggests that the activities
of subcellular fractions towards ganglioside G_M2 should be investigated.

REFERENCES

1.   Schneider, J.A., Bradley, K.H., & Seegmiller, J.E.,
      Transport and intracellular fate of cysteine - ^{35}S in
      leucocytes from normal subjects and patients with
      cystinosis, Pediat.Res., 2, 441, 1968.

2.   Brett, E.M. et al, Late-onset G_M2 - gangliosidosis,
      Arch. Dis. Childh, 48, 775, 1973

3.   Young, E.P., Ellis, R.B., & Patrick, A.D., Leukocyte
      β-galactosidase activity in G_M1-gangliosidosis,
      Pediatrics, 50, 502, 1972.

4. Fiske, C.H. & SubbaRow, Y., J. Biol. Chem., 66, 375, 1925.

5. Lowry, O.H., Rosebrough, N.J., Farr, A.L., & Randall, R.J.,
    Protein measurement with the Folin phenol reagent, J.Biol.
    Chem., 193, 265, 1951.

6. Ellis, R.B., Ikonne, J.U., & Masson, P.K., DEAE-cellulose
    microcolumn chromatography coupled with automated assay:
    application to the resolution of N-acetyl-β-D-hexosaminidase
    components, Anal. Biochem., 63, 5, 1975.

7. De Duve, C., Lysosomes, a new group of cytoplasmic particles.
    In: Subcellular Particles. T. Hayashi (Ed.), New York,
    Ronald Press, 1959, 128 - 159.

8. De Duve,C., The lysosome concept. In: Ciba Found. Symp.
    Lysosomes, de Reuck, A.V.S. & Cameron, M.P. (Eds.), London,
    J. & A. Churchill Ltd., 1963, 1 - 35.

9. Baggiolini, M., Hirsch, J.G., & de Duve, C., Resolution of
    granules from rabbit heterophil leukocytes into distinct
    populations by zonal sedimentation, J. Cell Biol., 40, 529, 1969.

10. Baggiolini, M., Hirsch, J.G., & de Duve, C., Further biochemical
    and morphological studies of granule fractions from rabbit
    heterophil leukocytes, J. Cell Biol., 45, 586, 1970.

11. Farquhar, M.G., Bainton, D.F., Baggiolini, M., & de Duve, C.,
    Cytochemical localization of acid phosphatase activity in
    granule fractions from rabbit polymorphonuclear leukocytes,
    J. Cell Biol., 54, 141, 1972.

12. Schulman, J.D., Bradley, K.H., & Seegmiller, J.E., Cystine:
    compartmentalization within lysosomes in cystinotic leukocytes,
    Science, 166, 1152, 1969.

13. Bretz, U. & Baggiolini, M., Biochemical and morphological
    characterization of azurophil and specific granules of human
    neutrophilic polymorphonuclear leukocytes, J. Cell Biol.,
    63, 251, 1974.

14. Kane, S.P. & Peters, T.J., Analytical subcellular fractionation
    of human granulocytes with reference to the localization of
    vitamin B12-binding proteins, Clin. Sci. and Mol. Med., 49,
    171, 1975.

15. Young, E.P., Ellis, R.B., Lake, B.D., & Patrick, A.D., Tay-
    Sachs disease and related disorders: fractionation of brain
    N-acetyl-β-hexosaminidase on DEAE-cellulose, FEBS Lett., 9, 1,
    1970.

16. Ikonne, J.U. & Ellis, R.B., N-acetyl-β-D-hexosaminidase
     component A: different forms in human tissues and fluids,
     Biochem. J., <u>135</u>, 457, 1973.

17. Beaufay, H., Methods for the isolation of lysosomes, In:
     Lysosomes, Dingle, J.T. (Ed.),London, North-Holland Publishing
     Co., 1972, 1 - 45.

18. Dewald, B., Rindler-Ludwig, R., Bretz, U., & Baggiolini, M.,
     Subcellular localization and heterogeneity of neutral proteases
     in neutrophilic polymorphonuclear leukocytes. J. Exp. Med.,
     <u>141</u>, 709, 1975.

19. Sandhoff, K., Andreae, U., & Jatzkewitz, H., Deficient
     hexosaminidase activity in an exceptional case of Tay-Sachs
     disease with additional storage of kidney globoside in visceral
     organs, Life Sci., <u>7</u>, 283, 1968.

20. Hayase , K. & Kritchevsky, D., Polyacrylamide gel electrofocusing
     of hexosaminidases, Clin. Chim. Acta, <u>46</u>, 455, 1973.

21. Bach, G. & Suzuki, K., Heterogeneity of human hepatic N-acetyl-
     β-D-hexosaminidase A activity toward natural glycosphingolipid
     substrates, J. Biol. Chem., <u>250</u>, 1328, 1975.

FETAL PATHOLOGY AND ULTRASTRUCTURE OF NEUROPATHIC

GAUCHER'S DISEASE

Shigehiko Kamoshita[1], Mariko Odawara[1],
Mariko Yoshida[2], Misao Owada[3], and
Teruo Kitagawa[3]

Department of Pediatrics, Jichi Medical School,
Tochigi-ken[1], Department of Biochemistry,
University of Tokyo School of Medicine, Tokyo [2],
and Department of Pediatrics, Nihon University
School of Medicine, Tokyo[3], Japan

Gaucher's disease results from genetically determined
abnormal metabolism of glucocerebroside, leading to its accumulation in tissue throughout the body.   It is not a common disease,
but is one of the more frequently encountered sphingolipidoses.
At least three different subtypes of Gaucher's disease are now
known.   Numerical nomenclature is sometimes confusing, but
according to Fredrickson (8), type I or adult form is to be
called a prototype of Gaucher's disease usually lacking a neurological impairment.   Type II or acute infantile form is characterized by a rapidly progressive neurological disorder.   The third
type is juvenile form, and, although less delineated, is known by
later onset and slower progressive course than type II.   As a
basic metabolic defect, the deficient activity of a specific
β-glucosidase is responsible for abnormal accumulation of glucocerebroside (3)

The application of enzyme studies on cultured amniotic fluid
cells makes the prenatal detection of genetic diseases possible
(4), and it has been successfully performed on various sphingolipidoses (6,11,13-18).   The fetal pathology of infantile (type II)
Gaucher's disease was reported by Schneider and associates (18).
The present report concerns a similar observation on a fetus of
20 weeks of gestational age.   Prior to this pregnancy, the
parents had a child who developed Gaucher's disease at 2 years of

age and died at 5 years. The clinical and enzymological data
will be reported in the separate paper (12). This paper concen-
trates on the pathological changes and ultrastructure of Gaucher
cells in the liver of the fetus.

MATERIALS AND METHODS

Because of clear deficiency of β-glucosidase of cultured
amniotic fluid cells, the pregnancy was terminated at request of
the parents at 20 weeks of gestational age.   Immediately after the
abortion, the body of the fetus was dissected, and small pieces of
liver, spleen, adrenal, kidney, testis, spinal cord, and hemisphere
of the brain were fixed in 10% neutralized formalin.   The rest of
the tissues were kept frozen for chemical analysis and enzyme
studies.

Paraffin sections were stained by hematoxylin-eosin, PAS,
luxol fast blue, and toluidine blue.   Sections of the brain were
taken from representative parts, including thalamus, basal ganglia,
Ammon's horn, midbrain, pons, cerebellum , and medulla oblongata.

For electron microscopy smaller cubic blocks measuring $1mm^3$
or less were cut from various tissues including above mentioned
parts of the brain, refixed in 1% osmic acid, and embedded in epon
according to usual procedure 48 hours after initial fixation in
10% formalin.   Thick sections were made by glass knives, and
stained by toluidine blue.   Ultrathin sections were cut by a
diamond knife, using MT2 Ultratome, stained by uranyl acetate and
lead citrate, and examined under JBM 100 electron microscope.

For chemical analysis of the brain, total lipids were extracted
from 1.0g of formalin fixed parietal lobe by chloroform-methanol
(2:1), and cholesterol, phospholipids, and N-acetyl neuraminic acid
were determined according standard procedures.   As controls two
unfixed frozen brains of 16 week old fetus were simultaneously
analysed.   The separation of gray and white matters was virtually
impossible at this fetal age.

OBSERVATIONS

Histopathology: Small numbers of multinucleated giant cells
measuring 20 to 40μ were scattered in the spleen and liver (Fig. 1,
3 & 4).   The cytoplasm of these giant cells was negative or very
weakly positive by PAS stain, and not stained by luxol fast blue.
These giant cells showed occasionally granular but not fibrillar
structure of cytoplasm.   They are apparently more abundant in
liver than in spleen, and most frequently seen in sinusoids.
Most parenchymal cells of the liver were unremarkable except for

some PAS positive granular materials in periportal areas (Fig. 2). Other organs examined were unremarkable, and such giant cells were not observed in the kidney, adrenal, and testis.

Neuropathology: The sections of various parts of the brain and spinal cord were essentially unremarkable. Fig. 5 and 6 may indicate that the nervous system of this fetus was quite well preserved. No evidence of neuronophagia, neuronal loss, or intra-neuronal storage was seen. Giant cells comparable with Gaucher cells were not observed in the central nervous system.

Electron Microscopy: In general the preservation of tissue was good. Although the cristae of mitochondria were not clear, other membranous component were pretty well preserved. Under the electron microscope liver cells showed round or oval nuclei with prominent nucleoli and abundant subcellular organelles (Fig. 7). Some liver cells especially those around portal regions showed multiple vacuoles, which contain flocky materials (Fig. 8). Occasionally, myelin figures up to 0.8μ were noted in the cytoplasm of liver cells (Fig. 9). No tubular structure consistent with glucocerebroside was noted in the liver parenchymal cells.

Multinucleated giant cells consistent with Gaucher cells in fetus were easily recognized under electron microscope. They were characterized by large size, eccentric nucleus, and scanty subcell-ular organelles (Fig. 10 & 11). The cytoplasm contained round dense bodies in variable amount, and occasionally showed erythro-phagocytosis. Multiple vacuoles containing myelin figures and ingested fragments of erythrocytes were often found adjacent the erythrophagocytosis (Fig. 12). Some tubular figures were noted, but any of them were typical as those described in postnatal Gaucher cells.

Ultrastructure of the brain was unremarkable. Any abnormal cytosomes including MCB were not found in the neurons of Ammon's horn, oculomotor, hypoglossal, and anterior horn nuclei.

Lipid Analysis of the Brain: The results were essentially unremarkable, and no definite difference was noted from two control brains (Table 1). No cholesterol ester was noted on thin layer chromatogram. Also, both gluco- and galacto- cerebrosides were undetectable on thin layer chromatogram.

DISCUSSION

Although it is not the purpose of this paper to discuss the classification of Gaucher's disease, it should be noted that the sibling of this fetus was atypical for infantile (type II) form,

simply because of later onset and subacute course. Yet the
patient had neurological manifestation including strabismus, which
seemed to justify to call "neuropathic Gaucher's disease".

The multinucleated giant cells in the spleen and liver were
considered to be Gaucher cells. We could not find such giant
cells in the liver of fetal Tay-Sachs disease with hexosaminidase
A deficiency. In agreement with Schneider and associates (18),
the Gaucher cells in the present fetus were apparently smaller
than those of postnatal cases. In addition, they were less PAS
positive, and had less delineated structure of cytoplasm. The
electron microscopic features appeared also somewhat different
from postnatal Gaucher cells (5,7,9). The major difference was
that the fetal Gaucher cells had not many tubular or crystaloid
inclusions comparable with glucocerebroside. It is curious that
in the post natal cases Gaucher cells are much more abundant in
the spleen than in the liver, while apparently the reverse is true
in fetal Gaucher's disease.

Table 1

Lipid Analysis of the Brain of Fetal Gaucher's Disease

	Control 1	Control 2	Gaucher
Water content (%)	92.51	89.11	92.67
(% of dry weight)			
Chloroform-methanol insoluble residue	69.03	80.97	73.32
Upper phase solids	4.69	2.46	4.26
Proteolipid protein	0.52	---	0.91
Total lipids	25.77	16.17	21.51
NANA (μg/mg dry weight)	69.31	44.43	34.05
(% of total lipids)			
Cholesterol	25.18	33.57	34.95
Phospholipids	75.56	84.77	66.23

The involvement of parenchymal cells of liver, lungs and adrenals are known in Gaucher's disease. In the present fetus we noted some PAS positive hepatic cells in periportal areas, and corresponding vacuolation by electron microscopy. It is not yet certain whether it represents the accumulation of some materials or it is just an artifact. We did not find such change of liver cells in a fetus of Tay-Scahs disease. Schneider and associates (18) described abnormal cytosomes in liver cells in their case, but they appear different from ours on electron micrographs.

The neuropathology of acute infantile Gaucher's disease has been well documented (2,10,19), and neurolipidosis does exist in infantile Gaucher's disease in a localized form mainly in the brain stem. In this fetus, careful microscopic examination as well as electron microscopic observation failed to find evidence of lipidosis in the neurons of thalamus, Ammon's horn, brainstem motor nuclei, and anterior horn of spinal cord. The simplest explanation for this is the brain is too young to show neurolipid-osis. Conventional lipid analysis also failed to find any abnorm-ality.

SUMMARY

Gaucher cells were found in the spleen and liver of 20 week old fetus with neuropathic Gaucher's disease. Ultrastructure of these Gaucher cells was presented. No definitive abnormality was noted in the brain pathologically as well as in lipid composition.

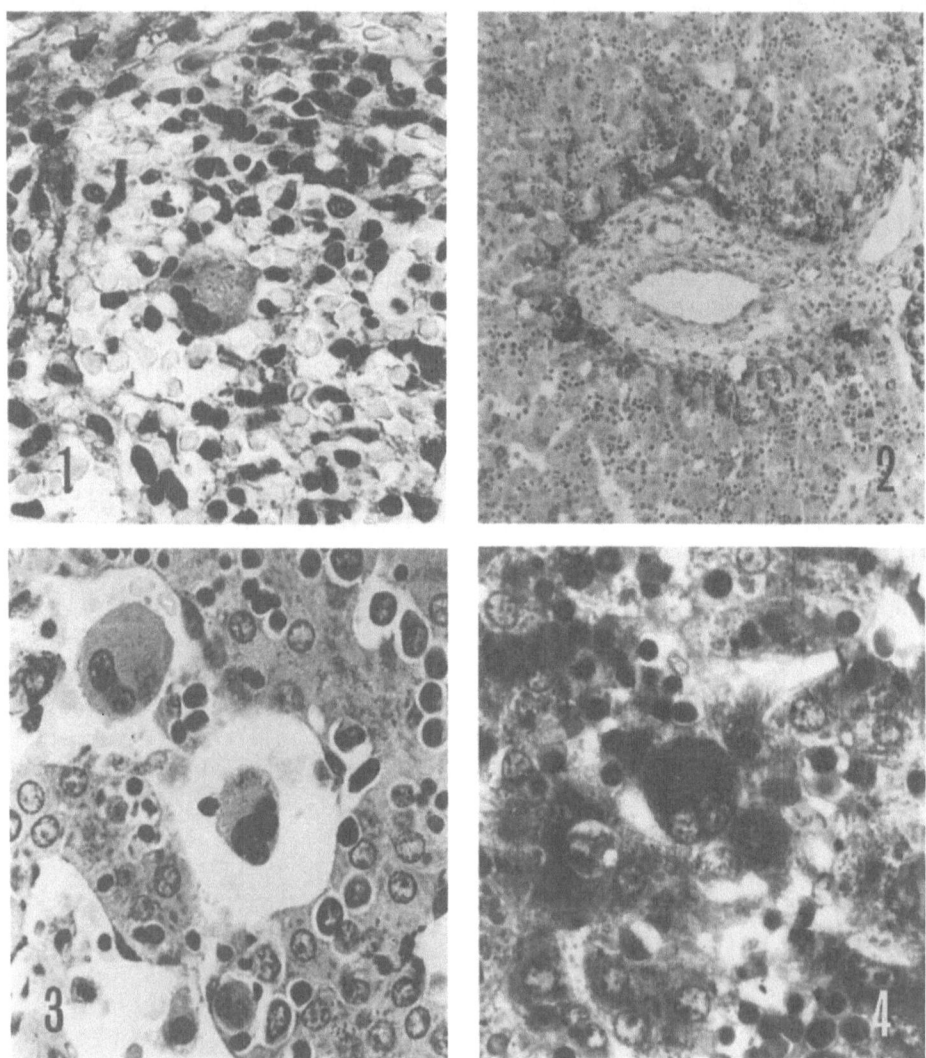

Fig. 1   A Gaucher cell in the spleen with multiple nuclei
and opaque granular cytoplasm. H & E stain, x 430

Fig. 2   General architecture of the liver. Some PAS positive
materials are noted in the periportal parenchymal cells. PAS
stain, x 120

Fig. 3   Gaucher cells in the liver. They appear frequently
in sinusoids. The cytoplasm is not or very weakly PAS positive.
PAS stain, x 470

Fig. 4   Gaucher cells in the liver. Note multiple and eccentric nuclei.   Toluidine blue stain of epon embedded section, x 470

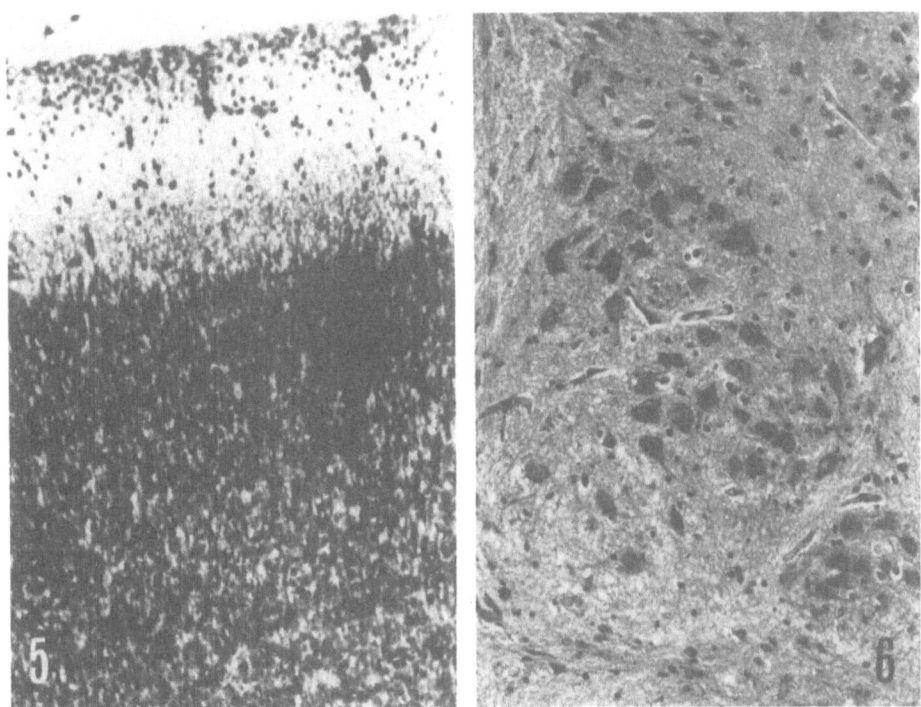

Fig. 5   Cerebral cortex from the frontal tip, showing normal architecture for this fetal age. Toluidine blue stain of epon embedded section, x 120

Fig. 6   Anterior horn of the spinal cord. All of the motor neurons appear normal, and no evidence of neuronophagia or intra-neuronal storage is noted.   H & E stain, x 240

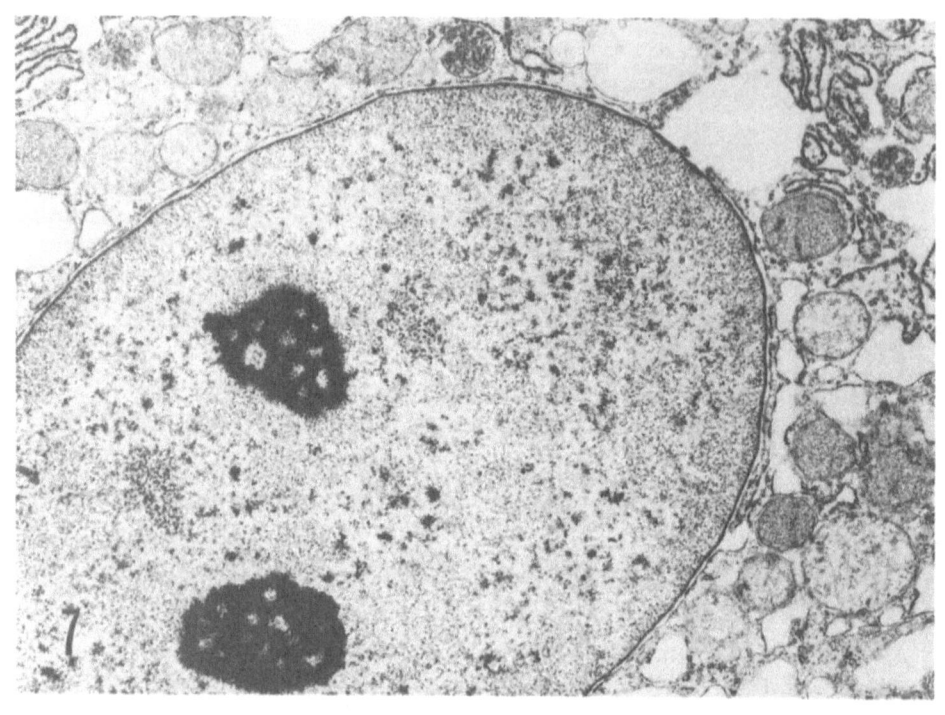

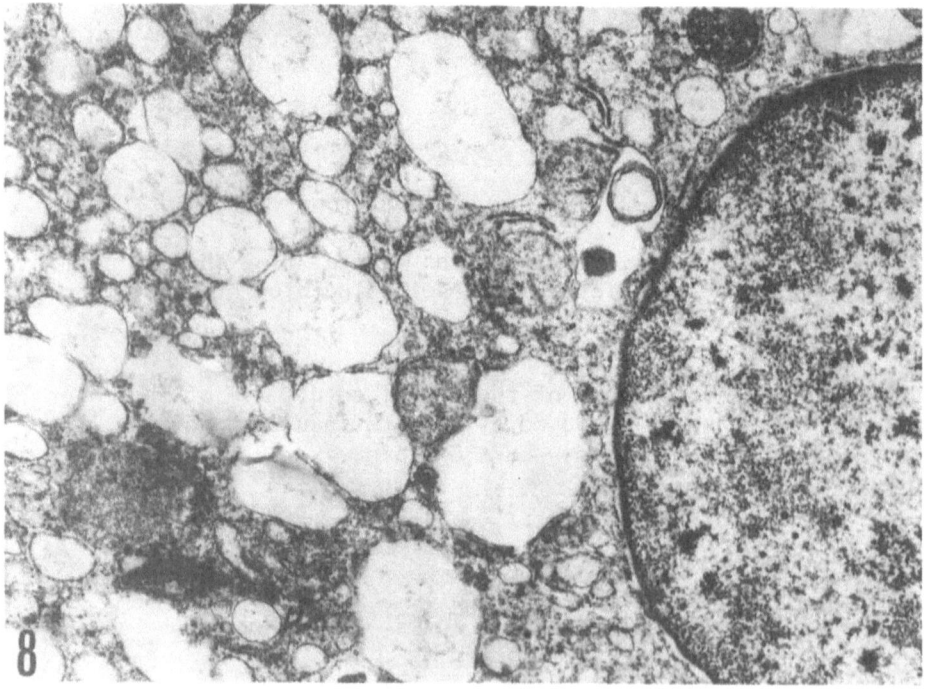

Fig. 7   Electron micrograph of a liver cell in the fetus of Gaucher's disease. In general, nucleoli are prominent. x 11,000

Fig. 8   Some liver cells around the portal areas show multiple vacuoles, which contain some residual material. x 16,000

Fig. 9   A part of liver cell cytoplasm showing myelin figures (arrow). x 34,000

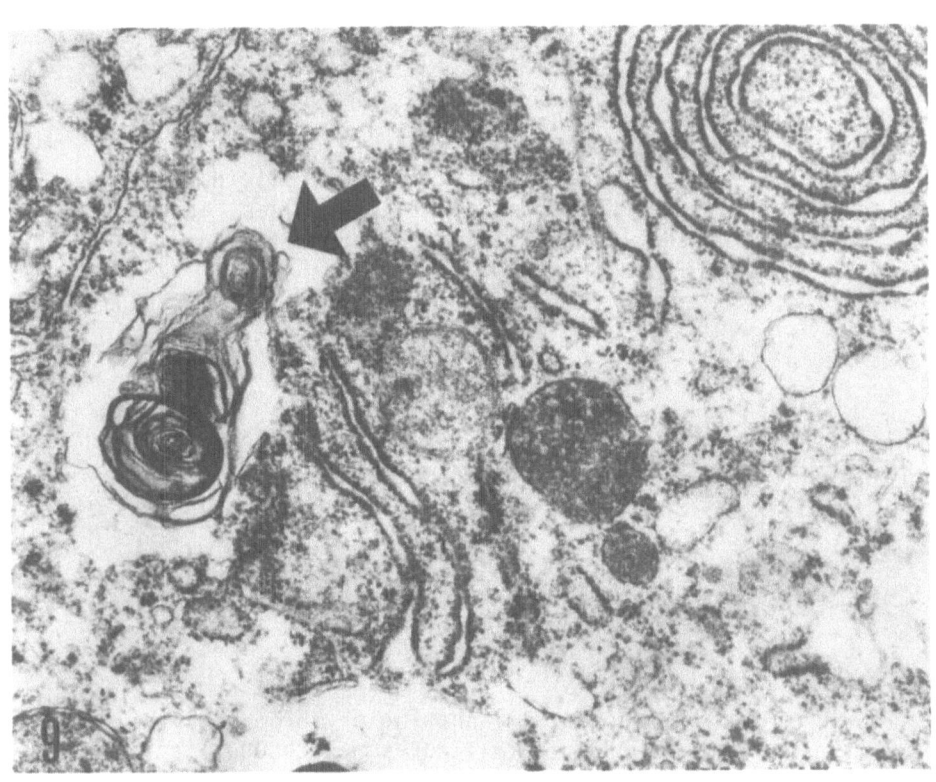

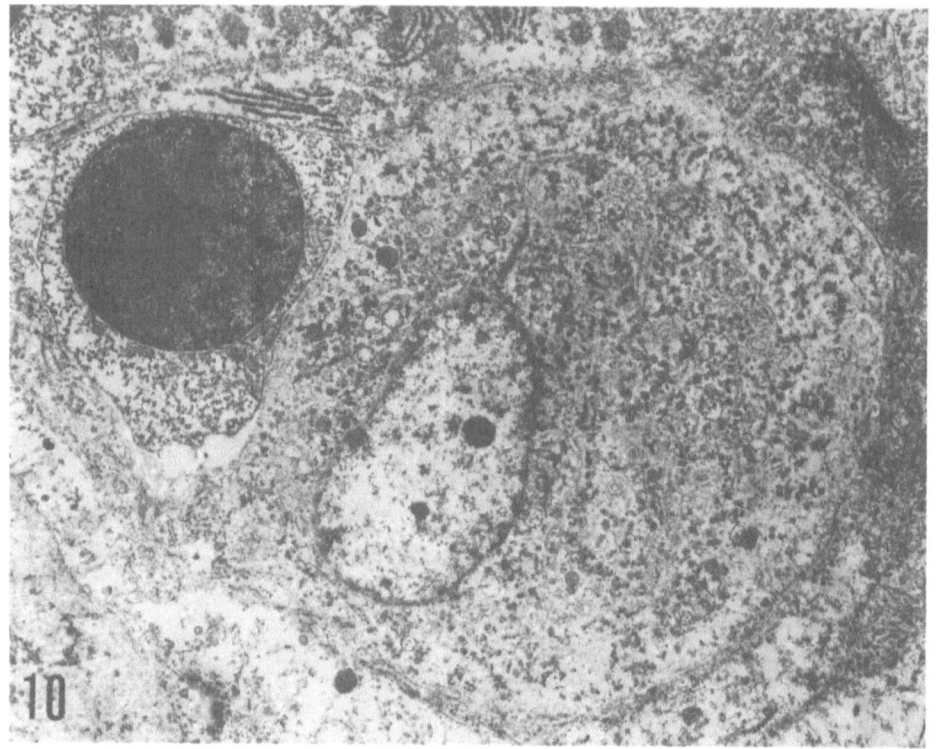

Fig. 10   Electron micrograph of a Gaucher cell in the liver
showing eccentric nucleus, rather scanty organelles, and many
dense bodies. The smaller cell in upper left with round dark
nucleus is an erythroblast. × 4,900

Fig. 11   Another Gaucher cell in the liver with multiple
nuclei, scanty organelles, and few dense bodies. × 14,500

Fig. 12   A liver Gaucher cell showing erythrophagocytosis
and multiple vacuoles with myelin figures. × 24,000

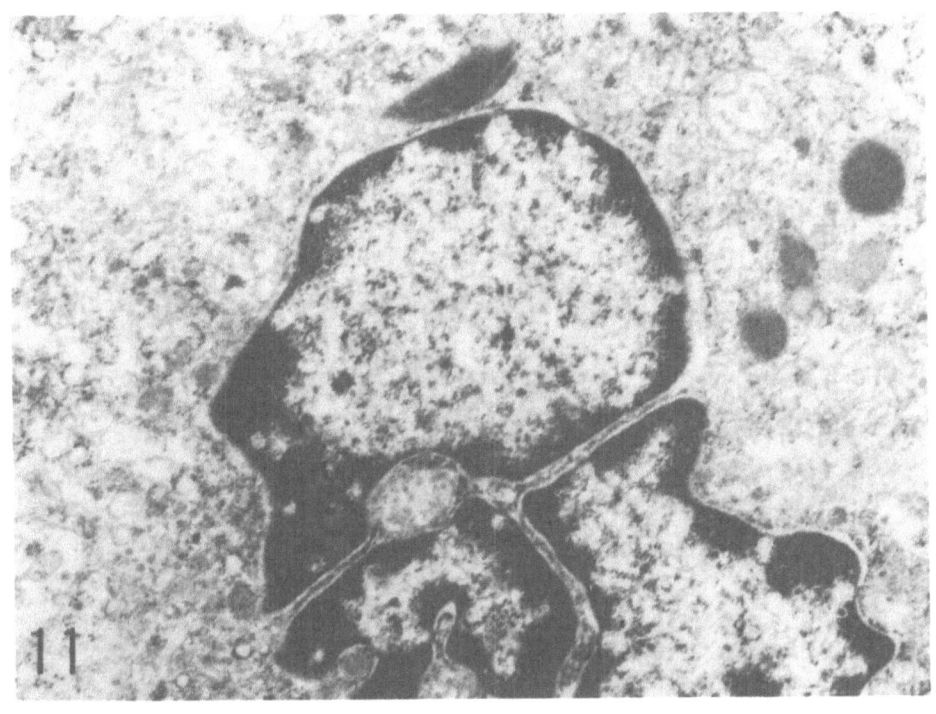

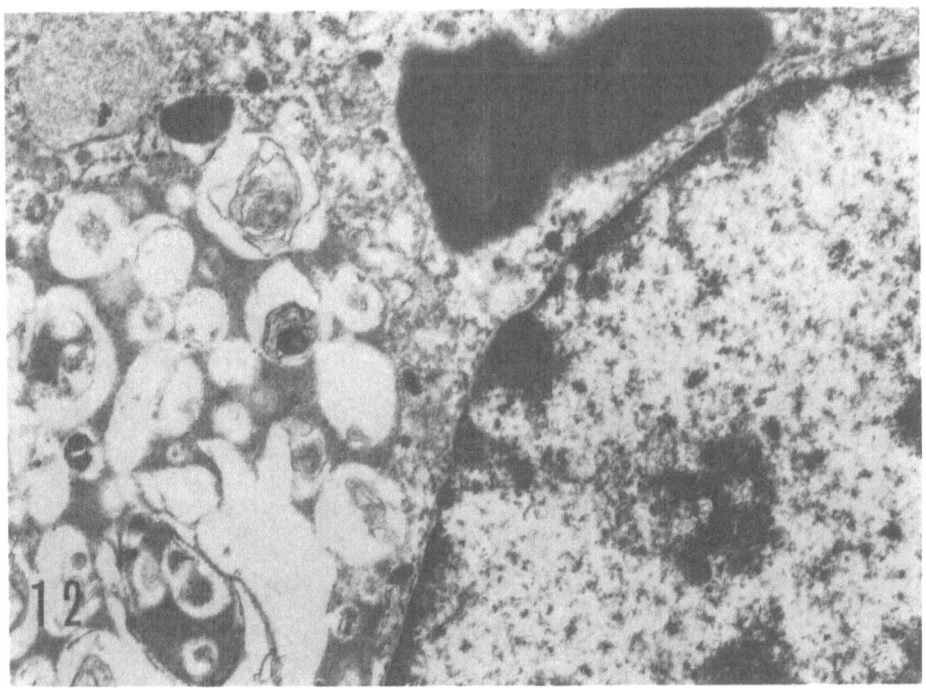

REFERENCES

1. Adachi, M., Wallace, B. J., Schneck, L., et al. : Fine structure of central nervous system in early infantile Gaucher's disease. Arch. Path. 83:513,1967.

2. Banker, B. Q., Miller, J. Q., and Crocker, A. C. : The cerebral pathology of infantile Gaucher's disease, in Cerebral Sphingolipidoses: A Symposium on Tay-Sachs' Disease and Allied Disorders, Aronson, S. M. and Volk, B. W. (eds.), New York: Academic Press, Inc., 1962, pp 73-99.

3. Brady, R. O., and King, F. M. : Gaucher's disease, in Lysosomes and Storage Diseases, Hers, H. G. and van Hoof, F. (eds.), New York and London: Academic Press, Inc., 1973, pp 381-394.

4. Dorfman, A. : Antenatal Diagnosis. University of Chicago Press, Chicago and London, 1972.

5. Eguchi, M., Komiyama, A., Tsukada, M., et al. : The electron microscopic observation of Gaucher cells - Ultrastructure and acid phosphatase activity -. Med. J. Shinshu Univ., 17:147,1973.

6. Ellis, W. G., Schneider, E. L., McCulloch, J. R., et al. : Fetal globoid cell leukodystrophy (Krabbe disease). Pathological and biochemical examination. Arch. Neurol. 29:253, 1973.

7. Fisher, E. R., and Reidbord, H. : Gaucher's disease: Pathogenetic considerations based on electron microscopic and histochemical observations. Am. J. Path. 41:679,1962.

8. Fredrickson, D. S., and Sloan, H. R. : Glucosyl ceramide lipidoses: Gaucher's disease, in The Metabolic Basis of Inherited Disease, Stanbury, J. B., Wyngaarden, J. B., and Fredrickson, D. S. (eds.), 3rd ed., New York etc., McGraw-Hill Book Co., 1972, pp 730-759.

9. Hibbs, R. G., Ferrans, V. J., Cipriano, P. R., et al. : A histochemical and electron microscopic study of Gaucher cells. Arch. Path. 89:137,1970.

10. Inose, T., Inoue, K., Sawaizumi, S. et al. : Beitrag zur Neuropathologie des Morbus Gaucher im Kindesalter. Acta Neuropath. 3:297,1964.

11. Kaback, M. M., Sloan, H. R., Sonneborn, M., et al. : G$_{M1}$-gangliosidosis type I: In utero detection and fetal manifestations. J. Pediat. 82:1037,1973.

12. Kitagawa, T., Owada, M., Sakiyama, T., et al. : Neuropathic Gaucher's disease: In utero diagnosis and fetal biochemistry and pathology. To be published.

13. Leroy, J. G., Van Elsen, A. F., Martin, J. J., et al. : Infantile metachromatic leukodystrophy. Confirmation of a prenatal diagnosis. New Eng. J. Med. 288:1365,1973.

14. Lowden, J. A., Cutz, E., Conen, P. E., et al. : Prenatal diagnosis of G$_{M1}$-gangliosidosis. New Eng. J. Med. 288:225, 1973.

15. O'Brien, J. S., Okada, S., Rillerup, D. L., et al. : Tay-Sachs disease: Prenatal diagnosis. Science 172:61,1971.

16. Schneck, L., Adachi, M., and Volk, B. W. : The fetal aspects of Tay-Sachs disease. Pediatrics 49:342,1972.

17. Schneider, E. L., Ellis, W. G., Brady, R. O., et al. : Prenatal Niemann-Pick disease: Biochemical and histological examination of a 19-gestational week fetus. Pediatr. Res. 6:720,1972.

18. Schneider, E. L., Ellis, W. G., Brady, R. O., et al. : Infantile (type II) Gaucher's disease: In utero diagnosis and fetal pathology. J. Pediat. 81:1134,1972.

19. Seitelberger, F. : Uber die Gehirnbeteiligung bei der Gaucher-schen Krankheit im Kindesalter. Archiv f. Psychiat. u. Zeitsch. ges. Neurol. 206:419,1964.

RECENT OBSERVATIONS ON GAUCHER'S DISEASE

J.N. Kanfer, S.S. Raghaven, R.A. Mumford,
J. Sullivan, and C. Spielvogel
Eunice Kennedy Shriver Center
200 Trapelo Road
Waltham, Massachusetts, U.S.A.

G. Legler
Institut für Biochemie der Universität Köln
Köln, Germany

R.S. Labow, D.G. Williamson, and D.S. Layne
Department of Biochemistry
University of Ottawa
Ottawa, Ontario, Canada K1N 9A9

Gaucher's disease has been classically defined biochemically as having an accumulation of glucosylceramide in concert with a decreased associated hydrolytic enzyme activity (1) in tissues from affected individuals. This reduced enzymatic activity was originally demonstrated using glucosylceramide as substrates (2) however, p-nitrophenol (pNP) or 4 methylumbelliferyl (4MU) β-glucose (3) and glucosylsphinogosine (4) cleavage are also reduced in tissue samples from affected individuals.

Lysosomal β-glucosidase

We decided several years ago that although glucosylceramide: β-glucosidase had been purified previously and some of its properties examined (5), a systematic study of substrate specificity and inhibitors of this enzyme still

Table I: Ability of Purified Calf Spleen β -glucosidase to
          hydrolyze various β -glucosides

	% Activity
Glucosylceramide	100
Deoxycortcosterone β -D-glucoside	80
Cellobiose	28
Gentiobiose	28
Methyl β -glucoside	26
Salicin	28

appeared warranted. We reasoned that the proper understanding of the disease would ultimately require a
complete understanding of the enzyme which was affected.

The enzyme was eventually purified from calf brain
(6) and spleen (7) by a reproducible affinity column
chromatographic procedure developed in this laboratory
(8). Substrate specificity is a constant problem when
studying hydrolytic enzyme deficiencies which are demonstrable with "artificial" substrates. Therefore, it
appeared desirable to investigate the hydrolysis of
several glucosides which might be potential substrates,
and the results of such an examination for the spleen
enzyme are shown in Table I. It is obvious that in
addition of glucosylceramide only deoxycosticosterone
(DOC)- β-D-glucoside was hydrolyzed to an appreciable extent by the purified enzyme preparations. In order to
further examine the role of these compounds as substrates, we reasoned that if they are substrates for
the same enzyme then they should also be competitive
inhibitors. A typical result which we obtained with
the spleen enzyme for DOC-β -D-glucoside inhibition of
both 4-MU- β-D-glucoside and glucosylceramide hydrolysis
is illustrated in Fig. 1 and the data obtained for both
the purified brain and spleen enzymes are summarized in
Table II. The inhibitors obtained with the first four
compounds were all of the competitive type and are consistent with the results from studies on the substrate
specificities.

Most acid hydrolases prepared from bacterial and
plant sources have been shown to catalyze a "transglycosylation" reaction, and this activity is believed to
be associated with the usual hydrolytic activity of
those enzymes. Thus, it is assumed that substrates for
the hydrolytic activity are also donors for the "trans-
glycolytic" activity of a given enzyme. We decided to
examine the possibility that this generalization also
held true for these mammalian β-glucosidases. The test
system employed (^{14}C)-ceramide as the acceptor molecules
and several β-glucosides as the potential donors (9).
The assay measured the formation of radioactive glucosylceramide, which is a substrate for the hydrolytic
activity of these enzymes.

Ceramide (^{14}C) + β-glucosides — glucosyl-ceramide (^{14}C)

As shown in Table III, only those compounds which had
been previously shown to be hydrolyzed by the enzyme and

Table II: Ki values for various inhibitors of 4 MU-β-D-glucoside and glucosylceramide hydrolysis by purified calf brain (6) and spleen β-glucosidase (7)

Inhibitor	4 MU-β-D-glucoside		Glucosylceramide	
	Brain	Spleen	Brain	Spleen
Glucosylceramide	1.0×10^{-3} M	1.8×10^{-3} M	--	--
4 MU-β-D-glucoside	--	--	3.4×10^{-3} M	2.8×10^{-3} M
Glucosylsphingosine	7.5×10^{-5} M	6.9×10^{-5} M	4.0×10^{-5} M	7.5×10^{-5} M
Deoxycorticosterone β-D-glucoside	2.1×10^{-4} M	4×10^{-4} M	4.2×10^{-4} M	4.3×10^{-4} M
Nojirimycine	1.2×10^{-5} M	1×10^{-6} M	5.8×10^{-5} M	1.5×10^{-6} M
Gluconolactam	2×10^{-4} M	4×10^{-4} M	4×10^{-4} M	2.0×10^{-4} M
Conduritol B expoxide	1.5×10^{-6} M	4.5×10^{-6} M	1.2×10^{-6} M	--

Table III: The ability of various glucosides to act as donors for the "transglucosylation" reaction of purified brain (6) and spleen (7) β-glucosidase with ceramide (^{14}C) as the acceptor

Donor	% Activity	
	Brain	Spleen
4 MU-β-D-glucoside	100	100
Glucosylceramide	44.7	-
Glucosylsphingosine	7.8	-
Deoxycorticosterone β-D-glucoside	17.9	27
Maltose	-	3
Gentiobiose	-	0
Cellobiose	2.7	5
Esculin	-	8
Salicin	-	3
Glucose	3.8	0
UDP-glucose	3.7	0.5

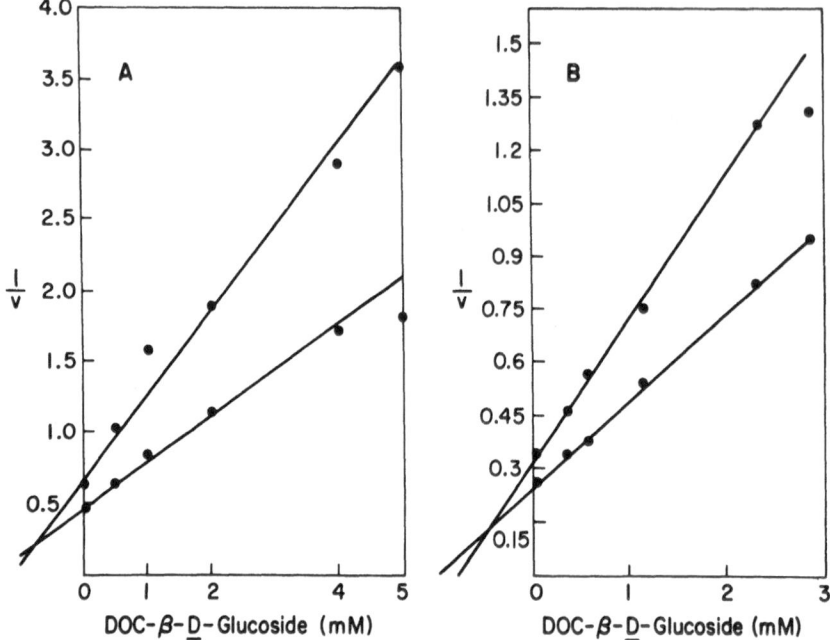

FIGURE 1: Effect of varying DOC- β-D-glucoside upon the hydrolysis of (a) 4 MU- β-D-glucoside and (b) glucosylceramide by the purified calf spleen β-D-glucosidase.

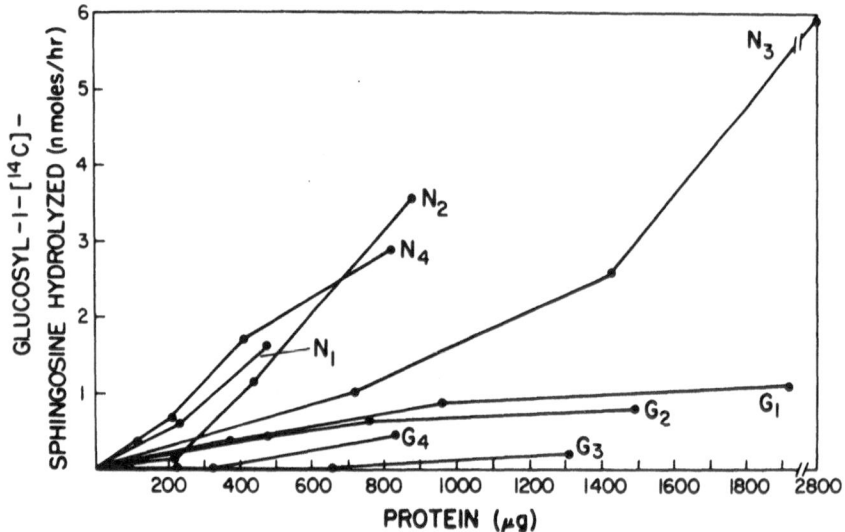

FIGURE 2: Effects of varying protein content from control and Gaucher fibroblast cell cultures upon the hydrolysis of glucosyl-sphingosine.

had been shown to be competitive inhibitors of the enzyme
were found to be active donors for this "transglucosylation" reaction. We concluded that based upon this evidence the purified lysosomal β-glucosidase which is
diminished in Gaucher's disease will hydrolyze pNP and
4 MU- β -D-glucosides, glucosylceramide, glucosylsphingosine and steroid β-glucosides.

Glucosylsphingosine and Gaucher's Disease

Since it appeared that glucosylsphingosine was a substrate for this β-glucosidase, we decided to examine the
hydrolysis of this substrate in Gaucher tissue samples.
This seemed a useful way to obtain supportive evidence for
glucosylsphingosine being a substrate and to possibly
document further deficiencies in Gaucher's disease in an
attempt at understanding both the enzyme and this disease.
The information presented in Fig. 2 is illustrative of
these results (10). It is apparent that the fibroblasts
from Gaucher individuals when compared to controls have
decreased hydrolytic activity towards glucosylsphingosine.
Similar observations were obtained with homogenates of
solid spleen tissue samples. This observation suggested
that perhaps we might be successful in detecting the presence of glucosylsphingosine in Gaucher's spleen tissue.
The information upon the isolation of glucosylsphingosine
and structural proof has already been published (11).

Steroid β-glucosides and Gaucher's Disease

As indicated from the studies on specificities
(Table I) and its ability to act as a competitive inhibitor (Fig. 2), it appeared that deoxycorticosterone-β
-D-glucoside was a substrate for the purified calf spleen
and brain enzyme. Therefore, it seemed appropriate to
examine the hydrolytic capacity of Gaucher tissues towards
such compounds. The 17 α(^{3}H)-estradiol-3 and 17 β-D-
glucosides were prepared by published methods (12) and
their hydrolysis determined as previously described (13).
It was readily apparent from such a study that there is a
significant decrease in the hydrolysis of these 2 compounds
by Gaucher spleen samples (Table IV). There is no demonstrable decrease in samples from either metachromatic
leukodystrophy or Niemann-Pick diseases, two other sphingolipidoses.

Studies in the metabolism of steroid β-glucosides
have suggested that these are both soluble and particulate
forms of this enzyme (14). We have reported that the

Table IV: 17α-Estradiol-17β-D-glucoside: β-glucosidase: 17α-estradiol-3-β-D-glucoside:
β-glucosidase 4-MU-β-D-glucosidase, β-galactosidase and β-N Acetyl hexosaminidase
activities in human spleen samples

Sample	17α-Estradiol 17β-glucoside	17α-Estradiol 3β-glucoside	4-MU-β-glucoside	4MU-β-galactoside	4MUβ-N-Acetyl-glucosaminide
Gaucher	0.015	0.086	0.94	126.3	27,950
Gaucher	0.010	0.046	0.66	74.8	12,360
Normal	0.079	0.278	30.7	53.7	4,300
Normal	0.087	0.18	33.1	132.8	6,490
MLD	0.119	0.194	57.2	95.2	7,200
Nieman Pick	0.074	0.164	28.3	101.3	8,300

Activities expressed as nmoles of substrate hydrolyzed per h per mgm protein except
17 -α3H(β-Estradiol-3-17β-glucoside which were incubated 17 h.

Table V: The hydrolysis of 4MU-β-D-glucoside, glucosyl ceramide and 17α-estradiol-3-β-D-glucoside by the soluble and particulate fraction of infantile and adult Gaucher tissues *

	4-MU-β-Glucoside		Glucocerebroside		Steroid β glucoside	
	Soluble	Particulate	Soluble	Particulate	Soluble	Particulate
INF. Control Spleen (1)**	16	27.5	6.6	215.2	9.4	13.1
INF. Gaucher Spleen (2)	1.5	0.3	4.4	18.2	NDH	NDH
INF. Gaucher Spleen (3)	NDH	0.4	2.6	0.9	1.6	0.8
INF. Control Liver (1)	72.6	32.5	5.5	204.7	11.8	12.1
INF. Gaucher Liver (2)	51.6	2.6	13.2	27.1	29.7	1.7
INF. Gaucher Liver (3)	77.6	1.2	3.8	10.9	21.5	.6
INF. Gaucher Liver (4)	NDH	1.0	4.9	17.3	13.8	.6
INF. Control Brain (1)	2.26	93.3	0	773.1	7.2	30.55
INF. Control Brain (11)	3.8	27.9	0.7	679.4	7.5	27.1
INF. Gaucher Brain (2)	0	7.2	2.0	96.9	0.2	3.5
INF. Gaucher Brain (3)	0.7	2.1	2.5	24.1	2.1	1.2
Control Adult Spleen (5)	5.5	44.3	61.2	260.0	4.7	6.7
Control Adult Spleen (6)	32.5	43.4	9.5	248.1	9.3	25.5
Adult Gaucher Spleen (7)	2.2	1.0	3.8	12.1	2.5	NDH
Adult Gaucher Spleen (8)	5.5	3.3	9.2	33.7	9.5	1.6
Adult Gaucher Spleen (9)	8.8	3.0	9.1	27.5	7.4	1.4
Adult Gaucher Spleen (10)	12.9	5.2	6.3	51.8	15.3	3.1

*Activities expressed as nmoles cleaved/mg protein/unit time.
**Numbers in parenthesis designate tissues from different individuals.

NDH = no detectable hydrolysis

purified bovine brain and spleen β-glucosidase cleaves
DOC- β-D-glucoside and have also found that these enzymes
effectively hydrolyzed both of the estradiol β-glucosides.
These particular enzymes are bound to the lysosomal particles. A soluble rabbit liver steroid β-glucosidase has
been highly purified (13) and we have recently shown that
this enzyme preparation does not hydrolyze glucosylceramide. We have also purified a soluble pig kidney β-glucosidase which hydrolyzes 4-MU- β-D-glucoside and the
steroid β-D-glucosides but not glucosylceramide. A
particulate enzyme simultaneously isolated from the same
source has the capacity to cleave all 3 of these substrates (15). Therefore, we decided to assay Gaucher
tissue samples for soluble and particulate β-D-glucosidase activities and these data are presented in Table V.

It is evident that the particulate enzyme activity
towards cerebroside, steroid β-glucoside and 4 MU- β -D-
glucoside was diminished in all Gaucher tissue samples
assayed. In the adult Gaucher spleens there was no
diminution of the soluble form. However, in infantile
Gaucher brain and spleen tissue samples there was a significant decrease in the soluble steroid β-glucosidase
activity. It should be noted that the infantile patient
#2 has reasonably active hydrolytic activity. This pa-
tient was the subject of CPC in 1963 since it appeared
clinically atypical at that time (16). In contrast to
most of the infantile patients the age of onset was 17
months rather than 6 months. This may represent a late
onset type of infantile Gaucher's disease.

In order to confirm this deficiency we decided to
investigate the possibility that this decreased hydrolytic enzyme activity may be demonstrable by measuring
the "transglucosylation" activity. The test system contained estradiol-(^{3}H) as the acceptor molecule and
4 MU-β-D-glucoside as the donor molecule. The assay de-
pended upon the thin layer separation of the product.,
estradiol β -glucoside, from the precursor. The areas
cochromatograming with authentic standards were scraped
from the plate and counted (Table VI). It is evident
that in adult Gaucher spleen particulates the activity
is reduced to 9% of control and in the infantile Gaucher
particulates it is reduced to 23% of control. The soluble fraction from the adult spleen is 150% of control.
In contrast, the infantile Gaucher soluble activity is
reduced to only 8% of the control value. This observation is in complete accord with the data presented in
Table V and supports our hypotheses that the absence of

Table VI: Estradiol β -glucoside formation in soluble and
           particulate fractions of Gaucher and control spleen
           samples

	Transglucosylation Activity	
	Soluble*	Particulate*
Adult Control	683	782
Adult Gaucher	859.6	118
Adult Gaucher	1204	27.6
Infantile Control	912	247.4
Infantile Gaucher	111.3	42.7
Infantile Gaucher	38.1	73.3

*Values expressed as p moles formed/mg protein/16 hrs.

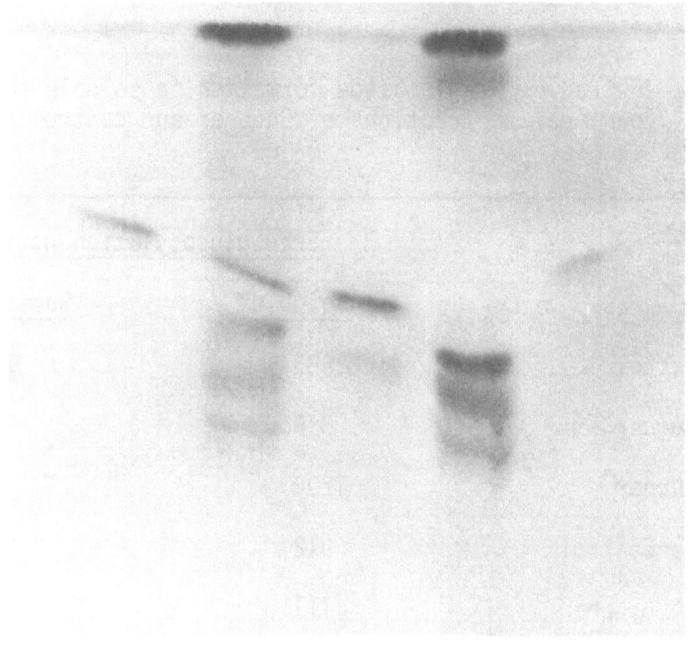

FIGURE 3: TLC of brain sphingolipids fraction from 3 month old of conduritol exposide treated and control mice. From left to right: lane 1 is a galactosyl ceramide, standard; lane 2 is a glucosyl ceramide standard; lane 3 is from the experimental animals; lane 4 is mixed cerebroside standard; lane 5 is from control animals; lane 6 is glucosylceramide standard. These were chromatogramed on a borate-treated plate with C-M-H2O (65:25:4) as solvent.

soluble β-glucosidase may distinguish the adult form from
the infantile form of this disease.

Therefore, it appears that there is an additional
lysosomal enzyme deficiency in Gaucher's disease which in-
volves the hydrolysis of steroid β-D-glucoside. This is
a reflection of the relative substrate non-specificity of
this particular enzyme towards the aglycone moiety.
Therefore, this enzyme deficiency observed in Gaucher's
disease should no longer be regarded as being specific
for glucosylceramide. The soluble, non-lysosomal form of
the steroid β-D-glucoside is not affected in the adult
Gaucher spleen samples, but is decreased in the infantile
tissues examined. This difference in soluble β-glucosidase activity may reflect the biochemical difference between these two forms of the disease. Studies are currently underway in an attempt to examine the steroid β-
glucoside content of Gaucher spleen tissue samples.

The Gaucher Mouse

Investigations on competitive inhibitors revealed
that conduritol- B -epoxide was very effective with a Ki
in the order of 10^{-6}M for the spleen and brain enzymes
(Table II). This compound has been extensively studied
and shown to be an effective inhibitor of non-mammalian
β-glucosidase (17). We thought that this compound might
be potentially useful in an attempt to produce an animal
model for Gaucher's disease. We used as criteria of
success the biochemical definition of the disease which
is increased tissue glucosylceramide levels in concert
with a diminished detectable β-glucosidase activity. In
the first study we injected 90 day old mice subcutaneously on a daily basis for 3 weeks with a dose of 100
mg/kg body weight. There were no obvious clinical differences between the experimental and the control group
during the course of this experiment. The glucosylceramide levels were quantitated according to published
procedures (18). A typical thin layer chromatogram of
the brain lipids is shown in Fig. 3 and the comparable
analytical data presented in Table VIIa. It is evident
that in both brain and peripheral tissues there was an
increased glucosylceramide content. The level of several hydrolytic enzymes in homogenates prepared from
these organs from experimental and control animals is
shown in Table VIIIa and the most dramatic decrease was
found in β-glucosidase activity.

In the next experiment the animals were injected

Table VII: Tissue levels of glucosylceramide in experimental
            and control mice *

A. 3 month animals	Tissue	Glucosylceramide (nmoles/gr wet wt)
Experimental	Spleen	138
Control	Spleen	74
Experimental	Liver	127
Control	Liver	75
Experimental	Brain	33
Control	Brain	6.9
B. Infant Animals		
Experimental	Brain	60
Control	Brain	21
Experimental	Liver	49.3
Control	Liver	32.2

*Each value is the average of analysis of at least 3 tissue
 samples from separate animals.

Table VIII: A comparison of tissue levels of several hydrolytic enzyme activities from experimental and control animals *

	α-mannoside	β-glucoside	β-hexosaminide	β-galactoside	α-glucoside	β-glucuronide
A. 3 month animals						
Experimental liver	17.6	2.24	278	5.84	2.57	5.49
Control liver	20.1	67.8	287	6.6	3.22	8.24
Experimental brain	13.11	0.1	2016	17.8	4.45	5.4
Control brain	8.66	9.49	966	16.47	4.12	3.09
B. Infant Mice						
Experimental spleen	86.2	1.49	1483	53.8	2.24	56.6
Control spleen	60.13	21.0	1858	55.3	5.79	80.2
Experimental brain	24.4	1.25	1896	22.26	1.52	15.18
Control brain	11.4	17.84	781	28.1	1.79	5.11

*All values expressed as nmoles substrat hydrolyzed/mg protein/hr. Tissues from 3 different 3 month old animals, 8 experimental infant mice or 16 control mice were assayed.

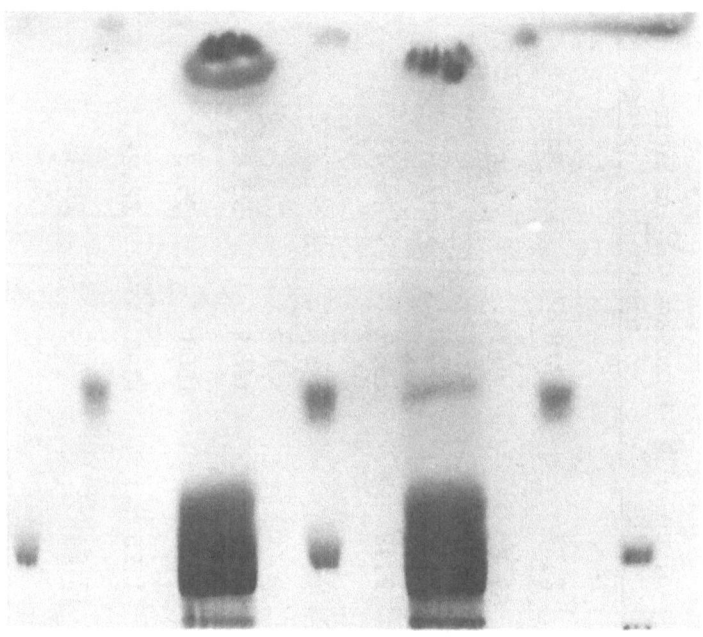

FIGURE 4: TLC of brain sphingolipid fraction from 28 day old experimental and control animals. From left to right: lane 1 is galactosyl ceramide standard; lane 2 is glucosyl ceramide standard; lane 3 is from control mice; lane 4 is mixed standards; lane 5 is from experimental animals; lanes 6 and 7 are glucosyl and galactosyl ceramides standards, respectively.

daily from birth to 28 days of age. A typical TLC of the
brain sphingolipids from this study is shown in Fig. 4.
The analysis of tissue glucosylceramide levels is present
in Table VIIb and the lysosomal enzyme activities in
Table VIIIb. In this case also there is a remarkable decrease in the detectable β-glucosidase activity and increase in glucosylceramide content of brain and peripheral
organs. These animals were evaluated independently by
Drs. V. Caveness and E. Kolodny of this institution who
concurred in their opinion that the experimental animals
appeared to show principally a gray matter disorder.
These observations support our contention that we have
successfully produced an animal model for Gaucher's
disease through the use of a specific enzyme inhibitor.

The final studies have been an attempt to examine
the developmental aspects of the drug administration.
Animals were injected at 1 day after birth and sacrificed
at various time periods thereafter. The animals killed
at day 10 had received 6 injections, the 17 day olds had
received 11 injections, the 19 day olds had received 16
injections, the 21 day olds had received 15 injections
and the 25 day olds had received 15 injections. The
brain levels of glucosyl and galactosylceramide were determined and the analytical data obtained presented in
Fig. 5. It is obvious that glucosylceramide levels are
already elevated at 10 days, the earliest experimental
time point, and continue to increase during the course
of the experiment. Similar changes have been observed
in the splenic glucosylceramide levels. There appeared
to be smaller amounts of galactosylceramide in the brain
samples from the experimental animals, suggesting arrested myelination.

The progressive effect of conduritol B-expoxide on
the hydrolytic enzyme activities of brain is shown in
Fig. 6. It is readily apparent that at the earliest
time point after only 6 injections the level of β-gluco-
sidase has been greatly reduced. In homogenates of brain
from the control animals there was a nearly linear decline from 10 to 25 postnatal days in the specific activi-
ty of β-glucosaminidase, β-mannosidase and β-glucuronidase.
There were only small changes seen in α-glucosidase, β-
galactosidase and β-glucosidase during this time period.
In the experimental animals there is no change in α-gluco-
sidase specific activity and a nearly linear decline of
β-galactosidase specific activity. However, in these
experimental animals there is a nearly linear increase in
β-glucosaminidase and α-mannosidase specific activities.

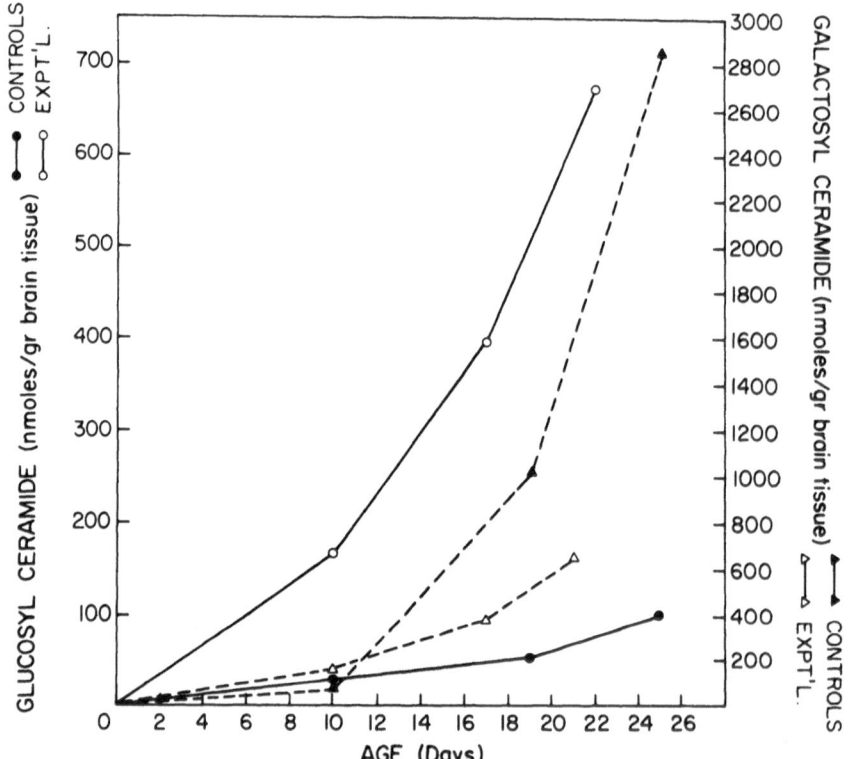

FIGURE 5: Levels of brain glucosylceramide and galactosyl ceramide in experimental and control mice as a function of age.

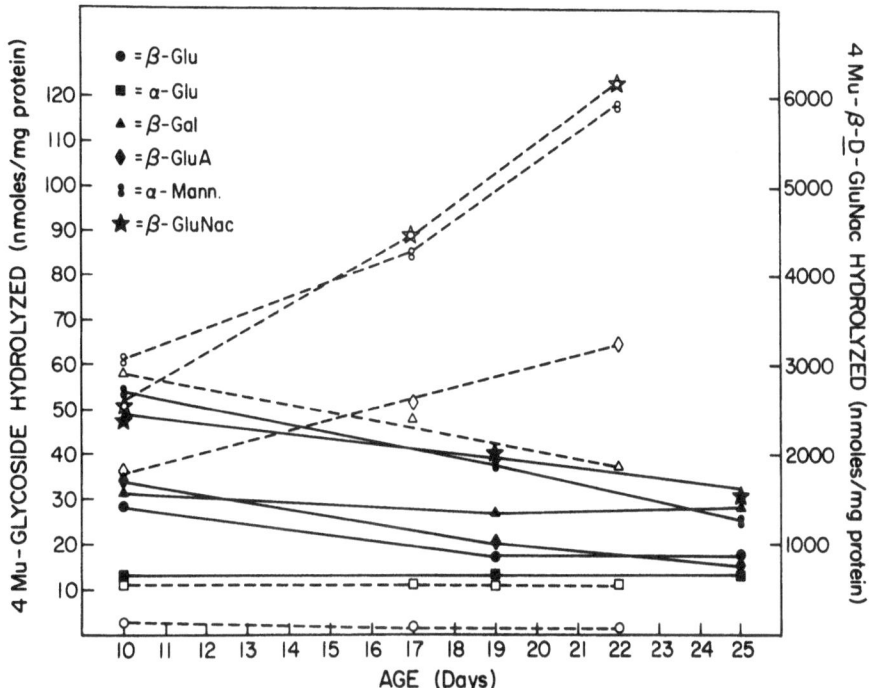

FIGURE 6: Levels of brain lysosomal hydrolases in experimental and control mice as a function of age. Closed symbols represent the control animals and the corresponding open symbols represent the experimental animals.

Table IX: Comparison of 6 lysosomal hydrolases in splenic
homogenates from control and experimental animals

	β-glu	α-glu	β-gal	β-glu-NAc	α man	β-glu A
Control (10)*	22.9	9.6	24.4	1654	92.2	84.4
Experimental(10)	5.7	6.9	36.7	1445	108.6	57.3
Control (25)	19.9	13.9	73.9	2407	102	173.3
Experimental(25)	2.81	12.3	175.9	7283	216	260

*Number in parenthesis is a postnatal age of animals at time of
sacrifice.

glu = glucosidase; gal = galactosidase; glu-NAc = -N-acetyl
hexosaminidase; man = mannosidase; glu A = glucuronidase.

Since only 3 of those enzyme activities increased while
1 remained unchanged and 1 decreased, it suggests that
perhaps each tissue may have lysosomes which do not contain an equally uniform distribution and complement of
acid hydrolases. Thus, in this particular experimental
condition only those lysosomes containing β-hexosaminidase, α -mannosidase and β-glucuronidase but not α -gluco-
sidase and β-galactosidase appear to be affected. The
data on the splenic acid hydrolases is presented in
Table IX.

Conclusion

These studies have documented the pharmacological
production of a Gaucher mouse which may prove to be very
useful for studying the pathogenesis of this disease in
humans. We have also demonstrated the reduced capacity
for Gaucher aisease tissue samples to hydrolyze estradiol
β-glucosides. In addition, a possible enzymatic difference between the adult and infantile forms of this disease is suggested.

Acknowledgements: Supported by Grants USPHS NS10330,
     HDo5515, HD04147 and M.R.C. of Canada MT 3287.

References

1. Fredrickson, D. S. and Sloan, H. R. in Metabolic Basis of
    Inherited Diseases. (ed. Stanbury, J. B., Wyngaarden, J. B.
    and Fredrikson, D. S.) McGraw-Hill, New York, 730,1972.

2. Brady, R.O., Kanfer, J. N. and Shapiro, D.B. Biochem. Biophys.
    Res. Commun. 18, 221 (1965).

3. Patrick, A. D., Biochem. J. 97, 17c (1965).

4. Raghavan, S. S., Mumford, R. A. and Kanfer, J. N. Biochem.
    Biophys. Res. Commun. 54, 256 (1973).

5. Brady, R. O., Kanfer, J. N. and Shapiro, D. J., Biol. Chem.
    240 , 39 (1965).

6. Mumford, R. A., Raghavan, S. S. and Kanfer, J. N., J. Neurochem.
    in the press.

7. Kanfer, J. N., Raghavan, S. S. and Munford, R. A., Biochem.
    Biophys. Acta 391, 129 (1975).

8. Kanfer, J. N., Mumford, R. A., Raghavan, S. S. and Byrd, J.,
    Anal. Biochem. 60, 200 (1974).

9. Raghavan, S. S., Mumford, R. A. and Kanfer, J. N., Biochem.
    Biophys. Res. Commun. 58, 99 (1974).

10. Raghavan, S. S., Mumford, R. A. and Kanfer, J. N., Biochem.
    Biophys. Res. Commun. 54, 256 (1973).

11. Raghavan, S. S., Mumford, R. A. and Kanfer, J. N., J. Lipid
    Res. 15, 484 (1974).

12. Collins, D. C., Williamson, D. G. and Layne, D. S., J. Biol.
    Chem. 245, 873 (1970),

13. Mallor, J. D. and Layne, D. S., J. Biol. Chem. 246, 4377 (1971).

14. Labow, R. S. and Layne, D. S., Biochem. J. 128, 491 (1972).

15. Mumford, R. A., Raghavan, S. S., and Kanfer, J. N., submitted
    for publication.

16. N. E. J. Med. Sept. 14, 1961, pg. 546.

17. Legler, G., H. S. Zeit. Physiol. Chem. <u>349,</u> 767 (1968).

18. Souami, E. D. and Agranoff, B. W., J. Lipid Res. <u>6</u>, 211 (1965).

STUDIES ON THE PATHOGENESIS OF KRABBE'S LEUKODYSTROPHY: CELLULAR
REACTION OF THE BRAIN TO EXOGENOUS GALACTOSYLSPHINGOSINE,
MONOGALACTOSYL DIGLYCERIDE, AND LACTOSYLCERAMIDE

Kinuko Suzuki, Harumi Tanaka and Kunihiko Suzuki

Department of Pathology (Neuropathology), The Saul S.
Korey Department of Neurology, Department of Neuroscience
and Rose F. Kennedy Center for Research in Mental
Retardation and Human Development, Albert Einstein
College of Medicine, Bronx, New York 10461

INTRODUCTION

Krabbe's leukodystrophy or globoid cell leukodystrophy (GLD)
is an autosomal recessive neurological disorder of infancy, affecting the central as well as peripheral nervous system. Tonic
seizures, generalized convulsions, spastic quadriplegia, optic
atrophy and deafness with rapid clinical progression are major
symptoms of the patient with GLD.

Neuropathologically, the lesion in the central nervous system
(CNS) is characterized by severe loss of oligodendroglia, myelin
and axons, dense fibrous astrocytic proliferation and prominent
presence of epithelioid and globoid cells in the white matter.
There is a concomittant loss of myelin which parallels the increased numbers of globoid cells when the disease process pro-
gresses (4). Isolated globoid cell rich fractions demonstrated
high cerebroside content (2) and injection of galactocerebroside
(galactosylceramide) in rat brain produced unique globoid cell
reaction (3,10). Ultrastructural morphology of such experimental
globoid cells are identical to that of GLD in man (12,1).

In 1970, deficiency of the enzyme, galactocerebroside
β-galactosidase (galactosylceramide β-galactosidase, galactosylceramidase) was discovered as a genetic defect in this disorder
(13). Subsequently, the tissue of patients with GLD was also
found to have deficient enzyme activity to cleave galactose from
three other lipids namely galactosylsphingosine (Psychosine) (8),
monogalactosyl diglyceride (17) and lactosylceramide (19) (Fig. 1).

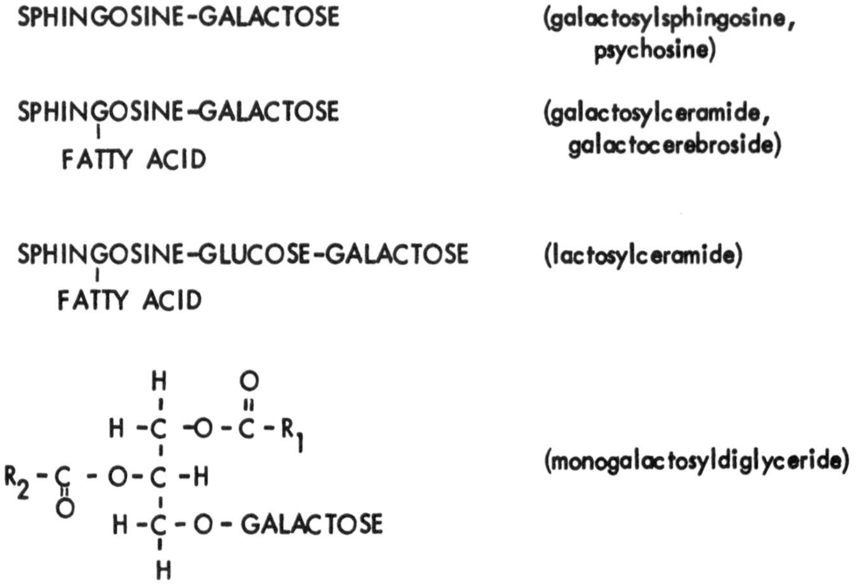

SPHINGOSINE-GALACTOSE   (galactosylsphingosine,
                                              psychosine)

SPHINGOSINE-GALACTOSE   (galactosylceramide,
      | galactocerebroside)
   FATTY ACID

SPHINGOSINE-GLUCOSE-GALACTOSE   (lactosylceramide)
      |
   FATTY ACID

$$
\begin{array}{c}
H \qquad O \\
| \qquad \;\; \| \\
H-C-O-C-R_1 \\
| \\
R_2-C-O-C-H \\
\| \qquad | \\
O \qquad H-C-O-GALACTOSE \\
| \\
H
\end{array}
$$
                                         (monogalactosyldiglyceride)

Fig. 1 Natural substrates of galactosylceramidase β-galactosidase.

Available data indicate that these enzymes are most likely
to be the same single enzyme, galactosylceramidase, acting on the
terminal galactose of these four natural substrates (7,8,9,15,17,
18,19).

Presence of excess galactocerebroside caused globoid cell
reaction in the brain of rats but did not produce other features
of GLD lesions (12,1). Therefore, the present investigation was
carried out to determine whether any of these other natural
substrates of galactosylceramidase may have a role in the histopathology of GLD.

MATERIALS AND METHODS

Source of commercial materials: Galactosylceramide from
bovine spinal cord and monogalactosyl diglyceride from plant
source were purchased from the Applied Science Laboratories
(State College, Pa.). Galactosylsphingosine was the product of
Supelco Inc. (Bellefonte, Pa.). Lactosylceramides (both stearoyl,
$C_{18:0}$, and lignoceroyl, $C_{24:0}$) were from Miles Laboratories, Inc.

(Elkhart, Ind.). Purity of these lipids was ascertained by thin-layer chromatography in appropriate solvent systems.

Wistar strain of rats were used for all the experiments. Intracerebral administration of the lipids were carried out in the right frontal cortex at 15 days of age.

Experiment I. Monogalactosyl diglyceride was given to experimental animals in two ways.
    A) 10mg of monogalactosyl diglyceride was suspended in 4 drops of 100% ethanol and 0.5cc of a 9% NaCl solution. 1/5 each of the solution was injected in the brain of test animals.
    Control rats received the same mixture without mono-galactosyl diglyceride.
    B) 10mg of monogalactosyl diglyceride was implanted as pellets in the test animals (approximately 1/5 each).

Experiment II. Lactosylceramide with long chain fatty acid ($C24:0$) and with short chain fatty acid ($C18:0$) was implanted in the test animals as a pellet.

Experiment III. Galactosylsphingosine (Psychosine) was given to experimental animals in two ways.

    A) Approximately 1mg each of psychosine was implanted in the brain in a pellet form.
    B) 10mg of psychosine was dissolved in physiologic saline and about 0.1 to 0.2mg each were injected into the brain of test animals.
    Controls received the injection of physiologic saline only.

Experiment IV. A mixture of galactocerebroside (galactosyl-ceramide) and psychosine (97:3v/v) was implanted in the experimental animals as a pellet.

The animals that received stab wounds in the cerebrum served as controls for Experiments 1B, II, IIIA, IV. All experimental and control animals were sacrificed by intracardiac perfusion of 2.5% glutaraldehyde in 0.1M phosphate buffer, pH 7.4 at 3,5, 8 and 15 days after injection. From each animal, coronal sections of the cerebrum through the sites of injection were submitted for light microscopic study. For electron microscopic study, small pieces of tissue were obtained around the site of injection. They were minced, post-fixed in Dalton's fixative and embedded in Epon 812 after a series of dehydration through graded ethanol. One micron thick sections of the tissue embedded in Epon were stained with toluidine blue and areas for electron microscopic study were selected. The thin sections were stained with lead citrate and uranyl acetate and examined with Siemens Elmiskop 101.

RESULTS

Light Microscopy

Light microscopic features of all the control animals including those that received a mixture of ethanol and physiologic
saline were essentially the same, consisting largely of collections
of lipid-laden macrophages with or without associated hemorrhage.
Degeneration of myelin, axons, neurons and glial cells were limited around the immediate vicinity of the site of injection.

The light microscopic features of animals that received
monogalactosyl diglyceride were essentially similar to those of
controls except for an occasional intracellular as well as
extracellular presence of homogenous osmiophilic material, pre-
sumabley monogalactosyl diglyceride (Fig. 2). Granulomatous
reaction was not present.

In the animals which received lactosylceramide, prominent
granulomatous lesions with formation of multinucleated giant cells
were observed at the site of injection (Fig. 3a,b). The reactive

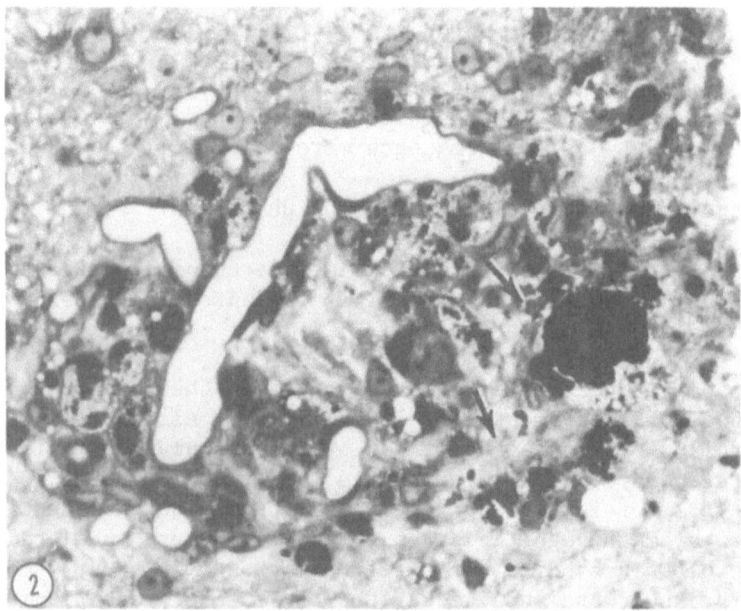

Fig. 2. Tissue reaction at the site of monogalactosyl diglyceride
injection. There are many lipid-laden macrophages around blood
vessels. Arrows indicate granular aggregates, presumably of
monogalactosyl diglyceride. X 640.

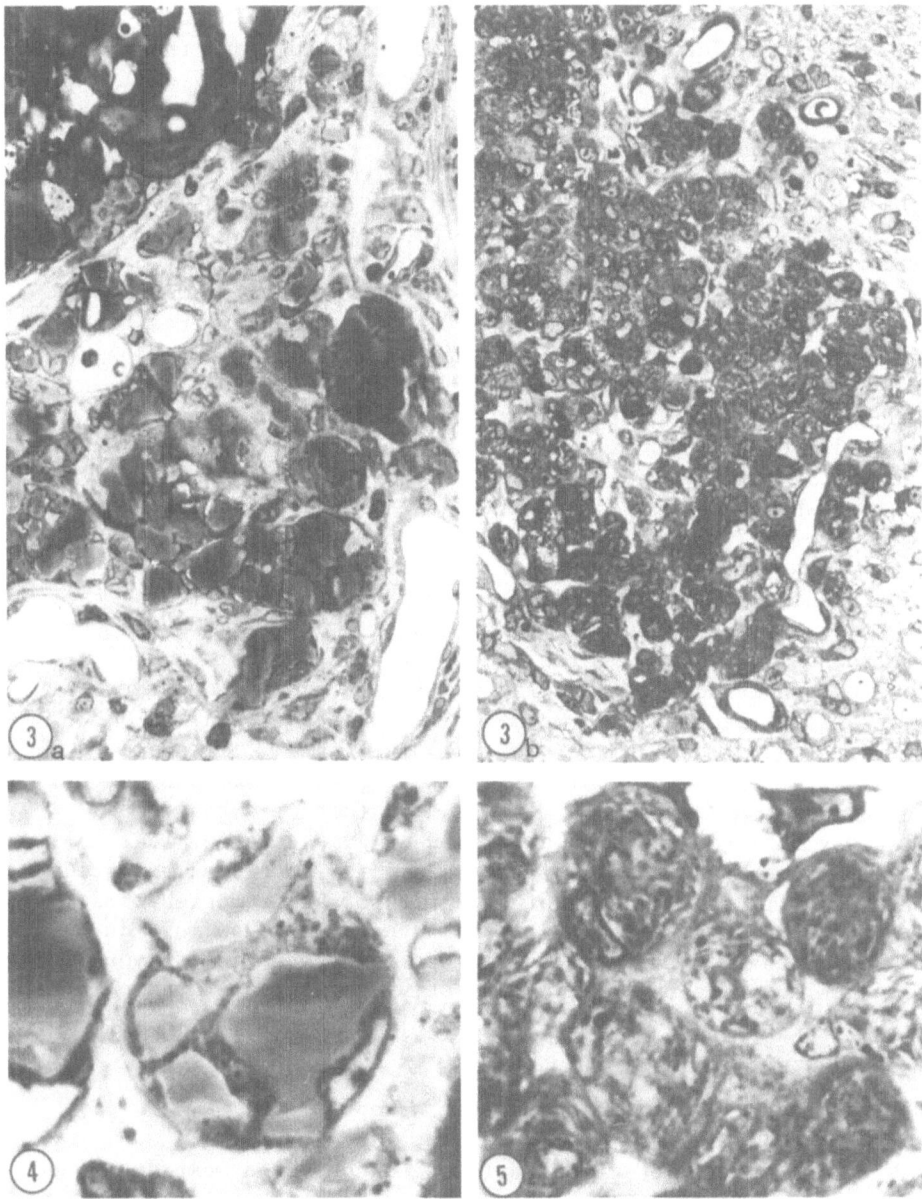

Fig. 3a. Granulomatous reaction following injection of lactosyl-
ceramide with $C_{18:0}$ fatty acid. X 400.
Fig. 3b. Granulomatous reaction following injection of lactosyl-
ceramide with $C_{24:0}$ fatty acid. X 400.
Fig. 4. Higher magnification of the macrophages seen in Fig. 3a.
X 1600.
Fig. 5. Higher magnification of the macrophages seen in Fig. 3b.
X 1600.

cells contained prominent intracytoplasmic inclusions. The
morphology of the inclusions differed considerably between those
found in lactosylceramide with a $C_{18:0}$ fatty acid and those with
a $C_{24:0}$ fatty acid. The former was homogeneously osmiophilic
and irregular in shape (Fig. 4). The latter was of more needle-
like crystalline appearance (Fig. 5).

Galactosylsphingosine was found to be very toxic in the
cerebral tissue. When pellets were implanted, the experimental
animals always developed acute subarachnoid, or intracerebral
hemorrhage at the site of implantation. When smaller amounts
(0.1 - 0.2mg) were injected with physiologic saline, focal areas of
acute edema and necrosis with or without associated hemorrhage
were observed around the site of injection. When galactosylsphingosine reached the white matter, diffuse prominent edema was
observed even apart from the site of injections (Fig. 6). Diffuse
degeneration of the ependymal and subependymal region were also
observed when galactosylsphingosine spread along the cerebrospinal
fluid pathways (Fig. 7).

In animals that survived more than two weeks following the
injection, diffuse or focal dilatation of ventricles were often
observed (Fig. 8). The white matter of these animals was edem-
atous with numerous degenerating myelin and axons. However, in
those animals sacrificed 4 weeks or more after the injection,
the white matter was thinner but well myelinated. In these
animals scattered dystrophic calcification was also observed.
The animals that received a mixture of galactocerebroside and
galactosylsphingosine revealed prominent granulomatous lesions
(Fig. 9) which were identical to those which have been reported
previously (12) at the site of injection of galactocerebroside
alone. Surrounding cerebral tissue appeared to show more degenerative changes than the lesions caused by the injections of
galactocerebroside only but quantitative estimates of the changes
were impossible.

Electron Microscopy

In the control animals, macrophages contained membrane-bound
moderately electron dense homogenous lipid droplets and granular
or lamellated dense bodies. Needle-like clear clefts were also
observed within some of them. The macrophages around the site of
implanted monogalactosyl diglyceride revealed, in addition, irregular shaped, packed or loose aggregates of electron dense
materials which were surrounded by single membrane (Fig. 10).
Upon higher magnification, they consisted of stacked alternate
electron dense and lucent lines of about 50 - 60Å in periodicity.

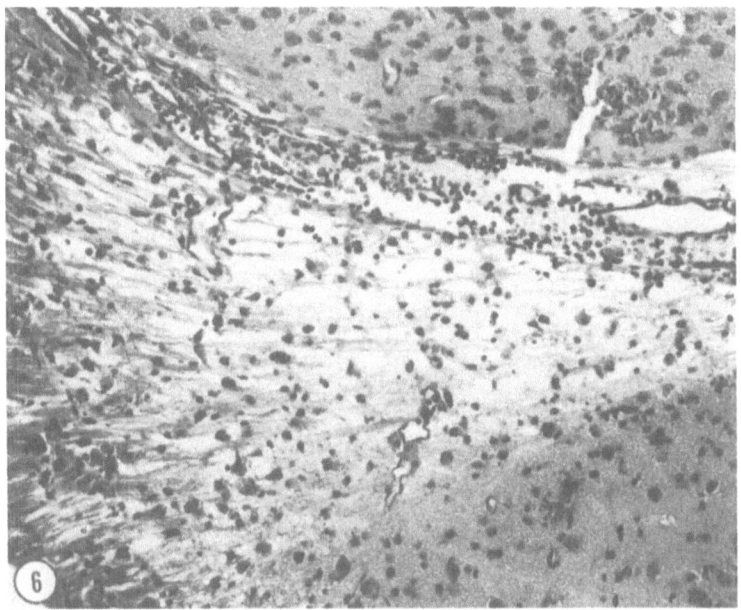

Fig. 6. Diffuse edema of cerebral white matter following injection of galactosylsphingosine. X 160.

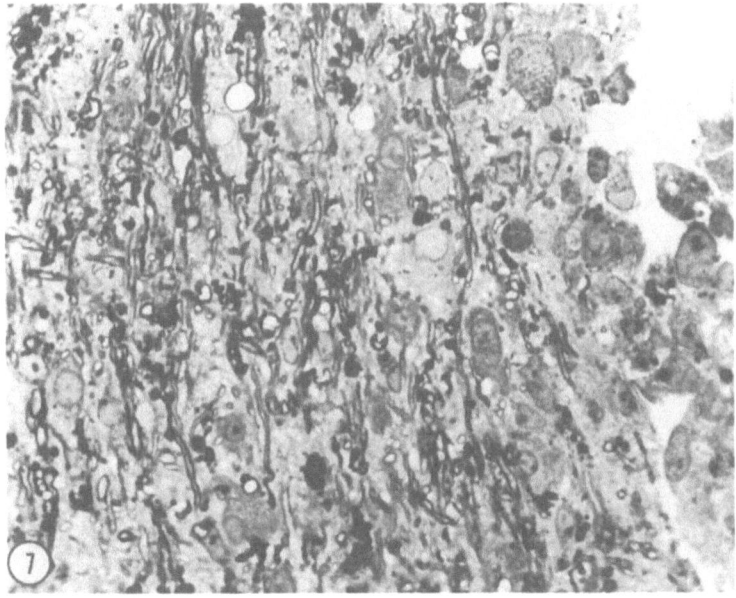

Fig. 7. Degeneration of white matter following injection of galactosylsphingosine. X 960.

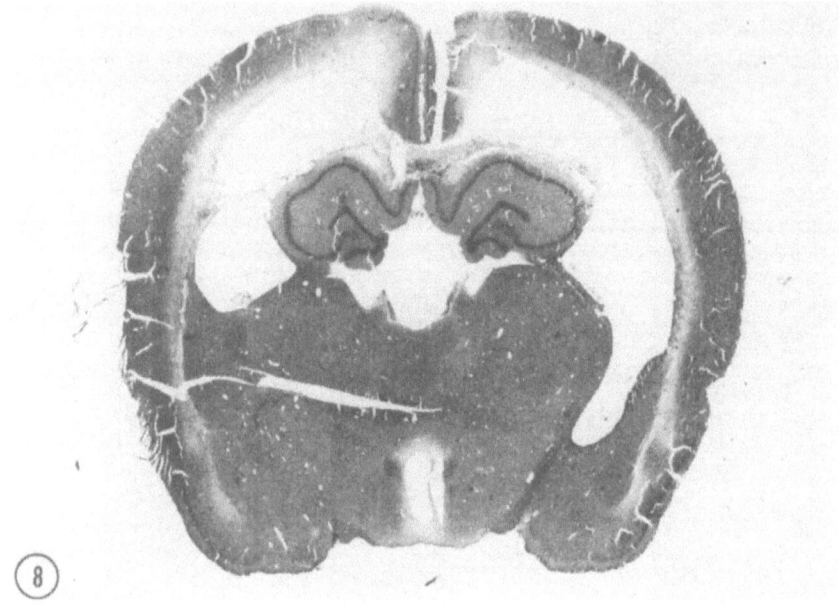

Fig. 8. Hydrocephalus ex vacuo caused by galactosylsphingosine
administration.

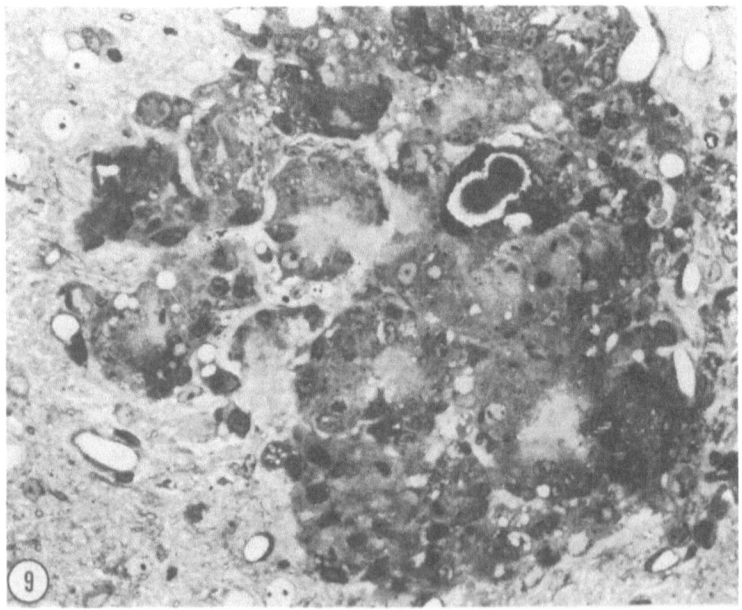

Fig. 9. Typical globoid cell reaction following galactocerebroside
administration. X 400.

Cytoplasmic inclusions in macrophages observed at or around the site of implanted lactosylceramide with the $C_{24:0}$ fatty acid were straight or stacked lamellae of alternate electron dense and lucent bands with a periodicity of 55 - 60Å (Fig. 11). They were randomly distributed within single membrane-bound electron lucent or densely granular areas within the cytoplasm of macrophages. Slender twisted tubules, which were morphologically indistinguishable from those seen in the macrophages following injection of galacto-cerebroside, were also observed, although far fewer in number, within the cytoplasm of the same macrophages (Fig. 12).

The cytoplasmic inclusions in the macrophages around the site of injection of lactosylceramide with the $C_{18:0}$ fatty acid revealed the inclusions to be moderately electron dense and homogenous in appearance. On higher magnification, however, they consisted of packed circular, semi-lunar or curved short lamellae (Fig. 13). The lamellae often consisted of three layers, namely one electron lucent zone in the center and two electron dense areas in each side but occasionally multilayered lamellae with alternate electron dense and lucent bands were observed. In some areas, however, straight or slightly curved stacked electron dense and lucent lamellae similar to those observed in lactosylceramide with $C_{24:0}$ fatty acide were observed (Fig. 14).

Following the injection of galactosylsphingosine alone, extensive degeneration of myelin and axons were produced and the macrophages that were present around the site of injection were identical to those observed in control animals without any specific inclusions.

When the mixture of galactocerebroside and galactosylsphingosine was given, granulomatous lesions composed of many macrophages, and giant cells were observed. The cytoplasmic inclusions in the macro-phages and giant cells were polygonal and crystalline in appearance on cross sections and appeared to be tubular on longitudinal sections (Fig. 15). They also were present within the single membrane-bound electron lucent spaces. These inclusions were identical to those found in the brains of animals that received galactocerebroside only. In addition, many cells - neurons, glia as well as endothelial cells - near these granulomatous lesions demonstrated completely different types of inclusions. They were spherical and often consisted of concentrically arranged lamellae (Fig. 16) but other more complicated inclusions composed of loosely packed irregular membranes were also found in some cells. Crystalline aggregates of calcium salts on the mitochondria within the degenerating axons were also a prominent feature within the vicinity of granulomatous lesions. The results of these experiments were summarized in Table 1.

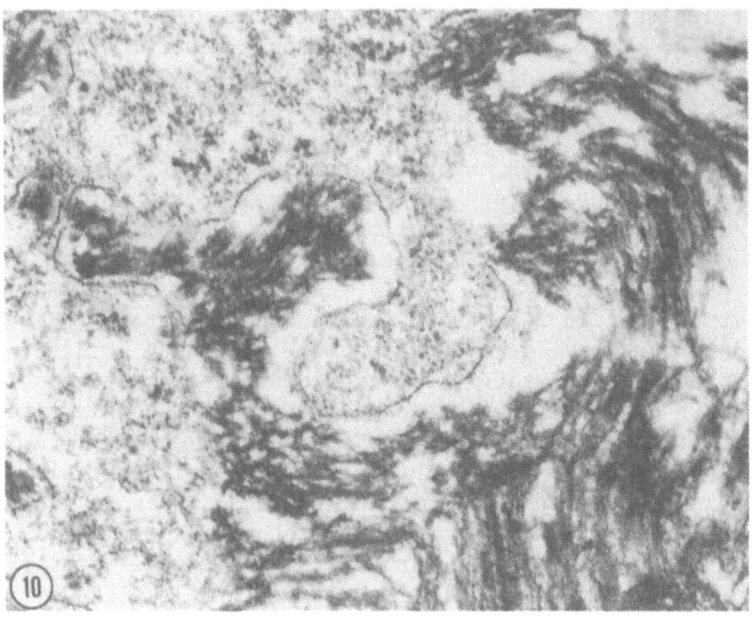

Fig. 10.   Electron micrograph of intracytoplasmic electron-dense
material, presumably monogalactosyl diglyceride in a macrophage.
X 60,000.

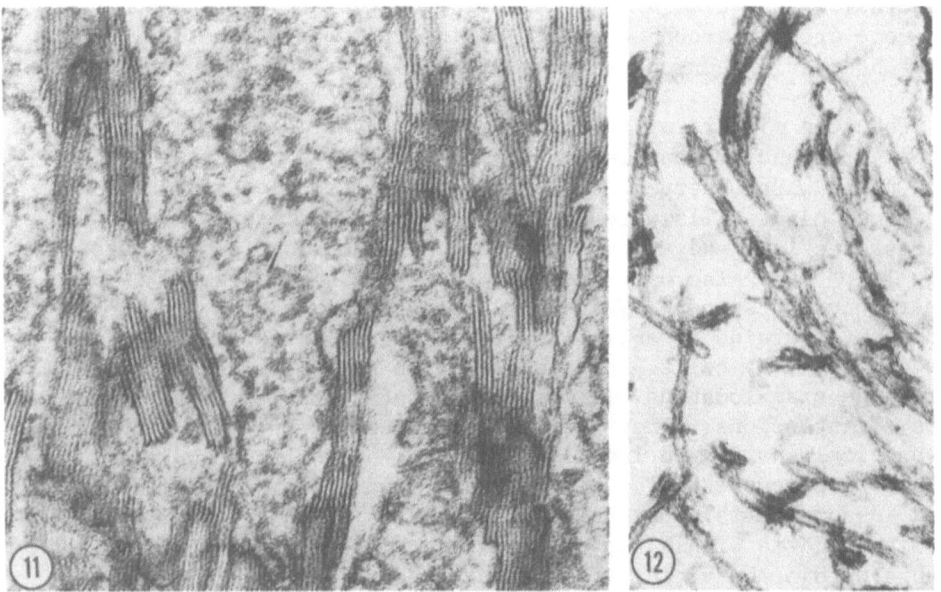

Fig. 11.   Inclusions seen within the macrophage following injection
of lactosylceramide with $C_{24:0}$ fatty acid. X 180,000.
Fig. 12.   Slender twisted tubules seen in lactosylceramide injection.
X 90,000.

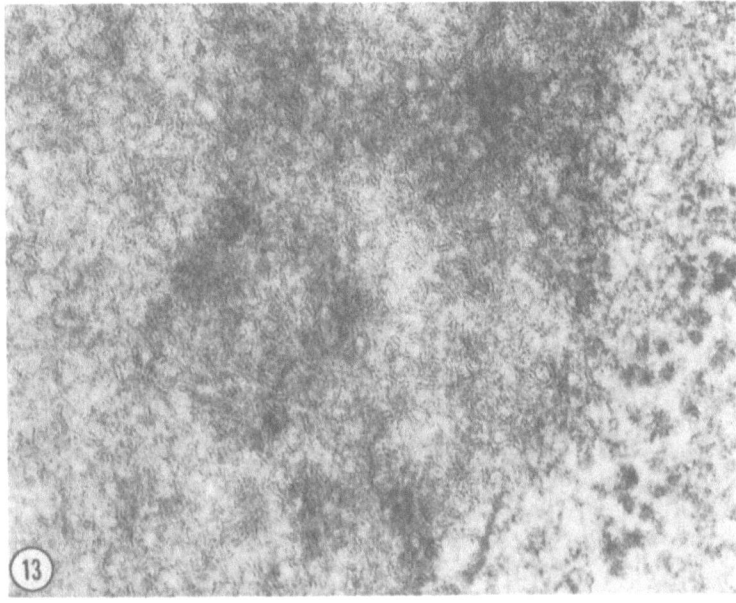

Fig. 13. Inclusion in macrophages following administration of lactosylceramide with $C_{18:0}$ fatty acid. X 120,000.

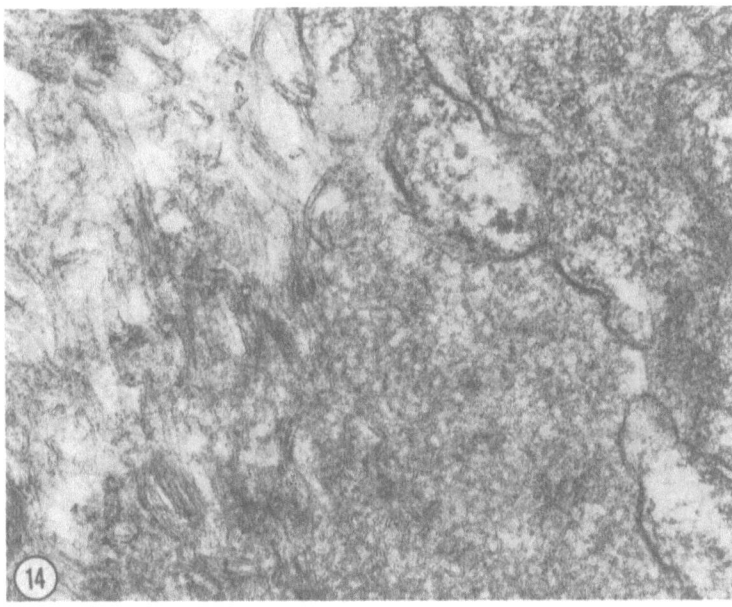

Fig. 14. Two types of different structures are seen within the same cytoplasmic inclusion, indicating possible transformation from one type to the other. X 80,000.

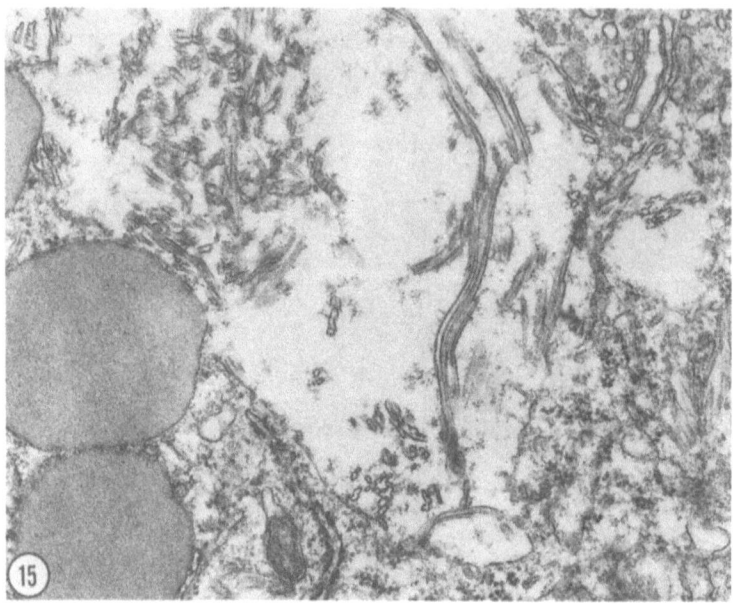

Fig. 15. Typical crystalline and tubular inclusions following injection of galactocerebroside. X 32,000.

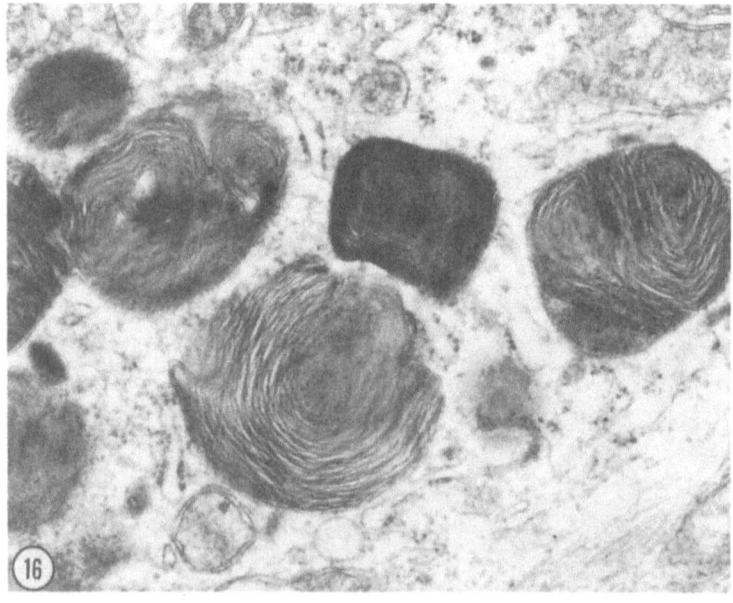

Fig. 16. Inclusions in an astrocyte following administration of a mixture of galactocerebroside-galactosylsphingosine. X 42,000.

TABLE I

	Granulomatous reaction	Tissue degeneration following administration	Nature of cytoplasmic inclusion in macrophages
galactosylceramide	+++ (globoid cell reaction)	±	1. polygonal crystalline inclusion 2. slender twisted tubules 3. straight flat forms
galactosylsphingosine	−	+++	no specific inclusions in macrophages
monogalactosyl diglyceride	±	+	loose aggregates of electron dense material
lactosylceramide			
C₁₈:₀	++	±	1. packed circular, semilunar or curved short lamellae 2. straight or slightly curved stacked lamellae
C₂₄:₀	++	±	1. straight or stacked lamellae 2. slender twisted tubules

DISCUSSION

From our results, it is clear that crystalline tubular inclusions, so characterisitic of globoid cells in GLD, were produced only by the presence of excessive galactocerebroside and not by any of the other three natural substrates of galactosyl- ceramidase, namely galactosylsphingosine, lactosylceramide and monogalactosyl diglyceride. However, the structures identical to the slender twisted tubules, first described by Yunis and Lee (20) in the biopsy specimen of the brain from a patient with GLD and later in experimentally produced globoid cells by injection of galactocerebroside (12) were observed in the macrophages following injection of lactosyl ceramide in the experimental animals. In the experimental condition the purity of both the galactocerebroside and lactosylceramide was tested with chromatograms prior to the experimental use. Therefore, it is very unlikely that these tubules were produced by contamination. Thus, we have to assume that morphologically identical inclusions were formed by two different compounds. The inclusions seen in the animals that received lactosylceramide with the long chain fatty acid are very closely similar to the "straight flat forms" described in GLD brain (21).

The inclusions found in the macrophages following injections of monogalactosyl diglyceride did not resemble any of the inclusions described in GLD and therefore it may not be too contributory to the production of the lesions in GLD.

Galactosylsphingosine, although structurally very similar to galactocerebroside, is found to be very toxic for the cerebral tissue. Diffuse cellular necrosis and hemorrhage as seen in the animal that received this compound only are very likely to be due to a non-specific toxic effect since there is no selective damage of any particular structure. Even when very minute amounts were given with galactocerebroside, the changes observed were not selective. Unlike complete tissue necrosis, when small amounts of psychosine were administered, many neurons, glia and endothelial cells in the adjacent tissue revealed accumulations of intracyto- plasmic inclusions. These inclusions were, interesting enough, identical to those found in neuro-glial and endothelial cells following administration of various drugs such as chloroquine, chlorphentermine, hypocholesterolemic drugs etc. (5,6,11,14) and therefore represent a rather non-specific reaction to the sub- lethal injury of cells.

In our preliminary in vitro study with CNS explant galactosyl- sphingosine also seems to affect all tissue elements. Galactosyl- sphingosine is present only in negligible amounts in normal brain but is increased at least 10 times in the brain of the patient with GLD (16). Therefore, it is still quite reasonable to postulate that this compound may have some role in degeneration of white matter although so far the results of our study are not conclusive.

ACKNOWLEDGEMENTS

This investigation was supported by the grants NS-03356, NS-10803, NS-10885 and HD-01799 from the National Institutes of Health, United States Public Health Service.

REFERENCES

1.   Andrews, J.M. and Menkes, J.H.: Ultrastructure of experimentally produced globoid cells in the rat. Exper. Neurol. 29:483, 1970.

2.   Austin, J.H.: Studies in globoid (Krabbe) leukodystrophy. II. Controlled thin-layer chromatographic studies of globoid body fraction in seven patients. J. Neurochem. 10:921, 1963.

3.   Austin, J.H. and Lehfeldt, D.: Studies in globoid (Krabbe) leukodystrophy. III. Significance of experimentally-produced globoid-like elements in rat white matter and spleen. J. Neuropathol. Exp. Neurol. 24:265, 1965.

4.   D'Agostino, A.N., Sayre, G.P. and Hagles, A.B.: Krabbe's Disease. Arch. Neurol. (Chicago) 8:82, 1963.

5.   Gleisen, C.A., Bay, W.W., Dukes, T.W., Brown, R.S., Read, W.K. and Pierce, K.K.: Study of chloroquine toxicity and drug-induced cerebrospinal lipodystrophy in swine, Amer. J. Path. 53:27, 1968.

6.   Lüllmann-Rauch, R.: Lipidosis-like alterations in spinal cord and cerebellar cortex of rats treated with chlorphentermine or tricyclic antidepressants. Acta Neuropath. 29:237, 1974.

7.   Miyatake, T. and Suzuki, K.: Galactosyl sphingosine galactosyl hydrolase: Partial purification and properties of the enzyme in rat brain. J. Biol. Chem. 247:5398, 1972.

8.   Miyatake, T. and Suzuki, K.: Globoid cell leukodystrophy: Additional deficiency of psychosine galactosidase. Biochem. Biophys. Res. Commun. 48:538, 1972.

9.   Miyatake, T. and Suzuki, K.: Galactosyl sphingosine galactosyl hydrolase in rat brain: Probable identity with galactosylceramide galactosyl hydrolase. J. Neurochem. 22:231, 1974.

10. Olsson, R., Sourander, P. and Svennerholm, L.: Experimental
studies on the pathogenesis of leucodystrophies. I. The effect of
intracerebrally injected sphingolipids in the rat's brain. Acta
Neuropath. 6:153, 1966.

11. Schutta, H.S. and Neville, H.E.: Effects of cholesterol
biosynthesis inhibitors on the nervous system. Lab. Invest.
19:487, 1968.

12. Suzuki, K.: Ultrastructural study of experimental globoid
cells. Lab. Invest. 23:612, 1970.

13. Suzuki, K. and Suzuki, Y.: Globoid cell leucodystrophy
(Krabbe's disease); deficiency of galactocerebroside β-galactosidase. Proc. Nat. Acad. Sci. U.S.A. 66:302, 1970.

14. Suzuki, K., Zagoren, J.C., Gonatas, J., and Suzuki, K.:
Ultrastructural study of neuronal cytoplasmic inclusions produced
by hypocholesterolemic drug AY 9944. Acta Neuropath. (Berl.)
26:185, 1973.

15. Tanaka, H. and Suzuki, K.: Lactosylceramide β-galactosidase
in human sphingolipidoses: Evidence for two genetically distinct
enzymes. J. Biol. Chem. 250:2324, 1975.

16. Vanier, M.T. and Svennerholm, L.: Chemical pathology of
Krabbe's Disease. III. Ceramide-hexosides and gangliosides of
brain. Acta Paediatr. Scand. 64:641, 1975.

17. Wenger, D.A., Sattler, M. and Markey, S.P.: Deficiency of
monogalactosyl diglyceride β-galactosidase activity in Krabbe's
disease. Biochem. Biophys. Res. Commun. 53:680, 1973.

18. Wenger, D.A.: Studies on galactosylceramide and lactosylceramide β-galactosidase. Chem. Phys. Lipids 13:327, 1974.

19. Wenger, D.A., Sattler, M. and Hiatt, W.: Globoid cell leukodystrophy: Deficiency of lactosyl ceramide beta-galactosidase.
Proc. Nat. Acad. Sci. 71:854, 1974.

20. Yunis, E.J. and Lee, R.E.: The ultrastructure of globoid
(Krabbe) leukodystrophy. Lab. Invest. 21:415, 1969.

21. Yunis, E. and Lee, R.E.: Further observations on the fine
structure of globoid leukodystrophy. Human Pathology 3:371, 1972.

CHEMICAL PATHOLOGY OF KRABBE DISEASE : THE OCCURRENCE OF PSYCHOSINE AND OTHER NEUTRAL SPHINGOGLYCOLIPIDS

Marie-Thérèse Vanier[¶] and Lars Svennerholm

Department of Neurochemistry, Psychiatric Research Centre
University of Göteborg, Göteborg, Sweden

In 1916, the Danish neurologist, Knud Krabbe (9), delineated a new type of infantile familial diffuse brain sclerosis and gave the first description of the characteristic giant cells, which are the histological hallmark of the disease. During the 60s, cumulative analytical and experimental findings resulted in the concept of Krabbe disease as galactosylceramidosis, a concept corroborated by the demonstration of a generalized deficiency of galactosylceramide β-galactosidase (21). But further investigations disclosed also additional enzymic deficiencies, involving the degradation of galactosylsphingosine (13), monogalactosyl diglyceride (37) and lactosylceramide (38), all substrates with a terminal β-galactosidic linkage. Though this does not imply the assumption of a multiple enzyme deficiency, since a single enzyme seems to catalyze the hydrolysis of galactosylceramide and of the three other substrates (12, 14, 32, 37), it does open up new approaches in our search for a better comprehension of the pathophysiology of Krabbe disease. The impaired degradation of galactosylceramide appears to be directly involved in the formation of the globoid cells (1, 15, 20), but it cannot by itself explain other characteristics of the disease, such as the lack of demonstrable accumulation of galactosylceramide in extra-neural organs or in brain outside the globoid cells.

Therefore, the finding of a broad specificity of the galactosyl-ceramide β-galactosidase, suggesting other causal mechanisms, roused renewed interest in detailed investigation of the sphingolipids and

---

[¶]Present address : Fondation Gillet, Hôpital Sainte-Eugénie,
69230-Saint Genis Laval, France

related compounds, particularly those involved in the enzymic defect, in tissues of patients who died from the disease.

The gangliosides and/or neutral sphingolipids have been studied in several previous investigations of Krabbe brains (2, 6, 7, 11, 16, 26, 29, 35), but only preliminary results have been reported on the levels of galactosylsphingosine in brains from patients who had died from Krabbe disease and from normal infants. Accumulation of glucosyl-sphingosine in spleens of patients with another form of sphingolipi-dosis, Gaucher disease, has recently been reported (17, 18). These are, to our knowledge, the only studies in which psychosine has, to date, been isolated from mammalian tissues.

MATERIAL AND METHODS

Brain Material

The material consisted of autopsy specimens of the brains from 16 subjects who had died from Krabbe disease at 7 to 32 months of age. The diagnosis was verified by histological examination and measurement of the cerebroside β-galactosidase activity. Data on the patients and their brain lipid composition have been reported previously (34).

For isolation of sphingolipids, the cerebral cortex and cere-bral white matter were carefully dissected and analysed separately. Three preparations were made with tissue specimens from 6-10 different brains in each batch, the size of which varied between 55 and 340 g. Whole cerebellar tissue (45 g) from 6 patients was also studied. Two of the preparations of cerebral white matter and that of cerebellum were investigated regarding their level of galactosylsphingosine (psychosine), and a parallel study was made on cerebral white matter (75-100 g) from three 2 to 4-month-old control infants. The sphingolipid composition of normal infant brain has been reported earlier from this laboratory (33).

Chemicals

The following material was obtained from commercial sources : silicic acid, < 100 mesh, Mallinckrodt A.R.; silica gel H and G, Fluka A.G., Buchs, Switzerland; DEAE-cellulose, Balston Ltd, England; Sephadex G-25, Pharmacia, Uppsala, Sweden. The organic solvents were of analytical grade and freshly distilled before use. The other chemicals were of analytical reagent quality.

Psychosine (galactosylsphingosine) and [^{3}H]- galactosylsphin-gosine were prepared by alkaline treatment (31) of galactosylcera-mide and [^{3}H]-galactosylceramide from human brain cerebrosides.

Isolation of Sphingolipids

The lipids were extracted according to the method elaborated for isolation of sphingolipids from normal infant brain (33). The total lipid extract was subjected to solvent partition, and the lower phase saponified overnight at room temperature with 10-20 ml of 0.5 M KOH in methanol-water (1:1, v/v). After neutralisation with 2 M HCl, salt was removed by chromatography on Sephadex G-25 (36) and the lipids were fractionated by column chromatography. Sulfatides were retained on a DEAE- or TEAE-cellulose column (28) and neutral glycolipids separated on a silicic acid column, developed with 10 vol. of chloroform, and afterwards with the same volume of chloroform-methanol mixtures (C-M) of increasing polarity, C-M (9:1), (4:1), (2:1), and (1:1) (all by vol.). The lipids were finally purified by preparative thin-layer chromatography (TLC) on silica gel G plates (23).

Isolation of Psychosine

The total lipid extract, dissolved in chloroform, was directly applied to a silica gel H column prepared in chloroform and developed successively with 10 vol. chloroform, 5 vol. C-M (19:1, v/v), 10 vol. C-M (4:1, v/v), 5 vol. C-M (2:1, v/v), 5 vol. C-M (2:1, v/v) and 10 vol. C-M (1:1, v/v), collected batchwise. The eluate from the first 5 vol. of C-M (2:1), which contained the psychosine, was applied to a silica gel H column prepared in C-M (9:1, v/v) and developed with 10 vol. of C-M-water (65:25:4, by vol.), using a fraction collector. After TLC-monitoring, suitable fractions were pooled, and subjected to mild alkaline hydrolysis, as described above. From normal brain, large aliquots were then tested by TLC together with authentic galactosylsphingosine as reference, in the solvent systems given below. Because of large amounts of globotriose and globotetraose, column chromatography on silicic acid had to be repeated on brain preparations from patients who had died from Krabbe disease before final purification by preparative TLC.

Identification and Quantitative Determination
of the Sphingolipid Fractions

Glycolipids were tested for purity by TLC on silica gel G plates together with authentic reference compounds in C-M-water (65:25:4, by vol.) and/or C-M-water (60:32:7, by vol.), and on borate-impregnated plates for glucosylceramide (39). The behaviour at TLC of psychosine was also tested in the following solvent mixtures : C-M-3 M ammonia (60:35:8, by vol.), C-M-0.1 M HCl (65:25:4, by vol.), C-M-water-glacial acetic acid (65:25:3:2, by vol.), and on borate-impregnated plates.

The carbohydrate structure was assayed by gas-liquid-chromato-graphy (GLC) of the alditol acetates (19), by sequential hydrolysis with specific hydrolases and by permethylation (M.T.Vanier, J.E. Månsson & L.Svennerholm, in preparation). Lipid hexose was measured with the orcinol method (24) and at the GLC procedure. The fatty acid and sphingosine compositions were analysed by GLC as previously described (27, 33).

RESULTS AND DISCUSSION

Neutral Glycosylceramides

The concentrations of the neutral glycosylceramides in normal infant brain and in brain tissue of patients who had died in Krabbe disease are given in Table 1. In normal controls, the largely dominating fraction was galactosylceramide, but also substantial amounts of lactosylceramide and glucosylceramide were found. Only traces of higher neutral glycosylceramides were observed.

The results obtained in Krabbe disease deviated in several respects from this pattern. The concentration of galactosylceramide was close to normal in cerebral cortex, but strikingly reduced in cerebral white matter. Values between 10 to 15% of normal had also previously been found at the analysis of the individual cases (34), and ever since first observed by Brante (3) the very low concentra-tion of cerebrosides has been a constant finding in all investiga-tions on Krabbe disease carried out with adequate methods. Glucosyl-and lactosylceramide showed common trends : a slight increase in cerebral cortex, and an approximately 50% decrease in the cerebral white matter, where they normally constitute much larger fractions than in cortex. Another dihexosylceramide fraction migrating slight-ly slower than lactosylceramide was also isolated from cerebral white matter and cerebellum, in which it constituted 13 and 10 nmol/g, respectively. It contained exclusively hydroxy fatty acids. Alditol acetate analysis and sequential hydrolysis by specific hydrolases revealed the uncommon structure of a digalactosylceramide with a β-linkage of the terminal galactose. Since we always found a glucose : galactose quotient slightly lower than 1.0 for lactosyl-ceramide, this fraction may have contained small amounts of digalactosylceramide with normal fatty acids.

In Krabbe disease, large amounts of several higher hexosyl-ceramides were found. After structural analysis, they were identified as globotriose, Gal α (1→4)Gal β (1→4)Glc-Cer, and globotetraose, GalNAc β (1→3)Gal α (1→4)Gal β (1→4)Glc-Cer. Another complex fraction, migrating at TLC as gangliotetraose G_{A1}, was shown to contain predominantly H-antigen, Fuc-Gal-GlcNAc-Gal-Glc-Cer. This fraction had probably been regarded as G_{A1} in previous studies (6, 29).

TABLE 1. CONCENTRATIONS OF THE NEUTRAL GLYCOSYLCERAMIDES OF BRAIN TISSUE IN KRABBE DISEASE

Values reported for Krabbe disease are means of results obtained in two different preparations of cerebral cortex and in three preparations of cerebral white matter

c.c. = cerebral cortex ; wh.m. = cerebral white matter

| | CONTROLS 2-27 months | | KRABBE DISEASE 7-32 months | | |
| | Cerebrum | | Cerebrum | | Cerebellum |
	c.c.	wh.m.	c.c.	wh.m.	total
	(nanomoles/g fresh tissue weight)				
Galactosylceramide	975	21400	715	3350	3700
Glucosylceramide	5	110	17	62	
Lactosylceramide	30	273	44	140	195
Globotriose	<1	<1	14	45	18
Globotetraose	1	1	14	76	
H-antigen	<1	<1	8	19	28

The ceramide portion was analysed, and the fatty acid compositions are reported in Table 2. A characteristic feature of galactosylceramide was the very high ratio of 24:0/24:1, previously reported by Svennerholm (25) and also found by others (6, 11). In all other glycolipids, the content of 24:0 was much lower. Stearic acid was the dominating fatty acid and constituted 40 to 50% of the total fatty acids except in glucosylceramide and lactosylceramide of white matter. In these two lipids the content of 18:0 was lower, and that of all fatty acids above C_{24} higher, than in the other glycolipids. Globotriose, globotetraose and H-antigen showed very similar patterns.

Globotriose, globotetraose and a glycolipid, which was most probably H-antigen, were also found in brain tissue in Tay-Sachs disease (29) and are thus not specific to Krabbe disease. Eto & Suzuki (6) were the first to suggest that these fractions were components of the globoid cells. One may generalize and say that they are witnesses of an invasion of brain tissue by cells of mesenchymal origin.

A close relationship between the glucosyl- and lactosylceramide of normal cerebral cortex and the gangliosides has been suggested (25, 26), while these lipids of white matter had fatty acid patterns indicating that they were formed in the same metabolic compartment

TABLE 2. FATTY ACID COMPOSITION OF NEUTRAL GLYCOSYLCERAMIDES OF CEREBRUM IN KRABBE DISEASE

Mean values of results obtained with two different preparations, expressed in molar percentage. Fatty acids 16:1, 22:1 and 23:1 were also detected but constituted less than 1%   c.c. = cerebral cortex; w.m. = white matter

		FATTY ACID							
		16:0	18:0	20:0	22:0	23:0	24:0	24:1	>24 C
Galactosylceramide	w.m.	1	11	2	6	6	42	19	13
Glucosylceramide	c.c.	7	40	4	8	10	17	11	3
	w.m.	6	24	3	10	13	23	17	3
Lactosylceramide	c.c.	10	52	3	5	4	9	11	5
	w.m.	8	27	3	7	8	18	22	5
Globotriose	c.c.	7	51	3	8	4	8	17	1
	w.m.	6	55	3	6	4	6	19	1
Globotetraose	c.c.	6	40	3	9	4	10	24	1
	w.m.	4	50	3	6	4	6	25	1
H-antigen	w.m.	3	51	3	6	4	6	26	1

as galactosylceramide, and that they were localized in the myelin
(33). Further evidence in support of the latter hypothesis is the
rapid increase in the concentration of lactosylceramide in infant
cerebral white matter during the early phase of myelination (L.
Svennerholm & M.T.Vanier, unpublished data). The ceramide composition of these glycolipids in brains from infants died in Krabbe
disease also disclosed similarities with the ceramide pattern of
globotriose and globotetraose, similarities suggesting that glucosyl-
and lactosylceramide had a partially non-neural origin. But the most
striking feature - and perhaps the most relevant for the understanding of the disease - was the low level of these lipids, particularly
lactosylceramide, in the cerebral white matter of patients who had
died from Krabbe disease. Concentrations of lactosylceramide similar
to those found in this study have previously been reported by Eto
& Suzuki (6) and Svennerholm & Vanier (29) but the lack of normal
values for lactosylceramide at that time led to the erroneous
conclusion of an increase of this lipid in white matter of Krabbe
disease. A decrease of lactosylceramide - as that of galactosylceramide - is more in line with the extensive demyelination, but
fits in badly with a galactosyl- and lactosylceramide β-galactosidase
deficiency.

Psychosine

In the elaboration of the procedure, endeavours were made to
avoid two of the most obvious pitfalls : the solvent partition step,
which incurs the risk of a loss of psychosine in the upper phase,
and the possible hydrolysis of cerebrosides to psychosine during
the alkaline hydrolysis of the phosphoglycerides. Mild alkaline
treatment should not release the fatty acid moiety of a cerebroside.
However, hydrolysis of 0.01 to 0.1% of the cerebrosides would be
enough to lead to the formation of more psychosine than the
naturally existing amount of this substance.

In order to optimize the isolation procedure, the chromatographic behaviour of [^{3}H]-labelled galactosylsphingosine (psychosine)
was carefully studied. It was not retained by DEAE-cellulose. At
silicic acid chromatography with C-M mixtures, [^{3}H]-psychosine
added to a total lipid extract was not eluted in the C-M (4:1)
eluate, but 90% of the [^{3}H]-psychosine was recovered in the C-M
(2:1) eluate. On silica gel columns developed with C-M-water
(65:25:4), psychosine was eluted after 5 to 8 column volumes of
solvent. At TLC on silica gel G plates, psychosine migrated slightly
ahead of globotetraose in neutral solvents, like globotriose in
acetic acid-containing solvents, and like lactosylceramide in
ammonia-containing solvents.

In preparations of brain tissue from patients who had died

from Krabbe disease, a substance with chromatographic properties
identical to those of galactosylsphingosine reference, was eluted
from the silicic acid column between globotriose and globotetraose,
with some overlapping. It was purified by repeated preparative TLC
using alternatively ammonia-containing and neutral solvents. Its
carbohydrate : sphingosine ratio was found to be I:I, with galactose
as the only sugar. The sphingosine composition was similar to that
of galactosylceramide, with 94% of $d18{:}I$ sphingosine and no detectable $d20{:}I$ sphingosine. Its concentration was I0 nmol/g in cerebral
white matter and 7 nmol/g in whole cerebellar tissue.

In preparations of normal infant brain run in parallel, faint
amounts of a substance with similar chromatographic behaviour were
obtained. By visual examination of TLC plates to which known amounts
of authentic galactosylsphingosine had been applied, it was
estimated to constitute at most 0.I nmol/g fresh tissue weight. No
further characterization was possible because of shortness of
material; however, our data support the idea that normal brain tissue
contains very small amounts of psychosine, at least during the period
of rapid myelination. A comparison of the findings in normal and
pathological tissues warranted the conclusion that the galactosylsphingosine concentration in brains of patients who have died from
Krabbe disease is approximately I00-fold normal.

Psychosine is a theoretical intermediate in the metabolism of
cerebrosides. However, all attempts to demonstrate an enzymic
degradation of cerebrosides to psychosine have failed (I0), and it
has not yet been unequivocally established whether or not psychosine
can act as a precursor for the formation of galactosylceramide. On
the other hand, *in vitro*, a galactosyltransferase catalyzing the
formation of psychosine from sphingosine and UDP-Gal has been
demonstrated (4, 5, 8), and a galactosylsphingosine β-galactosidase
has been purified (I2, I4). Both enzymic systems are most active
during the rapid phase of myelination (5, 8, I4). It has been
suggested that the same galactosyltransferase might catalyze the
galactosylation of ceramide and of sphingosine (8), and it has
now been reasonably well established that a single enzyme degrades
both galactosylceramide and galactosylsphingosine (I4). The
isolation of only trace amounts of psychosine from normal infant
brain and a I00-fold increase of psychosine in brain tissue in
Krabbe disease suggests that the degradation of galactosylsphingosine to galactose and sphingosine has a considerable
physiological significance.

But, especially, the finding of a psychosine accumulation in
brain from patients who have died from Krabbe disease raises the
question of its possible role in the pathogenesis of the condition.
Psychosine, with its free amino group, has been shown to be cyto-

toxic (30). Intracerebral injection into rats proved rapidly fatal, and its addition to cultured rat cerebellar explants led to degeneration of the cells (13). Its implication may cast new light on the comprehension of this paradoxal storage disease in which the net amount of the "accumulated" compound - galactosylceramide- is severely decreased in the target organ. This decrease has been attributed by Suzuki and coworkers (21, 22) to an early cessation of myelination as a consequence of the rapid and almost complete disappearance of the oligodendroglial cells, which is one of the striking morphological features of the disease. Our finding that lactosylceramide of cerebral white matter is diminished in spite of its impaired degradation, lends further support to this hypothesis. Of all compounds involved in the primary enzyme defect, psychosine is indeed the first substance that has been demonstrated to occur in strikingly increased concentration in Krabbe disease. Since there is experimental evidence that it is injurious to cells even in low concentrations, it might cause the death of oligodendroglial cells, as first suggested by Miyatake & Suzuki (13). The following hypothesis can be formulated : during the rapid phase of myelination, galactosylceramide, as well as allied glycolipids with a terminal β-linkage, monogalactosyldiglyceride, lactosylceramide, digalactosylceramide and psychosine, are formed. For obvious reasons, psychosine cannot be inserted in the plasma membrane, and is normally rapidly degraded. In Krabbe disease, however, the concentration of psychosine in the oligodendroglial cell gradually increases owing to the enzymic defect. Psychosine reaches a locally toxic level, which leads to the death of the oligodendroglial cell and an arrest of myelination. Thus, an accumulation of psychosine may be the primary lesion in Krabbe disease.

ACKNOWLEDGEMENTS

We thank Dr. Jan-Eric Månsson for the determination of the carbohydrate structure and for valuable advice at the determination of the ceramide composition, and Mrs. Birgitta Dellheden for skilful technical assistance. This investigation was supported by research grants from the Swedish Medical Research Council (project no. 3X-627).

REFERENCES

1. AUSTIN, J.H. & LEHFELDT, D.- Studies in globoid (Krabbe) leukodystrophy. III. Significance of experimentally produced globoid-like elements in rat white matter and spleen. *J.Neuropath.Exp. Neurol.*, 24: 265 (1965).

2. BERRA, B. & ZAMBOTTI, V.- Patterns of brain ganglioside fatty

acids in sphingolipidoses. *Adv.Exp.Med.Biol.*, 25: 311 (1972)

3. BRANTE, G.- Studies on lipids in the nervous system with special
    reference to quantitative chemical determination and topical
    distribution. *Acta Physiol.Scand.*, 18: Suppl. 63, 1-189 (1949).

4. CLELAND, W.W. & KENNEDY, E.P.- The enzymatic synthesis of psy-
    chosine. *J.Biol.Chem.*, 235: 45 (1960).

5. COSTANTINO-CECCARINI, E. & MORELL, P.- Biosynthesis of brain
    sphingolipids and myelin accumulation in the mouse. *Lipids*, 7:
    656 (1972).

6. ETO, Y. & SUZUKI, K.- Brain sphingoglycolipids in Krabbe's
    globoid cell leukodystrophy. *J.Neurochem.*, 18: 503 (1971).

7. EVANS, J.E. & Mc CLUER, R.H.- The structure of brain dihexosyl-
    ceramide in globoid cell leukodystrophy. *J.Neurochem.*, 16: 1393,
    (1969).

8. HILDEBRAND, J., STOFFYN, P. & HAUSER, G.- Biosynthesis of
    lactosylceramide by rat brain preparations and comparison with
    the formation of ganglioside G_{M1} and psychosine during develop-
    mant. *J.Neurochem.*, 17: 403 (1970).

9. KRABBE, K.- A new familial, infantile form of diffuse brain-
    sclerosis. *Brain*, 39: 74 (1916).

10. LIN, Y.N. & RADIN, N.S.- Alternate pathways of cerebroside
    catabolism. *Lipids*, 8: 732 (1973).

11. MENKES, J.H., DUNCAN, C. & MOOSY, J.- Molecular composition of
    the major glycolipids in globoid cell leukodystrophy. *Neurology*,
    16: 581 (1966).

12. MIYATAKE, T. & SUZUKI, K.- Galactosylsphingosine galactosyl
    hydrolase. *J.Biol.Chem.*, 247: 5398 (1972).

13. MIYATAKE, T. & SUZUKI, K.- Globoid cell leukodystrophy: addi-
    tional deficiency of psychosine galactosidase. *Biochem.Biophys.
    Res.Commun.*, 48: 538 (1972).

14. MIYATAKE, T. & SUZUKI, K.- Galactosylsphingosine galactosyl
    hydrolase in rat brain: probable identity with galactosyl-
    ceramide galactosyl hydrolase. *J.Neurochem.*, 22: 231 (1974).

15. OLSSON, Y., SOURANDER, P. & SVENNERHOLM, L.- Experimental studies
    on the pathogenesis of leukodystrophies.I. the effect of intra-
    cerebrally injected sphingolipids in the rat's brain. *Acta
    Neuropath.* , 6: 153 (1966).

16. PHILIPPART, M.- Glycolipid, mucopolysaccharide and carbohydrate distribution in tissues, plasma and urine from glycolipidoses and other disorders. *Adv.Exp.Med.Biol.*, 25: 231 (1972).

17. RAGHAVAN, S.S., MUMFORD, R.A. & KANFER, J.N.- Deficiency of glucosylsphingosine β-glucosidase in Gaucher disease. *Biochem. Biophys.Res.Commun.*, 54: 256 (1973).

18. RAGHAVAN, S.S., MUMFORD, R.A. & KANFER, J.N.- Isolation and characterization of glucosylsphingosine from Gaucher's spleen. *J.Lipid Res.*, 15: 484 (1974).

19. SAWARDEKER, J.S., SLONEKER, J.K. & JEANES, A.- Quantitative determination of monosaccharides as their alditol acetates by gas-liquid chromatography. *Anal.Chem.*, 37: 1602 (1965).

20. SOURANDER, P., HANSSON, H.A., OLSSON, Y. & SVENNERHOLM, L.- Experimental studies on the pathogenesis of leukodystrophies. II. The effect of sphingolipids on various cell types in culture from the nervous system. *Acta Neuropath.*, 9: 231 (1966).

21. SUZUKI, K. & SUZUKI, Y.- Globoid cell leukodystrophy (Krabbe's disease). Deficiency of galactocerebroside β-galactosidase. *Proc.Nat.Acad.Sci.USA*, 66: 302 (1970).

22. SUZUKI, K. & SUZUKI, Y.- Galactosylceramide lipidosis: globoid cell leukodystrophy (Krabbe's disease). In *The Metabolic Basis of Inherited Disease*, J.B.Stanbury, J.B.Wyngaarden & D.S. Fredrickson (eds.), New York, Mc Graw Hill Inc., 1972, pp.760- 782.

23. SVENNERHOLM, E. & SVENNERHOLM, L.- The separation of neutral blood-serum glycolipids by thin-layer chromatography. *Biochim. Biophys.Acta*, 70: 432 (1963).

24. SVENNERHOLM, L.- The quantitative estimation of cerebrosides in nervous tissue. *J.Neurochem.*, 1: 42 (1956).

25. SVENNERHOLM, L.- The distribution of lipids in the human nervous system. I. Analytical procedure. Lipids of foetal and newborn brain. *J.Neurochem.*, 11: 839 (1964).

26. SVENNERHOLM, L.- The metabolism of gangliosides in cerebral lipidoses. In *Inborn Disorders of Sphingolipid Metabolism*, S.Aronson & B.W.Volk (eds.), Oxford, Pergamon Press, 1967, pp. 169-186.

27. SVENNERHOLM, L. & STÄLLBERG-STENHAGEN, S.- Changes in the fatty acid composition of cerebrosides of human nervous tissue with age. *J.Lipid Res.*, 9: 215 (1968).

28. SVENNERHOLM, L. & THORIN, H.- Quantitative isolation of brain sulfatides. *J.Lipid Res.*, 3: 483 (1962).

29. SVENNERHOLM, L. & VANIER, M.T.- Brain gangliosides in Krabbe disease. *Adv.Exp.Med.Biol.*, 19: 499 (1972).

30. TAKETOMI, T. & NISHIMURA, H.- Physiological activity of psychosine. *Jap.J.Exp.Med.*, 34: 255 (1964).

31. TAKETOMI, T. & YAMAKAWA,T.- Immunochemical studies of lipids. I. Preparation and immunological proporties of synthetic psychosine-protein antigens. *J.Biochem.(Tokyo)*, 54: 444 (1963).

32. TANAKA, H. & SUZUKI, K.- Lactosylceramide β-galactosidase in human sphingolipidoses. Evidence for two genetically distinct enzymes. *J.Biol.Chem.*, 250: 2324 (1975).

33. VANIER, M.T., HOLM, M., MÅNSSON, J.E. & SVENNERHOLM, L.- The distribution of lipids in the human nervous system. V. Gangliosides and allied neutral glycolipids of infant brain. *J.Neurochem.*, 21: 1375 (1973).

34. VANIER, M.T. & SVENNERHOLM, L.- Chemical pathology of Krabbe's disease. I. Lipid composition and fatty acid patterns of phosphoglycerides in brain. *Acta Paediatr.Scand.*, 63: 494 (1974).

35. VANIER, M.T. & SVENNERHOLM, L.- Chemical pathology of Krabbe's disease. III. Ceramide hexosides and gangliosides of brain. *Acta Paediatr.Scand.*, 64: 641 (1975).

36. WELLS, M.A. & DITTMER, J.C.- The use of Sephadex for the removal of nonlipid contaminants from lipid extracts. *Biochemistry*, 2: 1259 (1963).

37. WENGER, D.A., SATTLER, M. & MARKEY, S.P.- Deficiency of monogalactosyl diglyceride β-galactosidase activity in Krabbe's disease. *Biochem.Biophys.Res.Commun.*, 53: 680 (1973).

38. WENGER, D.A., SATTLER, M. & HIATT, W.- Globoid cell leukodystrophy : deficiency of lactosylceramide β-galactosidase. *Proc.Nat. Acad.Sci.USA*, 71: 854 (1974).

39. YOUNG, O.M. & KANFER, J.N.- An improved separation of sphingolipids by thin-layer chromatography. *J.Chromatog.*, 19: 611 (1965).

GLYCOLIPID METABOLISM IN THE CANINE FORM OF GLOBOID CELL LEUKODYSTROPHY

Elvira Costantino-Ceccarini,*   Thomas F. Fletcher, ** and Kunihiko Suzuki*

*The Saul R. Korey Department of Neurology, Department of Neuroscience, and the Rose F. Kennedy Center for Research in Mental Retardation and Human Development, Albert Einstein College of Medicine, Bronx, N.Y. 10461; and **Department of Veterinary Biology, University of Minnesota, St. Paul, Minnesota 55108

The underlying cause of globoid cell leukodystrophy (Krabbe's disease) is a genetic deficiency of galactosylceramide β-galactosidase (galactosylceramidase, E.C. 3.2.1.46) which normally degrades galactosylceramide (21,22). In principle, the disease belongs to the so-called sphingolipidoses in which acidic lysosomal hydrolases are genetically deficient resulting in abnormal accumulation of sphingolipids specific in respective disorders. Unlike in other sphingolipidoses, abnormal accumulation of galactosylceramide does not occur in globoid cell leukodystrophy despite the block in its degradative pathway (22, 26). The only logical explanation for this unusual phenomenon appears to be that, sometime along the course of the disease, biosynthesis of galactosylceramide is terminated. Galactosylceramide is highly concentrated in the myelin sheath which is a specialized extension of the oligodendroglial plasma membrane. It is, therefore, reasonable to assume that the oligodendroglial cell is the major site of galactosylceramide biosynthesis in the brain. Since early and almost complete destruction of oligodendroglia is one of the characteristic morphological features of the disease, cessation of galactosylceramide biosynthesis may merely be a secondary result of the abnormal histology. However, it is also possible that biosynthetic abnormality may precede death of oligodendroglia, both due to the same as yet unidentified pathogenetic mechanism. Galactosylsphingosine (psychosine) has been proposed as a possible toxic metabolite responsible for the destruction of oligodendroglia (14). In the present study we attempted to evaluate biosynthetic capacity of globoid cell leukodystrophy tissues both in vitro and in vivo at different stages of the disease. Particular attention was directed to galactosylceramide and other myelin components.

The rarity of the disease and ethical considerations make it almost impossible to carry out the experiments of this type with human patients with globoid cell leukodystrophy. We utilized the enzymatically authentic animal model of globoid cell leukodystrophy occurring in the dog (9,19). Although certain subtle differences have been recognized between the two forms of the disease (20,23), the canine form of the disease is an excellent model to study consequences of the genetic galactosylceramidase deficiency and allows much better controlled experiments than are possible with human patients.

MATERIALS AND METHODS

The strain of Cairn terriers carrying the mutant gene for globoid cell leukodystrophy is being maintained in the University of Minnesota, St. Paul. For in vitro assays of lipid glycosyltransferases, the entire litter of a carrier to carrier breeding was sacrificed for an experiment at an appropriate stage of the disease. The brain and other organs were immediately removed and frozen. They were shipped to New York within 24 hours and tissues were dissected within 48 hours. For the in vivo experiment, one affected and one unaffected control dog were injected with an isotopic precursor and were killed 24 hours later. The brain was always cut longitudinally in the midline before freezing and the half brain was fixed for histological examination with hematoxylin-eosin and myelin stains.

In Vitro Experiments: Gray and white matter was dissected from the cerebral cortex and the centrum semiovale respectively, weighed, homogenized in 4 vols of water and lyophilized. The dry tissue was weighed and suspended in benzene. Activities of UDP-galactose: ceramide galactosyltransferase and UDP-glucose:ceramide glucosyltransferase were assayed according to the standard assay procedures of our laboratory in which a benzene suspension of the enzyme source was first dried together with a benzene solution of appropriate acceptor ceramide before addition of aqueous solutions of other assay components

(3,5)$_2$. The radioactive precursors, UDP-[U-^{14}C]galactose and UDP-[U-^{14}C]glucose, were purchased from New England Nuclear Corp., Boston, Mass. Protein determination was by the method of Lowry et al. (11).

In Vivo Experiment: A 17-week old affected dog and its littermate control dog were used for this experiment. The control dog was a heterozygous carrier according to the activities of galactosylceramide β-galactosidase of peripheral leukocytes determined prior to the experiment. [U-^{3}H]Galactose from New England Nuclear Corp. was diluted with non-radioactive galactose to 5 mCi/100 mg. Each dog received a saline solution of 5 mCi of the precursor intrathecally. Body weights were 2.93 kg for the affected, and 3.19 kg for the control dog. Blood samples were drawn at intervals after the injection of the isotope. The dogs were killed at 24 hours after injection, organs removed, and they were shipped to New York in dry ice. A half brain was set aside as usual for histological examination. The weight of the brains were 57.1 g for the affected and 54.6 g for the control dog.

Because of the nature of the isotope (tritium) and the relatively low incorporation in vivo (a few thousand counts per min per mg lipid), it was possible to determine activities of the two lipid glycosyltransferases in vitro. The assays were carried out in the same manner as described for the in vitro experiment. The final radioactivity determination was done with appropriate channel settings for the double isotope technique. In practice, it could be estimated from the in vivo incorporation data and from the amount of tissue used for the in vitro assays that the maximum spill-over of tritium activity into the ^{14}C channel was much less than one percent of the total activity in the channel. The only necessary correction was for the lower counting efficiency for carbon-14 in the double isotope mode.

The blood samples were centrifuged and serum separated. An equal volume of 10% trichloroacetic acid was added and the precipitate removed by centrifugation. Trichloroacetic acid was removed from the supernatant by repeated extraction with ethylether, and aliquots counted in a toluene-based scintillation solvent containing 10% Bio-Solv BBS-3 (Beckman Instr., Fullerton, Calif.).

To examine incorporation of the injected galactose into brain constituents, cerebral cortex was dissected as the gray matter sample, and the brain stem and medulla as the white matter sample. This choice was dictated by the histological finding that the cerebral white matter was already severely affected but that the brain stem and the medulla were still essentially normal with respect to the myelin and oligodendroglial population. The weighed tissues were extracted with chloroform-methanol (2:1, v/v) and the major tissue components -- chloroform-methanol insoluble residue, chloroform-methanol soluble protein, total lipid, and upper phase solids -- were determined gravimetrically according to our standard procedure which is based on the method of Folch et al. (10). The potassium citrate procedure of Webster and Folch (28) was used to accelerate denaturation of chloroform-methanol soluble protein.

Both chloroform-methanol insoluble residue and soluble protein were further extracted extensively with chloroform-methanol (2:1, v/v) and dried with acetone and ether. They were dissolved in Soluene 300 (Packard Instr., Downers Grove, Ill.) and radioactivity determined. The upper phase solid fraction was dissolved in 10 ml of water and dialyzed against 100 ml of water. An aliquot of 0.5 ml was taken from the dialysate to determine the radioactivity in the dialyzable upper phase fraction. The dialysis was then continued against a larger volume of water with frequent changes. The exhaustively dialyzed upper phase was lyophilized, dissolved in 5 ml of water, and appropriate aliquots used for determination of total ganglioside N-acetyl-neuraminic acid (NeuNAc) with the resorcinol method (13,25) and for determination of radioactivity. The protein-free lipid fraction was dissolved in chloroform-methanol (2:1, v/v) and an aliquot was taken to estimate radioactivity in the total lipid fraction. The total lipid fraction was analyzed for cholesterol (17), total lipid phosphorus (12), and total lipid hexose (24). Appropriate conversion factors were used to obtain approximate estimates for total phospholipids (P x 25) and for total galactolipids (galactose x 4.65). The general lipid pattern was examined semi-quantitatively by thin-layer chromatography with silica gel G plates developed in chloroform-methanol-water (70:30:4, v/v/v) and visualized by 50% sulfuric acid spray and heating. For determination of radioactivity in individual lipids, the same thin-layer chromatography was run with wider lanes so that each lane could accommodate up to 1 mg of total lipid without overloading. The separated spots were visualized by iodine vapor, each marked, and, after iodine was completely sulimed, scraped into counting vials. The powder was wet with the addition of 0.5 ml of water, and then the scintillation solvent containing Bio-Solv BBS-3 was added. Preliminary experiments as well as the estimates on the actual samples indicated essentially quantitative recovery of radioactivity from the thin-layer

Table 1.   Stages of Canine Globoid Cell Leukodystrophy
Examined for Glycolipid Biosynthesis

Age (weeks)	Clinical Picture	Histology
7	preclinical, diagnosis by enzyme assay.	early lesions, myelin and oligodendroglia normal.
17	7 weeks after onset, fairly advanced, used for both in vitro and in vivo studies.	advanced lesions in centrum semiovale but normal in brain stem and medulla.
22	full-fledged clinical signs	moderately advanced with myelin and oligodendroglial loss.
22	littermate of above but clinically more advanced.	severe pathology, loss of myelin and oligo-dendroglia

plate.   Thin-layer chromatographic separation of sulfatide and lecithin was incomplete and these two compounds were counted together.   In order to obtain quantitative estimate of galactosylceramide and sulfatide separately and to obtain radioactivity in sulfatide, appropriate amounts of the total lipid fraction were subjected to the mercuric chloride-saponification procedure (1) which eliminates almost all glycerophospholipids.   After saponification, the lipid mixture was chromatographed on a silicic acid (Unisil, Clarkson Chemical Co., Williamsport, Pa.) column according to Norton and Autilio (15).   For quantitative determination of galactolipids, fractions containing galactosylceramide and sulfatide were pooled separately, and galactose content determined (24).   For determination of radioactivity, galactosylceramide and sulfatide were eluted together with chloroform-methanol (1:1, v/v) after discarding the earlier fractions eluted with chloroform-methanol (98:2, v/v) and (96:4, v/v) which contained cholesterol and a small amount of liberated free fatty acids.   The galactolipid fraction was then subjected to the same thin-layer chromatography used for the total lipid fraction.   Radioactivity of galactosylceramide and sulfatide spots were determined as described above.   Radioactivity of galactosylceramide indicated that recovery of galactosylceramide after the mercuric chloride-saponification procedure was better than 95%.   From the radioactivity ratio of

galactosylceramide and sulfatide it was possible to calculate the radioactivity of sulfatide and lecithin separately in the mixed spot in the
thin-layer chromatogram of total lipids.

RESULTS

Altogether four dogs affected by globoid cell leukodystrophy
were included in the present study, representing different stages of the
disease (Table 1). There were a total of twelve control dogs, seven
of which were heterozygotes for the globoid cell leukodystrophy mutant
gene.

Galactosylceramide β-galactosidase: Brain tissues of all dogs
were assayed for activity of galactosylceramide β-galactosidase except
for the two dogs which received in vivo injection of the radioactive
precursor. Not only the affected homozygous dogs but heterozygous
carrier dogs could also be readily distinguished from normal dogs (Table
2). The assay procedure was essentially that of Bowen and Radin (2)
with minor modifications.

Lipid Glycosyltransferases: Preliminary experiments had shown
that activities of UDP-galactose:ceramide galactosyltransferase and
UDP-glucose:ceramide glucosyltransferase remained stable for at least
a few days postmortem when the tissue was kept frozen at the dry ice
temperature. When activities of the two glycosyltransferases were
examined in white and gray matter of 7 week-old control dogs,

Table 2.   Galactosylceramide β-Galactosidase in Canine Brain

Tissue	Genetic status	Galactosylceramide β-galactosidase
GRAY	affected (n=3)	3.07 ± 1.01
	carriers (n=6)	19.1 ± 2.1
	normal (n=5)	32.1 ± 6.1
WHITE	affected (n=3)	4.40 ± 0.96
	carriers (n=6)	43.6 ± 8.8
	normal (n=5)	89.2 ± 17.5

Activities are in nmol/hr/g wet weight ± S.D.
Age differences were insignificant between 6 to 30 weeks.

Table 3.   Lipid Glycosyltransferases in 7 Week-Old Carrier
and Normal Dogs

Tissue	Genetic status	UDP-gal:ceramide galactosyltransferase	UDP-glc:ceramide glucosyltransferase
GRAY	carriers (n=4)	0.21 ± 0.12	1.43 ± 0.15
	normal (n=5)	0.24 ± 0.03	1.42 ± 0.19
WHITE	carriers (n=4)	2.64 ± 0.41	0.49 ± 0.11
	normal (n=5)	2.84 ± 0.45	0.44 ± 0.10

Activities are expressed in nmol/hr/mg protein.

several important conclusions emerged (Table 3).   UDP-galactose:cera-
mide galactosyltransferase which catalyzes the last step of galactosylceramide biosynthesis is normally ten times more active in white matter
than in gray matter.   In contrast, UDP-glucose:ceramide glucosyltransferase, an enzyme for synthesis of glucosylceramide which is the basic
building block of gangliosides, is approximately three times more active
in gray matter.   These findings are consistent with localization of
galactosylceramide primarily in white matter and that of ganglioside in
gray matter.   The results also indicated that, despite the reduced
activity of galactosylceramide β-galactosidase in the carrier dogs, there
are no differences in the activities of the two lipid glycosyltransferases
between the normal homozygous, and the heterozygous carriers.   This
finding provided assurance that in vitro data for the glycosyltransferases
for normal and carrier dogs can be combined as the control data for
affected dogs.

The results of the in vitro assays of the two lipid glycosyltransferases are summarized in Fig. 1.   The control activities of the glycosyltransferases varied substantially during development.   Generally the
changes were similar to those observed in rodent brains (3,4,18).
UDP-galactose:ceramide galactosyltransferase showed the highest activity
at 7 weeks.   Its activity was almost as high at 17 weeks but declined
to one-third of the activity of 7 weeks by 22 to 30 weeks of age.   On
the other hand, UDP-glucose:ceramide glucosyltransferase showed a
gradual decline as the animal matured.   In order to simplify presentation
of the data, it was necessary to normalize the data at 17 and 22 weeks
of age to the value at 7 weeks.   The averages and scatters of the
control values at 17 and 22 weeks were compared with those at 7 weeks
and the normalization factors were developed for these ages.   This

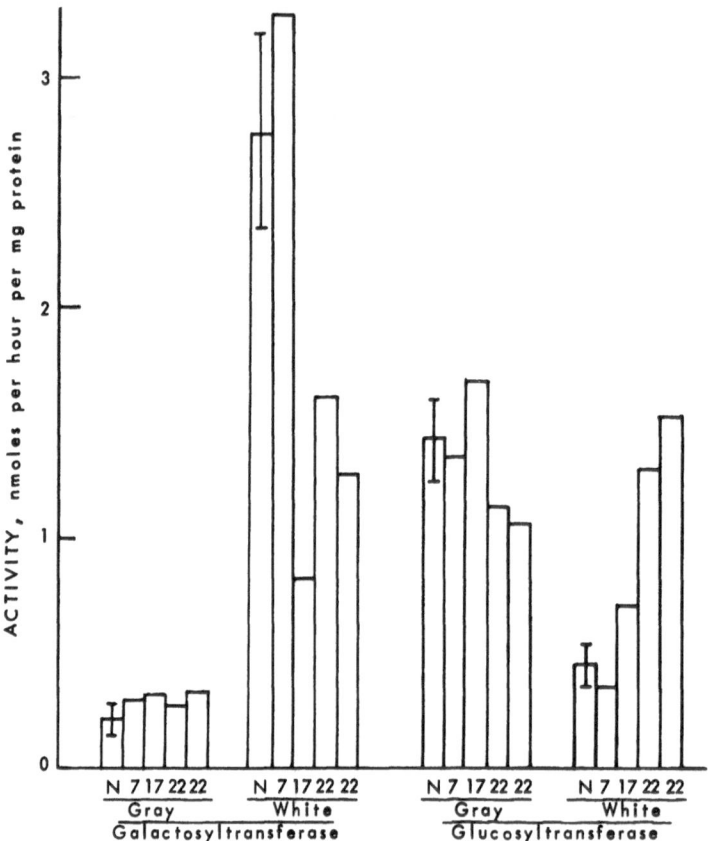

Fig. 1. Lipid glycosyltransferases assayed in vitro. The columns N represent the control activities normalized for the activity at 7 weeks, with standard deviations. Other bars represent individual affected dogs with the age given in weeks. Both enzymes are normal in gray and white matter at 7 weeks, but they develop abnormalities in later stages of the disease particularly in white matter.

manipulation permits comparison of the data on affected dogs of different ages against a single control value. In gray matter of affected dogs, UDP-galactose:ceramide galactosyltransferase showed relatively little changes. If anything, there was a tendency to increases in the activity of the galactosyltransferase in gray matter. On the other hand, the galactosyltransferase activity was clearly reduced in the white matter of the three affected dogs with fully-developed histological lesions. The activity was on the average about half of the control, and generally the reduction was more severe when histological involvement was more severe. A similar reduction of this enzyme in affected dog brain was recorded by Radin et al. (16). The white matter of the 7 week-old affected dog was essentially normal histologically and activity of the galactosyltransferase was not reduced. UDP-glucose:ceramide glucosyltransferase gave a contrasting picture. In gray matter, changes were minor as in the galactosyltransferase. But in white matter, the glucosyltransferase was dramatically increased in affected dogs with advanced histological lesions, up to more than three times normal. Again there was no such increase in the white matter of the 7 week-old affected dog, too early for histological abnormality. These in vitro results can be summarized as follows. Both of the lipid glycosyltransferases showed only minor changes in the gray matter while, in white matter of affected dogs, the galactosyltransferase was reduced and the glucosyltransferase was markedly increased at advanced stages of the disease. Both enzymes were normal in the very early stage of the disease before the clinical onset when histological abnormality was still minimum.

In Vivo Study: Analyses of the samples of the cerebral cortex and the brain stem-medulla (white matter) showed that there were no significant differences in the composition of these tissues between the control and the affected dogs (Table 4). These findings were important for interpretation of the subsequent data in two respects. They chemically

Table 4.   Analysis of 17 Week-Old GLD and Control Dog Brain

	Gray matter		White matter	
	affected	control	affected	control
Dry weight (% wet wt.)	16.2	16.7	23.4	25.4
	(% dry weight)		(% dry weight)	
C-M insoluble residue	59.9	56.7	39.0	35.7
C-M soluble protein	1.7	1.7	5.3	4.7
Total lipid	28.3	28.9	48.3	52.5
Upper phase solid	9.4	10.4	5.8	5.3
	(% lipid)		(% lipid)	
Cholesterol	25.2	27.8	27.5	27.5
Total phospholipid	68.4	71.9	47.3	46.8
Galactolipids				
cerebroside	2.07	2.67	17.3	18.4
sulfatide	0.68	0.61	1.2	0.9
Ganglioside NeuNAc	866	978	407	458
(μg/g)				

confirmed the morphological finding that the tissue samples taken from
the affected dog were histologically still normal. We can compare
the data of radioactivity incorporation in the two dogs on the basis of
wet weight, dry weight, protein weight, lipid weight, or any other
parameters without significantly altering the conclusions. These points
were further supported by the identical lipid patterns in both gray and
white matter between the affected and the control dog (Fig. 2).

After intrathecal injection of 100 mg of tritium-labelled galactose,
radioactivity in serum increased rapidly during the first three hours and

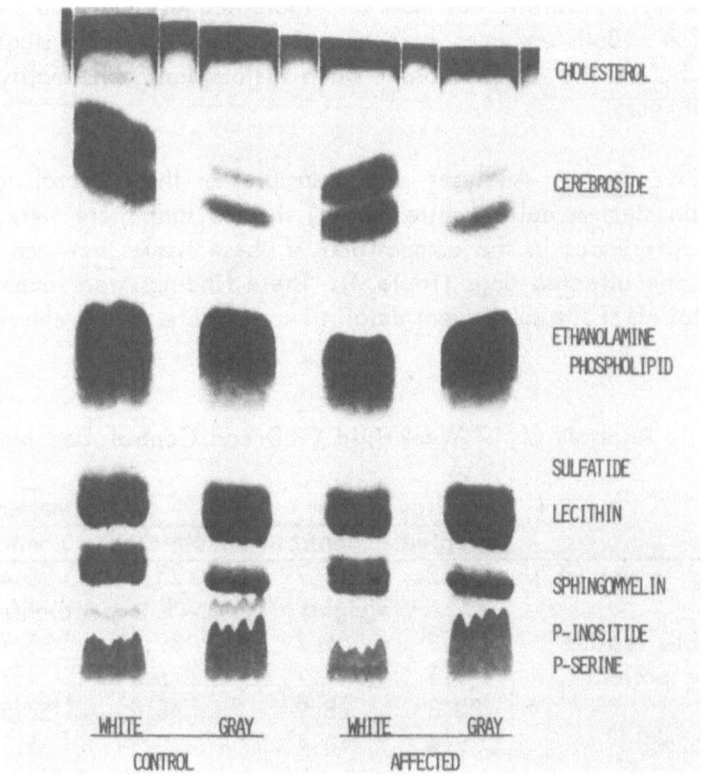

Fig. 2.   Thin-layer chromatogram of the total lipid fraction.
Approximately 500 µg of total lipid was chromatographed on silica gel
G plate in the solvent system of chloroform-methanol-water (70:30:4,
v/v/v).   Spots were visualized by 50% sulfuric acid spray and heating.
The lipid patterns are identical between the affected and control dogs,
both in gray and white matter. Sulfatide and lecithin are poorly separated.

then was maintained at relatively high and stable levels with only minor
and gradual decline (Fig. 3). Small systematic differences aside, the
time course was identical in the two dogs. The total radioactivity in the
dialyzable upper phase fraction was generally similar in all samples
except for the gray matter sample of the affected dog (Table 5). With
the rationale that this fraction represents the soluble precursor pool
available to the tissue, we normalized all subsequent incorporation data
for the activity of the dialyzable upper phase fraction using the normalization factors as indicated in Table 5.

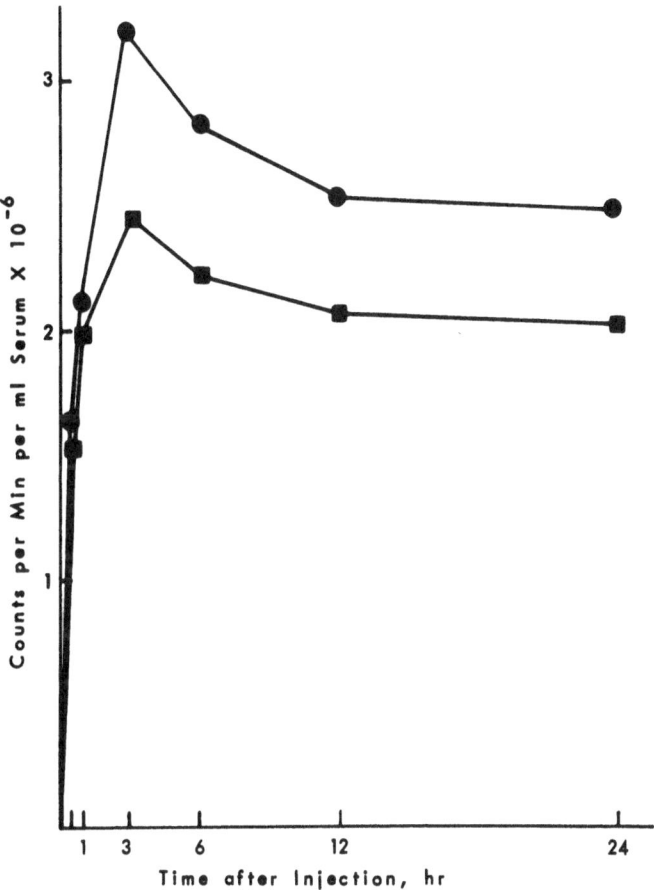

Fig. 3. Radioactivity in serum. Blood samples were drawn at
intervals after intrathecal injection of 5mCi (100 mg) of tritium-labelled
galactose. The graphs represent radioactivity in the trichloroacetic
acid nonprecipitable fraction of the serum. The round dots are from
the affected dog and the squares from the control dog. Note the qualitatively identical time course in the two dogs.

Table 5. Radioactivity in the Dialyzable Upper Phase Fraction

Specimen		cpm/g x 10^{-5}	normalization factor
affected,	gray	3.42	1
	white	4.83	0.71
control,	gray	4.48	0.76
	white	4.59	0.75

Among the four major tissue fractions, there were no differences between the affected and the control dogs in incorporation of radioactivity from the injected galactose into gangliosides and chloroform-methanol insoluble residue (Table 6). On the other hand there were substantial differences in the synthetic capacity for total lipid and chloroform-methanol soluble protein (Table 6). The gray matter of the affected dog incorporated approximately 80% of the control radioactivity into the total lipid fraction, and 90% of the control activity into the chloroform-methanol soluble protein. The differences were much greater in the white matter samples. Only 60% of the control activity was incorporated into the total lipid fraction, and only half normal activity into the chloroform-methanol soluble protein. Ganglioside is primarily a neuronal constituent and the chloroform-methanol insoluble residue represents the general cerebral protein, while lipid synthesis at this developmental stage heavily reflects myelin formation, and the chloroform-methanol soluble protein of brain tissue consists mostly of proteolipid protein of the myelin sheath. Therefore, the above data suggest that there is a substantial and selective reduction in the capacity to synthesize myelin components in the white matter of the affected dog.

Reflecting the finding in total lipid, none of the individual lipids in the gray matter of the affected dog showed dramatic differences from the control dog tissue. Most of them showed 10 to 20% reduction in incorporated radioactivity compared to the normal control (Table 7). Only sulfatide showed slightly higher activity for the affected dog, although this observation should be viewed with caution because of the very low activity in sulfatide in gray matter. In the white matter lipids, there were clearly two classes of lipids with respect to incorporation of radioactivity from the injected galactose. Cholesterol, galactosylceramide and sphingomyelin were most severely affected, all showing approximately half normal synthetic activity. Other lipids, such as

Table 6. Radioactivity in Major Tissue Fractions

Fraction	Gray Matter		White Matter	
	control	affected	control	affected
Ganglioside (cpm/μg NeuNAc)	29.8	27.8	32.6	29.5
C-M insoluble residue (cpm/mg $\times 10^{-3}$)	2.7	2.5	2.5	2.7
Total lipid (cpm/mg $\times 10^{-3}$)	1.98	1.59	3.45	2.37
C-M soluble protein (cpm/mg)	489	443	896	437

ethanolamine phospholipids, lecithin, and phosphatidylserine indicated relatively well preserved synthetic activity. If we assume that the total galactosylceramide in the tissue acts as the precursor pool for sulfatide synthesis, then the last step of biosynthesis of sulfatide, sulfation of galactosylceramide, is not affected in the white matter of the sick dog, because the acceptor pool has a lower specific activity to begin with in the affected dog white matter. The assumption itself may be incorrect, and in any case the overall synthesis of sulfatide from galactose is reduced. Summarizing the data from the in vivo experiment, we can conclude that the synthetic capacity of gray matter of the affected dog is relatively well-preserved while the synthetic capacity of white matter with respect to the tissue components primarily localized in the myelin sheath is substantially reduced in the affected dog, while components unrelated to myelin appear to be synthesized normally. It is important to add that these findings were obtained from affected white matter in which myelin and the oligodendroglial population were still well preserved.

DISCUSSION

In our in vitro studies we selected UDP-galactose:ceramide galactosyltransferase as the indicator enzyme for capacity of the tissue to make galactosylceramide. Reflecting the localization of galactosylceramide, the enzyme is highly localized in white matter, particularly in oligodendroglia (7,18). According to our preliminary data, bulk-isolated bovine oligodendroglia are enriched with this enzyme 10 to 20

Table 7. Radioactivity in Individual Lipids

Lipid	Gray matter			White matter		
	control	affected	%control	control	affected	%control
Cholesterol	111	102	92%	383	191	50%
Galactosylceramide	150	122	81%	1329	681	51%
Ethanolamine phospho-lipid	350	293	84%	454	349	77%
Sulfatide	17	21	123%	42	28	67%
Lecithin	1005	805	80%	766	649	85%
Sphingomyelin	81	74	91%	81	45	56%
Phosphatidylserine + P-inositide	99	77	78%	172	153	89%

Radioactivities are expressed in counts per min per mg of the total lipid mixture.

times over neuronal perikarya isolated from the same brain (Costantino-Ceccarini and Poduslo, unpublished observation). Furthermore, a portion of the galactosyltransferase appears to be an intrinsic constituent of the myelin sheath (6). On the other hand, UDP-glucose:ceramide glucosyltransferase has, although analogous biochemically, contrasting biological functions. It is enriched in gray matter and is primarily concerned with ganglioside synthesis in the brain. Changes in these two glycosyltransferases were minor, if any, in gray matter of affected dogs, and they were also normal even in white matter before the clinical onset and histological abnormalities. The two glycosyltransferases showed contrasting behavior in white matter of affected dogs in later stages of the disease; the galactosyltransferase decreased significantly and the glucosyltransferase increased dramatically. These observations are consistent with an interpretation that in vitro activities of the two lipid glycosyltransferases merely reflect the histological abnormalities. In advanced stages of the disease there are substantial reductions in oligodendroglia and myelin, resulting in similar loss of the galactosyltransferase normally highly localized in oligodendroglia. The marked increase in the activity of UDP-glucose:ceramide glucosyltransferase is likely to reflect the presence of globoid cells. Globoid cells are considered to be of mesodermal origin. Mesodermal cells are generally more active in synthesizing the globoside series of neutral glycosphingolipids with glucosylceramide as the starting building block. Eto and Suzuki (8) attributed the increased amounts of these glycolipids in white matter of a patient with globoid cell leukodystrophy to the massive infiltration of globoid cells. Since neither enzyme was abnormal in the white matter at an early stage of the disease, the data from the in vitro experiments provided no evidence that reduction in UDP-galactose:ceramide galactosyltransferase precedes destruction of oligodendroglia.

Unlike in assays of specific enzymes in vitro, results from in vivo incorporation experiments are always open to interpretative uncertainties. Injected precursors may well be metabolized and converted to other metabolites differently between experimental and control animals, resulting in different distribution of various immediate precursors for synthesis of tissue components. The size of immediate precursor pools may well be different. The relative distribution of the lable within the final product may vary -- for example, in sphingosine, fatty acid, and galactose, in the case of galactosylceramide. Although complete control of all possible variables is impractical, judicious control of some key parameters is essential.

The qualitatively identical time course of radioactivity in serum and the similar activity of the soluble precursor pool fraction of the brain (dialyzable upper phase) provided a reasonable assurance that there were no gross differences between the affected and the control dog in handling the injected galactose. The brain tissues of the affected dog, particularly white matter, showed selective reduction to synthesize tissue components that are enriched in the myelin sheath, while synthesis of constituents relatively unrelated to myelin was unaffected. While such results might merely be considered consistent with the in vitro results of galactosylceramide synthesis, they in fact provided significant additional information. It concerned the discrepancy between the biochemical data and the histological lesions. The brain stem-medulla was taken as the white matter sample. Despite extensive histological involvement in the cerebral white matter, the brain stem-medulla was still essentially normal histologically with respect to myelin and oligodendroglial population. Therefore, the selective reduction in the synthesis of myelin constituents observed in vivo in the white matter of the affected dog is not secondary to destruction of oligodendroglia. The data rather indicate that metabolic abnormalities precede the cellular destruction and that these oligodendroglia are in fact "sick" and unable to carry out myelin formation at the normal rate.

We do not yet know the precise biochemical mechanism as to how destruction of oligodendroglia is brought about. The presence of metabolic abnormality before cellular degeneration, as shown in our in vivo experiment, is consistent with the hypothesis that the eventual cellular destruction is due to accumulation of toxic metabolites within the oligodendroglia. One such hypothesis, the psychosine hypothesis (14), has recently received a strong support from analytical studies of Vanier and Svennerholm (27).

ACKNOWLEDGEMENT

This investigation was supported by research grants, NS-10885, NS-03356, and HD-01799 from the United States Public Health Service, and by RD-982-A-4 from the National Multiple Sclerosis Society.

REFERENCES

1. Abramson, M.B., Norton, W.T. and Katzman, R.: Study of Ionic Structures in Phospholipids by Infrared Spectra. J. Biol.

Chem., 240:2389, 1965.

2. Bowen, D.M. and Radin, N.S.: Cerebroside Galactosidase: A Method for Determination and a Comparison with Other Lysosomal Enzymes in Developing Rat Brain. J. Neurochem., 16:501, 1969.

3. Brenkert, A. and Radin, N.S.: Synthesis of Galactocerebroside and Glucocerebroside by Rat Brain: Assay Procedure and Changes with Age. Brain Res., 36:183, 1972.

4. Costantino-Ceccarini, E. and Morell, P.: Biosynthesis of Brain Sphingolipids and Myelin Accumulation in the Mouse. Lipids, 7:656, 1972.

5. Costantino-Ceccarini, E. and Morell, P.: Synthesis of Galacto-sylceramide and Glucosylceramide by Mouse Kidney Preparations. J. Biol. Chem., 248:8240, 1973.

6. Costantino-Ceccarini, E. and Suzuki, K.: Evidence for Presence of UDP-galactose:ceramide Galactosyltransferase in Rat Myelin. Brain Res., 93:358, 1975.

7. Deshmukh, D.S., Flynn, T.J. and Pieringer, R.A.: The Biosynthesis and Concentration of Galactosyldiglyceride in Glial and Neuronal Enriched Fractions of Actively Myelinating Rat Brain. J. Neurochem., 22:479, 1974.

8. Eto, Y. and Suzuki, K.: Brain Sphingolipids in Krabbe's Globoid Cell Leukodystrophy. J. Neurochem., 18:503, 1971.

9. Fletcher, T.F., Kurtz, H.J. and Low, D.C.: Globoid Cell Leukodystrophy (Krabbe Type) in the Dog. J. Am. Vet. Med. Assoc., 149:165, 1966.

10. Folch-Pi, J., Lees, M. and Sloane-Stanley, G.H.: Simple Method for the Isolation and Purification of Total Lipids from Animal Tissues. J. Biol. Chem., 226:497, 1957.

11. Lowry, O.H., Rosebrough, N.J., Farr, A.L. and Randall, R.J.: Protein Measurement with the Folin Phenol Reagent. J. Biol. Chem., 193:265, 1951.

12. Marinetti, G.V., Erbland, J. and Stotz, E.: The Quantitative Analysis of Plasmalogens by Paper Chromatography. Biochim. Biophys. Acta 31:251, 1959.

13. Miettinen, T. and Takki-Luukkainen, I.-T.: Use of Butyl Acetate in Determination of Sialic Acid. Acta Chim. Scand., 13:856, 1959.

14. Miyatake, T. and Suzuki, K.: Globoid Cell Leukodystrophy: Additional Deficiency of Psychosine Galactosidase. Biochem. Biophys. Res. Commun. 48:538, 1972.

15. Norton, W.T. and Autilio, L.A.: The Chemical Composition of Bovine CNS Myelin. Ann. N.Y. Acad. Sci., 122:77, 1965.

16. Radin, N.S., Arora, R.C., Ullman, M.D., Brenkert, A.L. and Austin, J.: A Possible Therapeutic Approach to Krabbe's Globoid Leukodystrophy and the Status of Cerebroside Synthesis in the Disorder. Res. Commun. Chem. Path. Pharmacol. 3:637, 1972.

17. Searcy, R.L. and Bergquist, L.M.: A New Color Reaction for the Quantitation of Serum Cholesterol. Clin. Chim. Acta 5:192, 1960.

18. Shah, S.N.: Glycosyltransferases of Microsomal Fractions from Brain: Synthesis of Glucosylceramide and Galactosylceramide During Development and the Distribution of Glucose and Galactose Transferase in White and Grey Matter. J. Neurochem. 18:395, 1971.

19. Suzuki, Y., Austin, J., Armstrong, D., Suzuki, K., Schlenker, J. and Fletcher, T.: Studies in Globoid (Krabbe) Leukodystrophy: Enzymic and Sphingolipid Findings in the Canine Form. Exp. Neurol., 29:65, 1970.

20. Suzuki, Y., Miyatake, T., Fletcher, T.F. and Suzuki, K.: Glycosphingolipid β-Galactosidases. III. Canine Form of Globoid Cell Leukodystrophy: Comparison with the Human Disease. J. Biol.Chem. 249:2109, 1974.

21. Suzuki, K. and Suzuki, Y.: Globoid Cell Leukodystrophy (Krabbe's Disease): Deficiency of Galactocerebroside β-Galactosidase.

Proc. Nat. Acad. Sci. (U.S.A.), 66:302, 1970.

22. Suzuki, K. and Suzuki, Y.: Galactosylceramide Lipidosis:
    Globoid Cell Leukodystrophy (Krabbe's Disease), in The
    Metabolic Basis of Inherited Disease, edited by J.B. Stanbury,
    J.B. Wyngaarden, and D.S. Frederickson, 4th Edition, McGraw
    Hill, New York, in press.

23. Suzuki, K., Suzuki, Y. and Fletcher, T.F.: Further Studies on
    Galactocerebroside β-Galactosidase in Globoid Cell Leukodystro-
    phy., in Sphingolipids, Sphingolipidoses and Allied Disorders,
    edited by B.W. Volk and S.M. Aronson, Plenum Press, New
    York, pp. 487–498, 1972.

24. Svennerholm, L.: The Quantitative Estimation of Cerebroside in
    Nervous Tissue. J. Neurochem. 1:42, 1956.

25. Svennerholm, L.: Quantitative Estimation of Sialic Acid. II.
    A Colorimetric Resorcinol Hydrochloric Acid Method. Biochim.
    Biophys. Acta 24:604, 1957.

26. Vanier, M.T. and Svennerholm, L.: Chemical Pathology of Krabbe's
    Disease. I. Lipid Composition and Fatty Acid Patterns of Phos-
    phoglycerides in Brain. Acta Paediat. Scand. 63:494, 1974.

27. Vanier, M.T. and Svennerholm, L.: Chemical Pathology of
    Krabbe's Disease. III. Ceramide Hexosides and Gangliosides
    of Brain. Acta Paediat. Scand. 64:641, 1975.

28. Webster, G.R. and Folch-Pi, J.: Some Studies on the Properties
    of Proteolipids. Biochim. Biophys. Acta 49:399, 1961.

FUCOSIDOSIS: CLINICAL, PATHOLOGIC, AND BIOCHEMICAL

STUDIES OF FIVE PATIENTS

Benjamin H. Landing (1,2), George N. Donnell (2),
Omar S. Alfi (2), Harry B. Neustein (1),
Fred A. Lee (3), Won G. Ng (1), William R. Bergren (1),
and Philip Sturgeon (4)

Departments of Pathology (1), Pediatrics (2),
  and Radiology (3)
Childrens Hospital of Los Angeles and
University of Southern California School of Medicine
and Brentwood Laboratories (4), Los Angeles, California

INTRODUCTION

Fucosidosis is an inherited metabolic disorder in which deficiency of a-1-fucosidase activity results in accumulation of fucosyl
compounds in lysosomes (6,7,24). Clinical manifestations reported
include progressive motor and mental deterioration, coarseness of
facial features, cardiomegaly, hepatomegaly, skeletal abnormalities
and short stature (1,5,6,8,13). Initially many of the patients exhibit hypotonia, but progressive spasticity develops with time.

The enzyme a-1-fucosidase is widely distributed in the body.
All patients with fucosidosis have very low a-1-fucosidase activity
in plasma, in leucocytes and in other tissues. However, some clinically normal individuals have low plasma activity as a hereditary
property, and assay of this enzyme in plasma is not a reliable cri-
terion for diagnosis of fucosidosis (16). Confirmation of diagnosis
thus depends on assay of enzyme activity in leucocytes, cultured
fibroblasts, or other tissues.

CLINICAL SUMMARIES: We have studied five patients with fucosidosis
from three families (Table 1). The first seen were two male siblings
(#s 1 and 2), whose parents are first cousins of Italian origin
(Formia, north of Naples). The elder, born in 1961, was first seen
at age 2 years because of muscular weakness. Muscle biopsy showed
small vacuoles or granules in the fibers, but no specific diagnosis
could be made. Rectal biopsy at 5½ years showed cytoplasmic granu-

147

lation of myenteric plexus neurons, and vacuolar histiocytosis of
colonic lamina propria and submucosa. Polyps removed from the right
antrum in 1971 showed vacuolate cytoplasm of epithelial and stromal
cells, again suggestive of lysosomal storage disease.

At age 12 years, he had his first grand mal seizure. At this
time, he could stand with support, but was unable to walk or talk.
He had marked kyphosis, dull facies, protruding tongue and heavy eyebrows. Punctate macular lesions which blanched on pressure were
present over the soles and the palms. Examination of lungs, heart
and abdomen was unrevealing. He had bilateral hamstring shortening
and diffuse muscle weakness, but the deep tendon reflexes were
hyperactive. Cranial nerve functions appeared intact.

The younger sibling, born in 1963, was first seen at 3 years of
age for generalized muscle weakness. Like his brother's, his course
was progressive. At 7 years of age, he had dull facies, protruding
tongue, open mouth with drooling, and mild kyphosis. All the
extremities were spastic, but he was able to walk with a scissor
gait when supported. By 10 years of age he required complete
nursing care.

The coarse features, progressive mental retardation, kyphosis,
and the presence of cytoplasmic vacuolation of a number of cell types
suggested fucosidosis, among other possible lysosomal storage diseases, in these children. The diagnosis of fucosidosis was established by demonstrating the absence of a-1-fucosidase activity in
plasma and in cultured fibroblasts (28, 29).

Patient #3 was found in a survey of patients in an institution
for the retarded. He was the product of young Mexican-American parents; the mother subsequently had two normal children by a second
marriage. Pregnancy was uncomplicated and delivery was described as
normal. He held his head up at 8 months and started to walk at 15
months. He was able to say a few single words at 18 months, but at
19 months retardation was suspected and at 2 years he did not speak
nor feed himself. At age 9, his IQ was less than 35. He was first
seen by us at age 17, with severe mental and physical retardation,
coarse features, thick eyebrows and very large tongue. The antero-
posterior diameter of the chest was increased, and dorsal kyphosis
was present. There were no skin lesions suggestive of angiokeratoma.
He could walk by himself, but with awkward gait. He was aggressive
and bit, scratched and pinched other patients.

In our third family there are two affected males (#s 4 and 5).
The parents are Mexican-American and there is no known consanguinity.
Each child had been the product of a normal pregnancy and delivery.
The elder was 3 9/12 years old when first seen for delayed speech
and abnormal gait. He had recurrent respiratory infections in
early life, and was developmentally slower than an older normal

sibling. He walked at 1½ years of age, but with an odd, tip-toe
gait. When first seen he had coarse facies, hoarse cry, umbilical
hernia, short stubby fingers and bilateral metatarsal adduction. He
now shows increasing spasticity, enlarged tongue, and flexion con-
tractures of wrists and knees. Initially no skin lesions were noted,
but subsequently telangiectasia of the ear lobes and hyperemia of
the proximal nail beds has appeared. There has been regression of
mental capacity. The younger sibling, when first seen at age 18
months, was considered normal by the parents, but did have mild
coarsening of facial features. Both children have deficient a-1-
fucosidase activity in leucocytes.

COMPARISON TABLE: Table I summarizes the clinical features of our
patients, in comparison with those reported in the literature. It
has been suggested that there may be two clinical forms of fucosidosis (8, 10, 15), one with rapidly progressive neurological signs and
death within the first 6 years (Type 1), and another with skin manifestations and much slower progression of disease (Type 2). Cutaneous angiokeratomata were originally proposed (10) to be found only
in Type 2 disease, and enlarged tongue is also more frequent in older
patients, but since both may be age-related, their absence in younger
patients may not indicate genetic heterogeneity. Hepatomegaly is
frequent in Type 1 patients, but rare in Type 2, and elevation of
sweat chloride may be more typical of Type 1 disease.

    This division of fucosidosis into two groups, on clinical
grounds, is useful, but whether the differences reflect genetic
heterogeneity awaits study of a larger number of patients and clari-
fication of possible differences in their enzyme defects.

RADIOLOGIC FINDINGS: Radiologic studies were carried out on four
patients. The calvaria were normal in size and shape. With age,
thickening of the diploe occurred, particularly of frontal bone and
supraorbital ridge. Prominent diploic venous channels were noted in
the thickened diploe of patient #3, and premature synostosis of
sagittal and coronal sutures (patient #3), and of sagittal and lamb-
doidal sutures (patient #4), were observed. The frontal sinuses were
undeveloped in all patients, and sphenoidal sinuses were either
absent or markedly hypoplastic. Mastoid air cells were poorly
pneumatized and diffusely cloudy, and the frontal incisors were
widely spaced.

    The vertebral columns of the four patients studied showed hypo-
plasia of the odontoid process and, to a mild degree, of cervical
vertebral bodies. Thoracic spine was relatively uninvolved, with
only mild central anterior beaking of the bodies of the lower two
or three thoracic vertebrae. Kyphosis, varying from mild to severe,
was present at the T 12 - L 1 region, and anterior inferior beaking
of lumbar vertebral bodies was apparent in all cases, mildly so in
patient #4, but severe in patients #s 2 and 5. In all, the L 5

TABLE I

Clinical Features of Five Patients With Fucosidosis in This Study, in Comparison With Those of Eleven Others

Patient #	1	S 2	3	4	S 5	6	S 7	8	9	10	S 11	12	S 13	14	15	16
Reference							-5,6,7-	13	24		-1-		-10-	18	20	15
Sex	M	M	M	M	M	M	F	M	M	M	F	M	M	M	M	F
Age onset disease	<2y	2y	?	1y	19m	$1\frac{3}{12}$	1y	$1\frac{4}{12}$	$\frac{6}{12}$	<2y	1y	1y	?	$1\frac{2}{12}$	?	?
Age as of report	12y	14y	17y	6y		$3\frac{3}{12}$(d)	$5\frac{2}{12}$(d)	5y(d)	$4\frac{1}{2}$	17y	5y	9y	$4\frac{1}{2}$	20y	9y	5y
Mental retardation	+	+	+	+	−	+	+	±	+	+	+	+	+	+	+	−
Growth retardation	+	+	+	−	−			+	+	+	+	+	+	+	+	+
Coarse facies	+	+	+	+	+		−	+	+	+	+	+	−	+	+	+
Clear corneas	+	+	+	+	+		−	+	+	+	+	+	+			+
Enlarged tongue	+	+	+	+	−	−	+	+	±	+	+	−	+	−		+
Enlarged liver	−	−	±	−	−	+	+	+	+	−	−	−	−	−		±
Enlarged spleen	−	−	±	−	−	+	+	+	−	−	+	−	−			−
Enlarged heart	−	−	−	+	−	+	+	−	+	+	+	+	+	+		−
Thick skin	+	+	+	+	−	+	+	?	−							+
Angiokeratomas	+	+	−	+	−	+	+	+	+	+	+	+	+	+		+
Recurrent respiratory infection	+	+	?	−	±	+	+	+	+					+		+
Early hypotonia	+	?	?	−		+	+	?	?					+		
Later spasticity		+	?	+		+	+	−	+	+	+					+
Vacuolate lymphocytes	+	+	?	+		+	+	+18%	+	+	1%	+	+			+
Vacuolate cells, bone marrow	+	+	?	+		−	?	−	+		−	+	+			+
Urine mucopolysaccharide	−	−	−	−	−	−	−	±	−	−	−	−	−		−	−
High sweat electrolytes	−	+	−	+		+	+		+	−	−	−	−			+

− not present or normal; ± doubtfully present; + present; blank--not stated, not determined or not determinable; (d) age at death; S siblings.

vertebra was hypoplastic and its pedicle was quite short, resulting in narrowing of the spinal canal at this level. The coccyx was absent or poorly developed in all (fig. 1). No calcification of intervertebral discs was found.

The rib cage was normal in contour, except that slight shortening of the clavicles and first ribs produced a slightly constricted thoracic inlet. There was slight widening of the medial ends of the clavicles, but the sternum was normal. Patient #2 had only 11 pairs of ribs, plus a rudimentary right 12th rib. The ribs become mildly broader with age, but do not develop the spatulate configuration seen in Hurler's disease. The heart was radiologically normal, and the lungs appeared normal except for the frequent presence of pneumonia.

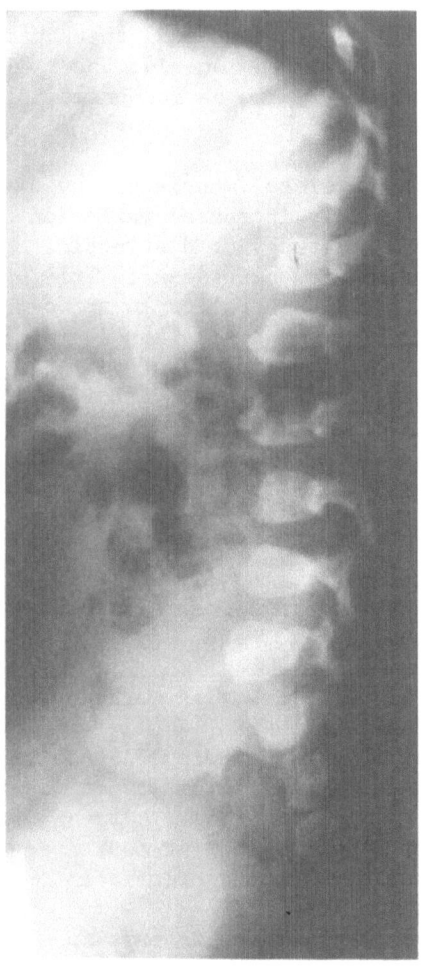

In the upper extremities, the glenoid fossae were broad and shallow. The long bones were initially normal, but with age there was relative overgrowth of the distal radii, with lateral bowing of the radial shafts. The distal radial-ulnar lines thus assumed a V-shape, with poor development of the medial aspect of the distal radial metaphysis and epiphysis, and of the lateral aspect of the distal ulnar metaphysis and epiphysis. Severe retardation of bone maturation was present in all, and mild deformities of the carpal bones were noted. Sclerotic epiphyseal ossification centers of the short tubular bones

Fig. 1 - Lateral X-ray view of lower thoracic and lumbosacral vertebral column of patient #2 at age 4½ years. Similar changes were seen in the four patients who had spinal X-ray studies (#s 1,2, 3,4), with slight kyphosis at the thoraco-lumbar junction, anterior inferior beaking of the upper lumbar vertebral bodies, hypoplasia of the fifth lumbar vertebra, and absence or severe hypoplasia of the coccyx. (Hypoplasia of the odontoid process is not visible in this X-ray.)

of the hands were present in patients #s 1 and 2, and peculiar taper-
ing of the distal ends of the proximal phalanges became more prominent
with age. The olecranon processes were hypoplastic. Progressive
demineralization and cortical thinning of all bones occurred with age.

The pelvis was initially normal but, with age, irregularity and
increased obliquity of the acetabular roofs occurred, and flattening
of the capital femoral epiphysis developed, affecting the medial
part particularly. Coxa valga thus developed with increasing age,
but femoral necks were otherwise normal.

In the lower extremities, demineralization of all bones progressed with age, and slight overtubulation of long bones was apparent.
Patellae were hypoplastic. The feet showed no gross deformity,
although slight irregularities of mid-tarsal bones were present.

Excretory urograms were normal in patients #s 1 and 2. Barium
esophogram showed dilatation of the esophagus, and unusual thickened
mucosal folds, in patient #2, but esophagram in patient #4, upper GI
and small bowel studies on patients #s 1 and 2, and barium enema in
patient #1, were normal.

PATHOLOGICAL AND HISTOCHEMICAL FINDINGS: Skeletal muscle biopsy
from patient #2, at age 2 years, showed mildly increased variation
in fiber size, but no apparent denervation atrophy or dystrophic
degeneration, and fine cytoplasmic vacuolation, best seen in Tri-
chrome stains. Small scattered or clustered, central or subsarcolemmal, granules stained more strongly with PTAH stain than do mitochondria (fig. 7); they were not PAS-positive. Tonsils of patient
#2, at 3 years, showed a moderate number of macrophages with vacuolo-

---

Fig. 2 - Nasal polyp of patient #2 at 12 years, showing cytoplasmic
vacuolation of respiratory epithelial cells and of stromal macrophages and fibroblasts. (H&E, X 500)
Fig. 3 - Acid phosphatase stain of same specimen as fig. 1, X 125,
showing strong finely granular stain, typical of lysosomal accumulation, in respiratory epithelium, stromal cells, and capillary
endothelium.
Fig. 4 - Skin biopsy of patient #2 at 13 years, showing marked cytoplasmic vacuolation of sweat gland epithelium. (H&E, X 315)
Fig. 5 - Rectal biopsy of patient #2 at 5 years, showing PAS-positi-
vity of macrophages in lamina propria (on left), and of stromal cells
in the submucosa (on right). (X 125)
Fig. 6 - Rectal biopsy of patient #1 at 3 years, showing positive
granular Sudan stain of PAS-positive cells of lamina propria
mucosae and submucosa. (Sudan black B, X 310)
Fig. 7 - Skeletal muscle biopsy of patient #2 at age 2 years,
showing occasional cytoplasmic vacuoles and a collection of
small subsarcolemmal granules. (H&E, X 500)

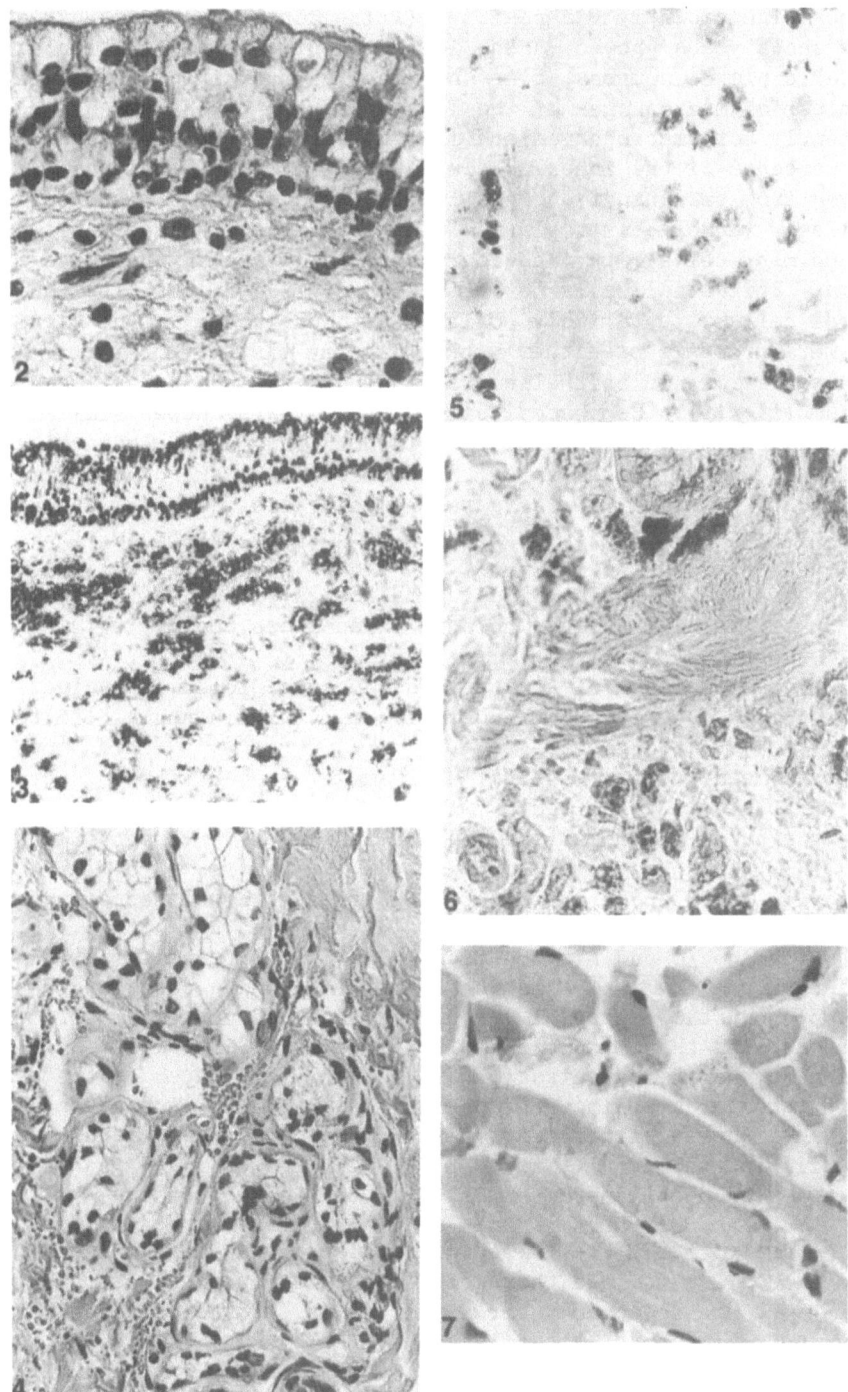

granular cytoplasm; their cytoplasm was often Sudan-positive, but
was not significantly PAS-positive (11). Rectal biopsy of patient
#2 at age 5 years showed PAS-positive cytoplasmic granulation of
myenteric plexus neurons, plus abundant PAS-positive material in
cytoplasm of macrophages of the lamina propria mucosae, and in cells,
apparently both macrophages and fibroblasts, in the submucosa and
fibrous septa of the inner muscle layer (fig. 5). Nasal polyps
removed from patient #2 at ages 10, 11, 12 and 13 years showed
strikingly vacuolate cytoplasm of respiratory epithelial cells (fig.
2), and many cells with vacuologranular cytoplasm in the loose myxoid
stroma. Epithelial cells were PAS, but not Sudan, positive, while
stromal cells were variably positive by both; there was no significant metachromasia of either with toluidine blue. Acid phosphatase
stain was strong in epithelium, stromal cells, and in capillary endothelium (fig. 3). Esophageal biopsy at 10 years showed similar PAS
and Sudan staining of stromal cells, which were also alcian blue
positive, and hyalinization of the connective tissue of the lamina
propria. Skin biopsy at 13 years showed hyalinization of the papillary layer of the dermis, markedly swollen pale cytoplasm of sweat
gland epithelial cells (fig. 4), and also cytoplasmic swelling of
dermal fibroblasts and basal epidermal cells. These cells showed
PAS, Sudan, toluidine blue and acid phosphatase positivity.

Microdissection of sweat glands gave the following values:
mean duct length (MSGDL)--1.8 mm. (within normal limits
for age)
"mean coil area" (MCA)--0.10 mm^2. (upper limit of normal
for age)
ratio MSGDL/MCA (sweat gland index)--19. (lower limit of
normal for age).
These values are those of sweat glands with enlarged secretory coils.

Microscopic and histochemical findings in rectal biopsies of
patient #1 and 3 at 4 years were similar to those described above
(fig. 6), but the degree of cytoplasmic storage in rectal stromal
cells was less than in patient #1 at 5 years. Skin biopsy at 11
years also showed hyalinization of the papillary layer of the dermis,
marked vacuolar swelling of sweat gland epithelium, and cytoplasmic
swelling of dermal fibroblasts. Microdissected sweat glands had
the following values:
mean duct length (MSGDL)--1.4 mm. (small for age)
"mean coil area" (MCA)--0.14 mm^2 (large for age)
ratio MSGDL/MCA (sweat gland index)--10 (low for age).
These values, again, are those of glands with enlarged secretory
coils. (We are indebted to Mr. T. R. Wells, Microdissection Laboratory, CHLA, for these determinations.)

Skin biopsy of patient #3, at age 17 years, showed increased
PAS and acid phosphatase staining of sweat-gland epithelium, but the
degree of cytoplasmic swelling was less marked than in the specimens
from patients #s 1 and 2.

ELECTRON MICROSCOPIC STUDIES: Electron microscopic studies have
been carried out on specimens from nasal polyps of patient #2, and
on skin biopsies and cultured skin fibroblasts from patients 1, 2
and 3. The tissues and tissue culture preparations were fixed and
processed for electron microscopy by standard methods. Nasal epithelial cells contained varying numbers of membrane-bound vacuoles
(lysosomes), which usually contained loose granular material suggestive of polysaccharide; in many, however, lamellar material consistent with lipid was present (fig. 8). Capillary endothelium in the
polyps, and also in the dermis, contained large numbers of smaller
storage-lysosomes, with both granular and lamellar content (fig. 9),
and similar material was present in perithelial cells' and fibroblasts. These findings support the histochemical demonstration of
both PAS and Sudan positivity of affected cells, and the abundant
acid phosphatase activity of epithelial, stromal and endothelial
cells in the nasal polyps. In the skin specimens, myoepithelial
cells of sweat glands contained many storage-lysosomes, smaller and
with more dense content than those in respiratory epithelium (fig.
10). Secretory and duct epithelium also were markedly involved (figs.
10,11), the material in the storage granules being more variable in
appearance, with a tendency to clearer matrix, than those of respiratory epithelium. No sebaceous glands were found in these specimens,
but epithelial cells of hair follicles contained a few storage-
granules. Cutaneous nerves, both myelinated and unmyelinated, showed no apparent abnormality of axons or Schwann cells, but nerve
sheath fibroblasts, and dermal fibroblasts generally, were markedly
affected, with large amounts of pale cytoplasmic storage-lysosomes
(fig. 14). In contrast, skin fibroblasts in tissue culture showed
abundant small granules with much electron-dense membranous material
(figs. 12,13). In peripheral blood specimens, lymphocytes contained
a small number of cytoplasmic vacuoles with pale granular polysac-
charide-type content (fig. 15). Occasional polymorphonuclear cells
contained a few much larger vacuoles, and rare cells of undetermined
type contained many cytoplasmic storage-lysosomes. No effect on the
size, number or content of the storage lysosomes in peripheral blood
white cells was noted following infusion of normal plasma in
patient #1.

GENETICS: It is accepted that fucosidosis is transmitted as an
autosomal recessive character, and this view is supported by the
data of our study. The a-1-fucosidase activity of mixed leucocyte
preparations from normal adults, obligate heterozygotes (parents)
and fucosidosis patients, summarized in Table 2, shows that adults
heterozyous for fucosidosis have approximately half (average 43%)
the normal enzyme level in white blood cells. We have found that
5-10% of normal individuals have extremely low plasma a-1-fucosidase
activity, and family studies indicate that this is an inherited
characteristic. The plasma enzyme activity of a person can be
classified as high, intermediate, or low (Table 3).

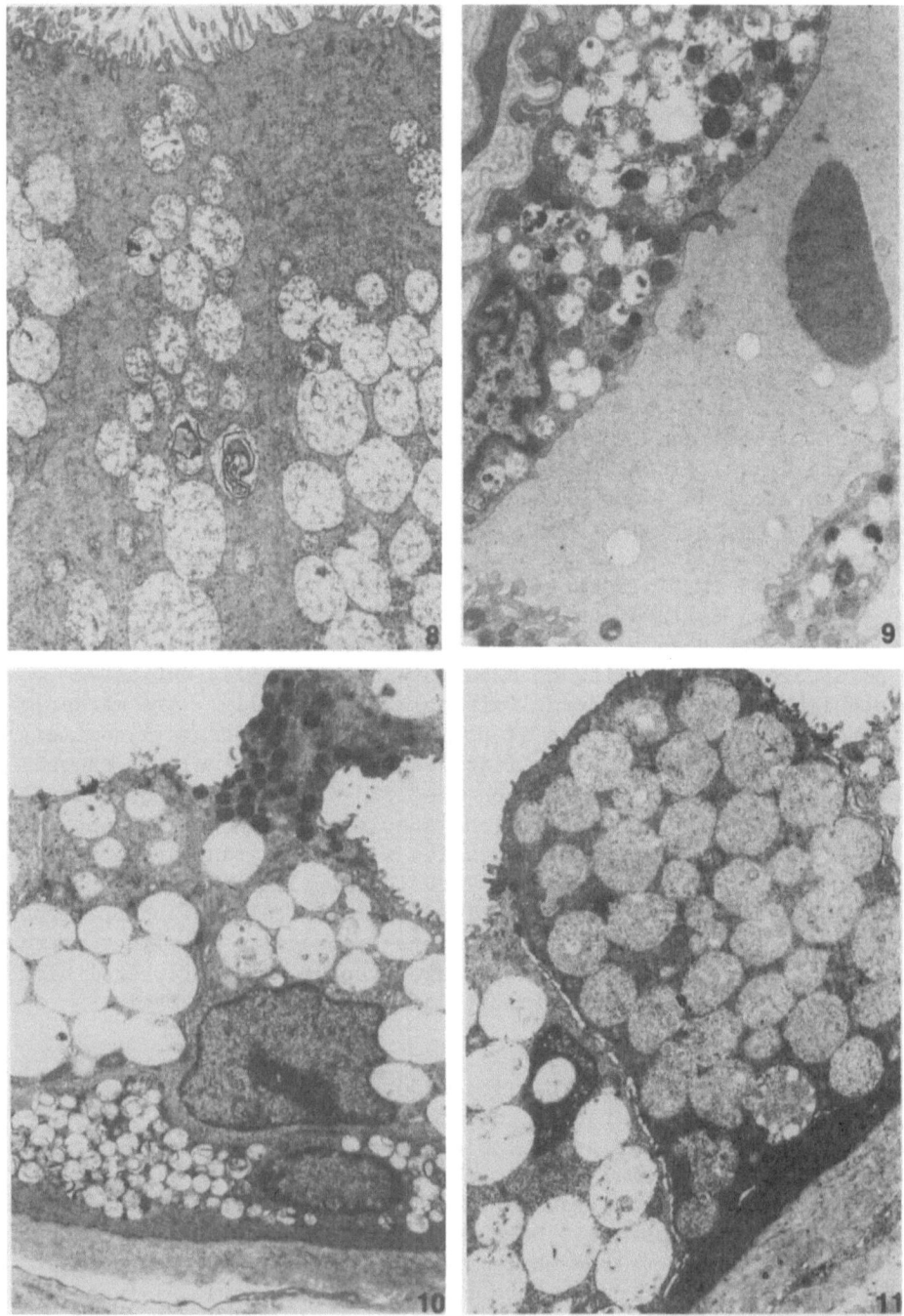

Fig. 8 - Nasal polyp of patient #2. The surface of the epithelial
cells shows cilia. The vacuoles (lysosomes) are of variable size,
and contain granular material and occasional membranes. (X 5600)
Fig. 9 - Capillary in dermis of patient #2. Endothelial cell cytoplasm shows abundant bodies, some containing granular and some
dense material. (X 7500)
Fig. 10 - Sweat gland of patient #2. The myoepithelial cell at the
base of the gland is filled with vacuoles which usually contain
some membranes. The secretory cell has mostly clear vacuoles.
Relatively few glands contained the normal dense secretory granules
noted in the upper center. (X 5000)
Fig. 11 - Sweat gland of patient #2. This gland shows various types
of vacuoles, one clear and the other containing granular material.
(X 5000)

TABLE 2

Alpha-1-fucosidase Levels of Peripheral Blood White Cells*

	Normal adults	Obligate heterozygotes for fucosidosis	Fucosidosis patients
Number studied	18	5	5
Mean activity	24.6	10.6	0
Range	18.2 - 32.4	6 - 12.5	
S.D.	4.2	2.6	

*Activity is expressed as nanomoles of p-nitrophenol formed per
hour per mg. protein, using p-nitrophenyl-a-1-fucoside as substrate.

TABLE 3

Plasma a-1-fucosidase Activities of Normal Persons*

Category	High	Intermediate	Low
Number studied	24	29	10
Mean activity	284	123	19
Range	196-477	85-181	4-32
S.D.	70	22	8

*Activity is expressed as nanomoles of p-nitrophenol formed from
p-nitrophenyl-a-1-fucoside per hour per ml.

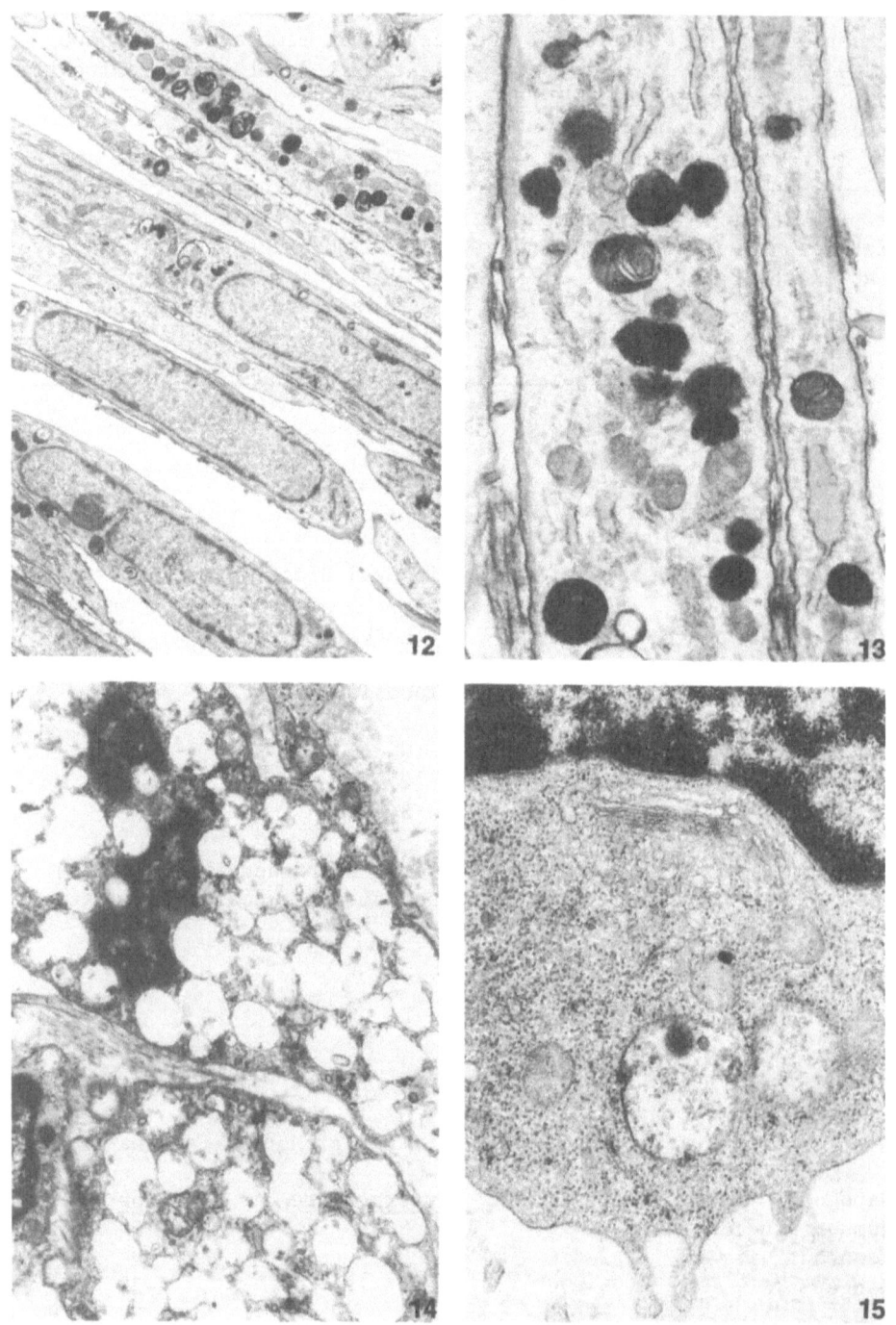

Fig. 12 - Skin fibroblast of patient #3, in tissue culture. This
low power view shows dense bodies, containing membranes, in the
cytoplasm, varying in number from cell to cell. (X4750)
Fig. 13 - Same specimen as fig. 5. Higher magnification shows the
dense granular and membranous character of the material in the
cytoplasmic bodies. (X 19,000)
Fig. 14 - Connective tissue cell of dermis of patient #2. The
cytoplasm is filled with clear vacuoles. (X 7500)
Fig. 15 - Lymphocyte of peripheral blood in patient #1. Two cytoplasmic bodies contain granular material somewhat similar to that
seen in sweat gland epithelium. (X 24,000)

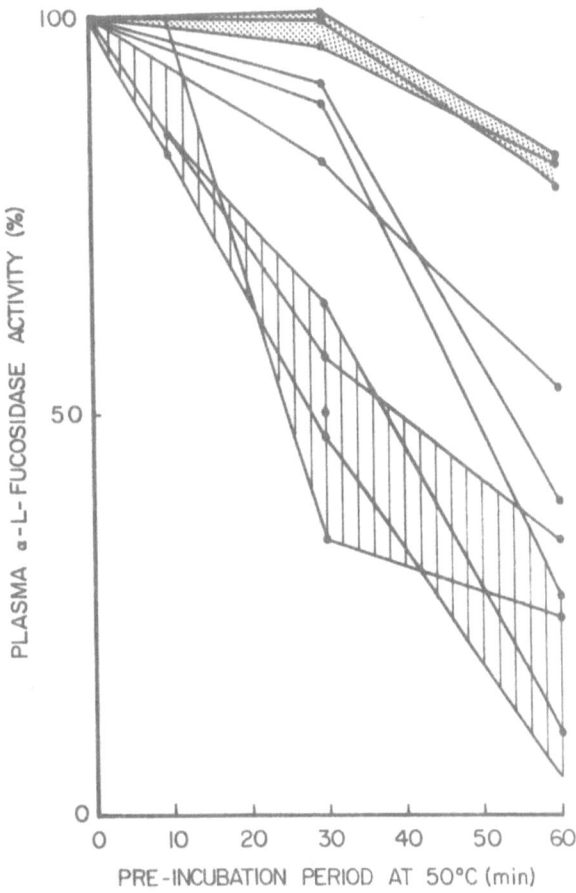

Fig. 16 - Thermostability of plasma a-1-fucosidase from persons
with high (upper curves), intermediate (middle curves) or low
(lower curves) enzyme levels.

In families in which both parents have high activity, the offspring have high activity. In families in which low and intermediate values occur, Mendelian segregation is suggested, and biochemical studies indicate that the enzyme with low activity is qualitatively different from those with high activity, based on heat stability and pH activity curves (17,27). The effect of pre-incubation of plasma from persons with normal, intermediate or low enzyme levels for varying periods of time at 50° C, with the assay performed at 37° C, is shown in fig. 16. Distinct thermolability of the fucosidase of persons with low plasma enzyme levels, and intermediate stability of that from persons with intermediate levels, is evident. Performance of assays at 50° C rather than at 37° C, without preincubation, however, gives increased activity (up to 200%) for both types of enzyme. With electrophoresis on cellulose acetate strips, the plasma enzyme from normal individuals migrates faster than that derived from urine, leucocytes, heart or liver. Whether the plasma enzyme is modified tissue (lysosomal) enzyme is not known. Thus leucocytes, urine, cultured skin fibroblasts, or other tissues, but not plasma, can be used to establish the diagnosis of fucosidosis.

PLASMA INFUSION: Plasma infusion studies (1 unit of fresh frozen plasma) were carried out on patients #s 1, 2 and 4. The enzyme from donor plasma persisted in the patients' circulation for an extended period, with decay curves exhibiting two different slopes (fig. 17). The early phase represents a half life of 8-9 hours, and the second phase one of approximately 22 hours. The plasma enzyme was not excreted into the urine, nor could it be demonstrated in patients' leucocytes tested at intervals up to 24 hours.

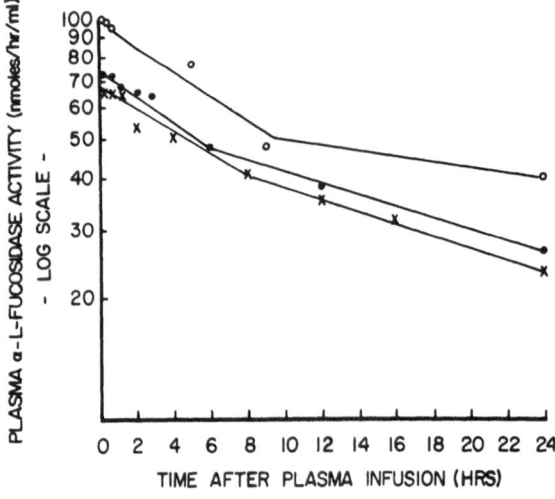

Fig. 17 - Plasma a-1-fucosidase activity after intravenous infusion of 1 unit of fresh frozen normal plasma. (Upper curve, patient #4; middle curve, patient #1; lower curve, patient #2.)

Borrone et al (1), (patients #s 10 and 11 of Table 1), whose serum
has unusually high levels of Le[a] substance. He also shows a high
titer of Le[x] and potent capacity to transform Le(a-b-x-) red blood
cells to Le(a+b-x+).

Our data, with those of Borrone et al (1), show that in fucosidosis there is abnormal expression of the Lewis blood group system.
ABH secretors normally have Le(a-b+x+) red cells, but the cells of
fucosidosis patients who are secretors react equally strongly with
anti-Le[a] and Le[b]. ABH non-secretors normally have Le(a+b-x+) red
cells, while the cells of non-secretors with fucosidosis also give
distinct, although weak, reaction with anti-Le[b].

DISCUSSION: Although only relatively recently (1968) described,
fucosidosis would appear to be a relatively common lysosomal storage
disease. At CHLA in the last decade it has compared in frequency
with Hurler's disease (MPS1), I-cell disease or generalized GM1
gangliosidosis type 1. Since the biochemical data indicate autosomal
recessive inheritance, an explanation for the striking (12 of 15)
male preponderance of reported patients is not apparent. Mediter-
ranean, especially Italian, ancestry of a high proportion of patients
suggests an epicenter, similar to those known for a number of other
lysosomal storage diseases. The implication of genetic homogeneity
of the disease in families derived from the epicenter may indicate
that the clinical dissimilarities among patients with fucosidosis
discussed above (type 1 and type 2 forms), and reported by others
(8,10,15), are not actually evidence for genetic heterogeneity.

Although fucose is an important component of the oligosaccharide
chains of glycolipids and glycoproteins of cell membrane (19), the
condition of hereditary low serum a-1-fucosidase level (17), which
causes no known clinical abnormalities, may suggest that hydrolysis
of such cell surface saccharides is not an important function of
serum a-1-fucosidase. Detailed study of blood group substances of
persons with this condition are needed, however. The fact that
persons with hereditary low serum a-1-fucosidase levels have no
obvious disease suggests that uptake of plasma enzyme into lysosomes
by pinocytosis does not make an important contribution to intracellular lysosomal fucosidase levels. The relatively long half-life of
infused plasma a-1-fucosidase, presented above, compared to half-
lives of 7.5-20 minutes for injected purified tissue lysosomal hydrolases (2), may support this, but the possibility that tissue fucosidase also enters cells poorly cannot be disproven at this time.
"Cross-correction" studies in tissue cultures would be of value in
this regard. The lack of obvious effect of infusion of normal plasma
on the storage-lysosomes in peripheral blood white cells in patient
#1 of this study also suggests that normal plasma a-1-fucosidase
enters at least some cell types poorly. Since normal plasma enzyme
does not appear therapeutically useful to patients with fucosidosis,
and since an appreciable amount of (? unmodified) tissue enzyme is

not normally present in plasma, transplantation of an organ, such as
kidney, which might release tissue enzyme, would not appear promising
for treatment of fucosidosis, but attempts to prepare and employ purified tissue enzyme(s) are certainly warranted.

The marked involvement of endothelial cells in fucosidosis may
reflect their normally high rate of pinocytosis, and it is possible
that the unhydrolyzed substrate which accumulates in their storage
lysosomes is derived from blood-group glycoproteins (85% carbohydrate), which are abundant on endothelial cells. Endothelial cell
involvement does not occur in the lysosomal storage diseases Hurler's
disease, Hunter's disease, and Sanfilippo disease (MPSs 1,2 and 3)
(12,21), but is seen in Sandhoff's generalized GM2 gangliosidosis (4).
Cardiac involvement is less impressive in fucosidosis than in I-cell
disease or Hurler's disease, for example, and the extent to which it
reflects endocardial versus myocardial damage is not certain. Brill
et al (3) compared the radiographic findings in two patients with
those of nine previously reported patients. Our findings are in
general accord with theirs, but the observations of premature fusion
of cranial sutures in two patients,of absent frontal and absent or
poorly developed sphenoid sinuses, of hypoplasia of the 5th lumbar
vertebra and its pedicle, of absence or severe hypoplasia of the
coccyx, and of minor dysplastic changes of hands and elbows are new.
Radiologic features do not appear to differentiate type 1 from
type 2 patients.

A number of the pathologic observations presented above offer
indications for further study. The apparent involvement of myenteric
plexus nerve cell cytoplasm, and the clinical findings of functional
deterioration in the central nervous system in patients with fucosidosis, are of interest, in view of the lack of abnormal findings in
peripheral nerves. More detailed analysis of the distribution of
nerve cell involvement, and of its severity in various areas of the
nervous system, would be of interest, and functional study of myenteric plexus neurons (e.g., by pressure tracing of peristaltic waves)
would be helpful. The muscular hypotonia which is a common early
feature of fucosidosis may reflect involvement of skeletal muscle
fibers, and the later feature of spasticity the progression of neuron
damage, but ultrastructural study of skeletal muscle is needed. Although the histochemical and clinical evidences of smooth muscle
involvement are slight, the striking changes in sweat gland myoepi-
thelium justify more detailed study of smooth muscle cells in a
variety of sites.

The striking involvement of respiratory tract epithelium, presented above, may, if also present in the lower respiratory tract,
explain the frequent occurrence of pneumonitis in patients with fucosidosis. The accessibility of nasal epithelium may suggest its
potential value for monitoring the effects of attempts at enzyme replacement. The underdevelopment of frontal and sphenoid sinuses,

and the recurrent maxillary sinus polyposis in patient #2 of this
series, may, in some way, reflect the nasal epithelial involvement.
Study of lower respiratory gland epithelium, and of salivary gland
epithelial structure and function, would be of interest. The marked
involvement of sweat gland epithelium described above can explain
the elevation of sweat electrolyte levels reported for some patients
with fucosidosis (see Table 1), but whether by direct effect on the
composition of primary sweat or by effect on electrolyte resorption
by duct epithelium requires further study. The hyalinization of
subepithelial connective tissue of skin and esophagus, at least,
suggest the skin lesions seen in Hurler's disease and I-cell disease,
for example. The mechanism by which lysosomal storage in fibroblasts apparently causes fibrosis is not known, but a comparable
disturbance of bone may explain the skeletal lesions described above.
The relatively slight involvement of white blood cells presented
above is in accord with the findings of Hansen (9). The histochemical and ultrastructural findings indicate that both fucose-containing
lipids and other fucose-containing compounds (? glycoprotein vs.
polysaccharide) normally serve as substrates for lysosomal a-1-fuco-
sidase, but their exact chemical structure is not yet known.

a-1-fucosidase activity can be demonstrated in cultured normal
amniotic cells, as well as in normal skin fibroblasts. Absence of
activity in cultured skin fibroblasts was demonstrated for four of
the five patients in this study. It is probable that pre-natal
diagnosis of fucosidosis can be made if enzyme activity is measured
in cultured amniotic cells, but probably not on the basis of levels
in amniotic fluid (14).

REFERENCES

1. Borrone, C., Gatti, R., Trias, X. and Durand, P.-Fucosidosis:
     Clinical, biochemical, immunologic and genetic studies in two
     new cases, J. Pediat. 1974, 84:727-730.
2. Brady, R.O., Pentchev, P.G. and Gal, A.E.-Investigations in
     enzyme replacement therapy in lipid storage diseases, Fed. Proc.
     1975, 34:1310-1315.
3. Brill, P.W., Beratis, N.G., Kousseff, B.G. and Hirschhorn, K.-
     Roentgenographic findings in fucosidosis type 2, Am. J. Roent-
     genol. 1975, 124:75-82.
4. Desnick, R.J., Snyder, P.D., Desnick, S.J., Krivit, W. and Sharp,
     H.L.-Sandhoff's disease: ultrastructural and biochemical studies
     in Sphingolipids, Sphingolipidoses and Allied Disorders, Ed.,
     B.W. Volk and S.M. Aronson, Plenum Press, 1972, pp. 351-371.
5. Durand, P. and Borrone, C.-Fucosidosis and mannosidosis, glyco-
     protein and glycosylceramide storage diseases, Helv. Paed.
     Acta 1971, 26:19-27.
6. Durand, P., Borrone, C. and Della Cella, G.-Fucosidosis, Lancet
     1968, 1:1198.

7. Durand, P., Borrone, C. and Della Cella, G.-Fucosidosis, J. Pediat. 1969, 75:665-674.

8. Gatti, R., Borrone, C., Trias, X. and Durand, P. - Genetic heterogeneity in fucosidosis, Lancet 1973,2:1024.

9. Hansen, H.G. - Hematologic studies in mucopolysaccharidoses and mucolipidoses, in Birth Defects: Original Article Series 1972, Vol. 8, #3, pp. 115-128.

10. Kousseff, B.G., Beratis, N.G., Danesino, C. and Hirschhorn, K. - Genetic heterogeneity in fucosidosis. Lancet, 1973, 2:1387-1388.

11. Landing, B.H., Neustein, H.B. and Kamoshita, S. - Biopsy diagnosis of lipidoses: background considerations, general concepts and practical aspects, in Sphingolipids, Sphingolipidoses and Allied Disorders, Ed., B.W. Volk and S.M. Aronson, Plenum Press, 1972, pp. 15-35.

12. Lasser, A., Carter, M. and Mahoney, M.J. - Ultrastructure of the skin in mucopolysaccharidoses. Studies performed before and after plasma infusion therapy, Arch. Path. 1975, 99:173-176.

13. Loeb, H., Tondeur, M., Jonniaux, G., Mockel-Phol, S. and Vamos-Hurwitz, E. - Biochemical and ultrastructural studies in a case of mucopolysaccharidosis "F" (fucosidosis). Helvet. Paed. Acta 1969, 36:519-537.

14. Matsuda, I. - Personal communication.

15. Matsuda, I., Arashima, S., Anakura, M., Ege, A. and Hayata, I. - Fucosidosis. Tohoku J. Exp. Med. 1973, 109:41-48.

16. Ng, W.G., Donnell, G.N. and Koch, R. - Serum a-1-fucosidase activity in the diagnosis of fucosidosis. Pediat. Res. 1973, 7:391.

17. Ng, W.G., Donnell, G.N., Koch, R. and Bergren, W.R. - Biochemical and genetic studies of human plasma a-1-fucosidase. XIII International Congress of Genetics, Berkeley, California, August, 1973.

18. Patel, V., Watanabe, I. and Zeman, W. - Deficiency of a-1-fucosidase. Science 1972, 176:426-427.

19. Roseman, S. - Sugars of the cell membrane, in Cell Membranes: Biochemistry, Cell Biology and Pathology, Ed. G. Weissmann and R. Claiborne, HP Publishing Co., 1975, pp. 55-64.

20. Schafer, I.A., Powell, D.W. and Sullivan, I.C. - Lysosomal bone disease. Pediat. Res. 1971, 5:391-392.

21. Spicer, S.S., Garvin, A.J., Wohltmann, H.G. and Simson, J.A.V. - The ultrastructure of the skin in patients with mucopolysaccharidoses. Lab. Invest. 1974, 31:488-502.

22. Sturgeon, P. and Arcilla, M.B. - Studies on the secretion of blood group substances. 1. Observations on the red cell phenotype Le(a+b+x+), Vox. Sang. 1970, 18:301-322.

23. Sturgeon, P. and Arcilla, M.B. - Le^x, the spurned antigen of the Lewis blood group system. Vox. Sang. 1974, 26: 425-438.

24. Van Hoof, F. and Hers, H.G. - Mucopolysaccharidosis by absence of a-1-fucosidase. Lancet 1968, 1:1198.
25. Voelz, C., Tolksdorf, M., Freitag, F. and Spranger, J. - Fucosidosis. Monatsschr. Kinderheilk 1971, 119:352-355.
26. Watkins, W.M. - Blood group substances. Science 1966, 152: 172-181.
27. Wood, S. - A sensitive fluorometric assay for a-1-fucosidase. Clin. Chem. Acta 1975, 58:251-256.
28. Zielke, K., Okada, S. and O'Brien, J.S. - Fucosidosis: diagnosis by serum assay of a-1-fucosidase. J. Lab. Clin. Med. 1972, 79:164-169.
29. Zielke, K., Veath, M.L. and O'Brien, J.S. - Fucosidosis: deficiency of alpha-1-fucosidase in cultured skin fibroblasts. J. Exp. Med. 1972, 136:197-199.

The authors acknowledge the support of the General Clinical Research Centers Branch, NIH (RR-86).

VARIABILITY OF EXPRESSIVITY OF α-FUCOSIDASE DEFICIENCY

Vimalkumar Patel and Wolfgang Zeman

Division of Neuropathology
Indiana University Medical Center
Indianapolis, Indiana 46202

I. INTRODUCTION

Following its discovery by Durand, et al., (1966), fucosidosis has been defined as a grave disease of infancy and early
childhood with premature death. This concept had to be modified
when Patel, et al., (1972) observed hitherto unknown aspects of
this enzyme defect, namely the occurrence of angiokeratoma
corporis diffusum and extension of the lifespan into adulthood.
Nevertheless, their patient also had severe mental retardation,
was dwarfed, and exhibited gargoylian features.

The present communication further extends the clinical
spectrum by demonstrating an even greater degree of variability
of expressivity. We have not only observed a patient with profound defect of this enzyme who showed only minor manifestations
of the disease, but we also have found phenotypically normal
blood relatives with an equally severe enzyme deficiency.

In view of this remarkable clinical heterogeneity, enzyme
studies were performed on three independent families which
suggest that the variability of expressivity might be controlled
again by genetic factors which code for blood group antigens,
glycolipids and glycoproteins. In other words, fucosidosis
appears to be an exceptional model for the study of the biochemical
basis of epistasis.

II. CLINICAL OBSERVATIONS

Proband Family S: J. S. was a full-term baby, although he
weighed only 5 lbs at birth. Two previous babies born to the
mother were also underweight but have since developed normally.
At the age of 3 months, the proband had his first convulsion
described by the parents as "pitching and jerking of the upper
and lower extremities with the eyeballs rolling". Electroen-
cephalograms revealed hypsarrhythmia and the patient was given
Valium to no avail. However, he improved on ACTH, as indicated
by an almost complete normalization of the EEG and a temporary
cessation of seizures.

Convulsions recurred at the age of 6 months, at which time
treatment with ACTH remained without success. At 12 months of
age, he suffered a spiral fracture of the midshaft of the right
femur, apparently without any trauma.

Physical examination at the age of 1 year revealed no
gargoylian features, no organomegaly, and no evidence of
skeletal abnormalities compatible with mucopolysaccharidoses
but corneal clouding was present. Dermatologic examination
revealed a roughening of the skin apparently due to "pili torti",
i.e. multiple twists along the longitudinal axis of the hair.
At the age of 14 months, he is cortically blind and severely
retarded, both mentally and physically.

Proband Family C: (previously reported (13)   M. C., a
23-year-old white male, was the product of an uneventful pregnancy and delivery. His parents are not known to be related to
each other by blood, nor are his grandparents. Early development was unremarkable, but at the age of 18 months mental and
motor retardation became obvious by his failure to walk and
talk; nor did he learn to understand the spoken word. At the
age of 24 months, muscular weakness and hypotonia were noted,
and his physical growth, being within normal limits up to this
time, began to slow down. Since that time the patient has
been bedridden, and has experienced frequent episodes of respiratory tract infections.

At age 4 years, he developed blue-brown, pinhead-sized,
raised skin lesions, first over the abdomen and back, and then
involving the lower, and finally the upper extremities, producing the characteristic picture of angiokeratoma corporis
diffusum. Histological examinations revealed multiple tele-
angioectasias. Anhydrosis and inability to control body
temperature developed synchronously with the skin lesions and
necessitated confinement in an air-conditioned room. Since
age 18 years, the patient has suffered from convulsions at the

rate of approximately one per month. The electroencephalographic
tracings showed low voltage activity throughout with occasional
paroxysms of 3- to 4-hz rhythmic waves, but no spike-wave
discharges.

As of the time of this report he weighs only 75 lbs, is 4 ft
tall, and shows severe kyphoscoliosis and pigeon chest. He never
displayed organomegaly nor did he present radiographic evidence
of skeletal abnormalities compatible with mucopolysaccharidoses.

Proband Family M: P. C. M., a 27-year-old white male, is a
successful journalist. He was a product of a normal pregnancy
and delivery and developed normally until the age of 18 years,
when macular, purpuric lesions were first noticed over the lower
torso and legs. Later on angiokeratoma corporis diffusum appeared
over abdomen and genitalia. No other signs of fucosidosis have
been uncovered by medical examinations.

III. ENZYME STUDIES

A. MATERIALS AND METHODS

Since all three probands exhibited a marked deficiency of α-
fucosidase but were clinically quite dissimilar, it was deemed
necessary to investigate the enzymes further. Towards this end,
the following studies were performed.

Sources of α-Fucosidase: Tissues from normal human individuals were obtained at autopsy (3 to 5 hours after death) and
stored at -70°C. Peripheral leukocytes from the probands, their
blood relatives, and normal control individuals were prepared according to previously reported procedures (16, 17). Blood sera
were collected by routine methods.

The tissues, including leukocytes, were homogenized in 1 mM
sodium phosphate buffer pH 6.8 and the supernatant concentrated
by lyophilization. These were fractionated on DEAE-cellulose or
Sephadex G-200 columns as previously described (2, 12).

Heat Inactivation: Aliquots of serum, leukocyte and tissue
extracts, and DEAE-cellulose and Sephadex G-200 fractions in
acetate buffer with pH 5.0, were kept at various temperatures
for 10 minutes and then rapidly cooled in crushed ice.   -fuco-
sidase activity was measured at 37°C.

Isolation of Fucose-Containing Glycolipids and Glycoproteins:
Two liters of urine from proband M. C. were filtered through fluted
paper, prewashed with chloroform-methanol (2:1). The filtrate was
assayed for enzymes, glycopeptides and glycoproteins. Soluble

glycolipids retained on the filter paper were extracted with 85%
ethanol (8). The extracts were flash-evaporated and the residue
dissolved in water for the determination of fucose. Dialyzable
and undialyzable fractions were prepared according to Lundblad
(10) and Brunngraber, et al. (3).

Enzyme Determinations: α-fucosidase and other lysosomal
enzyme activities were measured as previously described (13, 15).
Both p-nitrophenyl-α-L-fucoside and 4-Methylumbilliferyl-α-L-fuco-
side were used as substrates. Enzyme activity with fucose-
containing glycoprotein and undialyzable glycopeptides obtained
from M. C.'s urine was measured as follows: the enzymatic digest
was deionized and freed from unreacted substrates and proteins as
described by Bahl (1). The enzymatically liberated fucose was
assayed after Dische and Shettles (4).

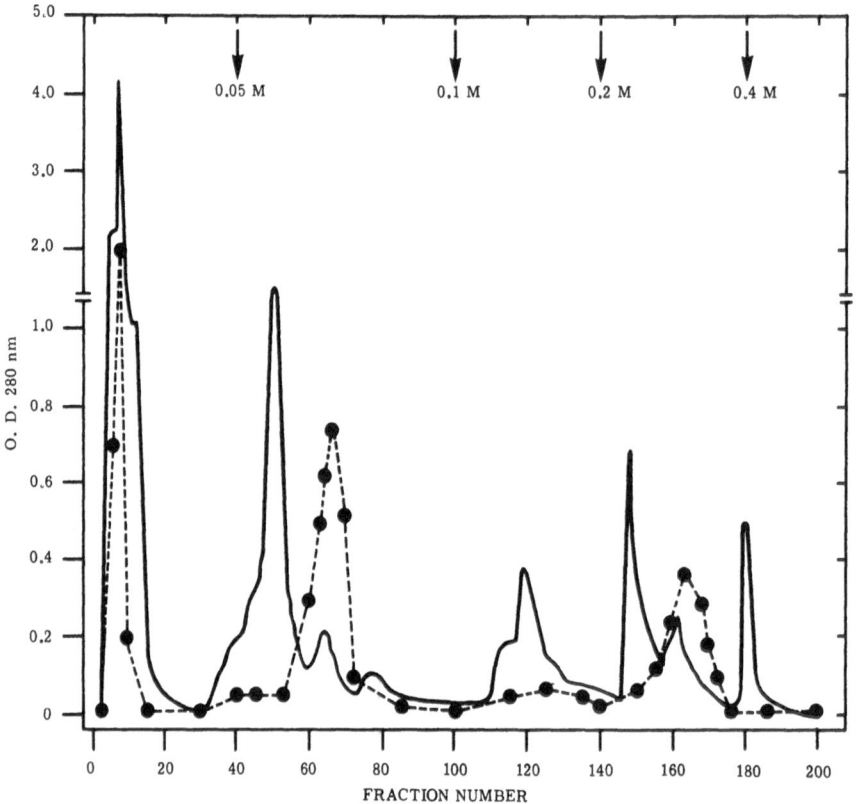

Fig. 1. DEAE-cellulose chromatography of lyophilized kidney extract at pH 6.8. The proteins (——) were eluted stepwise with
increasing concentration of NaCl. α-fucosidase activity was
measured with p-nitrophenyl-α-fucoside as substrate at pH 5.2.

B. RESULTS

DEAE-Cellulose Chromatography: Figure 1 shows proteins and
α-fucosidase fractions obtained from lyophilized kidney extracts.
Three separate peaks of enzyme activity are observed. Since the
unabsorbed fraction and the fraction eluted by .05 M NaCl exhibit
similar pH profiles and heat-lability, the unabsorbed fraction
was not studied further. The fractions eluted by 0.05 M and 0.2
M NaCl differ ·considerably with respect to pH profiles and stability toward heat (Fig. 2). The component eluted by 0.05 M NaCl

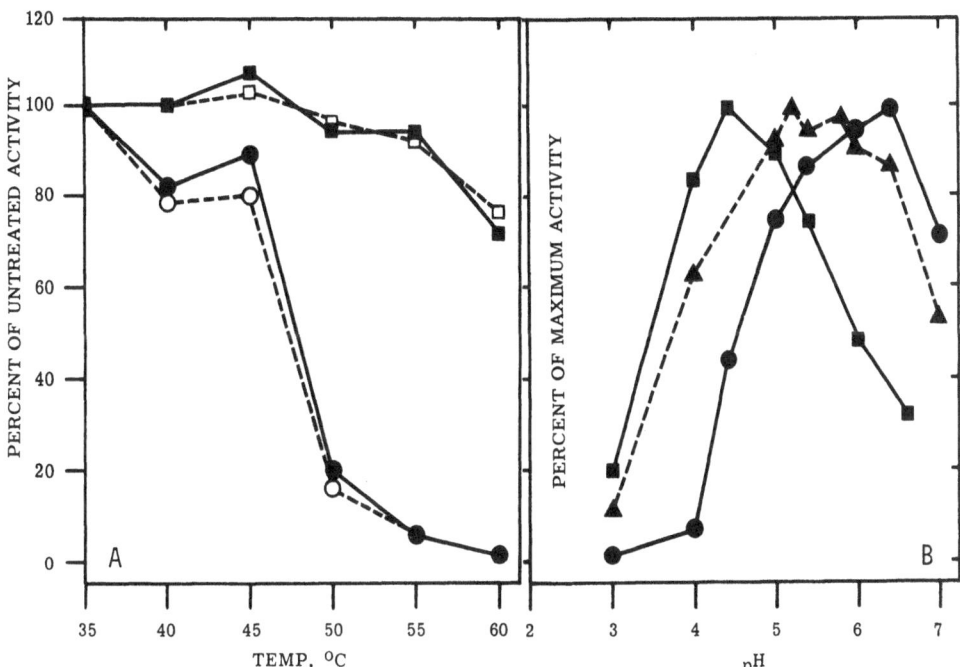

Fig. 2. A. Effect of temperature on kidney (——) and leukocyte
(—-—) α-fucosidase components. Circles and squares represent the
components eluted by 0.05 M and between 0.15 and 0.2 M NaCl,
respectively, from DEAE-cellulose column. Each component was
heated at a given temperature for 10 minutes (kidney) or 2 minutes
(leukocyte), and the activity measured at pH 5.2 where both components have approximately 80% of maximum activity.
B. Profiles of α-fucosidase components eluted by 0.05 M (●), 0.2 M
(■) and unfractionated kidney extract (▲). The activity was
measured in citrate-phosphate buffer.

is heat-labile and has a pH optimum of 6.5, the other component
has a pH optimum of 4.4 and is heat-stable. In contrast, whole
unfractionated kidney extract from which these components were obtained has a broad pH optimum as seen in Fig. 2B.

Activity of unfractionated leukocytic enzyme, though not
shown in the figure, behaves similarly to the crude kidney preparation, whereas fractionated leukocyte and liver extracts also
showed 2 α-fucosidase components as described above. More specifically, the leukocytic heat-labile component is eluted with 0.05
M NaCl and has a broad pH optimum of 4.4 (Fig. 2A). The liver
components were unstable and no detailed studies could be performed

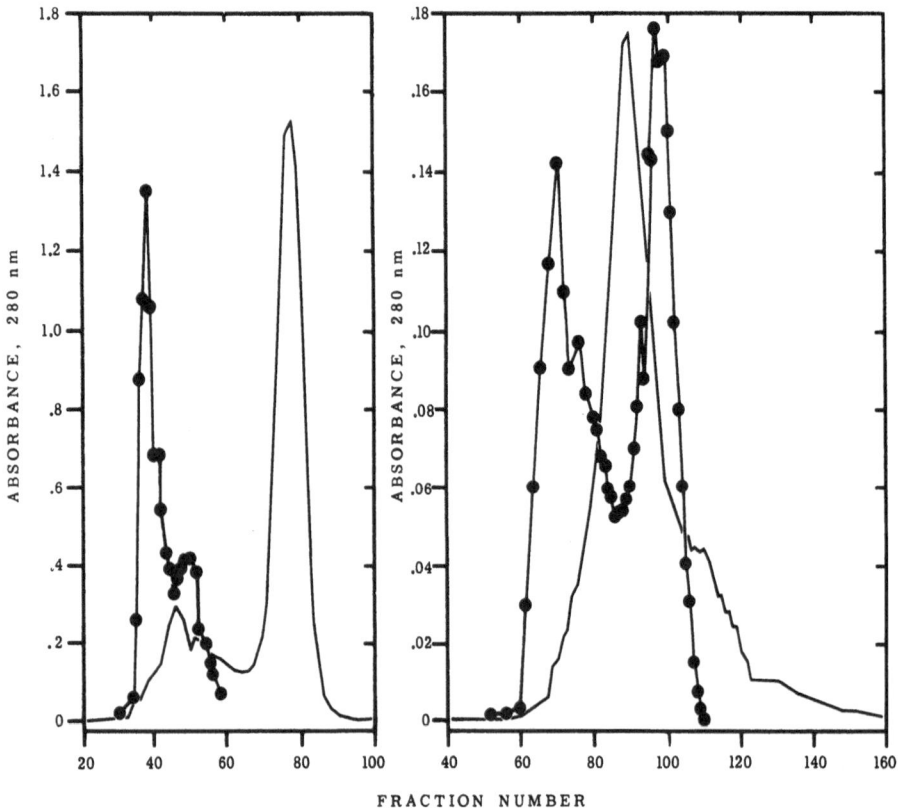

Fig. 3. Sephadex G-200 chromatography of lyophilized kidney extract
at pH 5.0. Elution of protein (——) was achieved by .05 M acetate
buffer containing 1 mM EDTA. The fractions containing α-fucosidase
activity (o——o) (left) were pooled and concentrated by lyophilization and rechromatographed (right). 2.5 ml fractions were
collected with a flow rate of approximately 10 ml/hr.

on these fractions.

   Sephadex G-200 Chromatography: The two components of kidney
derived α-fucosidase could also be separated on Sephadex G-200
(Fig. 3). The high molecular weight component is heat-labile,
with a pH optimum of 6.5, similar to that eluted by 0.05 M NaCl on
DEAE-cellulose. Conversely, the component with low molecular
weight has a pH optimum of 4.4 and is heat-stable.

   Other Lysosomal Hydrolases: The activity of several hydrolases determined on leukocytes and urine are shown in Tables I and

Table I

Hydrolase activity in leukocytes expressed
in nmoles of liberated p-nitrophenol per mg
protein per hour

Enzyme	Patient		Controls (10)
	J. S.	M. C.	
α-fucosidase	1.5	1.8	25 (19-37)
α-galactosidase	20.2	11.7	12 (11-18)
α-mannosidase	63.5	59.0	57 (45-67)
β-galactosidase	278.8	215.7	169 (130-215)
β-hexosaminidase	2120.5	1350.0	1275 (1000-1800)
acid phosphatase	-	5300.0	4500 (3500-6500)

II, respectively. Patients M. C. and J. S. show less than 10%
activity of α-fucosidase than controls. All other hydrolases determined are normal in range. Neither leukocytes nor urine was
available from patient P. C. M.

   Activity of serum hydrolases are shown in Table III. Again,
the activity of α-fucosidase is markedly reduced in the three probands and measures less than 10% of control values. All other
hydrolases studied were within normal range, which is particularly
significant with respect to α-galactosidase, which is deficient in

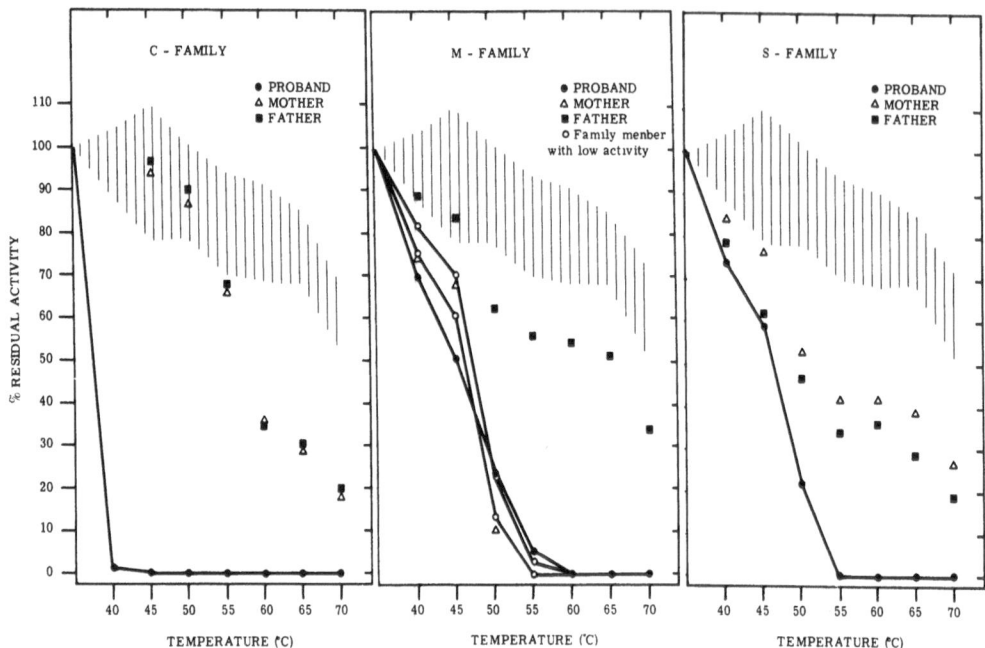

Fig. 4. Heat inactivation profile of serum α-fucosidase activity.

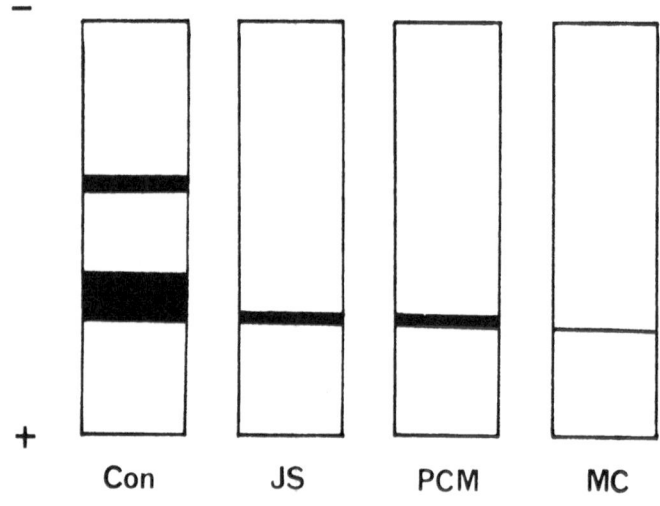

Fig. 5. Preliminary schematic presentation of electrophoretic
separation of Serum α-fucosidase activity. Con, control P. C. M.,
proband from M-family, J. S., proband from S-family, and M. C.,
proband from C-family.

Fabry's disease, a condition invariably associated with angiokeratoma corporis diffusum.

Heat Inactivation of Serum α-Fucosidase: The effect of heating on enzyme activity is shown in Fig. 4. The shaded areas
represent the variations in the control group. Even after heating
for 20 min at 70°C, the control group retains about 65% of initial
activity. In contrast, no measurable activity remains in any of
the patients after this treatment. Proband M. C. had no activity

Table II

Urinary hydrolase activity expressed in nmoles of
liberated p-nitrophenol per mg protein per hour

Enzyme	Patient		Controls (15)
	J. S.	M. C.	
α-fucosidase	8.2	6.0	88 (68–130)
α-galactosidase	78.7	66.0	58 (35–90)
α-mannosidase	98.5	87.0	56 (41–68)
β-hexosaminidase	2350.0	1680.0	1400 (850–1650)

left at 45° whereas P. C. M. and J. S. retained some activity up
to 55°C. The inactivation profiles for parents in the C- and S-
families, and the father in the M-family were intermediate between the controls and the patient. However, the mother and two
brothers of proband P. C. M. who all had initially less than 10%
of control activity, showed an almost identical inactivation profile as did the patient.

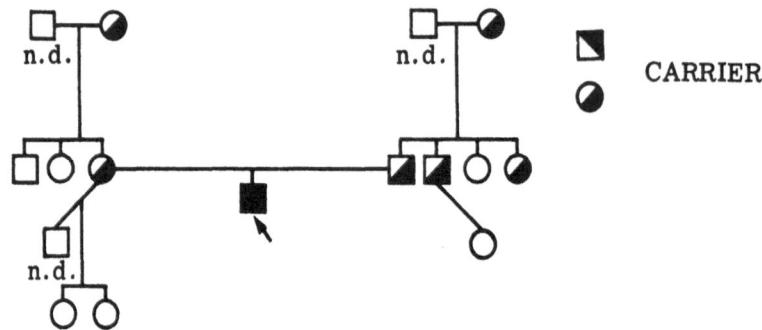

Fig. 6.   Pedigree of S-family.   Arrow indicates the proband.

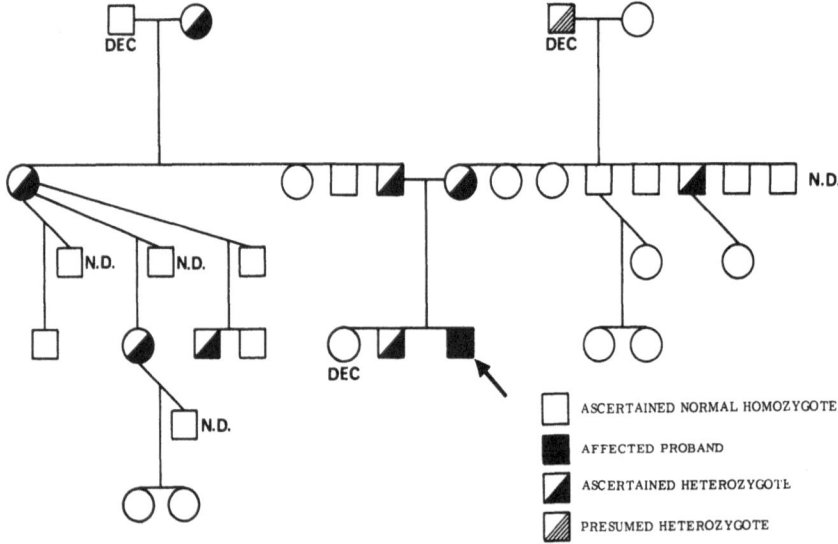

Fig. 7.   Pedigree of C-family.   Arrow indicates the proband.

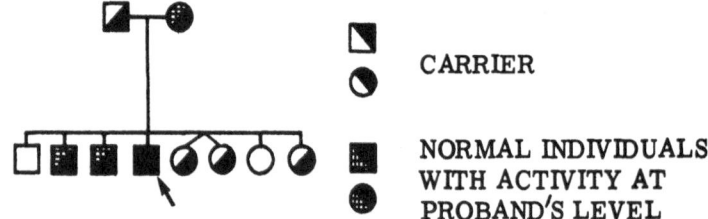

Fig. 8.   Pedigree of M-family.   Arrow indicates the proband.

Table III

Lysosomal glycosidases in human serum. The
activity is expressed as ng of 4-methylumbel-
iferyl released per mg protein per hour

Enzyme	Patients			Controls
	J.S.	M.C.	P.C.M.	
α-fucosidase	83.0	5.4	102.0	1320 (740-2450)
β-galactosidase	18.0	15.0	13.0	16 (8-38)
β-hexosaminidase	3700.0	3800.0	2800.0	3400.0 (1220-9900)

It appears from these studies that the heat-labile α-fucosidase component accounts for only 20% of initial activity in normal
controls, whereas this component represents the main activity in
the patients and also in the mother and two brothers of patient
P. C. M.

Electrophoretic Separation of Serum α-Fucosidase: A preliminary schematic representation of α-fucosidase components separated by electrophoresis is shown in Fig. 5. It is evident that
the anodal component is markedly reduced. Quantitative differences among the three patients were found, but were of minor magnitude.

Enzymatic Ascertainment of Heterozygotes: Leukocytic extracts
and/or sera of blood relatives of the probands were assayed for
α-fucosidase activity. Formerly, we had considered arbitrarily an
activity lower than 60% ofcontrols to indicate the carrier state.
(Figs. 6 to 8) This interpretation has now been confirmed by
determining the heat inactivation profiles which substantiated
the former assumption by being grossly abnormal as shown in Fig. 4.

Mixing Experiments: Sera of the three patients, their parents
and siblings as well as appropriate controls, were paired and mixed
in all possible combinations as shown in Table IV. No evidence for
compensation, nor activation or inhibition was produced, indicating
that the defective α-fucosidase component is probably identical or
at least near identical in all three families.

TABLE IV

Mixing Experiment: Determination of α-fucosidase activity in paired serum samples

	Initial Activity →	Proband M.C.	Proband P. C. M.	Proband J. S.	G. C. M.*	D. C. M.*	Control
		2.8	51.0	45.0	48.0	43.0	600.0
C-Mother	350.0	354.0	405.0	393.0	401.0	389.0	948.0
C-Father	300.0	301.0	350.0	347.0	351.0	345.0	903.0
M-Mother*	51.0	54.0	103.0	92.0	97.0	97.0	650.0
M-Father	250.0	256.0	307.0	301.0	302.0	298.0	853.0
S-Mother	300.0	301.0	358.0	342.0	346.0	343.0	898.0
S-Father	375.0	376.0	430.0	421.0	418.0	420.0	983.0
M. C.	2.8	-	52.0	48.0	49.8	45.0	601.5
P. C. M.	51.0	54.0	-	97.0	100.0	96.0	653.0
J. S.	45.0	47.5	98.0	--	101.0	89.0	643.5
G. C. M.*	48.0	50.0	97.8	97.0	-	88.0	648.5
D. C. M.*	43.0	46.0	96.0	88.0	90.0	-	640.0
Control	600.0	605.0	658.0	650.0	640.0	649.0	-

* Mother and two brothers (G.C.M. and D. C. M.) from M-Family show similar
  deficiency as does the Proband P. C. M.

Table V

Fucose content of substances isolated from the
M.C.'s urine, expressed in mg per g dry weight

Fraction	Control*	Patient
Non-dialyzable	40.5 (27-51)	65.7
Dialyzable glycopeptide	8.1 (6-11)	23.3
Non-dialyzable Fraction (containing glycoproteins and glycopeptides)	15.3 (10-23)	78.2
Water-soluble glycolipid	53.4 (23-60)	130.5

* Average of 5 controls; the figures in parenthesis indicate the
  range in controls.

Accumulation and Degradation of Fucose-containing Substances:
From the general concept of lysosomal diseases one would expect
lysosomal accumulation of fucose-containing biological species in
individuals with α-fucosidase deficiency. Unfortunately we were
unable to obtain tissue from any patient other than a skin punch
biopsy. Accordingly, we could not determine the noncatabolizable
biochemical species in the patients' tissues. However, we did
isolate fucose-containing compounds from the urine of M. C. as
shown in Table IV. All fractions which presumably harbor glycopeptides, glycoproteins, and water-soluble glycolipids, contained
markedly higher concentrations of fucose than homologue fractions
from age-matched normal controls. The greatest relative concentration of fucose was found in the nondialyzable fractions containing glycoproteins and glycopeptides, which revealed five times
as much fucose on a percentage basis as that of age-matched control preparations. These studies confirm the not unexpected conclusion that in α-fucosidase deficiency the degradation of fucose-
containing glycoproteins is also disturbed and that these compounds
accumulate in tertiary lysosomes, presumably those of the renal
tubular epithelium.

Although we observed a marked reduction of the heat-labile
component of α-fucosidase in the carriers, the deficient enzyme

nevertheless degraded the glycoproteins isolated from the patient's urine with a rate similar to that of whole enzyme extracts obtained from normal controls (Fig. 9). These observations suggest that the heat-labile component may not be strategically involved in the degradation of fucose-containing glycoproteins.

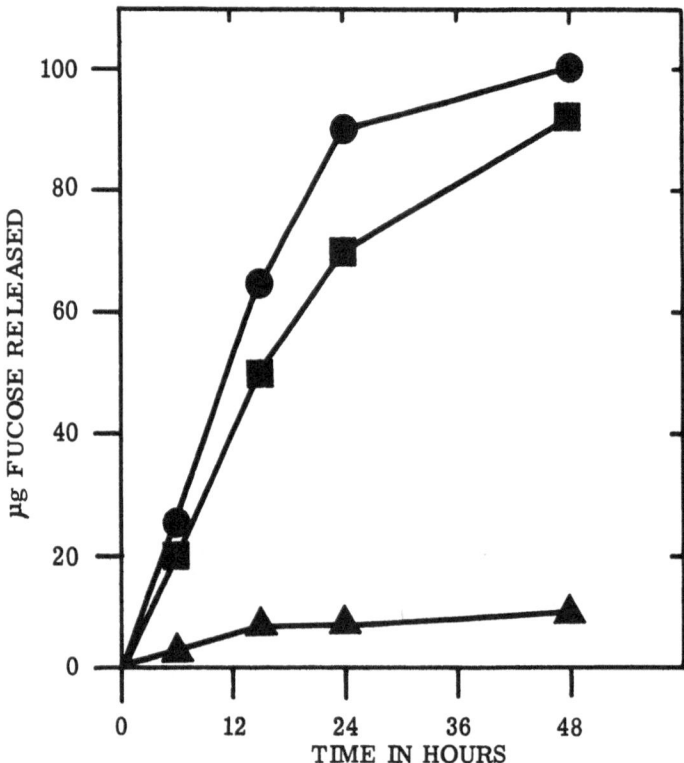

Fig. 9. Degradation of glycoprotein by leukocytic α-L-fucosidase. The reaction mixture contained 15 mg of glycoprotein (isolated from the patient M. C.'s urine) and 10-15 mg leukocytic proteins in 0.01 M acetate buffer. The total volume was 1.5 ml. Aliquots of 0.3 ml were withdrawn at 12 hour intervals in which the released fucose was measured. Appropriate substrate and enzyme blanks were included. The values for the controls represent averages of three individuals and those for the carriers the averages for mother and father of patient M. C. ▲, patient, ■, carrier, and ●, controls.

IV. DISCUSSION

a. Clinical Aspects

Obviously patient J. S. suffers from the disease which was first discovered by Durand, et al. (5), and subsequently termed fucosidosis as reviewed by Van Hoof (18). This condition is characterized by infantile onset, usually in the form of mental retrogression and arrested motor development, complicated by convulsions, leading to death during early childhood.

A second phenotype of this enzyme deficiency, also referred to as fucosidosis, was delineated by Patel, et al. (13) after a comprehensive examination of proband M. C. and his family. In this phenotype, the onset is during early childhood but the disease is much milder, both with respect to signs and progressions. Accordingly, such patients survive into adulthood. One important feature of this condition is the occurrence of angiokeratoma corporis diffusum which is usually manifested between the ages of 5 and 7 years. To date, five such cases have been reported (6, 9, 13). A similar case has recently been reported (11) affecting a woman with mental retardation, progressive motor degeneration, gargoylian features, skeletal abnormalities, and "lymphangioma" of the skin. However, a review of the original publication (14) clearly shows that this woman also has angiokeratoma corporis diffusum which began probably at age 5 years but was definitely present at age 11 years. Thus, of this phenotype, at least 6 cases are known, 4 being males, and 2 females. The signs of this particular disease are severe mental retardation, gargoylian features, skeletal abnormalities, and most important for differentiation, the occurrence of angiokeratoma corporis diffusum. It might be argued that the original patients of Durand, et al., and the patients with infantile onset might have developed similar skin lesions although this argument cannot be settled because of death during early childhood.

Yet another phenotype of α-fucosidase deficiency is exemplified by the proband in Family M. This 27 year-old male developed angiokeratoma corporis diffusum at age 18 years, but does not show any of the other manifestations of fucosidosis. He is eminently successful as a journalist and lives an entirely normal life. Even more significant is the fact that two of his brothers show the same degree of enzyme deficiency as does his mother, but none of these three individuals has any physical abnormality. Since one of the brothers with the enzyme defect is only 15 years old, it can be argued that he may yet develop the skin lesion.

It follows that α-fucosidase deficiency does not necessarily produce the disease fucosidosis as defined by Van Hoof (1973).

b. Biochemical Considerations

α-Fucosidase was first shown to consist of two components by Wiederschain and Rosenfeld (19) as obtained by gel filtration on Sephadex G-200 from pig kidney extract. These two components have also been demonstrated in human kidney and in liver. (20).

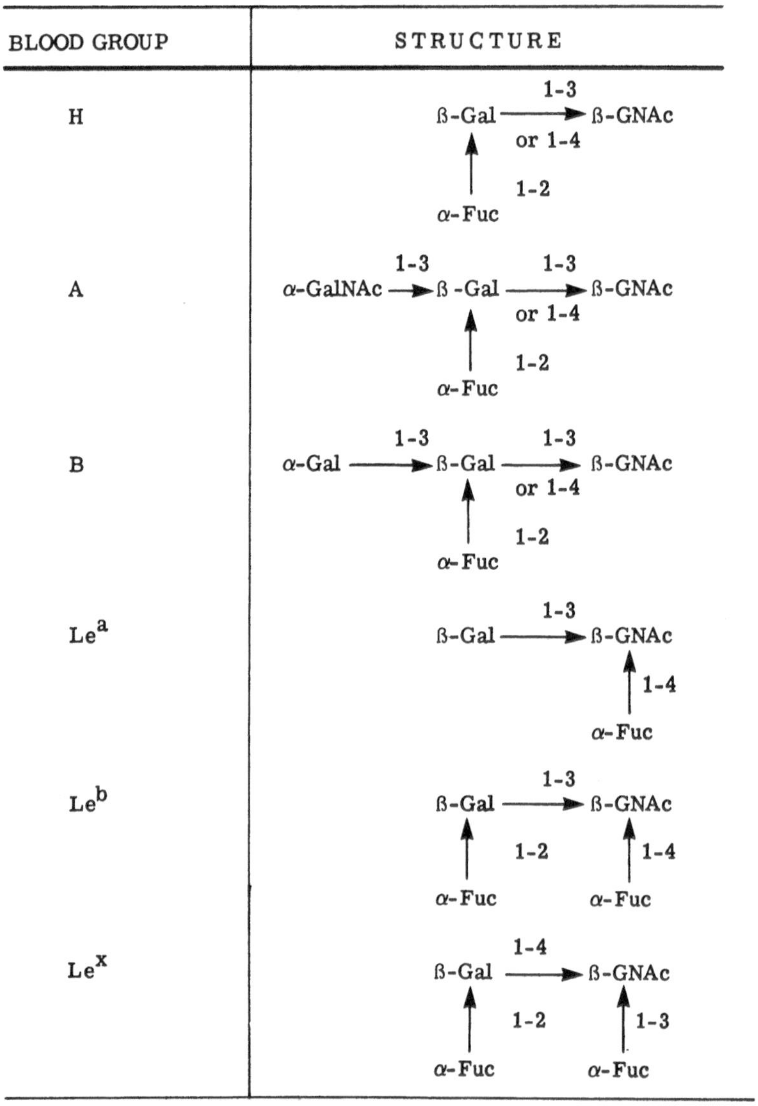

BLOOD GROUP	STRUCTURE
H	β-Gal $\xrightarrow{1-3}$ β-GNAc, or 1-4, $\uparrow$ 1-2, α-Fuc
A	α-GalNAc $\xrightarrow{1-3}$ β-Gal $\xrightarrow{1-3}$ β-GNAc, or 1-4, $\uparrow$ 1-2, α-Fuc
B	α-Gal $\xrightarrow{1-3}$ β-Gal $\xrightarrow{1-3}$ β-GNAc, or 1-4, $\uparrow$ 1-2, α-Fuc
Le^a	β-Gal $\xrightarrow{1-3}$ β-GNAc, $\uparrow$ 1-4, α-Fuc
Le^b	β-Gal $\xrightarrow{1-3}$ β-GNAc, $\uparrow$ 1-2, $\uparrow$ 1-4, α-Fuc, α-Fuc
Le^x	β-Gal $\xrightarrow{1-4}$ β-GNAc, $\uparrow$ 1-2, $\uparrow$ 1-3, α-Fuc, α-Fuc

*Modified from Watkins, W. M.: Science 152:172, 1966.

Fig. 10. Oligosaccharides of ABH blood group and Lewis specificities.

We have confirmed these findings on normal human kidney and liver extracts. However, owing to the fact that we had access only to live patients and their blood relatives, we have studied the characteristics of the enzyme mainly in serum and in leukocytes of patients, heterozygotes and controls. As reported here, both the serum and the leukocytic enzyme also consist of two components, α-fucosidase I which is thermo-stable and α-fucosidase II which is thermo-labile. The important finding of the present study is that all our probands with different phenotypes revealed very similar enzymatic defects, namely virtual absence of α-fucosidase I. The same component was absent in the mother and in two brothers of the patient in the M-family so that it appears rather conclusive that α-fucosidase I deficiency results in a variety of different phenotypes, spanning the range from normalcy to a very severe disease with infantile onset and premature death during early childhood.

c. Considerations on Phenotypical Variability

The fact that two phenotypes of fucosidosis have been found has been interpreted as evidence of genetic heterogeneity (6, 9), an erroneous conclusion in our opinion. Genetic heterogeneity is a conceptual term which expresses the fact that similar phenotypes are due to different genotypes but our studies seem to show rather conclusively that we have a specific genotype, namely α-fucosidase I deficiency which results in different phenotypes. This would then constitute genetic pleomorphism. It is our current opinion, though we do not have the data to support it, that this genetic pleomorphism is actually an example of epistasis, the result of the interaction of different genes at different loci.

This is a difficult concept and information on the subject is limited. Nevertheless, Wiederschain, et al. (20) could show that α-fucosidase II efficiently catalyzes 1--2 and 1--4 glycosidically linked fucose. That leads to the conclusion that α-fucosidase I deficiency can be expressed as a lysosomal disease mainly if the organism contains substances with a fucose in a 1--3 glycosidic linkage. Since these substances are genetically controlled, for instance with respect to the Lewis antigens (Fig. 10), it becomes clear that the enormous range of clinical manifestations of this enzyme defect has a genetic basis of its own. Obviously, many other fucose-containing compounds occur in the body in the form of oligosaccharides, glycolipids and glycoproteins (Fig. 11), and one may assume that each of these is somehow or other determined by genetic factors. Therefore, we would advance the hypothesis that the severity of the manifestations of α-fucosidase I deficiency is canonically conjugated with the genetically determined concentration and respective turnover of substrates which contain a terminal fucose in a 1--3 glycosidic linkage. Obviously

this is not an all-or-none situation and the relative deficiency
of α-fucosidase II observed in our patient may be an additional
pathogenetic factor, at least in the sense that the overall reduced catabolism of fucose-containing substances additionally
facilitates their respective lysosomal accumulation. Since the
sheer lysosomal accumulation of noncatabolizable products in

TRIVIAL NAME	STRUCTURE
2-Fucosyllactose	Galß1-4Glc 2 | Fucα 1
3-Fucosyllactose	Galß1-4Glc 3 | Fucα 1
Lacto-difucotetraose	Galß1-4Glc 2 3 | | Fucα 1 Fucα 1
Lacto-N-fucopentaose I	Galß1-3GlcNAcß1-3Galß1-4Glc 2 | Fucα 1
Lacto-N-fucopentaose II	Galß1-3GlcNAcß1-3Galß1-4Glc 4 | Fucα 1
Lacto-N-fucopentaose III	Galß1-4GlcNAcß1-3Galß1-4Glc 3 | Fucα 1
Lacto-N-difucohexaose I	Galß1-3GlcNAcß1-3Galß1-4Glc 2 4 | | Fucα 1 Fucα 1
Lacto-N-difucohexaose II	Galß1-3GlcNAcß1-3Galß1-4Glc 4 3 | | Fucα 1 Fucα 1

*Modified from Ginsburg et al.: In Glycoproteins of Blood Cells
and Plasma (Jamieson and Greenwalt, eds.) J. B. Lippincott Co.
p. 114, 1971.

Fig. 11.   Fucose-containing oligosaccharides of human milk.

lysosomal diseases is not per se damaging but rather the amount
of accumulation and perhaps its rate, it becomes clear that with
varying substrate concentration a wide spectrum of clinical manifestation is produced by an identical enzyme defect in different
individuals.

REFERENCES

1. BAHL, O. P.: Glycosidases of Aspergillus Niger, II Purifica-
    cation and general properties of 1,2, -α-L-fucosidase. J.
    Biol. Chem., 245: 299 (1970).

2. BECK, C., MAHADEVAN, S., BRIGHTWELL, R., DILLARD, C., and
    TAPPEL, A. L.: Chromatography of lysosomal enzymes. Arch.
    Biochem. Biophys., 128: 369 (1968).

3. BRUNNGRABER, E. G., BROWN, B. D., and HOF, H.: Determination
    of gangliosides, glycoproteins and glycosamine. Clin. Chem.
    Acta, 32: 159 (1971).

4. DISCHE, Z., and SHETTLES, L. B.: A specific color reaction
    of methylpentoses and a spec-rophotometric micromethod for
    their determination. J. Biol. Chem., 175: 595 (1948).

5. DURAND, P., BORRONE, C., and DELLA CELLA, G.: A new mucopoly-
    saccharide lipid storage disease? Lancet 2: 1313 (1966).

6. GATTI, R., BORRONE, C., TRIAS, X., and DURAND, P.: Genetic
    heterogeneity in fucosidosis. Lancet 2: 1024 (1973).

7. HOOGWINKEL, J., VELTKAMP, W., OVERDIJK, R., and LISMAN, J.:
    Electrophoretic separation of β-N-acetylhexosaminidases of
    human and bovine brain and liver and of Tay-Sachs brain tis-
    sue. Hoppe-Seyler's Z. Physiol. Chem. 353: 839 (1972).

8. KOSCIELAK, J.: Blood group A specific glycolipids from human
    erythrocytes. Biochim. Biophysic. Acta 78: 313 (1963).

9. KOUSSEFF, B., BERATIS, N., DANESINO, C., and HIRSCHHORN, K.:
    Genetic heterogeneity in fucosidosis. Lancet 2: 1387 (1973).

10. LUNDBLAD, A.: An ultrafilterable non-dialyzable fucose-rich
    glycopeptide fraction in normal human urine. Biochim. Bio-
    phys. Acta 101: 177 (1965).

11. MACPHEE, G., LOGAN, R., and PRIMROSE, D.: Fucosidosis: How
    many cases undetected? Lancet 2: 462 (1975).

12. PATEL, V., and TAPPEL, A.L.: Lysosomal β-galactosidoses of
    rat kidney. Biochim. Biophys. Acta 220: 622 (1970).

13. PATEL, V., WATANABE, I., and ZEMAN, W.: Deficiency of α-fuco-
    sidase. Science 176: 426 (1972).

14. PRIMROSE, D.: Mucopolysaccharidosis: A new variant? J.
    Ment. Defic. Res. 16: 167 (1971).

15. ROBINSON, D. and THORPE, R.: Fluorescent assay of α-fucosi-
    dase. Clin. Chim. Acta 55: 65 (1974).

16. SNYDER, R. and BRADY, R.: The use of white cells as a source
    of diagnostic material for lipid storage diseases. Clin.
    Chim. Acta 25: 331 (1969).

17. SUZUKI, Y., BERMAN, P., and SUZUKI, K.: Detection of Tay-
    Sachs disease heterozygote by assay of hexosaminidase A in
    serum and leukocytes. J. Pediat. 78: 634 (1971).

18. VAN HOOF, F.: Fucosidosis. in "Lysosomes and storage dis-
    eases". (H.G. HERS and F. VAN HOOF, Eds.). Academic Press,
    p. 277 (1973).

19. WIEDERSCHAIN, G.Y. and ROSENFELD, E.L.: Two forms of α -
    L-fucosidase from pig kidney and their action on natural oli-
    gosaccharides. Biochem. Biophys. Res. Comm. 44: 1008 (1971).

20. WlEDERSCHAIN, G., KOLIBABA, L., and ROSENFELD, E.: Human α-
    L-fucosidases. Clin. Chim. Acta 46: 305 (1973).

FUCOSIDOSIS

Glyn Dawson and Grace Chen Tsay

Departments of Pediatrics and Biochemistry
Joseph P. Kennedy, Jr., Mental Retardation
Research Center, University of Chicago
Chicago, Illinois 60637

Fucosidosis is an autosomally recessive inherited neurovisceral storage disease which has been attributed to a specific deficiency of the lysosomal hydrolase α-L-fucosidase (1,10,13,25). Onset of clinical symptoms occurs during the first two or three years of life, but the rate of progression of neurological degeneration to the decerebrate state may be variable. A considerable degree of clinical heterogeneity has been reported amongst fucosidosis patients (3,12). Thus, at least five patients (11,13,14) exhibited coarse facial features and skeletal abnormalities typical of the mucopolysaccharidoses, together with hepatosplenomegaly, cardiomegaly, thickening of the skin and repeated respiratory infections. A second group, characterized by the index case (10), rapidly progressed to spastic quadriplegia and bore less clinical resemblance to the mucopolysaccharide storage disorders; an intriguing finding in these patients was the abnormal sweat electrolyte levels, loss of gallbladder function and fibrotic degeneration of the pancreas. A third group showed a much more progressive cerebral degeneration (3,12,17) (with the oldest known patient in his late twenties) associated with skeletal abnormalities and angiokeratoma corporis diffusum. As yet there is no biochemical basis on which to differentiate the clinical variants of fucosidosis.

Neuropathological studies on fucosidosis tissue have revealed the presence of storage bodies filled with finely granular material in neurons, astrocytes and oligodendrocytes (10,13). Neurons were grossly distended and some lamellar inclusion bodies were observed. Evidence of extensive Wallerian degeneration of myelin sheaths was prominent and the appearance was likened to that of sudanophilic leukodystrophy. Similar investigation of liver revealed the cytoplasm of parenchymal cells to be filled with various forms of membranous storage bodies up to 3μ in diameter which appeared to be of lysosomal origin, together with Kupffer cells containing numerous clear inclusions (10,11,13,17).

Preliminary biochemical studies indicated the storage of "fucolipid" in liver, but not in brain, together with storage of other fucose-rich complex carbohydrate material (10,13,18) in both organs. Dawson (6,7) reported the characterization of the major stored glycosphingolipid in fucosidosis liver as H-antigen (Fuc $\alpha(1\longrightarrow2)$Gal $\beta(1\longrightarrow3)$ GlcNAc $\beta(1\longrightarrow4)$ Gal $\beta(1\longrightarrow4)$ Glc-Ceramide). Immunological studies have indicated that in addition to H-antigen, some patients have abnormally high titres to Le[a] and Le[b]-specific antibodies (3,10,18) indicating the possible additional storage of glycolipids containing Fuc $\alpha(1\longrightarrow3)$GlcNAc and Fuc $\alpha(1\longrightarrow4)$GlcNAc linkages. We have recently characterized two further major storage materials from patients with fucosidosis (21). The first is an oligosaccharide containing ten sugar residues, Fuc $\alpha(1\longrightarrow2)$ Gal $\beta(1\longrightarrow4)$ GlcNAc $\beta(1\longrightarrow2)$Man $\alpha(1\longrightarrow3)$ [[Fuc $\alpha(1\longrightarrow2)$Gal $\beta(1\longrightarrow4)$GlcNAc $\beta(1\longrightarrow2)$ Man $\alpha(1\longrightarrow6)$] Man $\beta(1\longrightarrow3)$ GlcNAc, which is structurally related to the oligosaccharide storage material in both G_{M1}-gangliosidosis (24) and the Sandhoff variant of G_{M2}-gangliosidosis (15) and is presumably derived from impaired glycoprotein catabolism. The second occurs either as a disaccharide (Fuc $\alpha(1\longrightarrow6)$ GlcNac) or a glycopeptide (Fuc $\alpha(1\longrightarrow6)$ GlcNAc-Asn) (21) and appears to be derived from a defect in the catabolism of the linkage region of a number of glycoproteins. The relative distribution of the three types of complex carbohydrate storage material in fucosidosis tissue and the insights this affords into complex carbohydrate catabolism will be the subject of this report.

MATERIALS AND METHODS

Autopsy samples of spleen, pancreas, lymph node, kidney and lung from patient 1 were provided by Dr. P. Durand, Gaslini Institute, Genoa, Italy, a skin biopsy from patient 2 by Dr. H. Loeb, University of Brussels, Belgium, liver and skin and urine biopsies from patient 3 by Dr. J. W. Spranger, University of Mainz, Germany,

an autopsy brain sample from patient 4 and urine from
patient 5 by Dr. D. Wenger, University of Colorado Medical School, Denver, U.S.A., urine and skin biopsy samples
from patient 6 by Dr. W. Zeman, University of Indiana
Medical School, Indianapolis, U.S.A., cultured skin
fibroblasts from patients 7 and 8 by Dr. J. S. O'Brien,
University of California, San Diego, La Jolla, U.S.A.,
and urine from patient 9 by Dr. Y. T. Li, University of
Tulane, New Orleans, U.S.A. and Dr. P. Durand. We are
deeply grateful for all these donations. Fucosidosis
fibroblast strains GM291 and GM292 from patients 10 and
11 were obtained from the human mutant cell collection,
Camden, New Jersey, U.S.A. A summary of the eleven
patients studied is presented in Table 1.

Isolation of Glycosphingolipids

Tissue samples (1-2 g fresh wt) were homogenized in
5 vols of 0.9% NaCl and extracted initially with 100 ml
of methanol, followed by two further additions of chloroform (100 ml). The mixture was filtered, 0.2 volumes of
0.9% KCl added and upper and lower phases separated as
described previously (8,23). Gangliosides were purified
and quantitated by gas-liquid chromatography (GLC) as
described previously (4,8,23). Total lipids were fractionated into neutral, glyco- and phospholipids by a modification (8) of the Vance and Sweeley silicic acid procedure (23). Glycosphingolipids were separated by thin-
layer chromatography and quantitated as described previously (8).

Isolation of Oligosaccharides and Low Molecular Weight
Storage Material

Tissue samples (10^7 cultured cells or 0.5-1.0 g
fresh wt of tissue) were sonicated in 2-5 vol. of distilled water, centrifuged to remove cell debris and
fractionated on Bio-Gel P-10 (21,22). The low molecular
weight fraction was pooled, concentrated, and the whole
sample applied to a column (180 x 1 cm) of Bio-Gel P-2.
An aliquot of each major fraction was then subjected to
total monosaccharide analysis by gas-liquid chromatography (4). Urine was subjected to an initial treatment
with 5 volumes of ethanol to precipitate glycoprotein
and high molecular weight oligosaccharide material (22).
Aqueous extracts of this precipitate and concentrated
fractions of the ethanol supernatant solution were then
subjected to column chromatography in a similar manner
to tissue extracts. Final purification was achieved by

Table 1. Patients with Fucosidase Deficiency (Fucosidosis) Studied*

No.	Patient	(Ref)	Sex	Hepato-spleno-megaly	Angio-keratoma#	Onset	Death§	Storage Material Reported
1	R.F.#	10	F	Yes	No	1	5	H, Le^a and Le^b GSL: polysaccharides
2	S.S.	13	M	Yes	No	3	7	Fucose-containing GSL and "mucopoly-saccharides"
3	M.S.	11	M	Yes	No	2-1/2	10§	H-antigen
4	B.L.	1	M	Yes	No	–	7	H-antigen
5	J.G.	1	M	No	No	–	§	not reported
6	M.C.	17	M	No	Yes	1	22§	not reported
7	G.Z.#	25	M	Yes	No	2	7§	not reported
8	M.Z.#	25	M	Yes	No	1	9§	not reported
9	A.Z.#	3	F	No	Yes	1	7§	Fucose-containing GSL in plasma
10	#	12	M	No	Yes	2-1/2	9§	not reported
11	#	12	M	No	Yes	2	11§	not reported

* All patients showed progressive psychomotor degeneration with varying degrees of skeletal dysmophism.

§ Still living as of 10-1-75

Similarly affected sibling

GSL = Glycosphingolipid

descending paper chromatography using the solvent system
n-butanol-acetic acid-water (12-3-5 v/v) (5); pure oligosaccharide, disaccharide or glycopeptide material was
eluted from paper strips with water and aliquots analysed
for monosaccharide content (5,22).

The Brain in Fucosidosis

Autopsy brain from patient 4 was analysed for glycosphingolipid abnormalities. Apart from a small amount
of H-antigen glycosphingolipid (Table 2, Fig. 1), which
could have been of extraneural origin, no major abnormalities were found. There was little chemical evidence
for extensive demyelination since levels of GalCer and
sulfatide were normal and there was only a slight increase
in cholesterol esters. Ganglioside content was essentially normal although GLC analysis indicated the presence of fucose in the G_{D1a} region (Fuc:Gal:Glc:GalNAc:
NeuNAc = 0.2:2.0:1.0:1.0:1.8) which could be interpreted
as storage of small amounts of monofucosylated-G_{M1}-
ganglioside. A dekasaccharide containing 2 moles of
fucose was the major storage compound in fucosidosis
brain (Table 3, Fig. 1) together with lesser amounts of
the Fuc-GlcNAc disaccharide.

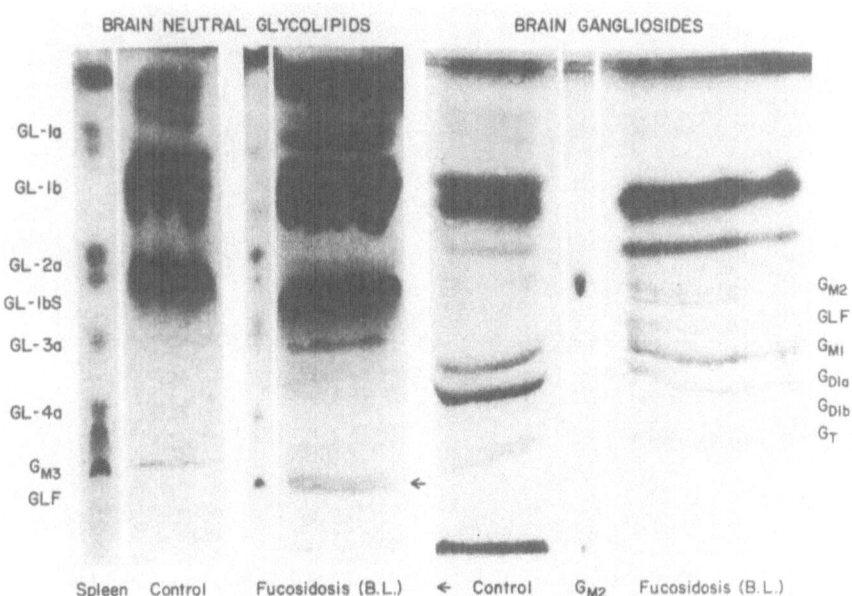

Fig. 1.   Brain glycosphingolipids in Fucosidosis Patient 4

The Pancreas in Fucosidosis

Analysis of normal human pancreas has revealed the
presence of a large number of glycosphingolipids, including the neutral glycolipids, glucosylceramide (GL-la),
GL-2a, GL-3a and GL-4a, galactosylceramide (GL-lb),
GL-2b and sulfatide (GL-lbS), gangliosides G_{M3}, G_{M2} and
G_{M1} together with at least two fucoglycosphingolipids
(H-antigen and Gal αGal [Fuc] GlcNAc-Gal-Glc-Cer)
(Table 2). Fucoglycosphingolipids were also found in
human intestine and appear restricted to secretory tissue.
Analysis of autopsy pancreas from a single case (Patient
1) of fucosidosis revealed a massive (400-fold) elevation
of H-antigen (Table 2) (Fig. 2) together with substantial
amounts of dekasaccharide and disaccharide in the ratio
3.7:1 (Table 3).

Other Tissues (Liver, Spleen, Kidney, Lymph Node and
Lung) in Fucosidosis

A biopsy liver sample from patient 3 was found to
contain large amounts of H-antigen glycosphingolipid;
oligosaccharides were not investigated at this time. Of
the tissues examined from patient 1, only lymph node and

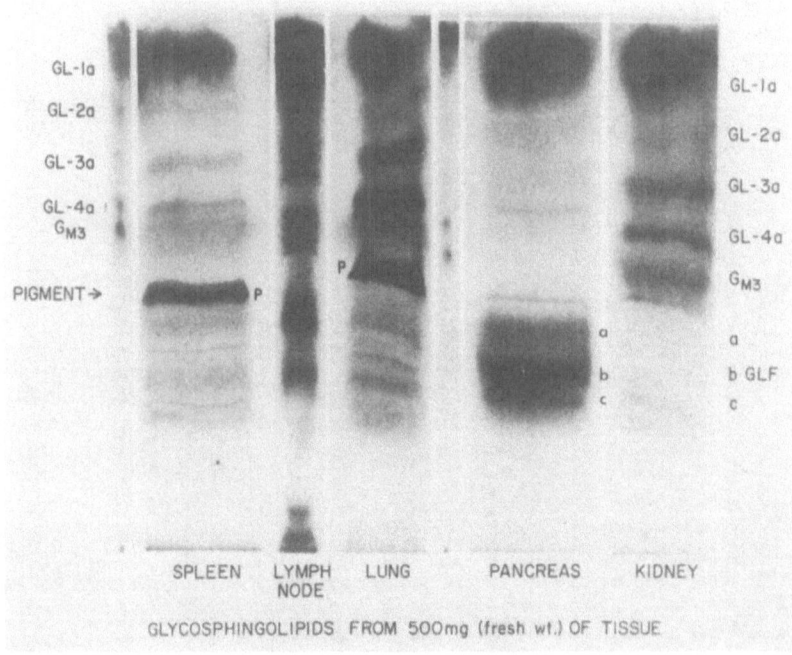

Fig. 2. Tissue glycosphingolipids in Fucosidosis Patient 1

Table 2. Glycosphingolipids in Normal and Fucosidosis Brain and Pancreas

Glycosphingolipids	Brain		Pancreas	
	Control	Fucosidosis Patient 4	Control	Fucosidosis Patient 1
	μmoles/100 g fresh wt			
Glc-Cer	2	4	1.6	1.5
Gal-Cer	600	595	2.8	3.0
Lac-Cer	1	10	4.3#	4.0#
Sulfatide	200	220	1.7	1.0
Trihexosylceramide	<0.1	<0.1	3.1	3.0
Tetrahexosylceramide	<0.1	3	2.8	2.5
G_{M3}	1	2	4.7	3.3
H-antigen*	0	15	1.0	400.0
G_{M2}	1	8	1.2	<0.1
G_{M1}	15	33	–	–
G_{D1a}	26	18§	<0.1	<0.1
G_{D1b}	10	5	<0.1	<0.1
G_{T1a}	18	10	<0.1	<0.1

* Includes H-antigen and uncharacterized fucoglycosphingolipids

§ 10% was a fucoglycosphingolipid

\# Also contains 1.0 mole/100 g of digalactosyl ceramide

lung contained appreciable levels of H-antigen (Fig. 2).
This was comparable to the low level in brain but much
less than liver or pancreas. In general, kidney contained little storage material, lung and spleen contained
mainly oligosaccharide whereas lymph node contained an
equal mixture of dekasaccharide and disaccharide (Table 3).
Of the tissues examined, substantial fucoglycosphingolipid
storage was only found in pancreas and liver.

Urine of Patients with Fucosidosis

     Analysis of urine sediment from patients 3, 6 and 9
revealed no glycosphingolipid storage, which is consistent
with analyses on kidney from patient 1 (Table 3). Urine
from patients 3, 5, 6 and 9 was rich in fuco-oligosac-
charides and glycopeptides and urine analysis represents
a simple chemical approach to the diagnosis of fucosidosis. The major component was the dekasaccharide which
could be conveniently precipitated with 5 volumes of
ethanol. No significant relationship between the amount
of this material excreted/24 hrs and the severity of the
clinical symptoms was established. Large amounts of the
Fuc $\alpha(1\longrightarrow 6)$GlcNAc disaccharide were also isolated from
urine; about half of this material was still attached to
the asparagine residue from the polypeptide chain with
only trace amounts (less than 0.1 mole/mole Asn) of other
amino acids present. Urine also contained significant
amounts of fucose-rich low molecular weight material
which remains to be completely characterized.

Structural Studies

     The fuco-oligosaccharide was sequenced by the use
of purified exo-glycosidases and the position of the
anomeric linkages determined by a combination of peri-
odate oxidation-GLC and permethylation-GLC-mass spectrometry (details to be published elsewhere). The structure
elucidated from these studies is shown in Table 3.

Cultured Skin Fibroblasts from Patients with Fucosidosis

     Fibroblasts were cultured from patients 2, 3, 6, 7,
8, 10 and 11. The results of enzymic and chemical
analysis were essentially the same from all 7 patients.
The glycosphingolipid fraction isolated from cell pellets
contained no fucoglycosphingolipids (9) and labelling

Table 3. Relative Amounts of Complex Carbohydrate Material in Fucosidosis Tissue

Tissue	High Molecular Weight "Glycoprotein"	Oligosaccharide*	Disaccharide§	GLF#
	μmoles/g fresh wt			
Brain	23	23	4	0.2
Spleen	21	24	6	0.05
Pancreas	13	22	6	4.0
Lung	12	15	2	0.2
Kidney	19	4		
Lymph node	42	6	5	0.3
Control range	0.5-4.0	<0.1	<0.1	<0.1

* Structure: Fuc $\alpha(1\rightarrow2)$ Gal $\beta(1\rightarrow4)$ GlcNAc $\beta(1\rightarrow2)$ Man $\alpha(1\rightarrow3)$

Man $\beta(1\rightarrow4)$ GlcNAc

Fuc $\alpha(1\rightarrow2)$ Gal $\beta(1\rightarrow4)$ GlcNAc $\beta(1\rightarrow2)$ Man $\alpha(1\rightarrow6)$

§ Structure: Fuc $\alpha(1\rightarrow6)$ GlcNAc; Fuc-GlcNAc-Asn-peptide

Structure: Fuc $\alpha(1\rightarrow2)$ Gal-GlcNAc-Gal-Glc-Ceramide

studies with [^{3}H]-fucose were also negative for fucolipid storage. Analysis of soluble storage material from
these cells revealed a single storage material, a simple
glycopeptide of the Fuc $\alpha(1\longrightarrow 6)$GlcNAc-Asn type (Table 4).
The absence of oligosaccharide or high molecular weight
glycopeptide storage material is in contrast to the situation in most other fucosidosis tissues (Table 3). Further, fibroblasts from patients with G_{M1}-gangliosidosis
stored a Gal-GlcNAc-Man-[Gal-GlcNAc-Man]-Man-GlcNAc-Asn
glycopeptide, those from G_{M2}-gangliosidosis Type II
patients stored a GlcNAc-Man-[GlcNAc-Man]-Man-GlcNAc-Asn
glycopeptide and those from a single patient with mannosidosis, a [Man]$_3$GlcNAc-Asn glycopeptide (21,22) (Table 4).
This suggests that glycoproteins in cultured skin fibroblasts contain oligosaccharide units of the NeuNAc
$\alpha(2\longrightarrow 6)$Gal-GlcNAc-Man-[NeuNAc $\alpha(2\longrightarrow 6)$Gal-GlcNAc-Man]-
Man [Fuc](GlcNAc)$_{1-2}$-Asn- and (Man)$_5$-GlcNAc-Asn type.
Fucose-rich glycoproteins of the Fuc-Gal-GlcNAc-Man ...
type have not been characterized as yet from any tissue
and the only evidence for their existence is the large
amounts of Fuc-Gal-GlcNAc oligosaccharide material stored
in fucosidosis tissue. This material is obviously quite
different structurally from the H-blood group glycoproteins and its abundance in certain types of tissue raises
intriguing questions as to its normal biological function.

Enzymology of Fucosidosis

    α-Fucosidase activity (as assayed with either p-
nitrophenyl-α-L-fucoside or 4-methylumbelliferyl-α-L-
fucoside) was always less than 1% of normal in the 7
strains of cultured fibroblasts from patients with fucosidosis examined in this study. We were unable to demonstrate a partial enzyme deficiency in any of the older
patients (for example, patient 6). Further, no electrophoretic differences in α-fucosidase, based on cellogel
electrophoresis, were found amongst the 7 strains examined
and it was concluded that use of 4-methylumbelliferyl-α-
L-fucoside is incapable of resolving the question of
clinical heterogeneity.

    Attempts to develop natural substrate assays for
α-L-fucosidase have been largely unsuccessful because of
technical problems in accurately measuring small amounts
of L-fucose. Further, there is no currently available
method for introducing [^{3}H] or [^{14}C] label into the fucose
moiety of substrates such as H-antigen, fucosyllactose
or lacto-N-fucopentaose. We have attempted to overcome

Table 4. Glycopeptide Fraction* from Cultured Skin Fibroblasts Obtained From Patients with Inborn Errors of Glycopeptein Catabolism

	G_{M1}-Ganglio-sidosis Type I (C.F.)	G_{M2}-Gangliosidosis Type II (D.B.)	Sandhoff's Disease (N.Z.)	Fucosidosis Pt-2	Fucosidosis Pt-3§	Fucosidosis Pt-6	Fuco-sidosis Pt-8§	Manno-sidosis# (M.G.)
				molar ratio				
Fucose	<0.1	<0.1	<0.1	0.8	0.8	1.2	1.0	<0.1
Mannose	2.8	1.8	2.7	<0.1	0.1	<0.5	<0.1	3.4
Galactose	1.8	<0.1	<0.1	<0.1	0.1	<0.1	<0.1	<0.1
GlcNAc	4.0	4.0	4.0	1.0	1.0	1.0	1.0	1.0
NeuNAc	<0.1	<0.1	<0.1	<0.1	<0.1	<0.1	<0.1	<0.1
Total μmoles/ 10^8 cells	1.85	1.60	1.65	0.42	0.92	0.14	1.85	0.50

* This low molecular weight fraction contains less than 0.1 μmoles complex carbohydrate in other normal and pathological fibroblasts.

§ Also contained Glu, Gly, Ser, Ala, Thr in the molar ratio 0.8:0.9:0.8:1.0:0.8 per mole of Asn

Gel filtration gave a molecular weight of 1100 which corresponded to a glycopeptide shown by analysis to contain - Man:GlcNAc:Asn:Glu:Gly:Ser:Ala:Thr in the ratio 3.0:1.0:1.0:1.0:0.8:0.8:0.5

these problems in two ways: (1) Small amounts of L-
fucose, in the presence of salt, detergent, etc., can be
estimated by incubating with purified porcine liver L-
fucose dehydrogenase (19) and NAD and recording the production of NADH spectrophotometrically at 340nm. The
reaction was linear over the range 10-200 nmoles. (2)
A labelled substrate [^{3}H] Fuc α(1$\longrightarrow$6)GlcNAc-Asn (Ser,
Thr, Glu, Ala)was prepared by culturing fucosidosis fibroblasts in medium containing [^{3}H] fucose and purifying the
storage material by a combination of Bio-Gel P-10, P-2
and paper chromatography (21). Extracts of fibroblasts
were incubated with the substrate at pH 4.9 for 20 hrs,
spotted on Whatmann-3MM filter paper and chromatographed
in n-butanol-acetic acid-water (12:3:5) for 20 hrs. The
area corresponding to free fucose was cut and subjected
to liquid scintillation counting. Activity in fucosidosis
fibroblasts (patients 3 and 6) was 10% of normal (Table 5)
but once again we were unable to demonstrate a partial
enzyme deficiency in the oldest patient, patient 6.

Table 5.   Fuc α(1$\longrightarrow$6) GlcNAc α-Fucosidase Activity
           in Human Skin Fibroblasts

Cell Strain	% of Radioactivity liberated as free fucose/mg protein/20 hrs
Normal	0.42 (400 cpm)
Batten's disease (D.W.)	0.41
Batten's disease (E. C.)	0.53
Hurler's disease	0.39
Fabry's disease	0.45
Sandhoff's disease	0.66
Fucosidosis (Patient 3)	0.04
Fucosidosis (Patient 6)	0.06

*   Treatment of [^{3}H] fucoglycopeptide with beef kidney
    α-fucosidase or 0.1M TCA at 100°C for 1-1/2 hrs re-
    leased 50% of radioactivity as free fucose.

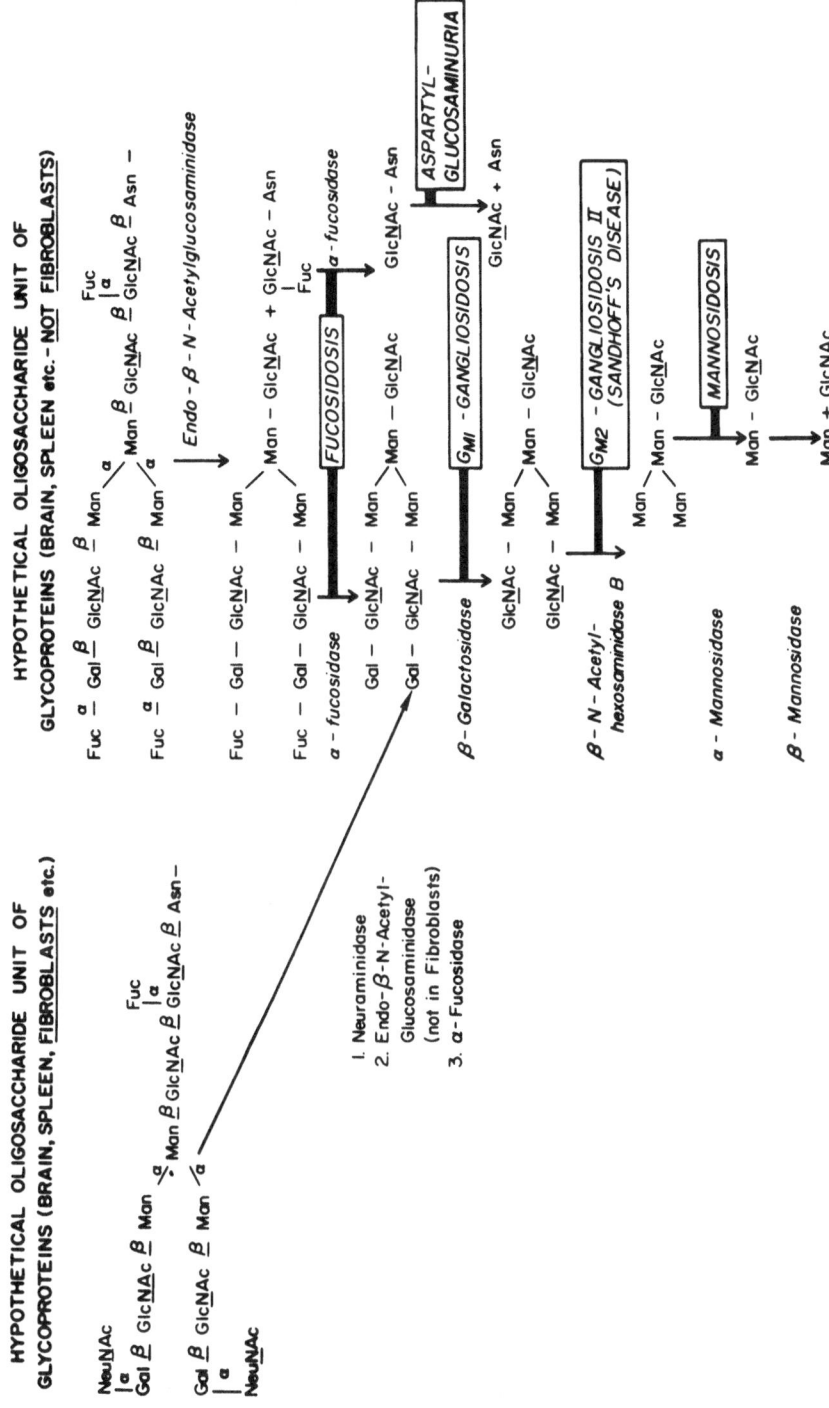

Fig. 3. Proposed scheme for the catabolism of glycoproteins showing location of known genetic disorders.

Conclusions

The major α-fucosidase deficient in fucosidosis is a soluble enzyme with a pH optimum consistent with a lysosomal subcellular localization (pH 4.9-5.2) (1,9,25). A membrane-bound form of α-L-fucosidase, with an optimum pH in the range 6.0-6.5 is also deficient in fucosidosis (G. Dawson, unpublished findings). As yet there is no evidence to explain the clinical heterogeneity in fucosidosis based on enzymic differences. It is possible that the blood group type or secretor status of an individual may represent a second degree of genetic control in this disease and explain why the disorder manifests itself quite differently in patients with a common ancestor (3). Our studies indicate that the α-fucosidase involved in fucosidosis normally hydrolyses Fuc $\alpha(1\rightarrow2)$ Gal and Fuc $\alpha(1\rightarrow6)$GlcNAc linkages in glycoproteins. Its reactivity towards Fuc $\alpha(1\rightarrow4)$GlcNAc and Fuc $\alpha(1\rightarrow3)$ GlcNAc linkages (Lewis antigens) remains to be clarified since we were unable to demonstrate storage of such compounds. The most abundant storage material is a dekasaccharide presumably liberated from a glycoprotein by the action of an endo-β-N-acetylglucosaminidase (20). Storage of a Fuc-GlcNAc disaccharide is also prominent and this may be still attached to a degraded peptide moiety through an asparagine residue. A third storage product is H-antigen glycosphingolipid. A scheme for the catabolism of both fuco- and sialo-glycoproteins is presented in Fig. 3, indicating the site of the enzyme block in fucosidosis, G_{M1}-gangliosidosis (24), G_{M2}-gangliosidosis Type II (15), mannosidosis (16) and aspartylglucosaminuria (2) - the inborn errors of glycoprotein catabolism.

ACKNOWLEDGEMENTS

We would like to thank Mr. John Oh for excellent technical assistance. Supported by USPHS Grants HD-06426, HD-04583 and AM-05996 and a Grant (I-340) from the National Foundation-March of Dimes. G.D. is a Joseph P. Kennedy, Jr. Scholar and the recipient of USPHS Research Career Development Award NS-00029.

REFERENCES

1. Alhadeff, J. A., Miller, A. L., Wenger, D. A. and
    O'Brien, J. S. Electrophoretic Forms of Human Liver
    α-Fucosidase and Their Relationship to Fucosidosis
    (Mucopolysaccharidosis F). Clin. Chim. Acta 57,
    307 (1974).

2. Aula, P., Nanto, V., Laipio, M. L. and Autio, S.
    Aspartylglucosaminuria: Deficiency of Aspartyl-
    glucosaminidase in Cultured Fibroblasts of Patients
    and Their Heterozygous Parents. Clin. Genet. 4,
    297 (1973).

3. Borrone, C., Gatti, R., Trias, X. and Durand, P.
    Fucosidosis: Clinical, Biochemical, Immunologic
    and Genetic Studies in Two New Cases. J. Pediat.
    84, 727 (1974).

4. Clamp, J. R., Dawson, G. and Hough, L. The Simul-
    taneous Estimation of 6-deoxy-L-galactose (L-fucose),
    D-mannose, D-galactose, 2-acetamido-2-deoxy-D-
    glucose (N-acetyl-D-glucosamine) and N-acetylneura-
    minic acid (sialic acid) in glycopeptides and glyco-
    proteins. Biochim. Biophys. Acta 148, 342 (1967).

5. Dawson, G. and Clamp, J. R. Investigations of the
    oligosaccharide units of an A myeloma globulin.
    Biochem. J. 107, 341 (1968).

6. Dawson, G. and Spranger, J. W. Fucosidosis: A
    Glycosphingolipidosis. New Eng. J. Med. 285, 122
    (1971).

7. Dawson, G. Glycosphingolipid Abnormalities in Liver
    from Patients with Glycosphingolipid and Mucopoly-
    saccharide Storage Diseases. In: Sphingolipids,
    Sphingolipidoses and Allied Disorders (B. W. Volk
    and S. M. Aronson, eds.) Plenum Publishing Co.,
    New York, p. 395 (1972).

8. Dawson, G. Glycosphingolipid Levels in an Unusual
    Neurovisceral Storage Disease Characterized by
    Lactosyl Ceramide Galactosylhydrolase Deficiency:
    Lactosylceramidosis. J. Lipid Res. 13, 207 (1972).

9. Dawson, G., Matalon, R. and Dorfman, A. Glyco-
    sphingolipids in Cultured Skin Fibroblasts. II.
    Characterization and Metabolism in Fibroblasts from

Patients with Inborn Errors of Glycosphingolipid and Mucopolysaccharide Metabolism. J. Biol. Chem. 247, 595 (1972).

10. Durand, P., Borrone, C. and Della Cella, G. Fuco-sidosis. J. Pediat. 75, 665 (1969).

11. Freitag, F., Küchemann, K., Blümcke, S. and Spranger, J. W. Hepatic Ultrastructure in Fucosidosis. Vir-chows Arch. Abt. Z. Zellpath. 7, 99 (1971).

12. Kousseff, B. G., Beratis, N. G., Danesino, C. and Hirschhorn, K. Genetic Heterogeneity in Fucosidosis. Lancet ii, 1387 (1973).

13. Loeb, H., Tondeur, M., Jonniaux, G., Mockel-Pohl, S. and Vamos-Hurwitz, E. Biochemical and Ultrastructural Studies in a Case of Mucopolysaccharidosis "F" (Fuco-sidosis). Helv. Paed. Acta 24, 519 (1969).

14. Matsuda, I., Arashima, S., Anakura, M., Ege, A. and Hayata, I. Fucosidosis. Tohoku J. Exp. Med. 109, 41 (1973).

15. Ng Ying Kin, N. M. K. and Wolfe, L. S. Oligosaccha-rides Accumulating in the Liver from a Patient with G_{M2}-Gangliosidosis Variant O (Sandhoff-Jatzkewitz Disease). Biochem. Biophys. Res. Commun. 59, 837 (1974).

16. Norden, N. E., Lundblad, A., Svenson, S. and Autio, S. Characterization of Two Mannose-Containing Oligo-saccharides Isolated from the Urine of Patients with Mannosidosis. Biochemistry 13, 871 (1974).

17. Patel, V., Watanabe, I. and Zeman, W. Deficiency of α-L-Fucosidase. Science 176, 426 (1972).

18. Philippart, M. Fucosidosis: A Novel Neurovisceral Sphingolipidosis. Neurology 19, 304 (1969) (Abstract).

19. Schachter, H., Sarney, J., McGuire, E. J. and Rose-man, S. Isolation of Diphosphopyridine Nucleotide-Dependent L-Fucose Dehydrogenase from Pork Liver. J. Biol. Chem. 244, 4785 (1969).

20. Tarentino, A. L. and Maley, F. Purification and Properties of an Endo-β-N-acetylglucosaminidase from Streptomyces griseus. J. Biol. Chem. 249, 811 (1974).

21. Tsay, G. C. and Dawson, G. Glycopeptide Storage in
    Fibroblasts from Patients with Inborn Errors of Glyco-
    protein and Glycosphingolipid Catabolism. Biochem.
    Biophys. Res. Commun. 63, 807 (1975).

22. Tsay, G. C., Dawson, G. and Matalon, R. Excretion
    of Mannose-Rich Complex Carbohydrates by a Patient
    with ⍺-Mannosidase Deficiency (Mannosidosis). J.
    Pediat. 82, 856 (1974).

23. Vance, D. E. and Sweeley, C. C. Quantitative Deter-
    mination of the Neutral Glycosylceramides in Human
    Blood. J. Lipid Res. 8, 621 (1967).

24. Wolfe, L. S., Senior, R. G. and Ng Ying Kin, N. M. K.
    The Structures of Oligosaccharides Accumulating in
    the Liver of G_{M1}-Gangliosidosis Type I. J. Biol.
    Chem. 249, 1828 (1974).

25. Zielke, K., Okada, S. and O'Brien, J. S. Fucosi-
    dosis: Diagnosis by Serum Assay of ⍺-L-Fucosidase.
    J. Lab. Clin. Med. 79, 164 (1972).

ALPHA-L-FUCOSIDASE IN NORMAL AND DEFICIENT INDIVIDUALS

Kurt Hirschhorn, Nicholas G. Beratis, and
Bryan M. Turner
Department of Pediatrics, Mount Sinai School of
Medicine of The City University of New York
Fifth Avenue & 100th Street, New York, N.Y. 10029

Fucosidosis is a mucolipidosis involving the accumulation in tissues of fucose-containing sphingolipids, glycoproteins and muco-polysaccharides (10,16). The disease is transmitted as an auto-somal recessive trait and the basic metabolic defect has been found to be deficiency of α-L-fucosidase (24). The enzymatic defect has been reported in various organs (25,16,14), serum (4,27), cultured skin fibroblasts (16,28) and peripheral blood leukocytes (16,7,4). Genetic heterogeneity of the disease has been identified and we have designated the two distinct forms as types 1 and 2 (13).

This report describes recent studies on two patients with fucosidosis type 2 and on clinically normal members of their family. (1) We have carried out comparative studies on the suita-bility of various cell types for diagnosis of the disease and heterozygote detection. (2) By following the segregation in this family, of two common alleles at the α-L-fucosidase gene locus, we have obtained evidence for the existence of a third, 'silent' allele at this locus. (3) Finally, we describe experiments on the uptake of purified placental α-L-fucosidase by skin fibroblasts from the two patients.

MATERIALS AND METHODS

Patients

We have discussed fucosidosis in two male siblings affected with mental retardation, neurologic signs, growth failure, coarse

facial features and angiokeratoma corporis diffusum (13), a skin
lesion previously considered as characteristic of Fabry's disease.
The age of the patients when we saw them last was 10 and 5 9/12
years. In both patients the first symptoms became apparent at the
age of 18 months when psychomotor regression was noticed. The
first angiokeratoma lesions on the skin appeared at the age of 5
years in the older brother (Case 1) and at 5 2/12 years on the
younger (Case 2). The angiokeratoma lesions were pinhead-sized,
red-brown to purplish, raised and did not blanch on diascopy.
They were mainly located on the penis and scrotum. The same
lesions, but more sparse, were also scattered over the buttocks,
abdomen and thighs. The gait of the patients was broad based,
there was stiffness of the joints and the muscle tone was generally increased. They could not use any words but they followed
simple instructions. The skin was thick and increased subcutaneous markings were present, most prominent on the chest, the
palms and the soles. Ten per cent of the peripheral lymphocytes
in Case 1 had vacuoles, but bone marrow smears were normal. The
sodium and chloride concentration in the sweat of both patients
was normal. Skeletal findings of mild dysostosis multiplex were
present in both patients. The spine, pelvis and femoral capital
epiphyses were predominantly involved.

Blood Typing

Quantitative typing of erythrocytes was carried out by the
method of Berkman et al. (6). Le^a, Le^b, H and A were measured in
saliva by an adaptation (13) of the same method for quantitative
inhibition of agglutination.

Cellular and Enzymatic Studies

Heparinized blood was obtained from the two patients, their
parents and 17 other family members, 15 of which were at risk for
carrying the fucosidosis gene, as well as 14 controls. Peripheral
leukocytes, lymphocytes and granulocytes were prepared as previously described(4).

Skin biopsies were obtained from the inner surface of the
forearm from the two patients, their parents, two family members
reliably identified as carriers by phenotyping (see below) and 10
normal donors. Skin fibroblasts grown from the biopsy tissue were
cultivated and harvested as previously described (5).

Long-term lymphoid cell lines were established from the two
patients and six normal controls. Lines were established as
described earlier (3) after stimulation with phytohemagglutinin.

Lines were multiplied in 75 cm^2 flasks and when the desired number
of cells was obtained, cultures were fed and 24 hours later cells
were harvested. Lymphoid cells were washed and stored at -85°C.

α-L-Fucosidase activity was determined by a modification of
the method of Zielke et al. (28). The concentration of the substrate p-nitrophenyl-α-L-fucoside (Sigma Chemical Co.) in the
reaction mixture was increased to 3.0 mM and the incubation time
was reduced to 2 hours. The assay was carried out at pH 5.8 in
peripheral leukocytes, lymphocytes and granulocytes and at pH 5.7
in cultured skin fibroblasts and lymphoid cell lines. α-L-Fucosidase activity was also measured by using the fluorogenic substrate
4-methylumbelliferyl-α-L-fucoside (Koch-Light). For peripheral
leukocytes the assay conditions were the same as previously
described (4). For cultured skin fibroblasts the substrate concentration in the reaction mixture was 0.8 mM and the pH of the
reaction was 4.5. α-D-Mannosidase activity was measured using the
4-methylumbelliferyl-α-D-mannoside as substrate (4). Protein was
determined according to the method of Lowry et al. (15). All
determinations were carried out in duplicate.

Electrophoresis and Isoelectric Focusing

Horizontal starch-gel electrophoresis was carried out using
phosphate buffer at pH 7.0 as previously described (20). Isoelectric focusing was carried out in thin-layer acrylamide gel
using a pH gradient of 3.5-9.0. The procedures used for isoelectric focusing and subsequent detection of enzyme activity with the
fluorogenic substrate 4-methylumbelliferyl-α-L-fucoside, have been
described in detail elsewhere (22).

Enzyme Purification and Cellular Correction

α-L-Fucosidase was purified from human placenta and serum by
ammonium sulphate precipitation and affinity chromatography. The
methods used were similar to those reported previously (1,18).
The purified enzyme was stored in 50% glycerol at -20°C. Prior to
addition of the enzyme to tissue culture medium for fibroblast
uptake experiments the concentration of glycerol and sodium was
reduced by dilution in distilled water and reconcentration through
an Amicon PM10 membrane. The supplemented medium was sterilized
by passage through a Millipore filter (0.45μ) and 5ml aliquots
were added to fibroblast monolayers in 25cm^2 plastic flasks. All
uptake experiments employed cells at the early confluent stage.
Cells were harvested by trypsinization and washed three times in
isotonic saline. Cell pellets were stored at -20°C prior to lysis

Table 1. Secretor status and Lewis activity on erythrocytes and
in saliva from fucosidosis patients and their parents.

Subject	Secretor Status	Lewis Status	Erythrocytes Lewis Activity*			Saliva Lewis Activity**		
			Le^a	Le^b	Total	Le^a	Le^b	Total
Case 1	H	ab	73.5	106.0	179.5	6	123	129
Case 2	H	ab	64.9	81.2	146.1	17	133	150
Father	No H	a	47.5	0.0	47.5	67	0	67
Mother	H	b	0.0	58.3	58.3	6	23	29

*In units, expressed as $\Delta \log_{10} OD \times 100$, adjusted for actual cell
  count and instrument performance.
**In units, expressed as reciprocal of salivary dilution required
  for 50 percent inhibition of Le-anti-Le agglutination.

by five cycles of freeze/thawing and assay of α-L-fucosidase
activity

RESULTS

Blood Grouping

    Table 1 lists the Lewis activity on erythrocytes and in saliva
obtained from the patients and their parents. Both patients showed
activity significantly higher than their parents and normal controls.
No difference was noted between the obligate heterozygous parents
and normal subjects. The H specificity, however, was normal in
both patients.

Cellular and Enzymatic Studies

    Figure 1 illustrates the α-L-fucosidase activity in purified
mononuclear cells. These cells showed the smallest variation in
enzyme activity of all the cell types tested. With both substrates
there was no overlap between patients, carriers and normal subjects.
The phenotypically normal family members were separated into two
clusters. In mixed peripheral leukocytes overlap occurred between
an obligate heterozygote and two normal subjects, when the fluoro-

Table 2. α-L-fucosidase and α-D-mannosidase activity in cultured skin fibroblasts.

Subject(No.)	Prepara-tions studied	α-L-Fucosidase		α-D-Man-nosidase**
		Mean ± SD*	Mean ± SD**	
Patients(2)	4	0	0	121.9
III.1	2	0	0	118.3
III.2	2	0	0	125.6
Heterozy-gotes(4)	12	32.9	38.1	57.1
II.1	3	44.2	44.5	67.3
II.4	3	35.9	47.0	41.2
II.5	3	27.2	27.2	44.9
II.6	3	24.3	33.8	74.9
Control(10)	20	75.5 ± 23.8	90.7 ± 22.8	46.5 ± 10.6
(Range)		(44.0-118.3)	(52.9-129.3)	

*nmoles p-nitrophenol/mg protein/hour
**nmoles 4-methylumbelliferone/mg protein/hour
For identification of family members see pedigree in Fig. 1

genic substrate was used. Although there was no overlap between normal subjects and carriers in the cases studied with the colori-genic substrate, the difference in activity between these two groups was too small to allow reliable identification of heterozy-gotes. In purified granulocytes, overlap between carriers and normal donors occurred with both substrates.

Table 2 lists the α-L-fucosidase activity and α-D-mannosidase activity in cultured skin fibroblasts obtained from the obligate heterozygous parents of the patients, two additional family members, II.1 and II.4, who were reliably identified as carriers by phenotyping (see below) and ten normal controls. No α-L-fuco-sidase activity could be measured in the patients' fibroblasts with either substrate, while the mean activity in the heterozygotes was lower than in the controls. All of the remaining family members, who were identified as heterozygotes in the lymphocytes, also showed activity within the carrier range in fibroblasts. However, some overlap between normal subjects and carriers was present when single enzyme determinations were considered. More-over, in 4 fibroblast cultures derived from normal donors, which appeared granular under the microscope, the α-L-fucosidase acti-

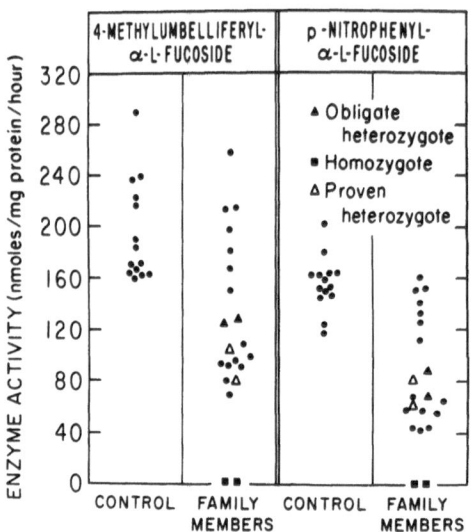

Fig. 1. α-L-Fucosidase activity in purified mononuclear cells.

vity was within the carrier range, while the activity of other
lysosomal enzymes was normal.

Table 3 shows the α-L-fucosidase activity and α-D-mannosidase
activity in lymphoid cell lines established from the two patients
with fucosidosis and six normal controls. No α-L-fucosidase activity could be detected in the fucosidosis lines, while the activity in the normal lines (mean ± SD) was 199.0 ± 79.9 nmoles
p-nitrophenol per mg of soluble protein per hour. No significant
difference in α-D-mannosidase activity was noted between the deficient and normal lines.

Polymorphism of Human α-L-Fucosidase

We have previously reported (20) that α-L-fucosidase from
peripheral leukocytes or cultured long-term lymphoid lines can be
resolved into six or more discrete isozymes by starch-gel electrophoresis. The enzyme from serum or plasma consisted of a diffuse
band with a greater anodal mobility than the cellular isozymes
(Fig. 2). Incubation of serum samples of cell extracts with purified bacterial neuraminidase prior to electrophoresis caused a
diminution in the staining intensity of the more anodal isozymes
and a parallel increase in activity of the less anodal forms
(Fig. 2). This observation suggests that the more anodal isozymes
are formed by attachment of sialic acid residues to the enzyme.

Table 3. α-L-Fucosidase and α-D-Mannosidase activity in long-term lymphoid lines established from patients with fucosidosis and normal subjects.

Line (No.)	α-L-Fucosidase*	α-D-Mannosidase**
Fucosidosis(2)	0.0	147.2
NB-39	0.0	70.9
NB-41	0.0	233.6
Normal(6)	$199.0 \pm 79.9^{+}$	$149.8 \pm 72.6^{+}$
NB-45	233.2	235.2
NB-47	243.1	249.4
NB-50	315.9	95.5
NB-57	156.2	97.7
NB-58	94.1	96.6
NB-61	151.4	124.3

*nmoles p-nitrophenol/mg protein/hour.
**nmoles 4-methylumbelliferone/mg protein/hour.
[+]Mean ± SD.

In subsequent studies (22) we have shown that isoelectric focusing in thin-layer acrylamide gel resolves the enzyme into a series of isozymes very similar to that seen after electrophoresis. Because of the greater resolving power of the isoelectric focusing technique, we used this method for further studies on the α-L-fucosidase isozymes in peripheral blood leukocytes.

Following simplification of the isozyme pattern by incubation with neuraminidase, three distinct α-L-fucosidase phenotypes are distinguishable in leukocytes from different individuals. These phenotypes are shown in Fig. 3 and have been designated Fu 1, Fu 2-1 and Fu 2. Phenotype Fu 1, which lacks the least acidic isozyme seen in Fu 2 and 2-1, is the most easily identifiable. The Fu 2 and 2-1 phenotypes can be distinguished by the relative staining intensities of the two least acidic bands. In the Fu 2 phenotype the least acidic of these two bands is the more prominent while in the 2-1 phenotype the more acidic is the more intensely staining. The 2-1 phenotype resembles a simple mixture of the isozymes present in the Fu 1 and 2 phenotypes.

Among 21 families tested (38 offspring) the inheritance of phenotypes was consistent with the segregation of two codominant

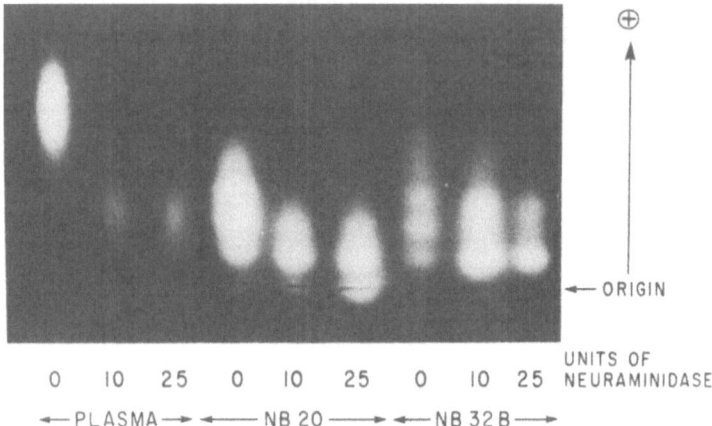

Fig. 2. Isozymes of α-L-Fucosidase in plasma and lymphoid lines
(NB 20 and NB 32B) separated by starch-gel electrophoresis.

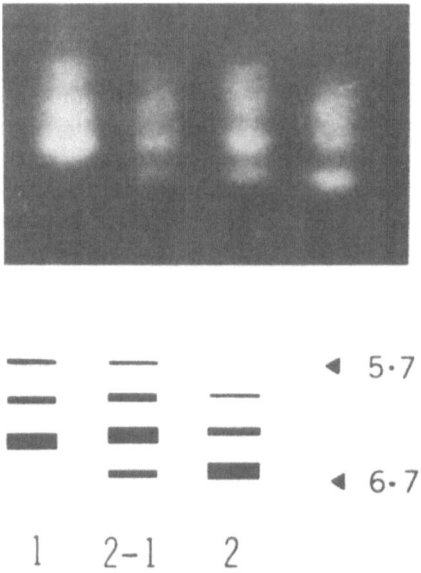

Fig. 3. Isozymes of α-L-fucosidase in neuraminidase-treated leukocyte extracts separated by isoelectric focusing in acrylamide
gel. (A) Photograph of a gel showing phenotypes (left to right)
Fu 1, Fu 2-1, Fu 2-1 and Fu 2. (B) Diagram showing the three
common phenotypes and the pH range in which the isozymes focus.

alleles at a single, autosomal gene locus. These alleles have
been designated $\underline{Fu^1}$ and $\underline{Fu^2}$. Thus, individuals with α-L-fucosidase
phenotypes 1, 2 and 2-1 are presumed to have the genotypes $\underline{Fu^1Fu^1}$,
$\underline{Fu^2Fu^2}$ and $\underline{Fu^2Fu^1}$, respectively. From a study of 194 unrelated,
white individuals (22) the frequencies of the $\underline{Fu^1}$ and $\underline{Fu^2}$ alleles
were calculated to be 0.753 and 0.247, respectively. The isozyme
pattern of α-L-fucosidase was examined in long-term lymphoid lines,
cultured skin fibroblasts, and extracts of human liver, spleen and
placenta. All these tissues showed similar isozymes to those seen
in peripheral leukocytes, although activity of the fibroblast
enzyme was comparatively low. Among the lymphoid line, fibroblast
and placental samples tested all three phenotypes were detected.
Among the liver and spleen samples tested so far, examples of the
Fu 1 and 2-1 phenotypes have been found. A single brain sample
has been examined and found to show a similar series of α-L-fucosidase isozymes to those found in other tissues. It seems likely
from these results that the same gene locus codes for α-L-fucosidase
in all these tissues. Whether or not the serum enzyme is also
coded by this locus remains to be established. We have been unable,
so far, to demonstrate consistent differences between the isozyme
patterns of serum samples from individuals of different α-L-fucosidase phenotypes.

We have been able to study (21) the segregation of the two
common alleles at the α-L-fucosidase gene locus in the family of
two brothers affected with fucosidosis 2 (Fig. 4). The three
phenotypes Fu 1, 2-1 and 2 were all observed in leukocytes from
family members. None of the α-L-fucosidase isozymes was detected
in leukocytes, long-term lymphoid lines, fibroblasts or serum from
the two affected children. With this exception, isozyme patterns
among family members did not differ from those seen in the general
population. However, there exist within this family two patterns
of inheritance of α-L-fucosidase phenotypes which are clearly not
consistent with the simple segregation of two codominant alleles.
The first incompatability is between the paternal grandmother
(I.5) of the two affected children and her daughter (II.4), with
the mother having the Fu 2 phenotype and the daughter the Fu 1
phenotype. In the normal course of events, the daughter would
inevitably have received an $\underline{Fu^2}$ allele from her mother and would
therefore have an Fu 2 or 2-1 phenotype, depending on whether she
received an $\underline{Fu^1}$ or $\underline{Fu^2}$ allele from her father. If one rules out
such unlikely events as fresh mutation or non-biological parent-
hood (particularly unlikely as it is mother and daughter who are
incompatible) then the presence of a silent (or "null") allele at
the α-L-fucosidase locus is the only satisfactory explanation for
the observed segregation of phenotypes. This allele, which we
will call $\underline{Fu^0}$, is silent in the sense that its product (if any) is
not detectable by the assay methods employed in this study.

Having introduced the $\underline{Fu^0}$ allele the explanation for the observed
pattern of inheritance becomes straightforward. The paternal
grandmother (I.5) has the genotype $\underline{Fu^2Fu^0}$ and consequently an Fu 2
phenotype. Her daughter (II.4) received an $\underline{Fu^0}$ allele from her
mother and a normal $\underline{Fu^1}$ allele from her father, resulting in the
genotype $\underline{Fu^1Fu^0}$ and an Fu 1 phenotype. This is shown in Fig. 4 in
which the symbols represent the proposed genotype for each family
member and the observed phenotypes are shown by the numbers, 1,
2-1 or 2.

The second example of apparent incompatability between parent
and child is between I.2, who has an Fu 2 phenotype, and his son
(II.1) who is Fu 1. This situation can also be resolved by proposing that a silent allele is present. In this case the father
must have the genotype $\underline{Fu^2Fu^0}$, resulting in an Fu 2 phenotype,
while the son has the genotype $\underline{Fu^1Fu^0}$, having received a normal
$\underline{Fu^1}$ allele from his mother (I.1) and an $\underline{Fu^0}$ allele from his father.

Because of the unusual inheritance of α-L-fucosidase phenotypes within this family we examined the segregation of phospho-
glucomutase (locus 1), esterase D and red cell acid phosphatase

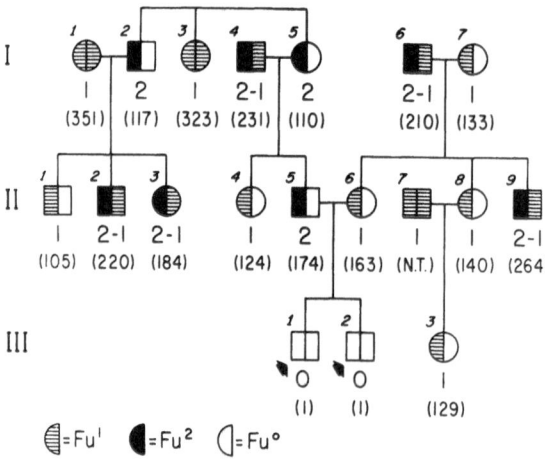

Fig. 4. Pedigree of two sibs (shown by arrows) with fucosidosis 2.
The numbers 1, 2-1 or 2 beneath each individual represent the
α-L-fucosidase phenotype determined by isoelectric focusing of
leukocyte extracts (see text). The specific activity (nmoles
4-methylumbelliferone/min/mg protein) of leukocyte α-L-fucosidase
is shown in parenthesis.

phenotypes. All these enzymes are coded by two or more common alleles in human populations (12). Throughout the family the inheritance of these polymorphic enzymes was completely normal and consistent with the relationships shown in Fig. 4.

If a silent allele is segregating at the α-L-fucosidase locus within this family it is likely that the two children affected with Fucosidosis and with virtual absence of α-L-fucosidase activity, are in fact homozygous for this allele. If this is so, then their parents must be carriers of $\underline{Fu^0}$ and must therefore have either an Fu 1 or Fu 2 phenotype. An Fu 2-1 phenotype is clearly impossible. The two parents (II.5 and II.6) have the phenotypes Fu 2 and Fu 1 respectively, presumably with the genotypes $\underline{Fu^2Fu^0}$ and $\underline{Fu^1Fu^0}$.

Based on the assumptions that the three alleles $\underline{Fu^1}$, $\underline{Fu^2}$ and $\underline{Fu^0}$ are segregating within this family and that individuals marrying into the family have two normal alleles, we have been able to derive unambiguous genotypes for most of its members. In three cases, however, it was not possible to do this on the basis of phenotyping alone. Individuals I.3, II.8 and III.3 all of whom have the Fu 1 phenotype, could be of genotypes $\underline{Fu^1Fu^1}$ or $\underline{Fu^1Fu^0}$, with equal probability. In these cases, the genotypes shown in the pedigree were assigned on the basis of the α-L-fucosidase activity of peripheral leukocytes, on the assumption that individuals carrying the silent allele should have a lower level of activity than individuals with two normal alleles. A comparison of obligatory carriers of $\underline{Fu^0}$ (i.e. I.2, 5, 7 and II.1, 4,5,6) with normals (i.e. I.1,4,6 and II.2,3,9) supports this assumption. Average α-L-fucosidase activity in obligatory carriers of $\underline{Fu^0}$ was 132 ± 27 nmoles/h/mg protein, while in normals the equivalent value was 243 ± 59. Leukocyte activities for individual members of the family are shown in Fig. 4.

In each branch of the family the $\underline{Fu^0}$ allele must have been passed down via the grandmother (I.5 and I.7) as both grandfathers are Fu 2-1 heterozygotes and must therefore have two normal alleles. It is of interest that while the two grandfathers are of Polish and German descent, the two grandmothers are both of Southern Italian parentage. Of six other families reported with Fucosidosis, (four with type 1 and two with the less severe type 2), three have been of Southern Italian origin (two type 1 and one type 2).

Enzyme Purification and Replacement Experiments

A method has recently been described for the purification in high yield of α-L-fucosidase from human placenta (1) and liver

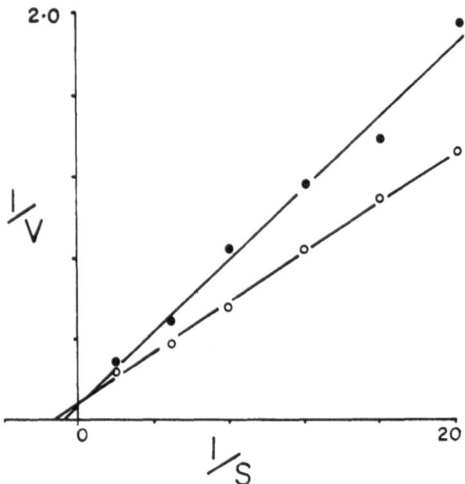

Fig. 5. Lineweaver-Burk plot showing competitive inhibition of placental α-L-fucosidase by 4-methylumbelliferyl-ß-L-fucoside. The concentration of substrate (4-methylumbelliferyl-α-L-fucoside) was varied in the presence (closed circles) or absence (open circles) of 0.45mM inhibitor. The K_1 value estimated from these results is 1.25mM.

(18). The procedure employs a commercially available affinity gel in which ß-fucosylamine is attached to Sepharose 4B via a spacer arm. α-L-fucosidase which binds to the column can be eluted with L-fucose, a competitive inhibitor of the enzyme (18). Single-step purifications of 300 (18) and 670 fold (1) have been reported. We have used a similar affinity gel (prepared in this laboratory) to purify α-L-fucosidase from human placenta to a specific activity of 5-10 I.U./mg protein with a 40% yield. The isozyme pattern of this preparation is similar to that of the original placental extract.

It is somewhat surprising that α-L-fucosidase binds to an affinity gel in which the ligand is in the ß-configuration. In fact it has been suggested that the enzyme may bind only to the small proportion of ligand molecules which have attached in the α-configuration (18). We have found that the placental enzyme is virtually incapable of hydrolysing 4-methylumbelliferyl-ß-L-fucoside. The reaction rate with this substrate is less than 0.3% of that with the α-anomer. However, the ß-derivative is a good competitive inhibitor of placental α-L-fucosidase, as shown in Fig. 5. This suggests that the active site of the enzyme is capable of binding ß-L-fucosides, but cannot catalyze their hydrolysis.

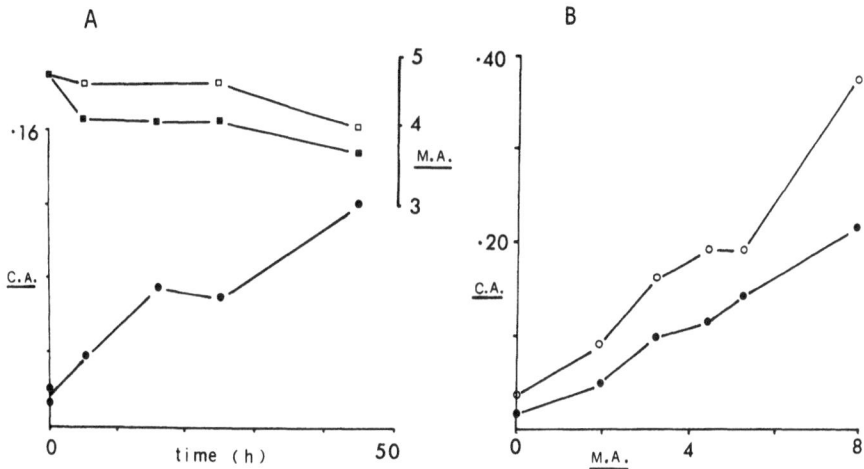

Fig. 6. Uptake of purified placental α-L-fucosidase by deficient skin fibroblasts. (A) lower part: increase in cellular α-L-fucosidase specific activity (C.A.) as a function of time of exposure to exogenous enzyme. Upper part: loss of activity from culture medium (M.A.) as a function of time in the presence (closed symbols) or absence (open symbols) of deficient fibroblasts. (B) Increase in cellular α-L-fucosidase specific activity (C.A.) as a function of the activity of the enzyme in the culture medium (M.A.). Open symbols: specific activity of 10,000g supernatant. Closed symbols: specific activity of whole homogenate. Activities are expressed as nmoles 4-methylumbelliferone per minute per mg protein (C.A.) or per ml medium (M.A.).

Our main objective in purifying α-L-fucosidase from human placenta was to assess the suitability of the enzyme preparation for enzyme replacement therapy. To this end, we have carried out some preliminary experiments on the uptake of this enzyme by skin fibroblast cultures from the two brothers with fucosidosis 2.

The purified enzyme preparation was added to fibroblast culture medium to a specific activity of 4.8 nmoles/min/ml and the cells harvested at intervals of 5,16,25 and 45 hours thereafter. As shown in Fig. 6A the specific activity of α-L-fucosidase in the cell pellet increased in an approximately linear fashion with time of exposure to enzyme. The specific activity of the enzyme taken up by the cells (over a 45 hour period) was also found to be directly proportional to the concentration of enzyme in the culture medium, over the range 0.0 to 7.8 nmoles/min/ml medium (Fig. 6B). To examine the stability of the enzyme following its uptake, five flasks of cells were incubated in supplemented medium (10.3 nmoles/min/ml) for 43 hours. The medium was then replaced by unsupple-

Table 4. Major findings in fucosidosis.

	Type 1 (5 Cases)	Type 2 (5 Cases)
Onset of Psychomotor Retardation (mos.)	12 - 16 (mean 12.8)	12 - 24 (mean 17.2)
Death (yrs.)	3 9/12 - 5 2/12 (3/5)	Alive (5/5)
Psychomotor Retardation	+ (5/5)	+ (5/5)
Neurologic Signs	+ (5/5)	+ (5/5)
Angiokeratoma Corporis Diffusum	- (5/5)	+ (5/5)
Splenomegaly	+ (1/5)	+ (1/5)
Kyphoscoliosis	+ (4/5)	+ (4/5)
Skeletal Abnormalities	+ (5/5)	+ (5/5)
Increased NaCl in Sweat	+ (4/4)	- (4/5)*

*One patient was anhydrotic
+ = symptom present   - = symptom absent

mented medium and the cells harvested after 0, 6, 24, 30, and 55
hours. The enzyme was quite stable within the cells with a loss
of activity of only 22% over the 55 hour period.

Isoelectric focusing of fibroblast extracts following incorporation of placental enzyme revealed a series of isozymes similar
to those seen in the original enzyme preparation. It was also
found that purified α-L-fucosidase from both placenta and serum
was incorporated by deficient cells with equal efficiency.

DISCUSSION

By comparing the findings of the two patients with fucosidosis
described here and those of eight other patients reported previously (7,11,14,16,17,26) it becomes apparent that there are two
types of the disease. In type 1 the onset of psychomotor regression

occurs in the beginning of the second year of life (mean age of onset 12.8 months). Severe neurologic signs also develop during the second year and the concentration of sodium and chloride in the sweat is increased. In type 2 psychomotor regression and neurologic signs develop during the second year of life (mean age of onset 17.2 months), but they are less severe than in type 1. Skin lesions of angiokeratoma corporis diffusion appear later in life and the concentration of sodium and chloride in the sweat is normal. Table 4 lists the major findings in fucosidosis types 1 and 2. The patient reported by Schafer et al., presented with unusual findings and, therefore, he is not included in Table 4.

Le[a] and Le[b] antigens were found significantly elevated on the erythrocytes and in saliva of both patients, while the H specificity was within the normal range. These findings suggest that the deficient fucosidase is an enzyme specific for α 1→4 linkages. This is because Lewis specific α-L-fucose is bound in α 1→4 linkage to N-acetyl-D-glucosamine, while H specific α-L-fucose is bound in α 1→2 linkage to β-galactose. It has previously been reported (11) that both H and Lewis activities are elevated in the more severe form of fucosidosis (Type 1). It is possible that the normal enzyme has the ability to cleave both α 1→2 and α 1→4 linkages, reminiscent of the double specificity reported for acid α-glucosidase (9). In that case, the mutation responsible for type 1 fucosidosis may destroy both specificities, while that in type 2 may disturb only the activity required for the hydrolysis of α 1→4 linkages.

The level of α-L-fucosidase activity observed in mixed leukocytes, mononuclear cells and granulocytes was most variable in the granulocytes and least variable in mononuclear cells. It appears that purified mononuclear cells are the best material for the identification of the carrier state of fucosidosis. No overlap was observed between patients, carriers, and controls.

The findings in cultured skin fibroblasts should be interpreted with caution when these cells are utilized for the detection of heterozygotes for fucosidosis. Enzyme activity within the carrier range may be found in fibroblasts obtained from normal subjects when the cells are not growing optimally.

The observation that long-term lymphoid cell lines established from patients with fucosidosis show absence of α-L-fucosidase activity, indicates that these lines express the genotype of the donor and, therefore, they can be used for the diagnosis of the disease. Moreover, since the lymphoid lines can be multiplied in large quantities and they have been found to maintain enzymatic stability over long periods in culture (2), it appears that these cells are the tissue of choice for the study of the basic metabolic defect in fucosidosis.

α-L-Fucosidase is polymorphic in the white population of
North America. The three common phenotypes distinguishable by isoelectric focusing were shown by family studies to be the result of
two autosomal alleles (designated $\underline{Fu^1}$ and $\underline{Fu^2}$). However, apparent
anomalies were observed in the inheritance of these two alleles in
the family of two brothers with fucosidosis 2. These unusual
patterns of inheritance could be explained by proposing that a
'silent' allele $\underline{(Fu^0)}$ was segregating at the α-L-fucosidase gene
locus within this family. These studies provide good evidence that
the mutation responsible for fucosidosis 2 is within the structural
gene locus for α-L-fucosidase, rather than at a second locus
responsible for activation, stabilization or regulation of the
enzyme. We have obtained preliminary evidence that the α-L-fucosidase structural locus is located on chromosome 1 (23).

Cultured skin fibroblasts from deficient individuals provide
a useful system for preliminary studies on the feasibility of
enzyme replacement therapy. We have shown that α-L-fucosidase
purified from placenta is taken up by skin fibroblasts from deficient individuals. Uptake is directly proportional to the time of
exposure of the cells to exogenous enzyme and to the concentration
of this enzyme. More importantly, the incorporated enzyme is
degraded relatively slowly. Serum α-L-fucosidase is incorporated
by deficient fibroblasts as efficiently as the placental enzyme
and we have no evidence so far for the existence of 'high' and
'low' uptake forms of the enzyme, analogous to those described for
β-glucuronidase (8). However, the various isozymes of α-L-fucosidase may well differ in their in vivo stabilities or in their
ability to hydrolyse the various fucose containing compounds which
accumulate in deficient individuals. Our experiments so far have
shown that cultured skin fibroblasts provide a suitable system
for the further investigation of these possibilities.

                              SUMMARY

Deficiency of the enzyme α-L-fucosidase has been demonstrated
in peripheral leukocytes, cultured skin fibroblasts and long-term
lymphoid lines from two sibs with fucosidosis 2. Reliable identification of heterozygotes for this disease was accomplished by
enzyme assay of mononuclear cells isolated from peripheral blood.
Isoelectric focusing of α-L-fucosidase isozymes in leukocyte
extracts from normal individuals revealed a common polymorphism
which was shown to result from two autosomal alleles at a single,
autosomal locus. Evidence was obtained for a third, 'silent'
allele segregating in the family of the two affected children.
It is probable that the disease fucosidosis type 2 results from

homozygosity for this 'silent' allele. Preliminary experiments have shown that cultured skin fibroblasts from deficient individuals can incorporate and retain purified α-L-fucosidase added to the culture medium.

This work was supported in part by U.S.P.H.S. Grant HD-02552 and Genetics Center Grant GM-19443.

REFERENCES

1. Alhadeff, J.A., Miller, A.L. and O'Brien, J.S.: Purification of human placental α-L-fucosidase by affinity chromatography. Anal. Biochem., 60:424, 1974.

2. Beratis, N.G., Danesino, C., and Hirschhorn, K.: Detection of homozygotes and heterozygotes for metachromatic leukodystrophy in lymphoid cell lines and peripheral leukocytes. Ann. Hum. Genet., 38:485, 1975.

3. Beratis, N.G., and Hirschhorn, K.: Establishment of long-term lymphoid cell lines. Mamm. Chrom. Newsl., 14:114, 1973.

4. Beratis, N.G., Turner, B.M., and Hirschhorn, K.: Fucosidosis: Detection of the carrier state in peripheral blood leukocytes. J. Pediat., in press.

5. Beratis, N.G., Turner, B.M., Weiss, R., and Hirschhorn, K.: Arylsulfatase B deficiency in Maroteaux-Lamy syndrome: Cellular studies and carrier identification. Pediat. Res., 9: 475, 1975.

6. Berkman, E.M., Nusbacher, J., Kochwa, S., and Rosenfield, R.E.: Quantitative blood typing. Transfusion, 2:317, 1971.

7. Borrone, C., Gatti, R., Trias, X., and Durand, P.: Fucosidosis: Clinical, biochemical, immunologic, and genetic studies in two new cases. J. Pediat., 84:727, 1974.

8. Brot, F.E., Glaser, J.H., Roozen, K.J. and Sly, W.S.: In vitro correction of deficient human fibroblasts by β-glucuronidase from different human sources. Biochem. Biophys. Res. Comm., 57:1, 1974.

9. Brown, B.I., Brown, D.H., and Jeffrey, P.L.: Simultaneous absence of α-1,4-glucosidase and α-1,6-glucosidase activities (pH 4) in tissues of children with type II glycogen storage disease. Biochemistry, 9:1423, 1970.

10. Dawson, G., and Spranger, J.W.: Fucosidosis: A glycosphin-
     golipidosis. New Engl. J. Med., 285:122, 1971.

11. Durand, P., Borrone, C., and Della Cella, G.: Fucosidosis.
     J. Pediat., 75:665, 1969.

12. Harris, H.: Principles of Human Biochemical Genetics, 2nd
     ed., Elsevier, Holland, 1975.

13. Kousseff, B.G., Beratis, N.G., Strauss, L., Brill, P.W.,
     Rosenfield, R.E., Kaplan, B., and Hirschhorn, K.: Fucosidosis
     Type 2. Pediatrics, in press.

14. Loeb, H., Tondeur, M., Jonniaux, G., Mockel-Pohl, S., and
     Vamos-Hurwitz, E.: Biochemical and ultrastructural studies in
     a case of mucopolysaccharidosis "F" (Fucosidosis). Helv.
     Paediat. Acta, 36:519, 1969.

15. Lowry, O.H., Rosebrough, N.J., Farr, A.L., and Randall, R.J.:
     Protein measurement with the Folin phenol reagent. J. Biol.
     Chem., 193:265, 1951.

16. Matsuda, I., Arashima, S., Anakura, M., Ege, A., and Hayata,
     I.: Fucosidosis. Tohoku J. Exp. Med., 109:41, 1973.

17. Patel, V., Watanabe, I., and Zeman, W.: Deficiency of alpha-
     L-fucosidase. Science, 176:426, 1972.

18. Robinson, D. and Thorpe, R.: Affinity chromatography of
     human liver α-L-fucosidase. FEBS Lett., 45:191, 1974.

19. Schafer, I.A., Powell, D.W., and Sullivan, J.C.: Lysosomal
     bone disease. Pediat. Res., 5:391, 1971 (abstr.).

20. Turner, B.M., Beratis, N.G., Turner, V.S., and Hirschhorn, K.:
     Isozymes of human α-L-fucosidase detectable by starch-gel
     electrophoresis. Clin. Chim. Acta, 57:29, 1974.

21. Turner, B.M., Beratis, N.G., Turner, V.S., and Hirschhorn, K.:
     Silent allele as genetic basis of fucosidosis. Nature, 257:
     391, 1975.

22. Turner, B.M., Turner, V.S., Beratis, N.G., and Hirschhorn, K.:
     Polymorphism of human α-fucosidase. Am. J. Hum. Genet., 27:
     651, 1975.

23. Turner, V.S., Turner, B.M., Kucherlapati, R., Ruddle, F., and
     Hirschhorn, K.: Localization of human α-L-fucosidase to
     chromosome 1 by the use of a 'clone panel'. Third Int. Work-

shop on Human Gene Mapping. Birth Defects: Original Article Series. The National Foundation, N.Y. (in press).

24. Van Hoof, F., and Hers, H.G.: Mucopolysaccharidosis by absence of α-fucosidase. Lancet, 1:1198, 1968.

25. Van Hoof, F., and Hers, H.G.: The abnormalities of lysosomal enzymes in mucopolysaccharides. Europ. J. Biochem., 7:34, 1968.

26. Voelz, C., Tolksdorf, M., Freitag, F., and Spranger, J.: Fucosidose. Mschr. Kinderheilk., 119:352, 1971.

27. Zielke, K., Okada, S., and O'Brien, J.: Fucosidosis: Diagnosis by serum assay of α-L-fucosidase. J. Lab. Clin. Med., 79:164, 1972.

28. Zielke, K., Veath, M.L., and O'Brien, J.S.: Fucosidosis: Deficiency of alfa-L-fucosidase in cultured skin fibroblasts. J. Exp. Med., 136:197, 1972.

STUDIES IN METACHROMATIC LEUKODYSTROPHY. XIII. PURIFICATION OF SULFATASE A FROM NORMAL HUMAN LIVER

Janet Collins, Warren Yamada, William Worth, and James Austin
Department of Neurology, University of Colorado Medical Center
4200 East Ninth Avenue, Denver, Colorado   80220

Metachromatic leukodystrophy (MLD) is a genetically-determined neurolipidosis characterized by deficient activity of sulfatase A (cerebroside sulfatase) and by the resultant accumulation of cerebroside sulfate. Immunological studies using a monospecific antibody to sulfatase A have shown that MLD patients do have the enzyme protein (7). The reason why this protein has little or no activity is not yet clear. The first step in such a study is to isolate and characterize the normal sulfatase.

Assay of Sulfatase Activity

Sulfatase A activity was determined colorimetrically against its substrate, nitrocatechol sulfate (NCS). The reagent system contained 10 mM NCS, 0.5 mM $Na_4P_2O_7$, and 1.7 M NaCl in 0.5 M sodium acetate - acetic acid buffer, pH 5.2. 0.2 ml of the reagent solution was added to 0.2 ml of enzyme sample and incubated at 37^0C for 30 min. The reaction was terminated by adding 0.6 ml of IN NaOH. The absorbance of liberated nitrocatechol was measured at 515 nm. Units of enzyme activity were expressed as umoles NCS hydrolyzed per minute. Protein was determined by the method of Lowry.

Supported by Grant # NS07701-09 from NINCDS.

Steps in the Isolation of Sulfatase A   (Table I)

Unless otherwise indicated, all steps were performed at 4°C. Centrifugations were at 10,000 X g for 20 min. Buffer pH was determined at room temperature. The entire procedure can be accomplished in 6 days.

Step I. 500 gm of normal human liver was obtained fresh at autopsy. Vessels and connective tissue were removed. Tissue was diced, washed twice with water, and homogenized in 3 vol. (vol/wet wt) of H_2O in a Waring blender. Lysosomes were disrupted by sonication for 2 min at 50 w. Insoluble material was removed by centrifugation.

Step II. Solid $(NH_4)_2SO_4$ was added to the supernatant to a concentration of 2.37 molal. The precipitate after centrifugation was resuspended in water and dialysed overnight.

Step III. Proteins were precipitated between 20 and 50% acetone at -5°C. Pellets were washed twice with 50% acetone, resuspended in 0.1 M sodium acetate buffer, pH 5.5, and dialysed extensively vs. this buffer. Material reprecipitating during dialysis was removed by centrifugation.

Step IV. The supernatant was applied to a 3 X 20 cm bed of CM-Sephadex (C-50-120) in 0.1 M sodium acetate buffer, pH 5.5 and the gel was subsequently washed with this buffer. Active fractions were combined, concentrated vs. dry polyethylene glycol, and dialysed extensively vs. 0.05 M Tris-HCl, pH 7.4.

Step V. The concentrated enzyme solution (5 ml or less) was applied to a Sephadex G-150 column (2.6 X 92 cm) previously equilibrated with Tris buffer and eluted. Peak fractions of sulfatase activity were pooled and dialysed vs. 0.1 M Tris-HCl pH 7.4.

Step VI. A 3 X 36 cm column of DEAE-Sephadex (A-50-120) was prepared and equilibrated with 0.1 M Tris-HCl, pH 7.4. Pooled fraction from the previous step was applied and the column was washed with 100 ml of buffer. Protein was eluted with a salt gradient formed from 200 ml of the above buffer and 200 ml of 0.4 M NaCl in buffer. Active fractions were pooled, concentrated as before, and dialysed vs. 0.05 M Tris-HCl, pH 7.4.

Step VII. The concentrated enzyme solution was applied to G-150

Table I. Steps of Sulfatase A Purification

Step	Protein (mg)	Total Units (umoles/min)	Yield %	Specific Activity (umoles/min/mg)
I	20,540	123.2	100	0.0060
II	5,200	93.6	76	0.018
III	2,000	66.4	54	0.033
IV	458	48.5	39	0.106
V	200	39.6	32	0.198
VI	44	23.8	19	0.541
VII	5.2	20.5	17	3.95

as in Step V. Active fractions, pooled and concentrated, are referred
to as the "purified enzyme preparation". The purified sulfatase A from
Step VII was rechromatographed on Sephadex G-150. A single protein
peak was observed at 280 nm that coincided with a single peak of arylsulfatase A activity (4.0 umoles/min/1.0 OD at 280 min).

Determination of the Molecular Size of Arylsulfatase A
by Gel Filtration

The partially purified material from Step VI was chromatographed
on a Sephadex G-150 column (44.5 X 1.5 cm), equilibrated with 0.1 M
Tris-HCl buffer, pH 7.4 (void volume 31 ml). The K_{av} value was calculated and compared to those of aldolase, ovalbumin, chymotrypsino-
gen, and ribonuclease chromatographed on the same column. The
molecular weight of sulfatase A was estimated as 134,000.

Determination of the Isoelectric Point

Isoelectric focusing was performed in polyacrylamide gels. Partially purified enzyme, Step VI, was applied at the top (cathode) of the
gel. 0.02 M NaOH was used as the cathodal solution, 0.01 M phosphoric
acid as anodal solution. Ampholyte range used was 3 - 6, and total
running time was 8 hours at 1 mA/gel. Sulfatase A activity focused at
pH 4.7.

Electrophoretic Studies

The electrophoretic pattern of the purified enzyme preparation,
Step VII, was determined by polyacrylamide disc electrophoresis at
pH 8.5 by the method of Davis (1), and at pH 4.5 by the method of
Reisfeld (3). The results are illustrated in Figs. 1 and 2. Gel 1A
shows the electrophoretic appearance at pH 8.5 and gel 2A the appearance at pH 4.5 of the enzyme preparation after it had been incubated for
30 min in substrate solution at 37°C and developed with IN NaOH. One
band of sulfatase A activity is seen on each gel. Immediately after isolation, material from Step VII was electrophoresed at pH 8.5 and stained
with 0.05% Coomassie blue (Fig. 1). The pattern of three protein bands
seen in 1 was observed. The band with the lowest electrophoretic mobility corresponded with sulfatase A activity and the second band with
greater mobility was only slightly active, whereas the band with the
greatest mobility had no sulfatase A activity. When the preparation was

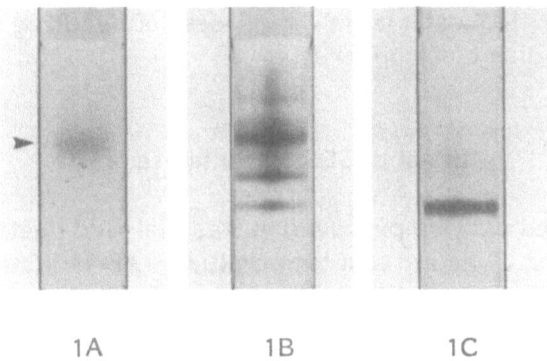

1A   1B   1C

Fig. 1. Disc electrophoresis at pH 8.5 of arylsulfatase A preparations. Gel 1A was developed for activity with NCS; 1B and 1C were
stained for protein with Coomassie blue. Enzyme applied to 1B was
freshly isolated whereas that applied to 1C had been stored for 1 - 2
weeks. Arrow indicates arylsulfatase A activity.

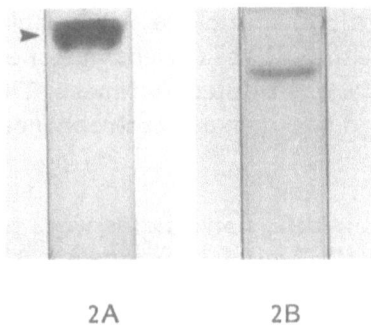

2A   2B

Fig. 2. Disc electrophoresis at pH 4.5 of arylsulfatase A preparations. Gel 2A was developed with NCS, whereas 2B was stained for
protein. 2B represents material stored for 1 - 2 weeks. Arrow indicates arylsulfatase A activity.

stored frozen for 1 - 2 weeks, thawed, and again electrophoresed in
each system, gels 1C (Fig. 1) and 2B (Fig. 2) were obtained. On this
occasion, only one band with high electrophoretic mobility could be
clearly seen, but slight sulfatase A activity was still found in the previously determined position, even though no protein band was revealed

there. Thus, it appeared that some breakdown of the enzyme had occurred in the purified material in the process of handling and/or during
the procedure of disc electrophoresis.

Effect of SDS on Sulfatase A

The purified enzyme preparation was dialysed against 1% sodium
dodecyl sulfate for 24 hr at room temperature. Arylsulfatase A activity
was destroyed and could not be regained by exhaustive dialysis. SDS
acrylamide gel electrophoresis gave a diffuse protein band the mobility
of which indicated that the enzyme had broken down. Gels were not
precisely calibrated due to the diffuse nature of the band.

Immunological Studies

Further to confirm the presence of pure enzyme, 100 micrograms
of the preparation was injected subcutaneously as previously described
(2) into two New Zealand white rabbits. Fourteen days after the initial
inoculation, the rabbits were again challenged. Two weeks later, sera
were obtained by femoral venepuncture. One rabbit yielded a high
antibody titer, precipitating 80% of the enzyme of a crude liver preparation when the antibody was diluted 16 times. This serum was then
used for double diffusion and immunoelectrophoresis studies shown in
Fig. 3.

Ouchterlony double diffusion studies were performed on microscope slides, covered with 2 ml of 1% agarose in 0.03 M phosphate buffer, pH 8.0, containing 0.1 M NaCl, 0.01 M EDTA, and 0.1% sodium
azide. Wells (0.2 mm diameter) were made and filled. Antiserum was
placed in the center well, and samples from various stages of purification were placed in the outer wells. A single line of identity seen after
24 hours, coincided with arylsulfatase A activity.

Microimmunoelectrophoresis slides were prepared (5) using 2%
agar in barbital buffer. Antibody was electrophoresed for 45 min, and
enzyme for 3 hours at a potential difference of 20 V/slide. Slides were
developed 48 hours, then washed and stained or developed for activity.
In each case a single precipitin line was seen. The enzyme migrated
8 mm towards the positive electrode, the antibody 6 mm towards the
negative, similar to gamma globulin. In each case arylsulfatase activity coincided with the precipitin band.

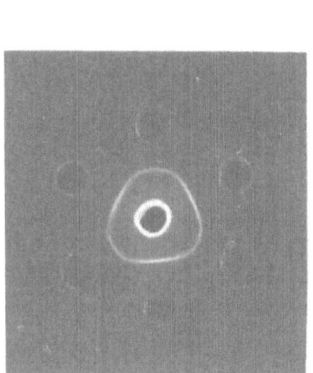
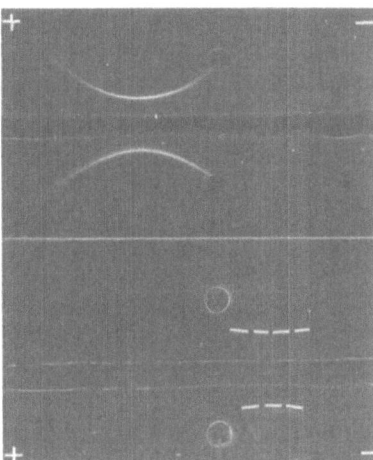

Fig. 3. Left: Immunodiffusion of sulfatase A at various stages of purification. Antibody was placed in center well. One precipitin line is seen. Right top: Immunoelectrophoresis of enzyme from Step VII run for 45 min. Antibody was placed in trough. Right bottom: Antibody was electrophoresed for 3 hours, and enzyme was placed in the trough. Dashed white line outlines single precipitin line. In both instances, only one precipitin band was seen coincident with arylsulfatase A activity.

Discussion

The procedure described takes 6 days and is a relatively simple way to isolate sulfatase A requiring no special equipment. The yield is substantial: over 5 mg of enzyme from 500 gm of liver. Evidence substantiating the purity and homogeneity of the preparation was obtained both from chromatographic, electrophoretic, and immunological techniques.

The apparent instability of the purified ASA is interesting and is in agreement with the observations of others. Thus, Stevens et al, observed spontaneous breakdown and loss of activity of the sulfatase A from human urine at a concentration of 100 ug/ml at pH 7.5 (6). Ox liver arylsulfatase A undergoes similar breakdown, but at more dilute concentrations (<.05 ug/ml) (4). The change observed in the present study might be due to dilution during G-150 chromatography, storage, or simple ageing. Enzyme instability has also been observed at a pH below 4.0, and during SDS treatment --- phenomena that are perhaps related. The purity resulting from the isolation procedure described and its milligram yield now make it possible to investigate these and other properties of the normal and abnormal sulfatase A more fully.

References

1)   Davis, B.J.: Disc electrophoresis. II. Method and application to human serum proteins. Ann N Y Acad Sci, 121, 404, 1964.

2)   Neuwelt E., Stumpf, D., Austin, J., Kohler, P.: A monospecific antibody to human sulfatase A: Preparation, characterization, and significance. Biochem Biophys Acta, 236, 333, 1971.

3)   Reisfeld, R., Lewis, U., Williams, D.: Disk electrophoresis of basic proteins and peptides on polyacrylamide gels. Nature, 193, 281, 1962.

4)   Roy, A.B., Jerfy, A.: The sulphatase of ox liver XIV. The subunit structure of sulfatase A. Biochem Biophys Acta, 207, 156, 1970.

5)   Scheidegger, J.: Une micro-methode de l'immuno-electrophorese. Intern Arch Allergy, 7, 103, 1955.

6)   Stevens, R.L., Fluharty, A.L., Skokut, M.H., Kihara, H.: Purification and properties of arylsulfatase A from human urine. J Biol Chem, 250, 2495, 1975.

7)   Stumpf, D., Neuwelt, E., Austin, J., Kohler, P.: Metachromatic leukodystrophy: X. Immunological studies of the abnormal sulfatase A. Arch Neurol, 25, 427, 1971.

p.NITROCATECHOL SULFATE FOR ARYLSULFATASE ASSAY :

DETECTION OF METACHROMATIC LEUKODYSTROPHY VARIANTS

Gisèle Dubois, Jean-Claude Turpin, Nicole Baumann

Laboratoire de Neurochimie, INSERM U.134, CNRS ERA 421

Hôpital de la Salpêtrière, 75634 Paris Cédex 13, France

Artificial substrates are being used routinely for the diagnosis of lipidosis. In the case of metachromatic leukodystrophy (MLD), p.nitrocatechol-sulfate (p.NCS) at acidic pH is the substrate for arylsulfatase A (ASA). Complete analogy of elution profile on column chromatography between ASA and cerebroside sulfate sulfatase (1) has secured in the use of the artificial substrate for MLD diagnosis. Although an activator protein is necessary for enzyme action on the natural substrate (2), only the ASA enzyme itself is deficient in MLD variant B (3). Another enzyme arylsulfatase B (ASB) reacts with p.NCS at less acidic pH ; together with ASA and other sulfatases, it is deficient in another type of sulfatidosis, Austin's disease or MLD variant O (3).

Although pH optimum are different, there is some interference for the colorimetric assay of ASA and ASB (4). Therefore an electrophoretic method was devised in our laboratory enabling separation of A and B isozymes (5). A third isozyme, reacting as ASA in relation to specific inhibitors, was also identified (6). Colorimetric assay and electrophoresis are run routinely when MLD is suspected.

We wish to report here two variants : cases 1 and 2 in which electrophoresis alone has allowed the diagnosis of MLD ; case 3 in which the healthy state of the patient was in contrast with the very low value of ASA. These facts will be discussed in relation to the genetic and the pathogeny of MLD.

METHODS

All studies have been made using techniques previously reported (7). Colorimetric assays and electrophoresis were always
performed on leukocytes isolated from freshly drawn blood, and
stocked at -30°C. Assay has been restandardised in leukocytes as
we found specific inhibitors different from those used in urine
(8). $AgNO_3$ inhibits specifically ASA and NaCl, ASB.

Electrophoresis is performed on polyacrylamide gels at acidic
pH with detection of enzyme activity after incubation of the gels
in the presence of the artificial substrate (7). The two upper
bands correspond to the two ASA isozymes and are deficient in MLD
variant B (Figure).

CASES 1 AND 2

The young girl C. started being ill at age 14 months, when
appeared for the first time signs of regression of mental and motor acquisitions. At age 2, the child had a quadriparesia ; there
were neither symptoms of decerebration nor extension to the peripheral nervous system. Nerve conduction was normal (40 m/sec.).
In CSF, protein concentration was 0.26 g/l. An intermittent sulfa-
tiduria was observed. A nerve biopsy showed no signs of demyelination but classical metachromatic deposits colored with cresyl-
violet were present. ASA level was 206 units (Normal 100-200
units). ASB level was 315 units (Normal 100-200 units). Electrophoresis showed the disappearance of only the upper band of ASA
(Figure) (6).

The young girl Y. was seen for the first time at 29 months of
age. The post-natal development was normal and the first symptoms
appeared at 22 months. When she was seen, she was in a state of
decerebration with pyramidal symptoms and complete loss of contact
with the outer world. There were no clinical peripheral symptoms.
CSF was normal. ASA level was 62 units. Peripheral nerve biopsy
visualized metachromatic deposits but no alteration of the myelin
sheaths. Electrophoresis showed the disappearance of the upper
band of ASA.

Both cases had a beginning at the same age as infantile MLD,
but evolution is less severe ; both children are still alive and
age 5 and 4. Although there was no peripheral clinical symptomato-
logy, metachromatic deposits were observed on nerve biopsy. Assay
for ASA was either normal or in the heterozygote range. Electrophoresis enabled the diagnosis of this variant as the upper band
of ASA was absent.

CASE 3

B. is the healthy father of ten children. 2 died before
birth ; another one died at age 4, after a convulsion. Two other
children who were heterozygote twins had a late infantile form of
MLD ; one died at age 3 ; the other, still living now, is 4 and a
half. All the other children are apparently healthy, and except
for one, well over the age of beginning of the disease. A survey
of the whole family was performed so as to determine ASA level.
The mother was in the heterozygote range (68 units) ; the father
and three children had levels analogous to those of the deceased
children, i.e. respectively 16, 11, 11 and 16 units. The values
previously observed in the children who died of MLD being 14 and
16 units. Electrophoresis confirmed the colorimetric assay ; in
all those having a low level of ASA, electrophoresis showed the
disappearance of the two ASA isozymes (Figure).

Therefore, even a healthy father and healthy children in a
MLD family may have an extremely low level of ASA as judged by
colorimetric assay and electrophoresis of enzyme activity (9).

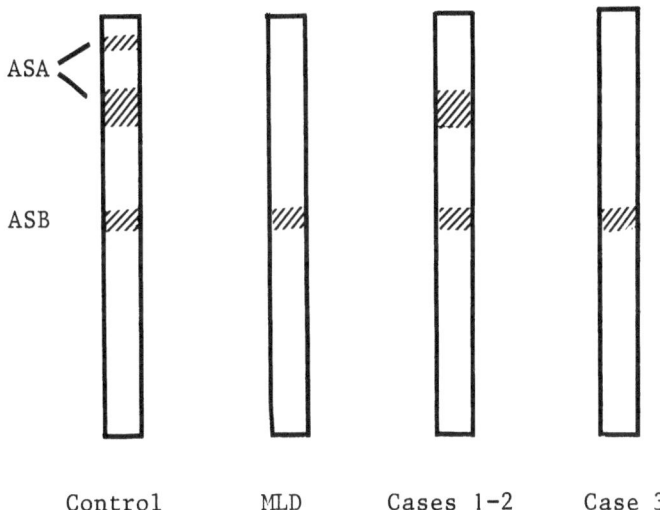

Figure 1. Electrophoregram of arylsulfatases of leukocytes from
different MLD cases. Enzymatic staining with p.NCS (5).

DISCUSSION

In MLD variant B, there is a deficiency in ASA as well as in cerebroside sulfate sulfatase ; this implies a common part, probably related to the active site, explaining the perfect correlation generally observed.

In the cases reported here, there is a discrepancy between the clinical states of the patients and the level of ASA. In cases 1 and 2, the metachromatic state is not correlated with a pathologic level of ASA as judged by the colorimetric assay. On the other hand, in case 3, a healthy condition is associated with a level of ASA identical to the one observed usually in MLD. These results would indicate a non complete identity between ASA and cerebroside sulfate sulfatase (CSS). The clinical differences observed in cases 1 and 2 compared to case 3 may be a reflexion of differences in the function of different subunits.

From the data reported here, at least two genes appear to be involved in controlling sulfatase activity : one related to the active site affecting both ASA and CSS activities, deficient in MLD variant B ; one affecting only ASA activity as in case 3. In case 2 leukodystrophy and metachromasy are present although ASA level is normal ; the upper band of ASA is a minor band in leukocytes but in brain it may be more important and essentially related to cerebroside sulfate sulfatase activity.

These hypothesis have been formulated by comparing ASA assays with the clinical state of the patients. Further studies are in progress which imply cerebroside sulfate sulfatase determinations. Data reported (10) in ox indicate that ASA is a tetramer composed of four presumably identical monomer. Cases reported here would indicate the presence of two different subunits. Studies are to be done implying the purification of normal and abnormal enzymes in leukocytes and in brain.

ACKNOWLEDGEMENTS

This investigation was supported by funds from CNRS and INSERM.

REFERENCES

1. Mehl E., Jatzkewitz H., Hoppe-Seylers Z. Physiol. Chem. <u>339</u>, 260-276, 1964.

2. Jatzkewitz H., Stinshoff K. F.E.B.S. Letters 32, 129-131, 1973.

3. Harzer K., Stinshoff K., Mraz W., Jatzkewitz H. J. Neurochem. 20, 279-287, 1973.

4. Dubois G., Baumann N. Biochem. Biophys. Res. Commun. 50, 1129-1135, 1973.

5. Dubois G., Turpin J.C., Baumann N. Compte-Rendu Acad. Sc. Paris 278,D, 1401-1403, 1974.

6. Turpin J.C., Dubois G., Baumann N. Compte-Rendu Acad. Sc. Paris 279,D, 2819-2822, 1974.

7. Dubois G., Turpin J.C., Baumann N. Biomedicine 23, 116-119, 1975.

8. Baum H., Dodgson K.S., Spencer B. Clin. Chim. Acta 4, 453-455, 1959.

9. Dubois G., Turpin J.C., Baumann N. New Engl. J. Med. 293 302, 1975.

10. Nichol L.W., Roy A.B. J. Biochem. 55, 645-651, 1964.

ARYLSULFATASES A AND B IN METACHROMATIC LEUKODYSTROPHY AND

MAROTEAUX-LAMY SYNDROME: STUDIES WITH 4-METHYLUMBELLIFERYL SULFATE

Edwin H. Kolodny and Richard A. Mumford

Eunice Kennedy Shriver Center for Mental Retardation,
Inc., at the Walter E. Fernald State School, Waltham,
Mass.; and Department of Neurology,
Massachusetts General Hospital, Boston, Mass.

Metachromatic leukodystrophy (MLD), a sphingolipidosis, and
Maroteaux-Lamy syndrome (MLS), a mucopolysaccharidosis, are
genetically distinct diseases which have in common a markedly
impaired ability to cleave the artificial substrate p-nitrocatechol
sulfate (NCS) under certain specified conditions. Numerous studies
employing this substrate have demonstrated deficiency of arylsulfatase A (AS-A) in MLD (1,6,7) and of arylsulfatase B (AS-B)
in MLS(3,4,7,13).However, several problems exist in connection
with its use.

The NCS method of assaying AS-A or AS-B, when they exist in
the same mixture, depends upon the differential inhibition of one
arylsulfatase while attempting simultaneously to maximize the
activity of a second arylsulfatase (2). Spillover of enzyme
activity probably occurs, particularly if the arylsulfatase
component to be measured comprises only a small proportion of the
total AS activity. Another difficulty is that the separate
delineation of MLD heterozygotes from homozygous normal and
homozygous affected individuals is not always certain with the
NCS method. Still another problem concerns the relative
insensitivity of assays employing NCS as the substrate. Because
the kinetics of the AS-A reaction are anomalous (12), short
incubation times are preferred necessitating high levels of enzyme
protein in the incubation mixtures to obtain measurable levels of
enzyme activity. Therefore, to improve the assay methods for AS-A
and AS-B, two modifications were needed, a method for the physical
separation of these two enzymes and a substrate which would permit
greater sensitivity in measuring enzyme activity.

The original intent in our study of the arylsulfatases was
to develop a method of enzyme analysis which would be useful for
the automated analysis of these enzymes in large numbers of
human specimens. This investigation led to the development of
a facile method for extracting the lysosomal arylsulfatases found
in leukocytes and fibroblasts and for separating them from each
other. By then assaying the separated enzyme fractions with the
fluorogenic substrate, 4-methylumbelliferyl sulfate, the activity
of the individual enzyme components could be determined with a
high degree of sensitivity.

MATERIALS AND METHODS

Substrate

4-methylumbelliferyl sulfate was purchased from Eastman Kodak
(Rochester, N.Y.) and further purified according to the technique
of Rinderknecht, et. al. (8). Modifications to the procedure
included repetition of the methanol-water crystallization four
times with adjustment to pH 9.0 using KOH and ommission of the
ethyl acetate extraction. The final substrate preparation contained
an amount of fluorescence equivalent to less than 0.025 nmoles
4-methylumbelliferone per mole MUS.

Electrophoresis

Sepraphore III cellulose acetate strips were utilized as the
support medium and 0.1M Tris-acetate pH 7.0 served as the running
buffer. Prior to sample application, the strips were soaked in
buffer containing 0.1% serum albumin (w/v). After 1 hour of
electrophoresis at 2.5 ma/strip, the strips were overlayed with a
second strip presoaked in 20 mM MUS- 6 mM lead acetate - 100 mM
sodium acetate pH 5.5 and incubated at 37°C for 1 hr in a sealed
moist chamber. Another strip presoaked in 0.25 M glycine-KOH pH
10.3 was then applied and the enzyme activity represented by the
fluorescence visualized under a long wavelength ultraviolet light.

Extraction of Leukocytes and Fibroblasts

Leukocytes were prepared from 10 ml of heparinized whole blood by differential dextran sedimentation (5). Skin fibroblasts were grown to confluency, harvested with trypsin and washed with 0.9% sodium chloride. Each pellet of leucocytes or fibroblasts was sonicated in 1.0 ml of 0.9% sodium chloride. The sonicate was centrifuged at 27,000 x g for 20 min. With this procedure more than 90% of the total arylsulfatase activity present was released into the supernatant.

Separation of Arylsulfatases A and B

Carboxymethylcellulose (CM-32) was prepared according to the manufacturer's instructions and then equilibrated with 0.05 M sodium acetate pH 6.0. Columns (0.5 x 8 cm) of CM-32 were used to separate leukocyte arylsulfatases while the fibroblast arylsulfatases were separated in a test tube containing a similar quantity (2 ml, in suspension) of CM-32. In the presence of 0.05 M sodium acetate pH 6.0, AS-A is not adsorbed on CM-32 but is recovered in the column eluates, or, if the test tube method is used, in the supernatant after centrifugation. AS-B is then obtained by treatment of the resin with 1-2 ml 0.3 M sodium chloride in 0.05 M sodium acetate pH 6.0.

Enzyme Assays

The reaction mixture for determination of arylsulfatase activity generally totaled 0.1 ml and included 0.02 ml enzyme, 0.02 ml 30 mM lead acetate and 0.05 ml 30 mM MUS in 0.1 M sodium acetate pH 5.5. The duration of incubations were 6 min for AS-A and 30 min for AS-B. The reaction was stopped by the addition of 2 ml of 0.25 M glycine-KOH buffer pH 10.3 and the amount of 4-methylumbelliferone liberated was determined fluorometrically in an Aminco-Bowman spectrofluorometer with an excitation wave length of 366 nm and an emission wavelength of 446 nm.

For the heat inactivation studies, 0.02 ml of the 27,000 x g supernatant enzyme was combined with 0.01 ml 1 M sodium acetate pH 5.5 and 0.05 ml distilled water and heated at 57° for specific periods of time. After cooling, 0.02 ml 30 mM lead acetate and 0.05 ml 20 mM MUS were added and the mixture incubated for 6 min at 37°. The reaction was then terminated and fluorometry conducted as described.

RESULTS

Separation of AS-A and AS-B

Cellulose acetate electrophoresis of leukocyte and fibroblast
extracts followed by incubation of the electrophoresis strips with
MUS disclosed the presence of two bands of enzyme activity in the
27,000 x g supernatants (Fig. 1, lane 1). The activity not adsorbed
by CM-32 migrated toward the anode (Fig. 1, lane 2) while that which
was adsorbed and then eluted with a concentrated salt solution moved
toward the cathode (Fig. 1, lane 3). Each of the CM-32 treated
fractions contained only one band of enzyme activity. The
designations shown in Figure 1 are based upon available information
about the relative net charge of AS-A and AS-B. The leukocytes
and fibroblasts of patients with MLD and MLS contained only one
band of enzyme activity corresponding in MLD cases to AS-B, and in
MLS cases to AS-A.

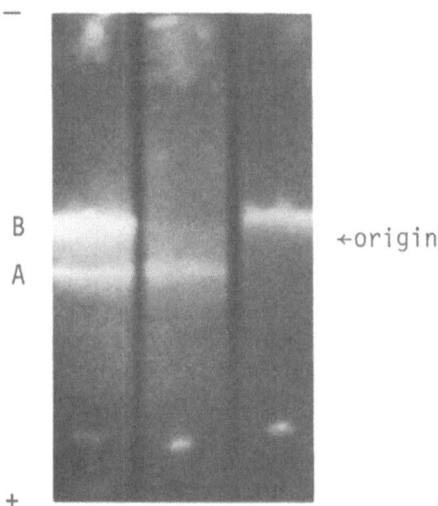

Figure 1. Arylsulfatase activity following electrophoresis on
cellulose acetate strips and incubation with MUS. Saline
supernatants of fibroblast sonicates were applied to 0.5 x 8 cm
columns of CM-32. Column elution was performed as described in
text. Origin = point of sample application. Lane 1 - activity
prior to CM-32 chromatography; lane 2 - unadsorbed activity;
lane 3 - adsorbed activity eluted with 0.3 M sodium chloride.

Properties of the Separated Enzymes

The properties of the leukocyte and fibroblast enzymes
separated with CM-32 and assayed with MUS are summarized in
Table 1. In an 0.1 M sodium acetate buffer, the optimum pH for
both enzymes was 5.5. The reaction velocity of AS-A was linear
only up to 10 minutes. After 10 minutes, the reaction slowed
progressively so that by one hour the amount of hydrolysis was
less than three times that observed at 10 minutes. The behavior
of AS-B with respect to time was quite different. Its reaction
with MUS was linear for periods greater than one hour. The
thermal stability of the two enzyme fractions also differed. The
separated AS-A lost 95% of its activity upon exposure to 60°
15 minutes while the activity of the AS-B fractions under these
conditions did not change.

TABLE 1

PROPERTIES OF ARYLSULFATASES A AND B SEPARATED FROM HUMAN LEUKOCYTES

AND FIBROBLASTS WITH CM-32 AND ASSAYED WITH 4-METHYLUMBELLIFERYL SULFATE

	AS-A	AS-B
pH optimum	5.5	5.5
Linearity with time	< 10 min.	> 60 min.
Heat stability at 60°	activity lost	stable
Effect of		
Lead acetate	3-fold stimulation	slight stimulation
Silver nitrate	80% reduction	no effect
Triton X-100	slight stimulation	3-fold stimulation

Different responses of the two enzyme fractions were also noted for lead and silver ions and for Triton X-100. Lead acetate, at a final concentration of 6 mM, stimulated leukocyte and fibroblast AS-A activity more than 3-fold whereas AS-B responded with only a slight increase in its MUS-cleaving activity. The presence of silver nitrate (0.24 mM) in the reaction mixtures caused an 80% reduction in AS-A activity but did not affect AS-B activity. The effect of 0.1% Triton X-100 was to stimulate the AS-B reaction three-fold. It also produced a slight stimulatory effect on AS-A activity. These effects of Triton X-100 were only observed with the separated enzyme fractions. The MUS-cleaving activity in the 27,000 x g supernatants of leukocyte and fibroblast sonicates was not altered by inclusion of Triton X-100 in the reaction mixture.

Arylsulfatase A Activities

The AS-A and AS-B activity of leukocytes and fibroblasts was determined with MUS after their physical separation with CM-32. Patients with MLD were markedly deficient in AS-A activity (Table 2). The mean specific activity in their leukocytes and fibroblasts was 11% of controls. All but one of the MLD homozygotes from whom the specimens were obtained carried a clinical diagnosis of infantile MLD. The single exception, a patient with the juvenile variant, had leukocyte and fibroblast AS-A values which were within the range of values obtained for the infantile MLD cases. In obligate heterozygotes for MLD, the mean specific activity of AS-A was approximately one-half of the mean control value. There was no overlap in the range of AS-A values for MLD homozygotes, heterozygotes and normals and the differences between these three groups were statistically highly significant for leukocytes. The difference in AS-A activity in fibroblasts between MLD patients and their parents was also highly significant, but that between parents and controls was only barely significant. The AS-A activity in MLS homozygotes and heterozygotes was within the range of values obtained for the control group.

TABLE 2

ARYLSULFATASE A ACTIVITIES IN HUMAN LEUKOCYTES AND FIBROBLASTS

Specimen	No.	Arylsulfatase A	t test
LEUKOCYTES			
MLD Homozygotes	5	2.8 ± 0.6	$p < 0.001$
MLD Heterozygotes	8	14.0 ± 4.7	
Controls	10	26.4 ± 6.4	$p < 0.01$
FIBROBLASTS			
MLD Homozygotes	4	9.6 ± 5.4	$p < 0.001$
MLD Heterozygotes	5	32.1 ± 6.4	
Controls	8	82.9 ± 54.7	$0.1 > p > 0.05$

Activities are expressed as nmoles/mg protein/hr. for leukocytes and as $nmoles/10^6$ cells for fibroblasts.

Arylsulfatase B Activities

A profound deficiency of AS-B activity was found in both leukocytes and fibroblasts from patients with MLS (Table 3). Three of four specimens (one leukocyte, two fibroblast) possessed virtually no AS-B activity while a trace amount of activity was detected in a second leukocyte sample. There was no statistical difference between the leukocyte AS-B values obtained in MLS heterozygotes and controls. The AS-B activity in leukocytes and fibroblasts of MLD patients and their parents was also not statistically different from that of controls.

TABLE 3

ARYLSULFATASE B ACTIVITIES IN HUMAN LEUKOCYTES AND FIBROBLASTS

Specimen	No.	Arylsulfatase B
LEUKOCYTES		
MLS Homozygotes	2	0.5 ± 0.7
MLS Heterozygotes	4	106.6 ±46.8
Controls	10	108.2 ±42.4
FIBROBLASTS		
MLS Homozygotes	2	0
Controls	8	63.9 ±43.9

Activities are expressed as nmoles/mg protein/hr. for leukocytes and as nmoles/10^6 cells for fibroblasts.

Thermal Inactivation

In leukocytes, AS-A accounts for only 20% of the total arylsulfatase activity while in fibroblasts approximately 55% of the total is AS-A activity. Therefore, the likelihood of demonstrating the differential effect of heat on AS-A and AS-B was deemed more likely to succeed with extracts of fibroblasts than of leukocytes. Preliminary results are promising (Fig. 2) and suggest that the four genotypes, MLD, MLS, MLD carriers and controls, can be distinguished from one another by heat inactivation of the 27,000 x g fibroblast supernatant for 5-10 minutes at 57°. The two extremes represented in Figure 2, MLD and MLS, bare out predictions based upon their relative content of the heat labile AS-A. No loss in total arylsulfatase activity is noted in MLD fibroblasts because the amount of AS-A in these cells is negligible, while exactly the opposite relationship holds for the MLS fibroblasts.

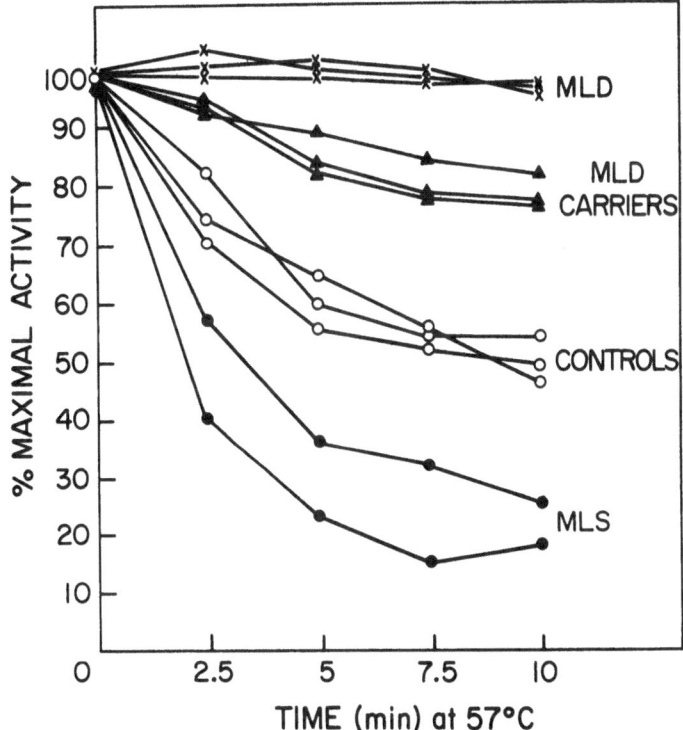

Figure 2. Aliquots of 27000 x g supernatants of fibroblast sonicates were mixed 1:3 with acetate buffer, heated for 2.5 to 10 minutes at 57°, and then assayed for their MUS-cleaving ability. The activity present in a non-heat treated sample was taken as 100%.

DISCUSSION

This investigation began as a search for a more sensitive
and specific tool to measure deficiencies of arylsulfatase activity
in human tissues. MUS was selected for study because, as a
fluorogenic substance, it provided the potential for a far greater
level of assay sensitivity than existed with the widely used
chromogenic substrate, NCS.

The use of MUS to measure arylsulfatase activity was first
reported in 1967 (11) yet NCS has remained the preferred substrate
for assay of arylsulfatases A and B. There are at least two
reasons for this. Commercially-available MUS is contaminated
with a significant amount of free 4-methylumbelliferone, producing
such a high level of baseline fluorescence that the amount of
superimposed fluorescence resulting from enzyme activity is in
comparison, insignificant. Another reason is that the conditions
which allow differential determination of AS-A and AS-B in
mixtures with NCS do not give the same results when used in
conjunction with MUS. As reported here, commercially-available
MUS can easily be purified to eliminate nearly all traces of free
4-methylumbelliferone and thus can serve as a very sensitive tool
for measurement of arylsulfatase activity. Also, the simple
separation technique described permits AS-A and AS-B to be assayed
separately without interfering with each other and therefore
without the need to utilize selective inhibitors.

Two limitations specifically affect accurate determinations
of AS-A activity in leukocytes, the very short time interval
during which the reaction is linear and the low ratio of AS-A to
total arylsulfatase activity characteristic of leukocytes.
However, with inclusion of lead acetate as a specific activator
of AS-A and with the use of highly purified MUS as substrate,
reliable measurements of leukocyte AS-A are possible utilizing
incubations as short as six minutes.

The nature of the residual AS-A activity in MLD and of
residual AS-B activity in MLS has been of considerable interest to
a number of investigators(2,3,10,14). The CM-32 separation technique
confirms the presence of "AS-A"- like material in MLD but suggests
that there is virtually no residual AS-B activity in MLS. Although
others have reported residual AS-B activity in MLS using NCS, the
results in Table 3 are probably more indicative of the true level
of residual AS-B activity in this disease. Use of the CM-32
technique to separate AS-A and AS-B activity in these diseases
should aid in further studies of their residual enzyme activity.

Heterozygote identification for MLD with the NCS assay is not always clearcut. The CM-32 method described here yielded levels of AS-A activity in patients, heterozygotes and controls approximating a 0.1:1:2 ratio without any overlap in individual values. It should be noted, however, that the p value for the differences between MLD carriers and controls in fibroblasts was greater than 0.05. However, it does appear to be a worthwhile alternative to the NCS method for the leukocyte detection of MLD heterozygotes and should receive a trial in a much larger population sample.

The heat inactivation method could simplify still further the diagnosis of MLD homozygotes and heterozygotes as well as of MLS homozygotes but it too must be examined in a much larger number of cases.

SUMMARY

Metachromatic leukodystrophy and Maroteaux-Lamy syndrome can be diagnosed by assay of leukocyte or fibroblast arylsulfatase A and B activity with the fluorogenic substrate 4-methylumbelliferyl sulfate. The arylsulfatases are extracted into a 27000 x g supernatant by sonication in 0.9% sodium chloride and then separated with CM-32 on columns or in test tubes. In 0.05 M sodium acetate pH 6.0, arylsulfatase A is not absorbed while arylsulfatase B is retained by the resin. The arylsulfatase B is then eluted from the resin with 0.3 M sodium chloride. The arylsulfatase A activity obtained from normal leukocytes and fibroblasts is linear for the initial 10 minutes of the reaction, is stimulated 3-fold by 6 mM lead acetate and inhibited 80% by 0.24 mM silver nitrate. After separation with CM-32, the arylsulfatase B activity is stimulated 3-fold by Triton X-100 (0.1%). Arylsulfatase A but not arylsulfatase B is destroyed by heat (60°). Both leukocyte and fibroblast arylsulfatase A activity was reduced to 11% of control values in metachromatic leukodystrophy. Essentially no arylsulfatase B activity was detected in cells from patients with Maroteaux-Lamy syndrome. Metachromatic leukodystrophy heterozygotes but not Maroteaux-Lamy syndrome heterozygotes can also be distinguished by this method. A heat inactivation technique utilizing the differential thermal stabilities of the two enzymes for diagnosis of patients and carriers of metachromatic leukodystrophy and of patients with Maroteaux-Lamy syndrome is also described. The advantages of these 4-methylumbelliferyl sulfate assay procedures over the p-nitrocatechol sulfate method of assay are greater sensitivity, selectivity for the desired enzyme and potential for use in large scale testing.

ACKNOWLEDGEMENTS

We are indebted to Drs. Jan Breslow, Allen Crocker, Richard
Hoefnagel, Aubrey Milunsky, Hugo Moser, Rudy Leibel and Ira Lott
for permitting us to study their patients.

This study was supported by grants from the U.S. Public Health
Service (HD-05515, HD-04147), the Massachusetts Developmental
Disabilities Council, the National Foundation - March of Dimes,
the Charles H. Hood Foundation and the Tay-Sachs Foundation of
New England, Inc.

REFERENCES

1. Austin, J.H., Balasubramanian, A.S., Pattabiraman, T.N.,
    Saraswathi, S., Basu, D.K. and Bachhat, B.K.: A controlled
    study of enzyme activities in three human disorders of gly-
    colipid metabolism. J. Neurochem., 10:805, 1963.

2. Baum, H., Dodgson, K.S. and Soencer, B.: The assay of aryl-
    sulfatases A and B in human urine. Clin. Chim. Acta, 4:
    453, 1959.

3. Beratis, N.G., Turner, B.M., Weiss, R. and Hirschhorn, K.:
    Arylsulfatase B deficiency in Maroteaux-Lamy syndrome:
    Cellular studies and carrier identification. Pediat. Res.,
    9:475, 1975.

4. Fluharty, A.L., Stevens, R.L., Sanders, D.L. and Kihara, H.:
    Arylsulfatase B deficiency in Maroteaux-Lamy syndrome cul-
    tured fibroblasts. Biochem., Biophys. Res. Commun., 59:
    455, 1974.

5. Kampine, J.O., Brady, R.O., Kanfer, J.N., Feld, M., and
    Shapiro, D.: Diagnosis of Gaucher's disease and Niemann-Pick
    disease with small samples of venous blood. Science, 155:
    86, 1967.

6. Percy, A.K. and Brady, R.O.: Metachromatic leukodystrophy:
    Diagnosis with samples of venous blood. Science, 161:594,
    1968.

7. Porter, M.T., Fluharty, A.L. and Kihara, H.: Metachromatic
    leukodystrophy: Arylsulfatase A deficiency in skin fibroblast
    cultures. Proc. Natn. Acad. Sci., U.S.A., 62:887, 1969.

8. Rinderknecht, H., Geokas, M.C., Cormack, C. and Haverback,
    B.I.: The determination of arylsulfatases in biological
    fluids. Clin. Chim. Acta, 29:481, 1970.

9. Shapiro, E., De Gregorio, R.R., Matalon, R. and Nadler, H.L.:
    Reduced arylsulfatase B activity of the mutant enzyme protein
    in Maroteaux-Lamy syndrome. Biochem., Biophys. Res. Commun.,
    62:448, 1975.

10. Shapiro, E. and Nadler, H.L.: The nature of the residual
    arylsulfatase activity in metachromatic leukodystrophy. J.
    Pediatr., 86:881, 1975.

11. Sherman, W.R. and Stanfield, E.F.: Measurement of the aryl-
    sulfatase of Patella vulgata with 4-methylumbelliferone
    sulfate. Biochem. J., 102:905, 1967.

12. Stevens, R.L., Fluharty, A.L., Skokut, M.H. and Kihara, H.:
    Purification and properties of arylsulfatase A from human
    urine. J. Biol. Chem., 250:2495, 1975.

13. Stumpf, D.A., Austin, J.H., Crocker, A.C. and La France, M.:
    Mucopolysaccharidosis type VI (Maroteaux-Lamy syndrome).
    I. Sulfatase B deficiency in tissues. Am. J. Dis. Child.,
    126:747, 1973.

14. Stumpf, D., Neuwelt, E., Austin, J. and Kohler, P.: Meta-
    chromatic leukodystrophy (MLD) X: Immunological studies of
    the abnormal sulfatase A. Arch. Neurol., 25:427, 1971.

IDURONATE SULFATASE DETERMINATION FOR THE DIAGNOSIS OF THE

HUNTER SYNDROME AND THE DETECTION OF THE CARRIER STATE

Elizabeth F. Neufeld, Ingeborg Liebaers and Timple W. Lim

National Institute of Arthritis, Metabolism and
  Digestive Diseases
National Institutes of Health, Bethesda, Maryland 20014

The research efforts of the last few years have clarified
the biochemical basis of the mucopolysaccharidoses (17). Some
practical benefits have emerged from this new knowledge - not
yet for the patients themselves, but for their families, who now
can be counseled accurately and offered the option of prenatal diagnosis.

It is particularly important to the families to discriminate
between the Hunter syndrome, an X-linked disorder, and the other
mucopolysaccharidoses, which are inherited in autosomal recessive
fashion (14). For several years, we have identified the Hunter
syndrome biochemically in fibroblasts cultured from the patients'
skin, on the basis of excessive ^{35}S-mucopolysaccharide accumulation
and the reduction of this accumulation (i.e., correction) in the
presence of highly-purified Hunter corrective factor (5,6). It is
now known that Hunter fibroblasts are deficient in the enzyme
iduronate sulfatase, and that the Hunter corrective factor has
iduronate sulfatase activity (1), and we surmise that correction
of the abnormal metabolism of Hunter fibroblasts results from the
introduction of exogenous enzyme into the cells. Enzyme uptake
into fibroblasts associated with correction has been experimentally
demonstrated in analogous deficiencies of α-L-iduronidase (2,19),
β-glucuronidase (4), and N-acetyl-α-glucosaminidase (20).

The accumulation-correction test for the Hunter syndrome is
simple, reliable and specific. Nevertheless, it has not been
widely adopted, perhaps because of the need for specialized techniques and for purified corrective factor. In addition, it has
two drawbacks: it cannot detect partial enzyme deficiency, such
as might occur in Hunter heterozygotes, and it entails a lengthy

interval between the time a biopsy is taken until a fibroblast culture is established and the test can be performed. There is a
clear need for a more rapid procedure, since the differential diagnosis of the Hunter syndrome is often urgently requested in connection with the pregnancy of a close relative of the patient.
Ideally, the same procedure should also be useful for detection
of heterozygotes.

We have developed a simple diagnostic test for use with
serum and lymphocytes, based on the assay for iduronate sulfatase
described by Lim et al. (12). The principle is illustrated in
Fig. 1. The radioactive substrate, O-(α-L-idopyranosyluronic acid
2-sulfate)-(1⟶4)-2,5-anhydro-D-mannitol 6-sulfate, prepared as
previously described (12) is hydrolysed by iduronate sulfatase to
yield a radioactive monosulfated disaccharide, product 1. Since
product 1 has a terminal iduronic acid residue, it can be further
hydrolysed by α-L-iduronidase to product 2, a radioactive monosulfated monosaccharide. After incubation, the products and
residual substrate are separated from each other by high-voltage
paper electrophoresis, located with the aid of a chromatogram
scanner, cut out and quantitated by counting, without elution, in
a scintillation spectrometer. The activity of iduronate sulfatase
is expressed in nmol of substrate hydrolysed per 24 hr per mg of
protein (13), and is calculated from the fraction of substrate
hydrolysed, the cpm included in the incubation mixture, and the
specific activity of the substrate. A detailed description of
the procedure will be given elsewhere (11).

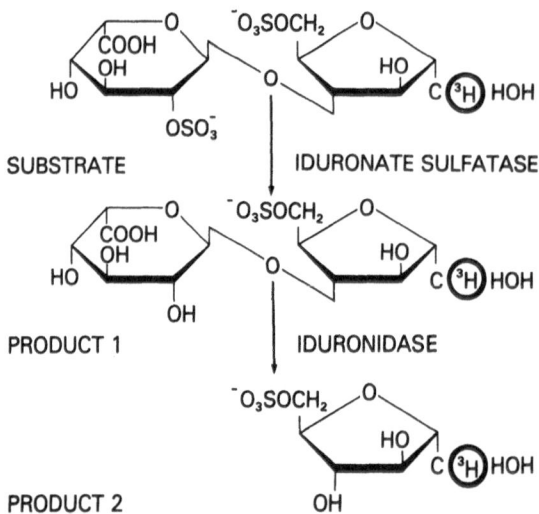

Fig. 1. Degradation of ³H-labeled substrate by the sequential
action of iduronate sulfatase and α-L-iduronidase.

Although it is not the primary purpose of the method to measure α-L-iduronidase activity, this additional information is obtained by taking the ratio of the radioactivity found in the second product to that found in the sum of products 1 and 2. It is obvious from Fig. 1 that such an estimate of iduronidase activity can be made only when iduronate sulfatase is present to generate product 1.

The test was first applied to acetone powders prepared from cultured fibroblasts (Table I). It confirmed results obtained by other procedures (1,2,10), showing an essentially total deficiency of iduronate sulfatase in fibroblasts from Hunter patients, an equally profound deficiency of iduronidase in fibroblasts from patients with mucopolysaccharidosis I (Hurler, Scheie and Hurler/Scheie syndromes) and a marked deficiency of both enzymes in fibroblasts from patients with mucolipidosis II or III. Cells from two patients with multiple sulfatidosis (9) were found to have only 12% of the normal iduronate sulfatase activity.

TABLE I: IDURONATE SULFATASE AND
IDURONIDASE ACTIVITIES OF FIBROBLAST EXTRACTS

Fibroblasts in confluent monolayers (3-4 weeks after trans-plantation) were converted to acetone powders in order to remove inhibitors of iduronate sulfatase. The powders were extracted with 0.9 NaCl (0.3 ml per 75 cm^2 Falcon flask) and dialysed. Twenty μl of the dialysed solution (10-20 μg of protein) was incubated for 24 hr at 37° with 15 μl of a mixture containing 0.27 M sodium acetate buffer, pH 4.0, 13.3 mM sodium azide, 0.75 mM substrate (specific activity, 14 μCi/μmol), and 1 mg/ml bovine serum albumin.

	N	Iduronate sulfatase nmol/mg/24 hr mean ± S.E.M.	Iduronidase Product 2 (products 1 + 2)
Normal	6	182 ± 28	0.95
Hunter	8	2 ± 1	not applicable
Mucopolysaccha-ridosis I	4	117 ± 24	0.02
Other Mucopoly-saccharidoses	6	144 ± 11	0.96
Mucolipidoses II and III	3	31 ± 11	0.31
Multiple Sulfatidosis	2	23 ± 3	0.93

TABLE II: IDURONATE SULFATASE ACTIVITY IN SERUM

Samples of serum were thoroughly dialysed against 0.9% NaCl
in order to remove inhibitors. Fifty μl aliquots were incubated for 6 hr at 37° with 30 μl of a mixture containing 0.27 M
sodium acetate buffer at pH 4.5, 13.3 mM sodium azide and 0.75mM
substrate.

	N	Iduronate sulfatase nmol/mg/24 hr mean ± S.E.M.
Normal	30	10 ± 0.5
Hunter	10	0.08 ± 0.03
Other Mucopoly-saccharidoses	5	12 ± 1.0
Mucolipidoses II and III	7	234 ± 43
Hunter mothers	7	8 ± 0.7

Normal serum contains appreciable iduronate sulfatase
activity (Table II), whereas serum from Hunter patients with
either the mild or the severe form of the disease has essentially
none. Iduronidase activity is not detected in serum by the present test, perhaps because the incubation conditions selected are un-
favorable. Mucolipidoses II and III can be distinguished by the
marked elevation of iduronate sulfatase activity; such elevation
is characteristic of a number of serum lysosomal enzymes in these
disorders (17).

Assay of iduronate sulfatase in serum is without doubt the
best method for the diagnosis of the Hunter syndrome. One ml of
serum is ample; the enzyme is very stable, so that serum kept frozen
for up to two years may be used, provided that similarly stored control samples are available. Plasma may be substituted for serum.
The total time required for the assay is three working days.

The high activity of iduronate sulfatase in serum was surprising, since serum has been previously found to contain negligible Hunter corrective factor activity (16). Preliminary
results suggest that the iduronate sulfatase of serum is not
corrective, in contrast to the analogous enzyme derived from
urine or fibroblasts. The existence of lysosomal enzymes in
corrective and non-corrective forms has been shown in other systems
(e.g., 19).

Useful as serum might be for diagnosing the disease itself, it proved disappointing for detecting heterzygotes (Table II). Lymphocytes, on the other hand, seemed promising: the mean activity for 11 Hunter mothers was half that of 30 normal controls (mean ± S.E.M., 24 ± 6 and 46 ± 4, respectively). These data are presented in Fig. 2. Data obtained from obligated heterozygotes (i.e., women with two affected sons, or one affected son and other family history of the Hunter syndrome) have been separated from data for women with only one affected son, among whom there might be cases of sporadic mutation (7).

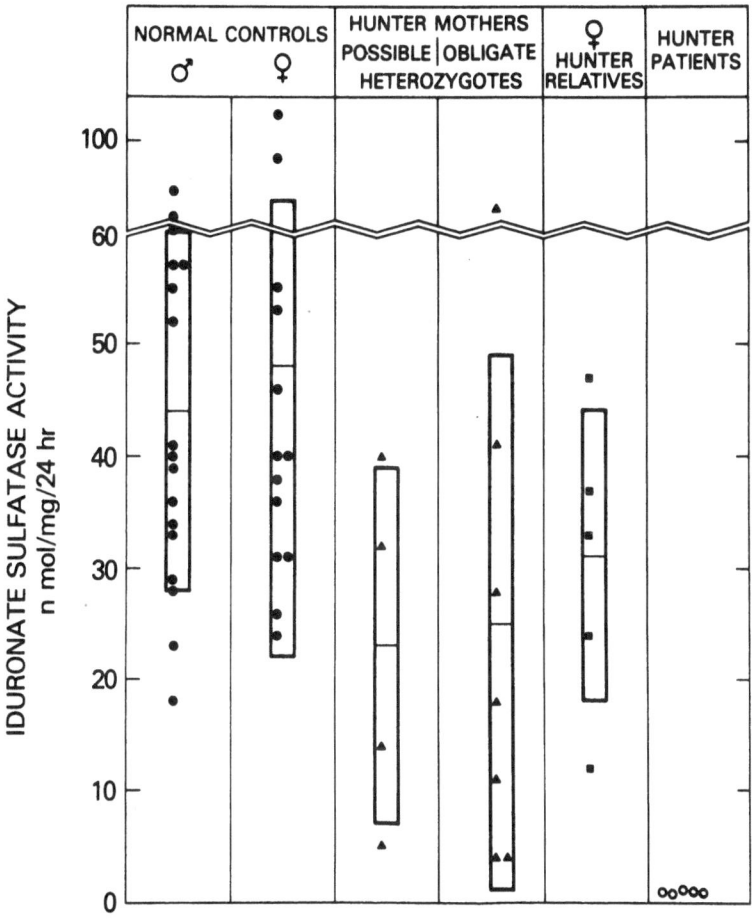

Fig. 2. Iduronate sulfatase activity of lymphocytes prepared by the Hypaque-Ficoll method of Böyum (3). The preparation includes monocytes and platelets in addition to lymphocytes. Bars indicate the standard deviation.

It can be seen that although the mean activity for obligate heterozygotes is half that for normal women, the scatter is very great, and half the obligate heterozygotes have enzymatic activity well within the normal range. Since some of this scatter may be due to experimental variables of the test, or to physiological variables in the activity of lymphocytes, it may be reduced as the variables become understood. Yet even with such improvements, it is likely that numerous heterozygotes would have relatively high enzyme activity. A better procedure would be one that incorporated an immunological assay for iduronate sulfatase protein; in those kindreds where the mutation resulted in an enzymatically inactive but cross-reactive protein, the heterozygote would have a reduced ratio of catalytic to antigenic activity. Analogous testing of the biological and antigenic activities of Factor VIII allows the detection of 70-90% of heterozygotes for classical hemophilia (18,21). However, a certain number of Hunter heterozygotes may still escape detection, if selection in vivo of cells with an active paternal X-chromosome had given them an essentially normal complement of somatic cells, instead of the random distribution predicted by the Lyon hypothesis (8,15).

CONCLUSION

Measurement of iduronate sulfatase activity in serum constitutes a rapid and simple diagnostic test for the Hunter syndrome. The same assay applied to lymphocytes may form the basis of a carrier detection test.

ACKNOWLEDGMENT

A United States Public Health Service International Fellowship and a Belgian "Nationaal Fonds voor Wetenshappelÿk Onderzoek" Fellowship to Ingeborg Liebaers are gratefully acknowledged.

REFERENCES

1. Bach, G., Eisenberg, F., Jr., Cantz, M., and Neufeld, E. F.:
    The defect in the Hunter syndrome: deficiency of sulfo-
    iduronate sulfatase. Proc. Nat. Acad. Sci. U.S. 70: 2134
    (1973).

2. Bach, G., Friedman, R., Weissmann, B. and Neufeld, E. F.:
    The defect in the Hurler and Scheie syndromes: deficiency
    of α-L-iduronidase. Proc. Nat. Acad. Sci. U.S. 69: 2048 (1972).

3. Böyum, A.: Isolation of mononuclear cells by one centrifuga-
    tion and of granulocytes by combining centrifugation and pedi-
    mentation at 1 g. Sand. J. Clin. Lab. Invest. 21: (suppl. 97)
    77 (1968).

4. Brot, F. E., Glaser, J. H., Roozen, K. J., and Sly, W. S.:
    In vitro correction of deficient human fibroblasts by
    β-glucuronidase from different human sources. Biochem.
    Biophys. Res. Commun. 57: 1 (1974).

5. Cantz, M., Chrambach, A., Bach, G. and Neufeld, E. F.:
    The Hunter corrective factor. J. Biol. Chem. 247: 5456 (1972).

6. Cantz, M., Kresse, H., Barton, R. W., and Neufeld, E. F.:
    Corrective factors for inborn errors of mucopolysaccharide
    catabolism. Methods in Enzymol. 28: 884 (1972). (V. Ginsburg,
    ed., Academic Press, New York)

7. Chase, G. A. and Murphy, E. A.: Risk of recurrence and carrier
    frequency for X-linked lethal recessives. Hum. Hered. 23:
    19 (1973).

8. Danes, B. S. and Bearn, A. G.: Hurler's syndrome: a genetic
    study of clones in cell culture with particular reference to
    the Lyon hypothesis. J. Exp. Med. 126: 509 (1967).

9. Eto, Y., Wiesmann, U. N., Carson, J. H., and Herschkowitz,
    N. N.: Multiple sulfatase deficiencies in cultured skin
    fibroblasts. Arch. Neurol. 30: 153 (1974).

10. Hall, C. W. and Neufeld, E. F.: α-L-Iduronidase activity in
    cultured skin fibroblasts and amniotic fluid cells. Arch.
    Biochem. Biophys. 158: 817 (1973).

11. Liebaers, I. and Neufeld, E. F.: Iduronate sulfatase activity
    in serum, lymphocytes and fibroblasts - simplified diagnosis of
    the Hunter syndrome. Submitted to Ped. Res.

12. Lim, T. W., Leder, I. G., Bach, G., and Neufeld, E. F.:
    An assay for iduronate sulfatase (Hunter corrective factor).
    Carbohyd. Res. 37: 103 (1974).

13. Lowry, O. H., Rosebrough, N. J., Farr, A. L., and Randall, R. J.:
    Protein measurement with the Folin phenol reagent. J. Biol. Chem.
    193: 265 (1951).

14. McKusick, V. A.: Heritable Disorders of Connective Tissue,
    4th Ed. C. V. Mosby, St. Louis, 1972, pp. 521-681.

15. Migeon, B. and Neufeld, E. F.: in preparation.

16. Neufeld, E. F.: Mucopolysaccharidoses, the biochemical
    approach. Medical Genetics (V. A. McKusick and R. Claiborne,
    eds.) H. P. Publishing Co., New York, 1973. pp. 141-147.

17. Neufeld, E. F., Lim, T. W., and Shapiro, L. J.: Inherited
     disorders of lysosomal metabolism. Ann. Rev. Biochem. 44:
     357 (1975).

18. Rizza, C. R., Rhymes, I. L., Austen, D. E. G., Kernoff, P. B. A.,
     and Aroni, S. A.: Detection of carriers of hemophilia: a
     "blind" study. Brit. J. Haematol. 30: 447 (1975).

19. Shapiro, L. J., Hall, C. W., Leder, I. G., and Neufeld, E. F.:
     The relationship of α-L-iduronidase and Hurler corrective
     factor. Arch. Biochem. Biophys. in press.

20. Von Figura, K., and Kresse, H.: Quantitative aspects of
     pinocytosis and the intracellular fate of N-acetyl-α-D-
     glucosaminidase in Sanfilippo B fibroblasts. J. Clin. Invest.
     53: 85 (1974).

21. Zimmerman, T. S., Ratnoff, D. D. and Littell, A. S.: Detection
     of carriers of classic hemophilia using an immunologic assay
     for antihemophilic factor (Factor VIII). J. Clin. Invest. 50:
     255 (1971).

THE ENZYMIC DEFECTS IN MORQUIO AND MAROTEAUX-LAMY SYNDROME

Albert Dorfman, Bradley Arbogast[+] and

Reuben Matalon[*]

Departments of Pediatrics and Biochemistry,
and the Joseph P. Kennedy, Jr., Mental
Retardation Research Center, Pritzker School
of Medicine, University of Chicago, Chicago,
Illinois 60637

The mucopolysaccharidoses are a group of heritable
diseases which result from defective degradation of
glycosaminoglycans. Since the original descriptions
of Hunter and Hurler (15,16), there has been an extensive clinical and biochemical literature. The earlier
studies have been reviewed elsewhere (10,25,33).
Studies during the last few years have elucidated the
enzyme defects in Hurler, Scheie, Hunter and Sanfilippo
A and B diseases (9,26). More recently, several reports
have appeared concerned with defects in Maroteaux-Lamy
and Morquio diseases (2,4,12,13,23,24,27,31). These two
syndromes are distinguished from the other mucopolysaccharidoses by lack of mental retardation in the
presence of severe somatic changes. Maroteaux et al.
(22) described a group of patients with marked somatic
defects and no mental retardation except that which
occurs secondary to the frequent hydrocephalus. In contrast to the excretion of heparan sulfate and dermatan
sulfate in Hurler disease, patients with Maroteaux-Lamy

[+] Present Address: General Clinical Research Center,
    Pennsylvania General Hospital, Philadelphia,
    Pennsylvania 19104

[*] Joseph P. Kennedy, Jr. Scholar

disease excrete only dermatan sulfate. Morquio disease
is manifested by spondoepiphyseal dysplasia and corneal
clouding. This syndrome was originally grouped with
what is probably a large number of other distinct heritable skeletal diseases. With the discovery of the
excretion of keratan sulfate (29) in the urine of one
group of patients, the definition of Morquio disease
became more clearcut. A detailed discussion of the
clinical distinctions has been presented by McKusick (25).

It is the purpose of this paper to present certain
studies conducted in our laboratories utilizing natural
substrates for the elucidation of the enzymic defects
in these two syndromes.

Initially we attempted to use keratan sulfate as a
substrate for the study of Morquio disease. It was
found difficult to prepare a radioactive keratan sulfate
from rabbit rib cartilage of sufficiently high activity
to demonstrate degradation by extracts of normal fibroblasts. Accordingly, we turned to the use of chondroitin
sulfate since several reports indicated that this polysaccharide is also excreted in Morquio disease (19).

For this purpose femoral and tibial epiphyses of
13 day old chick embryos were diced and incubated with
$H_2^{35}SO_4$ in Krebs-Ringer buffer for 2 hours. After digestion with papain, the $[^{35}S]$chondroitin sulfate was
isolated with cetylpyridinium chloride. Digestion with
chondroitinase ABC yielded a mixture of disaccharides
indicating that the original chondroitin sulfate contained 59.5% 4-SO_4 and 37.1% 6-SO_4 linkages. Attempts
to separate chondroitin 4-SO_4 from chondroitin 6-SO_4
in this preparation were unsuccessful suggesting that
the chondroitin sulfate isolated from the chick epiphyses
was probably a hybrid molecule rather than a mixture of
the two isomeric chondroitin sulfates. Assay for release
of $^{35}SO_4$ from the $[^{35}S]$chondroitin 4/6-SO_4 was carried
out by incubation with extracts prepared by sonication
of cultured fibroblasts. Studies were performed with
both the 10,000 x g supernatant solution and pellet.
Inorganic sulfate was determined by high voltage electrophoresis. The data in Table 1 present the results obtained from experiments with a number of different fibroblast strains. Of the extracts used, only those derived
from Morquio and Maroteaux-Lamy fibroblasts failed to
release significant quantities of $^{35}SO_4$. When a mixture
of pellets of the two types of preparation was used, the
amount of sulfate released was considerably greater than

Table 1. Degradation of Chick Embryo [^{35}S]Chondroitin 4/6-SO$_4$ by Fibroblast Extracts*

Cell Type	Supernatant		Pellet	
	cpm	%	cpm	%
Normal	8,410	7.6	15,400	14.4
Normal boiled	0	0	0	0
Hurler	11,050	8.5	10,900	8.1
Hunter	12,950	10.6	15,875	9.0
Sanfilippo A	6,520	5.8	11,775	10.0
Metachromatic Leukodystrophy	11,320	10.0	14,150	
Morquio	1,005	0.8	0	0
Morquio	1,243	1.1	1,017	0.9
Maroteaux-Lamy	456	1.4	94	0.9
Maroteaux-Lamy	115	0.2	61	0.6
Maroteaux-Lamy + Morquio[+]			318	6.7

*   Each incubation mixture containing 200,000 cpm [^{35}S]-chondroitin 4/6-SO$_4$ and 250 g protein was incubated for 18h. Percent sulfate released was calculated on the basis of inorganic ^{35}SO$_4$ divided by the total radioactivity of recovered undegraded material plus the inorganic sulfate recovered.

[+] This experiment was performed separately and counts are not comparable to others in this table.

the sum of that released from either individually. Since the two diseases are clearly different, it was concluded that two distinct enzymes are involved in the release of ^{35}SO$_4$ from this substrate. Since dermatan sulfate contains primarily 4-SO$_4$ linkages and keratan sulfate contains 6-SO$_4$ linkages, it seemed reasonable that degradation of chondroitin 4/6-SO$_4$ requires the action of two distinct sulfatases, N-acetylhexosamine 4-SO$_4$ sulfatase and N-acetylhexosamine 6-SO$_4$ sulfatase.

Because earlier studies by Tudball and Davidson (37) had suggested that oligosaccharides might serve as better substrates for chondroitin-SO$_4$ sulfatases and it was possible the sulfatases might act only on the sulfate group in a non-reducing terminal position, a heptasaccharide was prepared from [^{35}S]chondroitin 4/6-SO$_4$ by digestion of the chondroitin 4/6-SO$_4$ with testicular hyaluronidase and β-glucuronidase. The results of degradation by fibroblasts of this substrate are shown in Table 2. Striking is the release of $^{35}SO_4$ by Maroteaux-Lamy and normal extracts but only minimal release by extracts of Morquio fibroblasts. These findings were initially somewhat surprising. However, when the labeled heptasaccharide was digested with chondroitinase AC, it was found that it contained 59% 4-SO_4 and 37% 6-SO_4, a reversal of the ratio in the [^{35}S]chondroitin 4/6-SO_4 from which it was prepared. The explanation of this finding is not clear but may depend on the relative rates of hydrolysis and/or transglycosylation of $\underline{N}$-acetyl-galactosaminyl-4-SO_4 and $\underline{N}$-acetylgalactosaminyl-6-SO_4 linkages by testicular hyaluronidase.

The results became clearer when the products of digestion of the heptasaccharide after incubation with fibroblast extracts were analysed by digestion with chondroitinase AC. The results summarized in Table 3 indicate that $^{35}SO_4$ released by normal extracts from the [^{35}S]heptasaccharide is only minimally derived from the 4-SO_4 groups, therefore, the degradation of this substrate depends primarily on the presence of a 6-SO_4 sulfatase. Accordingly, the marked decrease of degradation by Morquio extracts (which presumably lacks the 6-SO_4 sulfatase) becomes reasonable. In contrast, Maroteaux-Lamy extracts (which presumably contain the 6-SO_4 sulfatase) shows degradation comparable to normal extracts.

Table 2. Degradation of [^{35}S]Heptasaccharide 4/6-SO_4 by Fibroblast Extracts*

Cell Type	$^{35}SO_4$ Released	$^{35}SO_4$ Released
	cpm	%
Normal	303	19.0
Morquio	113	4.6
Maroteaux-Lamy	821	20.6
Maroteaux-Lamy	438	20.0

* Each incubation mixture containing 5,000 cpm of [^{35}S]heptasaccharide 4/6-sulfate and 250 μg protein was incubated for 18h. Percent sulfate released calculated as in Table 1.

Table 3. Degradation of Ch-SO$_4$ and Heptasaccharides

Substrate	Normal	Morquio		Maroteaux-Lamy	
	cpm	cpm	% normal	cpm	% normal
Ch 4/6-SO$_4$	652	177	27	169	25
Ch 4-SO$_4$	2,913	1,176	40	363	12
Heptasaccharide 4/6-SO$_4$					
4-SO$_4$	150	160	110	180	120
6-SO$_4$	1,580	320	20	1,620	104
Heptasaccharide 4-SO$_4$	4,700	4,300	91	600	13

All values normalized to 10,000 cpm recovered.

Values averaged for results on 3-5 experiments.

Ch 4/6-SO$_4$	59%	4-SO$_4$	37%	6-SO$_4$
Heptasaccharide 4/6-SO$_4$	37%	4-SO$_4$	63%	6-SO$_4$

In order to pursue this question, further additional natural substrates were sought. For this purpose the Swarm rat chondrosarcoma was utilized for the preparation of [^{35}S]chondroitin sulfate. Previous studies by Choi et al. (7) had demonstrated that this tumor produces only chondroitin 4-SO$_4$, a fact that was verified by digestion with chondroitinase ABC of the polysaccharide isolated from the tumor. [^{35}S]Chondroitin 4-SO$_4$ was prepared by incubating trypsinized tumor cells in Eagle's medium with H$_2$^{35}SO$_4$. After 24 hours of incubation the mixture was treated with papain and free [^{35}S]chondroitin sulfate was isolated utilizing cetylpyridinium chloride. The use of this substrate clearly confirmed our suspicions. The data presented in Table 4 show the clearcut difference in degradation of chondroitin 4-SO$_4$ by extracts of a number of fibroblast lines derived from various mucopolysaccharidoses. Striking is the marked diminution of activity of Maroteaux-Lamy extracts. The moderate decrease in activity in Morquio extracts has been consistently observed.

When a heptasaccharide, prepared as described above from [^{35}S]chondroitin 4-SO$_4$, was utilized as substrate the results presented in Table V were obtained. Over 40% of the radioactivity was released by both the normal

Table 4.   Degradation of [^{35}S]Chondroitin 4-SO$_4$
           by Fibroblast Extracts*

Cell Type	^{35}SO$_4$ Released	^{35}SO$_4$ Released
	cpm	%
Normal	24,708	21.2
Hunter	25,084	20.2
Hurler	13,753	13.5
Sanfilippo A	23,130	19.8
Sanfilippo B	23,521	23.1
Morquio	10,977	13.2
Maroteaux-Lamy	1,642	1.4
Maroteaux-Lamy	1,107	0.8
Maroteaux-Lamy	1,887	1.5
Maroteaux-Lamy	1,462	1.2

* Each mixture containing 200,000 cpm [^{35}S]chondroitin
  4-SO$_4$ and 250 μg protein extracted with Triton X-100
  was incubated for 18h. Percent sulfate released calculated as in Table 1.

and Morquio extract, while only minimal release of
^{35}SO$_4$ was produced by Morquio extract. These results
confirmed the diminution of the activity of N-acetylgalactosamine 4-SO$_4$ sulfatase in Maroteaux-Lamy disease.

The amount of sulfate released from this substrate
is in excess of that anticipated if activity of the
appropriate sulfatase is limited to ester sulfate on

Table 4.   Degradation of [^{35}S]Heptasaccharide 4-SO$_4$
           by Fibroblast Extracts*

Cell Type	^{35}SO$_4$ Released	^{35}SO$_4$ Released
	cpm	%
Normal	967	47.0
Morquio	1,054	43.0
Maroteaux-Lamy	152	6.0
Maroteaux-Lamy	145	5.3

* Each mixture containing 4,000 cpm [^{35}S]heptasaccharide
  4-SO$_4$ and 250 μg protein extracted with Triton X-100
  was incubated for 18h. Percent sulfate released calculated as in Table 1.

the non-reducing N-acetylgalactosamine groups. This could be explained by the concerted action of N-acetyl-hexosaminidase, β-glucuronidase and the sulfatase or by the action of the sulfatase on internal esters. The latter explanation appears to be correct since we have found that extracts of fibroblasts obtained from a patient with Sandhoff disease (which lack both N-acetyl-hexosaminidase A and B) release as much sulfate from chondroitin 4-SO_4 as do normal fibroblasts.

Table 3 summarizes the degradation by normal, Morquio and Maroteaux-Lamy extracts of the four substrates that were used in these studies. In order to make the various studies comparable, all results were calculated as if 10,000 counts were recovered. The extent of degradation of the 4-SO_4 and 6-SO_4 linkages from the [^{35}S]heptasaccharide was calculated on the basis of the comparison of the composition of the substrate with the products remaining after treatment with fibroblast extracts (as determined by chromatography following chondroitinase AC hydrolysis). As indicated, the failure to detect 4-SO_4 sulfatase deficiency utilizing the heptasaccharide 4/6-SO_4 is probably due to low 4-SO_4 sulfatase activity on this substrate. Another disturbing anomaly illustrated in this table is the lower than normal activity of Morquio extracts on chondroitin 4-SO_4. The explanation of this finding is not clear. A mixture of Morquio and Maroteaux-Lamy extracts gave no evidence of an inhibitor in the Morquio extracts.

Several other recent studies have also been concerned with the enzymic defect in Maroteaux-Lamy disease. Prior to our studies, Austin et al. (2) have reported a diminution of arylsulfatase B in tissues of patients with Maroteaux-Lamy disease. This defect has also been found in fibroblasts by Fluharty et al. (13) and Beratis et al.(4). O'Brien et al. (27), utilizing a method of end group analysis, concluded that Maroteaux-Lamy disease was due to a deficiency of N-acetylhexosamine 4-SO_4 sulfatase. Utilizing the substrate uridine diphospho-N-acetylgalactosamine 4-SO_4, Fluharty et al. (12) reached a similar conclusion regarding the enzyme defect in Maroteaux-Lamy disease. Shapira et al. (31) showed that extracts of Maroteaux-Lamy fibroblasts contain a protein which reacts with antibodies to arylsulfatase B but shows no activity toward nitrocatechol sulfate.

Taken together these various studies appear to clearly indicate that Maroteaux-Lamy is characterized

by a structural mutation resulting in a protein which
is immunologically cross reactive with arylsulfatase B.
The natural substrate for this enzyme appears to be the
ester sulfate groups on the 4 position of N-acetylgalactosamine in chondroitin sulfate and dermatan
sulfate.

Pedrini et al. (30) have reported an increased
concentration of chondroitin 6-SO_4 but not chondroitin
4-SO_4 in cartilage of patients with Morquio disease.
These findings are in agreement with our conclusion
that Morquio disease results from defective activity
of an N-acetylhexosamine 6-SO_4 sulfatase which acts on
both keratan sulfate and chondroitin 6-SO_4.

These studies add to our understanding of the
mucopolysaccharidoses. Fig. 1 summarizes portions of
the structures of the various glycosaminoglycans, the
degradation of which is impaired in the mucopolysaccharidoses. The individual chemical linkages requiring specific enzymes for their hydrolysis and the
diseases which result from deficits of the specific
hydrolases.

Sufficient progress in the elucidation of the
deficient enzymes in the mucopolysaccharidoses has now
been made to delineate a pathway for their metabolism.
When this is done systematically, it becomes clear that
certain problems remain unsolved. It is likely that
solution of these problems will lead to the identification of other mucopolysaccharidoses.

The initial step(s) of heparan sulfate degradation
not depicted in Fig. 1 remain uncertain. Present evidence indicates that heparin and heparan sulfate are
initially synthesized as proteoglycans. It is possible
that heparin chains are split from the proteoglycan by
proteolytic enzymes or endoglycosidases before release
from cells. Ogren and Lindahl (28) have reported the
presence of a heparinase in transplantable mouse masto-
cytoma which apparently cleaves macromolecular heparin
by an endoglucuronidase activity. The existence of an
endoglycosidase which splits heparan sulfate has been
suggested by Hutterer (17). Further evidence of an
enzyme of this type was indicated by Knecht et al.
(20) since the degraded fragments of heparan sulfate
found in urine and tissues of Hurler patients were of
two types; one type was highly sulfated and contained
large amounts of N-sulfate but no linkage region com-

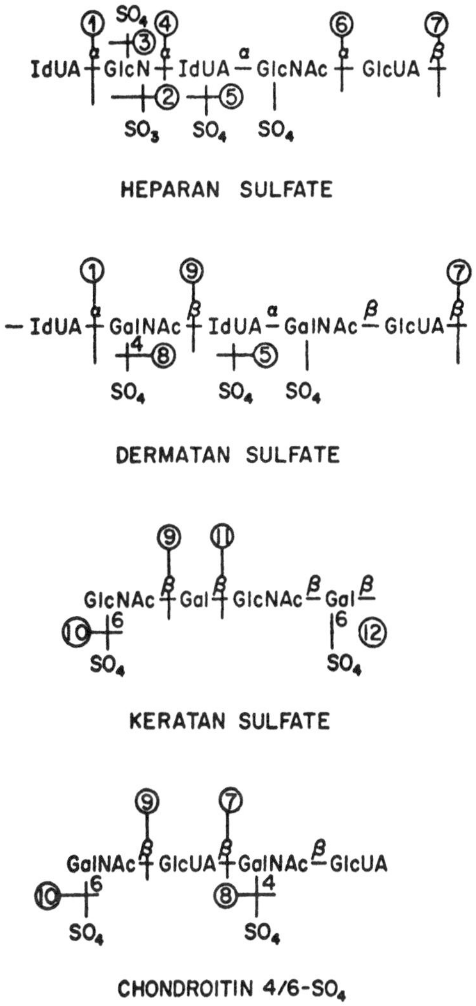

HEPARAN SULFATE

DERMATAN SULFATE

KERATAN SULFATE

CHONDROITIN 4/6-SO₄

Fig. 1.   Pathway of degradation of glycosaminoglycans
          stored in mucopolysaccharidoses. The defects
          in various syndromes are indicated by number
          steps with line across arrow. The known dis-
          eases of degradation are: 1. Hurler,Scheie
          diseases, 2. Sanfilippo A disease, 4. San-
          filippo C disease (?), 5. Hunter disease,
          6. Sanfilippo B disease, 7. β-Glucuronidase
          deficiency, 8. Maroteaux-Lamy disease, 9.
          Sandhoff disease, Tay-Sachs diseases, 10.
          Morquio disease, and 11. G_{M1}-Gangliosidosis.
          No known disease has been shown for step 3.
          The enzyme involved in step 12 is not clear.

ponents (xylose, galactose and serine), while the other
type contained low sulfate, high N-acetylglucosamine
and xylose, galactose and serine in molar ratios of
1:2:1. These findings suggested that the latter fragments derive from the portion of the chains proximal
to the protein while the former fragments derive from
the distal portions of the chain.

The pattern of further degradation of heparan
sulfate is now relatively clear. The removal of $N-SO_3$
groups by sulfamidase results in a terminal α-gluco-
saminide linkage which probably requires a specific
enzyme other than the α-N-acetylglucosaminidase. The
recent report by Kresse and von Figura (21) suggests
that such an enzyme is absent in Sanfilippo C disease.
Further data are required to characterize this step.

Studies on the structure of heparan sulfate indicate that a considerable number of $N-SO_3$-hexosamine
residues also contain $6-O-SO_4$ (8). Whether a critical
order exists between steps 2 and 3 (Fig. 1) is unknown.
In any case an enzyme must exist for the hydrolysis of
the glucosamine $6-SO_4$ groups. The studies reviewed
above demonstrated that an N-acetylhexosamine $6-SO_4$
sulfatase is deficient in Morquio disease. This enzyme
presumably acts on both N-acetylgalactosamine $6-SO_4$
linkages (that occur in chondroitin $6-SO_4$) and N-acetylglucosamine $6-SO_4$ linkages (that occur in keratan
sulfate). If this same enzyme is responsible for the
hydrolysis of the $6-SO_4$ linkage in heparan sulfate,
Morquio disease should be characterized by the excretion and storage of heparan sulfate. Increased quantities of heparan sulfate have never been reported in
Morquio urine. These facts suggest that yet another
sulfatase is required for the hydrolysis of the $6-SO_4$
groups in heparin and heparan sulfate. The requirement
for an enzyme which is different from that active on
chondroitin $6-SO_4$ (or keratan sulfate) may be due to
the presence of $N-SO_3$, a free amino group if $N-SO_3$ is
first removed, or a conformational difference that results from the α-glycoside bond.

Another possibility is that the enzyme deficient in
Morquio disease acts on the galactose $6-SO_4$ and is specific for the galactose configuration which also occurs
in the N-acetylgalactosamine in chondroitin $6-SO_4$. (The
authors are grateful to Dr. Elizabeth F. Neufeld for
this suggestion.)

Step 7 of Fig. 1 refers to the action of β-glucuronidase which would be required for the complete degradation of heparan sulfate. The available data are confusing regarding the storage or excretion of heparan sulfate in the published cases of β-glucuronidase deficiency (3,14,32).

The role of β-N-acetylhexosaminidases (Step 9) in degradation of glycosaminoglycans requires further investigation. Studies by Thompson et al. (35) indicated that extracts of fibroblasts derived from patients with Sandhoff and Tay-Sachs disease fail to remove the non-reducing terminal N-acetylhexosamine group of a heptasaccharide derived from chondroitin sulfate. Since β-N-acetylhexosaminidase A is absent in Tay-Sachs disease and β-N-acetylhexosaminidase A and B are absent in Sandhoff disease, these data indicate that β-N-acetylhexosaminidase A is required for the degradation of chondroitin sulfate and presumably dermatan sulfate. Cantz and Kresse (5) have recently reported the accumulation of glycosaminoglycans in fibroblasts of patients with Sandhoff disease but not Tay-Sachs disease. Despite this finding, the failure of either of these two syndromes to exhibit the characteristics of mucopolysaccharidoses remains unexplained. It is possible that chondroitin sulfate and hyaluronic acid are primarily degraded by the endohexosaminidase, hyaluronidase, in certain tissues, however, hyaluronidase appears to be absent from cultured skin fibroblasts (1); hyaluronidase has been reported in skin (6).

Step 11 refers to β-galactosidase activity. There is no evidence of more than one β-galactosidase involved in degradation of gangliosides (34). The β-galactosidase responsible for degradation of G_{M1}-ganglioside appears to be involved in the degradation of keratan sulfate in view of the storage and excretion of a keratan sulfate-like material in G_{M1}-gangliosidosis (36).

A number of problems remain concerning the degradation of keratan sulfate. There is no available evidence regarding the enzyme responsible for hydrolysis of the galactose 6-SO_4 linkage present in keratan sulfate. The large number of variants of spondoepiphyseal dysplasia offer many more disease possibilities for a deficiency of such an enzyme. The storage of mucopolysaccharides in the metachromatic leukodystrophy variant characterized by multiple sulfatase deficiencies has been observed. Fibroblasts from this unusual disease show reduced amounts or absence of arylsulfatases A, B, C, cholesterol sulfatase and dehydroepiandrosterone sulfate sulfatase. On the basis of correction studies there also appears to be a deficiency of iduronosulfate sulfatase and sulfamidase. The basis for this multiple sulfatase deficiency is unclear (11).

In addition, a number of problems regarding the pathogenesis of the mucopolysaccharidoses remain. It is still difficult to correlate the enzyme deficiencies with clinical manifestations of disease. Kaplan (18) originally suggested that increased excretion of heparan sulfate was correlated with mental retardation. This correlation is striking in Sanfilippo syndrome but is difficult to apply to the Scheie syndrome and the milder form of Hunter syndrome. Whether the clinical symptoms can be correlated with the extent of activity of different allelic mutant enzymes remains to be determined.

ACKNOWLEDGEMENTS

This work was supported by USPHS Grants AM-05996, HD-04583 and HD-09402.

REFERENCES

1. Arbogast, B., Hopwood, J. J. and Dorfman, A.
    Absence of Hyaluronidase in Cultured Human Skin
    Fibroblasts. Biochem. Biophys. Res. Commun.,
    in press (1975).

2. Austin, J. H. Studies in Metachromatic Leukodys-
    trophy. XII. Multiple Sulfatase Deficiency.
    Archiv. Neurol. 28, 258 (1973).

3. Beaudet, A. L., Di Ferrante, N. M., Ferry, G. D.,
    Nichols, B. L. and Mullins, C. E. Variation in
    Phenotypic Expression of β-Glucuronidase Defici-
    ency. J. Peds. 86, 388 (1975).

4. Beratis, N. G., Turner, B. M., Weiss, R. and
    Hirschhorn, K. Arylsulfatase B Deficiency in
    Maroteaux-Lamy Syndrome. Cellular Studies and
    Carrier Identification. Ped. Res. 9, 475 (1975).

5. Cantz, M. and Kresse, H. Sandhoff Disease:
    Defective Glycosaminoglycan Catabolism in Cultured
    Fibroblasts and Its Correction by β-N-Acetylhexo-
    saminidase. Europ. J. Biochem. 47, 581 (1974).

6. Cashman, D. S., Laryeu, J. U. and Weissmann, B.
    The Hyaluronidase of Rat Skin. Archiv. Biochem.
    Biophys. 135, 387 (1969).

7. Choi, H. U., Meyer, K. and Swarm, R. Mucopoly-
    saccharide and Protein-Polysaccharide of a Trans-
    plantable Rat Chondrosarcoma. Proc. Natl. Acad.
    Sci. USA 68, 877 (1971).

8. Cifonelli, J. A. and King, J. The Distribution of
    Sulfated Uronic Acid and Hexosamine Residues in
    Heparin and Heparan Sulfate. Conn. Tiss. Res. 3,
    97 (1975).

9. Dorfman, A. and Matalon, R. The Mucopolysacchari-
    doses. Proc. Natl. Acad. Sci. USA, in press (1975).

10. Dorfman, A. and Matalon, R. In: "The Metabolic
    Basis of Inherited Diseases". Eds: Stanbury,
    J. B., Wyngaarden, J. B. and Fredrickson, D. S.
    New York, McGraw Hill, Third Edition, 1972, p. 1218.

11. Eto, Y., Wiesmann, U. N., Carlson, J. H., Hersko-
     vitz, N. N. Multiple Sulfatase Deficiencies in
     Cultured Fibroblasts. Archiv. Neurol. 30, 153
     (1974).

12. Fluharty, A. L., Stevens, R. L., Fung, D., Peak,
     S. and Kihara, H. Uridine Diphospho-N-Acetyl-
     galactosamine-4-Sulfate Sulfohydrolase Activity of
     Human Arylsulfatase B and its Deficiency in the
     Maroteaux-Lamy Syndrome. Biochem. Biophys. Res.
     Commun. 64, 955 (1975).

13. Fluharty, A. L., Stevens, R. L., Sanders, D. L.
     and Kihara, H. Arylsulfatase B Deficiency in
     Maroteaux-Lamy Syndrome in Cultured Fibroblasts.
     Biochem. Biophys. Res. Commun. 59, 455 (1974).

14. Gehler, J., Cantz, M., Tolksdorf, M. and Spranger,
     J. Mucopolysaccharidosis. VII. β-Glucuronidase
     Deficiency. Humangenetik 23, 149 (1974).

15. Hunter, C. A Rare Disease in Two Brothers. Proc.
     Roy. Soc. Med. 10, 104 (1917).

16. Hurler, G. Uber Eninen Typ Multipler Abartungen,
     Vorwiegend am Skelettsystem. Z. Kinderheilk. 24,
     220 (1919).

17. Hutterer, F. Degradation of Mucopolysaccharides
     by Hepatic Lysosomes. Biochim. Biophys. Acta 115,
     312 (1966).

18. Kaplan, D. Classification of the Mucopolysacchari-
     doses Based on the Pattern of Mucopolysacchariduria.
     Am. J. Med. 47, 721 (1969).

19. Kaplan, D., McKusick, V. A., Trebach, S. and
     Lazarus, R. Keratosulfate in Chondroitin Sulfate
     Peptide from Normal Urines and from Urine of
     Patients with Morquio Syndrome (Mucopolysacchari-
     dosis IV). J. Lab. Clin. Med. 71, 48 (1968).

20. Knecht, J., Cifonelli, J. A. and Dorfman, A.
     Structural Studies on Heparitin Sulfate of Normal
     and Hurler Tissues. J. Biol. Chem. 242, 4652
     (1967).

21. Kresse, H. and von Figura, K. A New Biochemical
     Subtype of the Sanfilippo Syndrome: Sanfilippo C
     Disease. Third International Symposium of Glyco-

conjugates, Brighton, England (1975) (Abst.).

22. Maroteaux, B., Leveque, B., Marie, J. and Lamy,
     M. Une Nouvelle Dysostose Avec Elimination Urinaire
     de Chonddroitine Sulfate B. Presse Med. 71, 1849
     (1963).

23. Matalon, R., Arbogast, B. and Dorfman, A. Defi-
     ciency of Chondroitin Sulfate N-Acetylgalactosamine
     4-Sulfate Sulfatase in Maroteaux-Lamy Syndrome.
     Biochem. Biophys. Res. Commun. 61, 1450 (1974).

24. Matalon, R., Arbogast, B., Justice, P., Brandt, I.
     K. and Dorfman, A. Morquio's Syndrome: Deficiency
     of a Chondroitin Sulfate N-Acetylhexosamine Sulfate
     Sulfatase. Biochem. Biophys. Res. Commun. 61,
     759 (1974).

25. McKusick, V. A. Heritable Disorders of Connective
     Tissue. St. Louis, C. V. Mosby, 4th Edition, 1972.

26. Neufeld, E. F., Lim, T. W. and Shapiro, L. J.
     Inherited Disorders of Lysosomal Metabolism. In:
     "Annual Review of Biochemistry". Eds: Snell, E. E.,
     Boyer, P. D., Meister, A. and Richardson, C. C.
     Palo Alto, Annual Reviews, 1975, Volume 44, p. 357.

27. O'Brien, J. F., Cantz, M. and Spranger, J. Maro-
     teaux-Lamy Disease (Mucopolysaccharidosis VI), Sub-
     type A: Deficiency of a N-Acetylgalactosamine-4-
     Sulfatase. Biochem. Biophys. Res. Commun. 60,
     1170 (1974).

28. Ogren, S. and Lindahl, U. Cleavage of Macromolecular
     Heparan by an Enzyme from Mouse Mastocytoma. J.
     Biol. Chem. 250, 2690 (1975).

29. Pedrini, V., Lenzi, L. and Zambotti, V. Isolation
     and Identification of Keratosulfate in Urine of
     Patients Affected by Morquio-Ullrich Disease.
     Proc. Soc. Exp. Biol. Med. 110, 847 (1962).

30. Pedrini-Mille, A., Pedrini, V. A. and Ponseti, I. V.
     Glycosaminoglycans of Iliac Crest Cartilage in
     Normal Children and in Morquio's Disease. J. Lab.
     Clin. Med. 84, 465 (1974).

31. Shapira, E., DeGregorio, R. R., Matalon, R. and
     Nadler, H. L. Reduced Arylsulfatase B Activity of

the Mutant Enzyme Protein in Maroteaux-Lamy Syndrome. Biochem. Biophys. Res. Commun. $\underline{62}$, 448 (1975).

32. Sly, W. S., Quinton, B. S., McAlister, W. H. and Rimoin, D. L. Beta-Glucuronidase Deficiency: Report of Clinical, Radiologic and Biochemical Features of a New Mucopolysaccharidosis. J. Pediat. $\underline{82}$, 249 (1973).

33. Spranger, J. The Systemic Mucopolysaccharidoses. Ergeb der Inn. Med. Kinderhl. $\underline{32}$, 166 (1972).

34. Tanaka, H. and Suzuki, K. Lactosylceramide β-Galactosidase in Human Sphingolipidoses. Evidence of Two Genetically Distinct Enzymes. J. Biol. Chem. $\underline{250}$, 2324 (1975).

35. Thompson, J. N., Stoolmiller, A. C., Matalon, R. and Dorfman,A. $\underline{N}$-Acetyl-β-Hexosaminidase: Role in the Degradation of Glycosaminoglycans. Science $\underline{181}$, 866 (1973).

36. Tsay, G. C. and Dawson, G. Structure of the "Keratosulfate-Like" Material from a Patient with G_{M1}-Gangliosidosis (β-D-Galactosidase Deficiency). Biochem. Biophys. Res. Commun. $\underline{52}$, 759 (1973).

37. Tudball, N. and Davidson, E. A. Isolation of a Novel Sulphatase from Rat Liver. Biochim. Biophys. Acta $\underline{171}$, 113 (1968).

MANNOSIDOSIS: STUDIES OF THE α-D-MANNOSIDASE ISOZYMES IN HEALTH AND DISEASE

R.J. Desnick[1,2], L.L. Walling[2], P.M. Anderson[2],
M.K. Raman[2], H.L. Sharp[1] and J.U. Ikonne[2]

Departments of Pediatrics[1], Genetics and Cell Biology[2]
and The Dight Institute for Human Genetics[2]
University of Minnesota, Minneapolis, Minnesota 55455

INTRODUCTION

Mannosidosis, a systemic lysosomal storage disease first described by Ockerman (22), is characterized by psychomotor retardation, a facial dysmorphia resembling that of the Hurler syndrome, dysostosis multiplex, hepatosplenomegaly, hearing loss, recurrent infections and autosomal recessive inheritance. The primary metabolic defect responsible for these manifestations is the deficiency of the acidic α-mannosidase activity (α-D-mannoside mannohydrolase EC 3.2.1.24) (4,19,22) which results in the lysosomal accumulation of mannose-rich oligosaccharides in neural (23) and visceral tissues (1,22) and in the urine (1,20,21,32) of affected homozygous patients. Presumably this enzymatic defect also leads to the accumulation of other glycoconjugate substrates with terminal α-mannosyl residues as evidenced by the recent finding of abnormal glycopeptides, rich in mannose, in cultured skin fibroblasts from a homozygote with mannosidosis (33).

Originally, Ockerman (22) observed 21-36 percent of normal mean α-mannosidase activity in the liver, spleen and cerebral gray matter from an affected homozygote; Hultberg (13) later demonstrated that the residual activity in the liver of this patient had a lower apparent molecular weight and a more neutral pH optimum than the normal hepatic activity. Subsequently, normal human liver α-mannosidase activity was resolved into three components, A, B and C, by anion-exchange chromatography (4) and by electrophoresis on

cellulose acetate (26). The A and B isozymes both had an acidic
pH optimum whereas the more electronegative C isozyme was most
active at neutral pH. In hepatic tissue from two homozygotes with
mannosidosis, Carroll and coworkers (4) demonstrated that both A
and B isozymes were absent and that the residual α-mannosidase
activity represented normal levels of the C isozyme.

Recently, α-mannosidase, purified to homogeneity from the
jack-bean, was characterized as a zinc-metalloenzyme (29). In-
triguingly, zinc has also been found to stimulate the activities
of α-mannosidase A and B isolated from normal human liver (25).
Since no other lysosomal hydrolase is known to be a metalloenzyme
or a metal-dependent enzyme complex, and since the biochemical and
genetic interrelationships among these isozymes have not been resolved, studies were undertaken to further characterize the physical and kinetic properties of the human α-mannosidase isozymes in
health and disease.

CASE REPORT

Table 1 compares the major clinical and laboratory findings
in the patient described below with those of the 12 enzymatically
diagnosed homozygotes with mannosidosis reported in the world
literature (1,9,16,22,32).

Patient M.L. (UMH 1194722), a 2 2/12 year-old Caucasian female
was initially referred to the University of Minnesota Hospitals for
evaluation of recurrent infections. She was the first-born (6-6-
71) of unrelated parents following an uncomplicated pregnancy,
labor and delivery. Birth weight was 3.2 kg and the neonatal and
early infancy periods were unremarkable. At 6 months of age she
was noted to have a greater occipital-frontal circumference than
chest circumference and was hospitalized to rule-out hydrocephalus.
At that time, the diagnosis of arrested hydrocephalus was made.
During the next 19 months she had chronic otitis media and 8 episodes of upper respiratory tract infections, 4 of which required
hospitalization. In addition, a mild developmental delay was
noted; she rolled over at 4 months, sat at 8 months, crawled at 12
months, and walked with and without assistance at 18 and 23 months,
respectively.

On admission, physical examination revealed a well-developed
2 2/12 year-old female with a prominent forehead and a mild facial
dysmorphia resembling that of the Hurler syndrome. Her height was
91.5 cm (+1 SD), weight 14.9 kg (+1.7 SD), and occipital-frontal
circumference 54.0 cm (+3 SD). Pertinent physical findings included frontal bossing, dull-gray tympanic membranes and hepatosplenomegaly. The liver edge was firm, smooth and palpable 5 cm

TABLE 1.   MAJOR CLINICAL AND LABORATORY FINDINGS OF ENZYMATICALLY
CONFIRMED HOMOZYGOTES WITH MANNOSIDOSIS

Finding	World Literature*	Present Case
Facial Dysmorphia	12/12	+
Mental Retardation	8/10	+
Hearing Loss	2/4	+
Corneal or Lenticular Opacities	4/12	-
Hepatosplenomegaly	4/7	+
Recurrent Infections	6/6	+
Dysostosis Multiplex	12/12	+
Vacuolated Lymphocytes	11/12	+
Decreased Serum IgG	4/4	+
Mucopolysacchariduria	2/12	-

*Reported cases with markedly deficient acidic α-mannosidase
activity demonstrated in various sources (1,9,16,22,32).

below the right costal margin and the splenic tip was palpable 2
cm below the left costal margin. In addition, there was a small
reducible umbilical hernia, unusually thick-feeling skin without
lesions, and prominent lymphadenopathy. Cardiac examination and
EKG were normal. Neurologically, she had normal motor strength,
tone and sensory response. Cranial nerves were grossly intact
except for a severe 70 db hearing loss. Cerebellar function was
intact, although her gait was broad-based for age. Electroencephalographic studies were normal. Denver Developmental
Screening indicated gross motor, fine motor, language and personal-
social skills at 13, 21, 6 and 14 months of age, respectively. The
delay in language development presumably was related to her severe
hearing loss.

Radiologic examination revealed chronic pulmonary infiltrates
consistent with repeated infections. Extensive bony abnormalities
compatible with dysostosis multiplex were present, including a
"J-shaped" sella, a hypoplastic L-2 lumbar vertebra with anterior
beaking, tapered proximal metacarpals, mild flaring of the iliac
wings, and extensive sclerosis of the cranial vault, particularly

of the base of the skull. No corneal or lenticular opacities were
seen by slit-lamp microscopy; normal discs, retinae and maculae
were seen on fundiscopic examination.

Clinical laboratory studies included normal BUN, creatinine,
sodium, potassium, chloride, bicarbonate, calcium, phosphorous,
bilirubin, SGOT, alkaline phosphatase, serum protein electrophoresis, cholesterol, triglycerides and total phospholipids. Sweat
chlorides were normal and the quantitative immunoglobulins were
IgA, 157 mg%; IgG, 940 mg%; and IgM, 127 mg%. Coagulation studies
were within normal limits. The hemoglobin was 11.5 gm% and the
leukocyte count was 9200 per mm^3 with a normal differential. On
examination of a peripheral smear, approximately 90% of the lymphocytes were vacuolated. The urinary metabolic screen was normal,
including a Berry spot test.

Special studies included quantitative urinary amino acids and
mucopolysaccharides, which were within normal limits. Bone marrow
biopsy revealed foamy appearing macrophages similar to those seen
in Niemann-Pick disease as well as vacuolated lymphocytes. No
inclusion bodies were observed by phase microscopy in cultured skin
fibroblasts. Ultrastructural examination of hepatic tissue obtained by percutaneous biopsy showed numerous, enlarged lysosomes containing amorphous mucopolysaccharide- or glycoprotein-like material
as shown in Figure 1. Assays of various lysosomal hydrolase
activities were performed; the demonstration of deficient acidic
α-mannosidase activity in plasma and isolated peripheral leukocytes
established the diagnosis of mannosidosis.

At 3 1/2 years of age, the patient was transported to the
University of Minnesota Hospitals following 4 months of almost
continual hospitalization elsewhere for recurrent pneumonitis,
otitis and upper respiratory tract infections. Immunologic evaluation on admission revealed IgA, IgG, IgM and IgE values of 105,
576, 66 and 9 mg%, respectively. Lymphocyte transformation studies showed a 20% of normal response to PHA-M and a 50% of normal
response to purified PHA(HA-17). A profound defect in leukocyte
response to chemotactic attraction was observed whereas the
mechanism for random migration was intact. In addition, phagocytosis and bacterial killing studies revealed slow phagocytosis and
incomplete intracellular killing by her neutrophils. She was aner-
gic on skin testing to PPD, SK/SD, Candida and mumps antigens.

During this hospitalization she developed severe respiratory
distress with nasal flaring, intercostal retractions, diffuse
rhonchi and a temperature of 105°F. Chest X-ray revealed marked
bilateral basilar infiltrates. The patient's respiratory status
deteriorated rapidly over a week period despite intensive chemotherapy and respiratory support. She expired from respiratory
failure and disseminated intravascular coagulation. Adenovirus

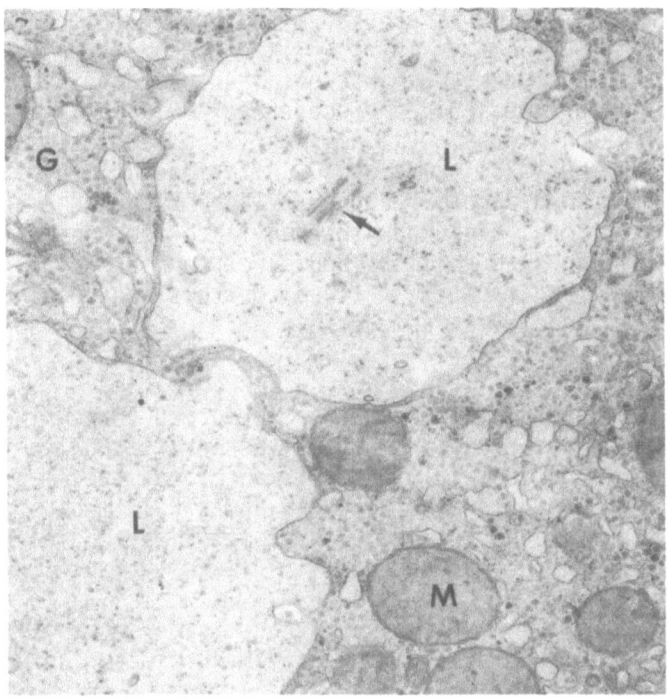

Figure 1. Electron micrograph of a portion of a hepatocyte containing two large, membrane-bounded vacuoles, presumably lysosomes (L), which contain a fine reticulogranular material similar to that seen in the Mucopolysaccharidoses. Occasional small, single membrane-lined vesicles and stacks of elongated structures consisting of very fine fibrils (←) are seen within the lysosomes. Other normal cytoplasmic structures include mitochondria (M) and glycogen (G) (X 15,700).

type 7 was subsequently cultured from urine, stool, throat, and lung. An autopsy was performed immediately after death and the histochemical, ultrastructural and biochemical findings will be reported elsewhere (7).

MATERIALS AND METHODS

Blood, Tissue and Cell Preparations

Plasma was obtained from heparinized blood by centrifugation at 2,000 X g for 10 minutes at 4°C; the buffy coat was removed and

the erythrocytes were washed twice with 0.9% sodium chloride.
Leukocytes were isolated as previously described (6).

Percutaneous liver biopsy was obtained with a 1.6 mm Menghini
needle by previously described procedures (28). The specimen was
fixed for electron microscopy in Millong's buffer containing 1.25%
glutaraldehyde and 1.25% osmic acid. After one hr, the tissue was
dehydrated in graded alcohols and propylene oxide and embedded in
Epon. Thin sections, stained with uranyl acetate and lead hydrox-
ide, were examined in a Phillips 200 electron microscope. Liver
from the patient and from age-matched controls was obtained within
15 min of death and frozen immediately at -70°C for subsequent
analyses.

Transabdominal amniocentesis was performed during the 14th to
16th week of gestation and the amniocytes were separated from the
fluid by centrifugation at 100 X g. Skin biopsy specimens and
amniocytes were grown to confluency in Ham's F-10 medium with 20%
fetal calf serum and harvested by trypsinization according to
standard tissue culture procedures.

Resolution and Purification of α-Mannosidase Isozymes

The α-mannosidase isozymes in normal human liver were resolved
by ion-exchange chromatography. Liver (2.0 gm) was homogenized in
distilled water (1:4, w/v), centrifuged at 30,000 X g for 25 min
and the supernatant (5 ml) was chromatographed on DEAE-cellulose
(Whatman DE-52, Reeve Angel, Clifton, N.J.), essentially by the
method of Ikonne et al. (15).

The α-mannosidase isozymes were purified from human liver
according to the following scheme. Liver (300 gm) was homogenized
in a Waring Blender for 4 minutes and in 2 volumes of distilled
water and then centrifuged at 30,000 X g for 25 min. Two steps of
ammonium sulfate fractionation were carried out on the supernatant
at 0-30% and 40-55% saturation, and the precipitated protein in
each fraction was dissolved in 100 ml of distilled water. The
40-55% fraction containing the acidic activity was subjected to
chromatography on Concanavalin-A Sepharose (Pharmacia, Uppsala,
Sweden). The α-mannosidase A and B isozymes were eluted together
and then separated and further purified by chromatography on DEAE-
cellulose. The 0-30% fraction containing the neutral α-mannosidase
C activity was chromatographed directly on DEAE-cellulose, since
this component did not bind to Concanavalin-A Sepharose. Details
of the purification procedure will be reported elsewhere (14).

Electrophoresis of α-Mannosidase Isozymes

Electrophoresis of partially purified α-mannosidases A, B and C and tissue extracts was performed on cellulose acetate gels (Cellogel, 350μ, 16 cm X 17 cm, Kalex Scientific, Manhasset, NY) according to general procedures (10) with the following modifications for these isozymes. Electrophoresis was carried out in 0.04 M potassium phosphate buffer, pH 7.3, at 4°C with the electrophoresis tank on ice. Gels were prerun at 0.88 mamps/cm, constant current, for 20 min; then samples (5-10 μl containing 3.5-6.5 nmoles/hr) were applied with capillary micropipets and allowed to equilibrate for 10 min. Constant current (0.88 mamps/cm) was applied and the duration of the electrophoretic run was 5 hours. The gel was removed from the tank and incubated for 1 min (face down) in 1.5 mM 4-methylumbelliferyl-α-D-mannopyranoside in 0.1 M citrate-phosphate buffer, pH 4.5. The gel was removed, gently blotted with filter paper, and placed (face up) in a moist chamber consisting of two glass plates separated by a border of felt strips saturated with water. The chamber was incubated at 37°C for 40 min. Bands of fluorescence were developed by placing the gel (face down) in 0.17 M glycine-carbonate buffer, pH 10.7, for 2 min. The gel was blotted with filter paper and again placed in the moist chamber; the bands of enzymatic activity were viewed under long wavelength UV light and photographed immediately.

Enzyme Assays

The acidic (pH 4.4) and neutral (pH 6.0) α-mannosidase activities in various sources were determined by the following methods. Plasma, amniotic fluid and leukocyte, erythrocyte, amniocyte and cultured skin fibroblast and amniotic cell extracts were diluted ten-fold in McIlvaine's citrate-phosphate buffer (11) at pH 4.4 and 6.0. Hepatic tissue was homogenized in distilled water (1:2, w/v), centrifuged at 30,000 X g for 25 min, and the supernatant assayed for enzymatic activity. The standard reaction mixture contained 300 μl of 1 mM 4-methylumbelliferyl-α-D-mannopyranoside (RPI, Inc., Elk Grove Village, IL) in citrate-phosphate buffer, pH 4.4 or pH 6.0 and 100 μl of enzyme source. Leukocytes, hepatic supernatants, amniocytes, cultured fibroblasts or amniotic cells and column fractions (100 μl of the 2.0 ml fractions) were incubated for 30 min, and erythrocytes, plasma and amniotic fluid for 1 hr at 37°C. The reactions were terminated by the addition of 4.6 ml 0.1 M ethylene diamine, pH 11.4, except for erythrocyte assays which were terminated by the addition of 50 μl of 21% TCA, centrifuged at 2000 X g for 10 min and then brought to 5.0 ml with 0.1 M ethylene diamine. Fluorescence was measured in a Turner Model 111 fluorometer with an excitation wavelength of 365 nm and an emission wavelength of 450 nm and compared to 4-methylumbelliferone as a standard. Under these assay conditions, the rates of the enzyme reaction were linear with respect to time and protein concentration for each enzyme source.

For studies with metal ions, the reaction mixture was modified to contain 50 μl of enzyme source, 50 μl of the appropriate metal ion ($CuSO_4$, $ZnSO_4$ or $MnCl_2$) in distilled water, and 300 μl of the appropriate substrate and then assayed as described above.

The activities of other lysosomal hydrolases were determined in various sources with the appropriate artificial substrate according to the following methods: total α- and β-galactosidases (6), β-glucuronidase (34), total β-hexosaminidase (8), α-L-iduronidase (12), arylsulfatase A (3), and α-L-fucosidase (17). Protein concentrations were determined according to the method of Lowry (18).

Trace Metal Determinations

Zinc and copper concentrations were determined in whole plasma, ashed liver, and liver extracts, the latter prepared as described for enzyme assay, according to standard techniques (29,30).

RESULTS

Diagnostic Studies

Table 2 shows the levels of acidic and neutral α-mannosidase activities in plasma, isolated peripheral leukocytes and cultured skin fibroblasts from the homozygote with mannosidosis, her obligate heterozygous parents and normal individuals. In each enzyme source from the homozygote, there was a marked deficiency of α-mannosidase activity at pH 4.4, whereas the activity at pH 6.0 was normal. The levels of acidic enzymatic activity obtained for the obligate heterozygotes were within the normal range; their ratios of acidic α-mannosidase activity to total β-hexosaminidase activity at pH 4.4 in plasma (15.6, 21.6) and leukocytes (16.9, 32.0) were within the respective ranges calculated for normal individuals and did not discriminate the heterozygous state (19). Table 3 shows the specific activities of seven other lysosomal hydrolases in leukocytes and cultured skin fibroblasts from the homozygote with mannosidosis. With the exception of the values ‘for β-galactosidase and β-glucuronidase in leukocytes and for α-L-fucosidase in cultured skin fibroblasts, the lysosomal hydrolase activities in these sources were within normal control ranges.

The levels of acidic and neutral α-mannosidase activities were determined in amniotic fluid, amniocytes and cultured amniotic

TABLE 2. ACIDIC AND NEUTRAL α-MANNOSIDASE ACTIVITIES IN VARIOUS SOURCES FROM HOMOZYGOTES AND HETEROZYGOTES FOR MANNOSIDOSIS AND NORMAL INDIVIDUALS*

Source	Plasma (nmoles/hr/ml)		Leukocytes (nmoles/hr/mg protein)		Erythrocytes (nmoles/hr/gm protein)		Cultured Fibroblasts (nmoles/hr/mg protein)	
	pH 4.4	pH 6.0	pH 4.4	pH 6.0	pH 4.4	pH 6.0	pH 4.4	pH 6.0
Homozygote								
M.L.	3.0	232	0.18	26.6	–	–	0.0	11.9
Heterozygotes								
J.L.	40.2	192	75.0	30.0	–	–	–	–
R.L.	53.4	170	125.0	39.2	–	–	–	–
Normal Mean	30.6	87.4	76.9	18.8	20.9	93.3	204.0	70.3
(and Range)	(13.2–64.2)	(39.6–214.0)	(22.8–135.0)	(9.6–28.8)	(17.1–27.0)	(69.2–120.0)	(40.4–483.0)	(14.3–184.0)
n =	10	10	7	7	6	6	16	16

*Enzymatic activities determined using 4-methylumbelliferyl-α-D-mannopyranoside as substrate as described in Materials and Methods.

TABLE 3. ACTIVITIES OF VARIOUS LYSOSOMAL HYDROLASES IN LEUKOCYTES AND CULTURED SKIN FIBROBLASTS FROM A HOMOZYGOTE WITH MANNOSIDOSIS AND NORMAL INDIVIDUALS

Lysosomal Hydrolase	Leukocytes			Cultured Skin Fibroblasts		
	Mannosidosis Homozygote	Normal Mean (n)	Normal Range	Mannosidosis Homozygote	Normal Mean (n)	Normal Range
	(nmoles/hr/mg protein)					
α-Mannosidase*						
pH 4.4	0.18	87.7 (6)	22.8- 135.0	0.0	204.0 (16)	40.4- 482.0
pH 6.0	26.6	20.4 (6)	9.6- 28.8	11.9	70.2 (16)	14.3- 184.0
α-Galactosidase*	27.6	39.3 (25)	23.0- 65.0	57.1	145.0 (24)	50.6- 292.0
β-Galactosidase*	95.1	170.0 (10)	134.0- 227.0	531.0	394.0 (50)	124.0- 646.0
β-Glucuronidase*	384.0	131.0 (3)	110.1- 162.0	116.0	112.0 (70)	28.0- 200.0
β-Hexosaminidase*	1470.0	1450.0 (81)	547.0-3260.0	4470.0	4160.0 (70)	2020.0-8920.0
α-L-Iduronidase**	242.0	180.0 (50)	111.0- 272.0	425.0	1590.0 (8)	684.0-2370.0
Arylsulfatase A**	-	183.0 (12)	96.2- 272.0	273.0	437.0 (50)	201.0- 784.0
α-L-Fucosidase**	-	-	-	49.0	20.0 (16)	7.0- 38.0

*Enzymatic activities determined using the *appropriate 4-methylumbelliferyl-glycopyranoside
**phenyl-α-L-iduronide, or p-nitrophenyl-α-L-fucopyranoside or p-nitrocatechol-sulfate as substrates as described in Materials and Methods.

TABLE 4. ACIDIC AND NEUTRAL α-MANNOSIDASE ACTIVITIES IN AMNIOTIC FLUID,
AMNIOCYTES AND CULTURED AMNIOTIC CELLS FROM NORMAL PREGNANCIES *

Source	Amniotic Fluid**		Amniocytes**		Cultured Amniotic Cells**	
	pH 4.4	pH 6.0	pH 4.4	pH 6.0	pH 4.4	pH 6.0
	(nmoles/hr/ml)				(nmoles/hr/mg protein)	
Mean	8.2	24.1	9.2	4.1	75.1	20.7
Range	2.8-13.6	18.3-26.5	5.0-19.6	2.2-7.2	10.8-178.0	5.7-42.8
n =	4	4	5	5	3	3

*Amniocentesis performed at 14-16 weeks of gestation in pregnancies at-risk
for chromosomal or neural tube defects; birth of normal infants confirmed
the prenatal diagnosis.
**Enzymatic activities determined using 4-methylumbelliferyl-α-D-mannopyrano-
side as substrate as described in Materials and Methods.

cells obtained from normal pregnancies as shown in Table 4. In contrast to normal amniotic fluid or amniocytes, cultured amniotic cells had greater levels of acidic than neutral α-mannosidase activity, providing a more reliable source of activity for prenatal diagnostic studies; the mean α-mannosidase activities at pH 4.4 and pH 6.0 in the cultured amniotic cells were 75.1 and 20.7 with ranges of 10.8-178.0 and 5.7-42.8 nmoles per hr per mg protein, respectively.

Characterization of the Acidic α-Mannosidase Activities

Effect of pH and Substrate Concentration. The effect of pH on total α-mannosidase activities in leukocytes and liver extracts from normal individuals revealed an optimum of pH 4.4 in both sources, in agreement with previously reported values (2,8,19,25). In contrast, a marked deficiency of activity at pH 3.5-5.0 was observed in these sources from the homozygote with mannosidosis.

Figure 2A shows the relationship between substrate concentration and α-mannosidase activities, assayed at pH 4.4, in leukocyte and liver extracts from a normal individual and the homozygote with mannosidosis. Using the synthetic substrate, 4-methylumbelliferyl-α-D-mannopyranoside, the acidic α-mannosidase activity was saturated at a substrate concentration of about 2.5 mM in both sources from the normal individual. A striking finding was the presence of detectable levels of acidic α-mannosidase activity in these sources from the homozygote with mannosidosis which could not be saturated within the solubility range of the substrate. Apparent Km values for α-mannosidase activity as determined from Lineweaver-Burk plots were 1.1 mM for normal liver (Figure 2B) and 0.9 mM for normal leukocytes (Figure 2C). In contrast, the apparent Km values in the homozygote with mannosidosis were extremely difficult to calculate; the apparent Km was estimated at 15.4 mM in liver extracts.

Effect of Inhibitors. To rule out the possible existence of endogenous inhibitors of acidic α-mannosidase activity in the homozygote with mannosidosis, the acidic α-mannosidase activity in 1:1 mixtures of both liver and leukocyte extracts from normal individuals and the patient with mannosidosis was determined. As shown in Table 5, the observed activity in each mixture approximated the expected average of the activities in the normal and enzyme-deficient sources.

Effect of $ZnSO_4$, $CoSO_4$ and $MnCl_2$. Figure 3A shows the differential effects of increasing concentrations of zinc and cobalt ions on the acidic α-mannosidase activity in liver extracts from the homozygote and an age-matched normal individual. Zinc

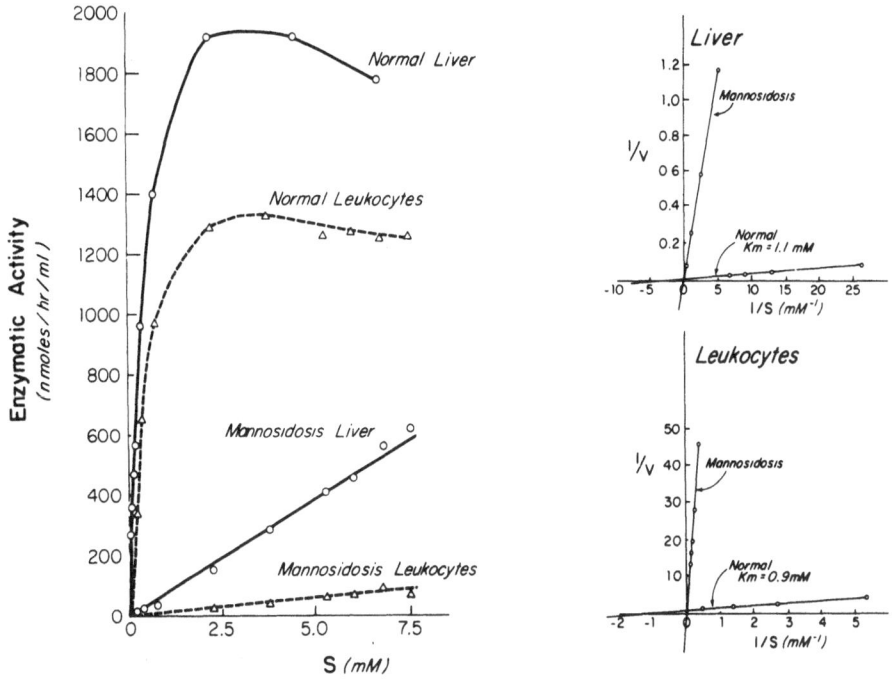

Figure 2. (A) Effect of substrate concentration on acidic α-mannosidase activities in liver and leukocyte extracts from a homozygote with mannosidosis and a normal individual. Lineweaver-Burk plots of acidic α-mannosidase activities in liver (B) and leukocyte extracts (C) from indicated sources.

TABLE 5. ACIDIC α-MANNOSIDASE ACTIVITIES IN EQUAL

MIXTURES OF LIVER AND LEUKOCYTE EXTRACTS FROM

A HOMOZYGOTE WITH MANNOSIDOSIS AND A NORMAL INDIVIDUAL

Source	Mannosidosis	Normal	Mixture	
			Observed	Expected
	(nmoles/hr/ml extract)			
Leukocytes	1.0	97.6	51.2	49.3
Liver	35.2	1520.0	805.0	778.0

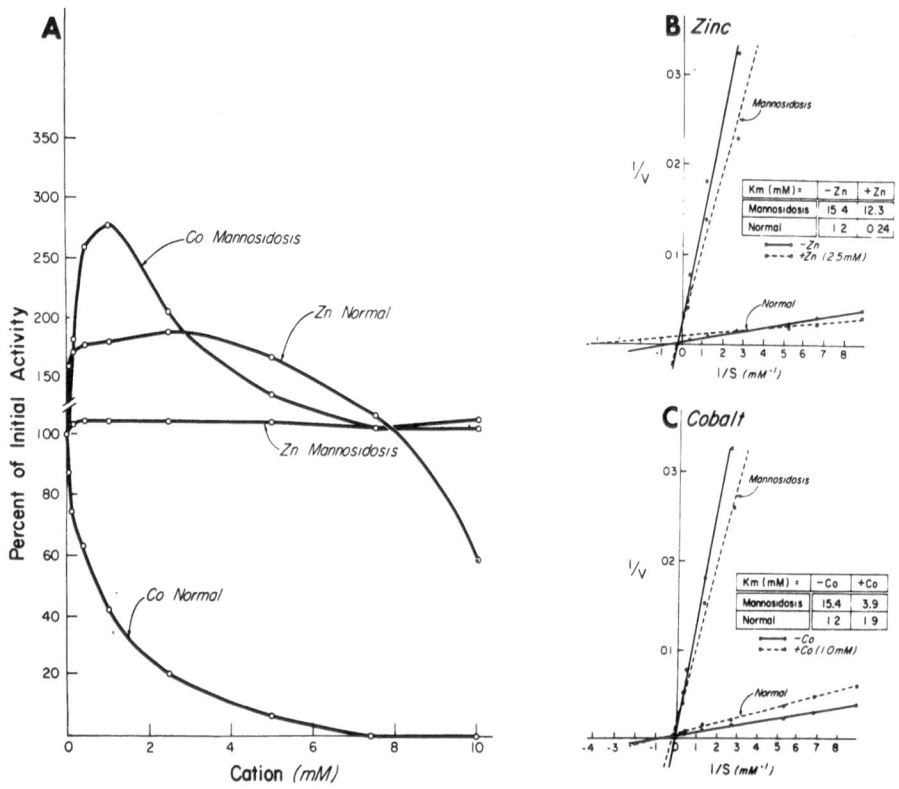

Figure 3.   (A) Effect of ZnSO₄ and CoSO₄ on acidic α-mannosidase
activities from indicated hepatic sources. Lineweaver-Burk plots
of acidic α-mannosidase activities in liver extracts from indicated
sources in the presence and absence of (B) 2.5 mM ZnSO₄ and (C)
1.0 mM CoSO₄.

stimulated the acidic activity in normal liver to about 150 to 190
percent of initial activity at ZnSO₄ concentrations between 0.01
to 5.0 mM with maximal stimulation at 2.5 mM.   In contrast, the
acidic α-mannosidase activity from the mannosidosis homozygote was
only slightly stimulated to approximately 115 percent of initial
activity at all concentrations from 0.01 to 10.0 mM ZnSO₄.   Whereas
cobalt inhibited acidic α-mannosidase activity in normal liver at
all concentrations studied, a marked stimulation of the residual
acidic activity in the homozygote was observed at final concentrations from 0.01 mM to 8.0 mM, with maximal stimulation, 280 percent
of initial activity, at 1 mM CoSO₄.   MnCl₂ was found to inhibit the
acidic activities in normal and mannosidosis liver extracts; at
5.0 mM, both activities were inhibited to approximately 30 percent
of initial activity.

Figures 3B and 3C show the effect of 2.5 mM $ZnSO_4$ and 1.0 mM $CoSO_4$ on the Vmax and apparent Km values of the acidic activity in the normal and mannosidosis liver extracts as determined by Lineweaver-Burk plots. Zinc significantly lowered the apparent Km value of the acidic activity in normal liver (1.2 to 0.24 mM) whereas this metallic ion had little effect on the values for mannosidosis hepatic activity (15.4 to 12.3 mM). Unlike zinc, cobalt had its major effect on the acidic activity in the mannosidosis liver extract, lowering the apparent Km from 15.4 to 3.9 mM, whereas the apparent Km for the normal activity was increased from 1.2 to 1.9 mM.

In order to ascertain the endogenous concentration of zinc in the assay mixtures, the levels of this metallic ion were determined by atomic absorption spectroscopy. Table 6 shows the concentrations of zinc and copper, as an internal control, in the liver extracts, ashed liver and plasma from the homozygote with mannosidosis and normal individuals. Compared to the concentrations in each of the normal sources, the levels of zinc were higher in the homozygote, especially in the liver extract. When expressed as the ratio of zinc to copper, the values for the mannosidosis and normal liver extracts were 15.8 and 6.9, respectively.

TABLE 6. CONCENTRATIONS OF ZINC AND COPPER IN VARIOUS SOURCES FROM A HOMOZYGOTE WITH MANNOSIDOSIS AND NORMAL INDIVIDUALS *

Source	Plasma			Ashed Liver			Liver Extract		
	Zn	Cu	Zn/Cu	Zn	Cu	Zn/Cu	Zn	Cu	Zn/Cu
	(µg/ml)			(µg/g wet weight)					
Mannosidosis Homozygote	2.11	1.87	1.17	56	1.75	32.0	30.0	1.90	15.8
Normal Control-1	1.66	1.76	0.94	43	3.0	14.3	10.0	1.44	6.9
Normal Control-2	1.34	1.45	0.92	44	7.22	6.1	-	-	-

*Concentrations of zinc and copper were determined by atomic absorption spectroscopy as described in Materials and Methods.

Resolution and Purification of α-Mannosidase Isozymes

     Three peaks of α-mannosidase activity, A, B and C, were ob-
served after chromatography of normal·liver extract on DEAE-
cellulose as shown in Figure 4. The A and B isozymes were maxi-
mally detected at pH 4.4, whereas the C isozyme was most active at
pH 6.5; low levels of A and B activity were also detected at pH
6.5. The A isozyme was eluted with the initial buffer wash and
the B and C isozymes at 0.06 M and 0.12 M concentrations, respectively, on the linear KCl gradient.

     Purification of the α-mannosidase isozymes was achieved by
differential ammonium sulfate precipitation followed by combined

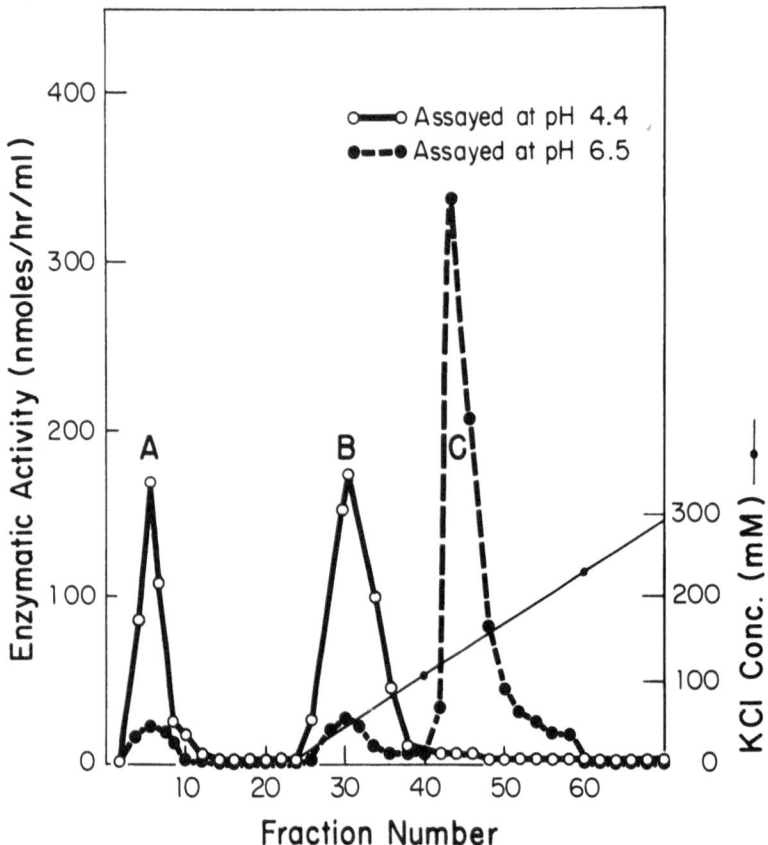

Figure 4. Elution profile from the DEAE-cellulose chromatography
of α-mannosidase A, B and C isozymes in normal liver. For details,
see Materials and Methods.

conventional and "oligo-affinity" (Concanavalin-A Sepharose) chromatography (14). By these procedures, the α-mannosidase A and B isozymes were purified about 15- and 550-fold with yields of 2 and 13 per cent, respectively, based on their initial pH 4.4 activities. The neutral α-mannosidase C was purified about 60-fold with a 31 per cent recovery based on the pH 6.5 activity in the crude extract.

   Electrophoresis of the α-Mannosidase Isozymes. Figure 5 shows that electrophoresis on cellulose acetate gel at pH 7.3 distinctly separated the α-mannosidase A, B and C isozymes which were partially purified from normal human liver. The B isozyme migrated between the A isozyme and the more electronegative C isozyme. In a liver extract from the homozygote with mannosidosis, a single band of activity was visible which was comparable in mobility to partially purified, normal hepatic α-mannosidase C, further documenting the deficient activity of the α-mannosidase A and B isozymes.

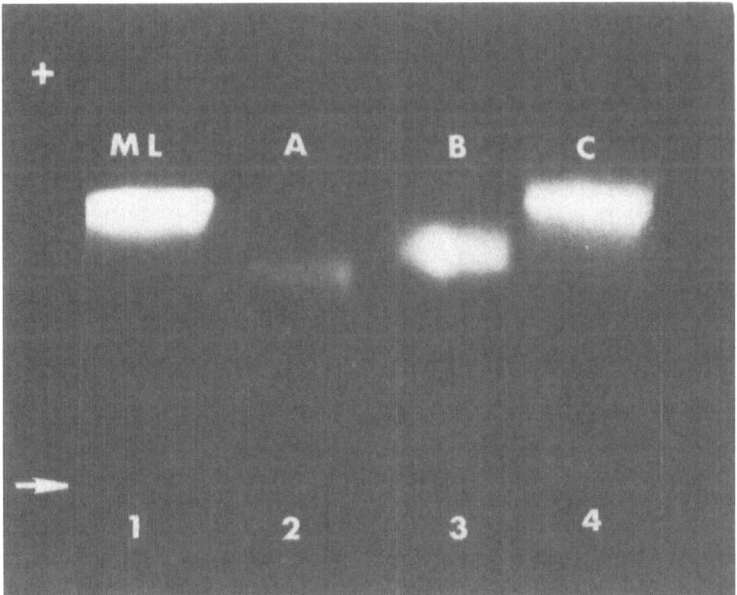

Figure 5. Fluorescent bands of enzymatic activity after electrophoresis on cellulose acetate gel and staining with 4-methylumbelliferyl-α-D-mannopyranoside. Lane 1 - liver from the homozygote with mannosidosis (1:3 w/v extract); lane 2, 3 and 4 - partially purified normal human liver α-mannosidase A, B and C isozymes, respectively. Arrow = point of application.

DISCUSSION

Since the original clinical and biochemical delineation of mannosidosis by Ockerman (22) in 1967, only twelve enzymatically diagnosed homozygotes have been reported in the world literature. Presumably, many patients have been misdiagnosed since the phenotypic features, as well as hematologic and radiologic findings, resemble those of the mucopolysaccharidoses. Thus, suspect patients should be confirmed biochemically. Our studies demonstrate that the enzymatic diagnosis of suspect homozygotes can be made reliably using plasma, isolated leukocytes, or cultured skin fibroblasts assayed carefully at the appropriate acidic pH (Table 2). The necessity to demonstrate deficient α-mannosidase A and B activities, rather than high levels of urinary mannose (21, 22), is further underscored by the recent demonstration that total urinary mannose may be unreliable due to the wide variability in glycoprotein excretion in normal individuals (32).

Unfortunately, the enzymatic identification of heterozygotes for mannosidosis has been difficult (1,9) as evidenced by our results (Table 2). Even when the ratio of α-mannosidase to total β-hexosaminidase activities at pH 4.4 is calculated, the values do not always discriminate heterozygotes as previously suggested (19). Thus, multiple determinations of acidic α-mannosidase activity in several different sources may be required for heterozygote identification. The difficulty in heterozygote detection is unusual among the lysosomal storage diseases and suggests a unique interaction of the mutant and active gene products or associated cofactors *in vivo*.

The occurrence of acidic α-mannosidase activities in amniotic fluid, amniocytes and cultured amniotic cells makes possible the prenatal diagnosis for pregnancies at-risk for mannosidosis. The observation of greater levels of acidic than neutral activity in the cultured amniotic cells indicates that these cells will provide the most reliable enzyme source for the detection of fetuses affected with mannosidosis. However, another lysosomal hydrolase (e.g., β-hexosaminidase) must be simultaneously determined as control for cell viability, etc.

The most intriguing aspect of our kinetic studies was the demonstration of residual acidic α-mannosidase activity in crude liver and leukocyte extracts from the homozygote with mannosidosis. Using the synthetic substrate, 4-methylumbelliferyl-α-D-mannopyranoside, this acidic activity could not be saturated in either enzyme source. The apparent Km values estimated from Lineweaver-Burk plots (Figure 2) were 1.1 and 15.4 mM for the hepatic activity and 0.9 and >20 mM for the leukocytic activity from a normal individual and the homozygote, respectively. The apparent Km values were about 15 times higher for the acidic activities in the homozygote compared to those calculated for the normal sources.

The effects of zinc (stimulation) and cobalt (inhibition) on acidic α-mannosidase activity in normal human liver have ›en reported previously (5,25). In addition, the specific activity of α-mannosidase at pH 5.0 was correlated directly with the zinc content of various rat tissues (30) and α-mannosidase purified to homogeneity from the jack-bean has been shown to be a zinc metalloenzyme (29), indicating the importance of zinc to this enzymatic activity. Our studies also demonstrated a stimulatory effect of zinc and an inhibitory effect of cobalt ions on acid α-mannosidase activity in normal liver extracts. In the presence of 2.5 mM $ZnSO_4$ and 1.0 mM $CoSO_4$, the Vmax and apparent Km values estimated for the acidic activity in normal liver extracts from Lineweaver-Burk plots were altered; the apparent Km values were decreased in the presence of zinc and slightly increased when cobalt was present in the crude extract. However, a differential effect was observed when these metal ions were incubated in the liver extracts from the homozygote with mannosidosis. The apparent Km values for the residual acidic activity were decreased slightly with zinc and markedly with cobalt. In contrast to the significant effect of zinc on the kinetics of normal acidic activity, the minimal effect of zinc on the residual acidic activity may be related to the physical properties of the mutant enzyme or possibly to the presence of higher endogenous concentrations of zinc in the extract as well as in other sources from the mannosidosis homozygote (Table 6). It is possible that a residual acidic activity in patients with mannosidosis might be increased following the administration of these trace metals; the effectiveness of this therapeutic approach should be evaluated in Angus calves with mannosidosis, an animal model of the human enzymatic deficiency disease (24) and in cultured skin fibroblasts obtained from the patient prior to *in vivo* trials.

Three major components of α-mannosidase activity in normal human liver were resolved by ion-exchange chromatography on DEAE-cellulose (Figure 4) and electrophoresis on cellulose acetate gels (Figure 5) in agreement with previously reported findings (4,5, 19,25,26,27). Two isozymes, α-mannosidases A and B, had optimal activities at pH 4.4 and the third isozyme, α-mannosidase C, had an optimum at pH 6.5. Differential ammonium sulfate precipitation followed by conventional and affinity chromatographic (27) procedures has already resulted in significant purification of these isozymes from normal human liver for subsequent physical and kinetic characterization.

Electrophoresis of the liver extract from the homozygote with mannosidosis revealed only one band of activity which co-electrophoresed with the α-mannosidase C isozyme partially purified from normal liver (Figure 5); similar results have been previously reported in tissues (26) and cultured skin fibroblasts (31) from homozygotes with mannosidosis. Although no residual acidic activities were detected electrophoretically in the mannosidosis liver extract, preliminary ion-exchange chromatrographic studies have revealed the presence of residual acidic activities eluted in positions corresponding to those of the normal α-mannosidase A and B isozymes. These studies tend to exclude the possibility that the residual acidic activity represents the recently described α-mannosidase component which is stimulated by cobalt and has an optimum at pH 5.5 (25). Experiments are now in progress to attempt to purify and characterize these residual activities.

Our studies of the acidic α-mannosidase isozymes in the crude tissue extracts have provided intriguing data, particularly the finding of residual acid activity in the leukocytes and liver from the homozygote with mannosidosis. These results suggest the possible occurrence of a missense mutation in the structural gene coding for the acidic α-mannosidase activity; it is tempting to postulate that the mutation in our patient resulted in a gene product with residual acidic activity but with altered kinetic properties.

Although this hypothesis is appealing, clearly, the implications of these studies with crude extracts are only suggestive. Further investigation of the kinetic and physical properties of highly purified α-mannosidase isozymes with natural as well as synthetic substrates will be required to elucidate the molecular and genetic interrelationships among the normal isozymes and especially the molecular pathology of the residual activity in mannosidosis.

ACKNOWLEDGMENTS

The authors wish to express their gratitude to Dr. J.G. Leroy for his expert clinical suggestions and fibroblast enzyme determinations, to Dr. P.G. Quie for the leukocyte function studies, and to Dr. L. Singer for the trace metal analyses and to Dr. G.A. Grabowski for his helpful clinical advice. We also wish to thank Ms. Debra Seehausen for her skillful technical assistance and Ms. Ardys Ferman for her expert clerical assistance.

This work was supported in part by a grant (1-273) from the National Foundation-March of Dimes; a grant (AM 15174) from the National Institutes of Health; a grant (RR-400) from the General Clinical Research Center Program of the Division of Research Resources, National Institutes of Health; and a grant (74-915) from the American Heart Association. R.J. Desnick is a recipient of a Research Career Development Award (K04 AM 00042) and P.M. Anderson is a recipient of a Predoctoral Fellowship (T1 MH 10679) from the National Institutes of Health.

REFERENCES

1. Autio, S., Norden, N.E., Ockerman, P.A., Riekkinen, P., Rapola, J. and Louhimo, T.: Mannosidosis: Clinical, fine-structural and biochemical findings in three cases. Acta Paediat. Scand. 62:555, 1973.

2. Avila, J.L. and Convit, J.: Characterization and properties of α-D-mannosidase of human polymorphonuclear leukocytes. Clin. Chim. Acta 47:335, 1973.

3. Baum, H., Dodgson, K.S. and Spencer, B.: The assay of aryl-sulfatases A and B in human urine. Clin. Chim. Acta 4:453, 1959.

4. Carroll, M., Dance, N., Masson, P.K., Robinson, D. and Winchester, B.G.: Human mannosidosis--the enzymatic defect. Biochem. Biophys. Res. Comm. 49:579, 1972.

5. Chester, M.A., Lundblad, A. and Masson, P.K.: The relation-ship between different forms of human α-mannosidase. Biochim. Biophys. Acta 391:341, 1975.

6. Desnick, R.J., Allen, K.Y., Desnick, S.J., Raman, M.K., Bernlohr, R.W. and Krivit W.: Fabry's disease: Enzymatic diagnosis of hemizygotes and heterozygotes. J. Lab. Clin. Med. 81:157, 1973.

7. Desnick, R.J., Brunning, R., Sung, J.H., Quie, P.G., Grabowski, G.A. and Ikonne, J.U.: Mannosidosis: Clinical ultrastructural, biochemical and immunologic studies. J. Pediat., in review.

8. Desnick, R.J., Krivit, W., Snyder, P.D., Desnick, S.J. and Sharp, H.L.: Sandhoff's disease: Ultrastructural and bio-chemical studies. In: Sphingolipids, Sphingolipidoses and Allied Disorders, edited by S.M. Aronson and B.W. Volk. New York, Plenum Press, 1972, p. 351.

9. Farriaux, J.P., Legoius, I., Humbel, R., Dhondt, J.L., Richard, P., Strecker, G., Fourmaintraux, A., Ringel, J. and Fontaine, G.: La mannosidoses. Nouv. Presse Med. 4:1867, 1975.

10. ⁻luharty, A.L., Lassila, E.L., Porter, M.T. and Kihara, H.:
     The electrophoretic separation of human β-galactosidases on
     cellulose acetate. Biochem. Med. 5:158, 1971.

11. Gomori, G.: Preparation of buffers for use in enzyme studies.
     Methods of Enzymol. 1:138, 1955.

12. Hall, C.W. and Neufeld, E.F.: α-L-iduronidase activity in
     cultured skin fibroblasts and amniotic cells. Arch. Biochem.
     Biophys. 158:817, 1973.

13. Hultberg, B.: Properties of α-mannosidase in mannosidosis.
     Scand. J. Clin. Lab. Invest. 26:155, 1970.

14. Ikonne, J.U. and Desnick, R.J.: Mannosidosis: Characteriza-
     tion of the enzymatic defect. in preparation.

15. Ikonne, J.U., Rattazzi, M.C. and Desnick, R.J.: Characteri-
     zation of Hex S, the major residual β-hexosaminidase activity
     in type O G_{M2} gangliosidosis (Sandhoff-Jatzkowitz Disease).
     Amer. J. Human Genet. 27:639, 1975.

16. Kjellman,B., Gamstorp, I., Brun, A., Ockerman, P.A. and
     Palmgren, B.: Mannosidosis: A clinical and histopathologic
     study. J. Pediat. 75:366, 1969.

17. Leroy, J.G., Ho, M.W., MacBrinn, M.C., Zielke, K., Jacob, J.
     and O'Brien, J.S.: I-cell disease: Biochemical studies.
     Pediat. Res. 6:752, 1972.

18. Lowry, O.H., Rosebrough, N.J., Farr, A.L. and Randall, R.J.:
     Protein measurement with the Folin phenol reagent. J. Biol.
     Chem. 193:265, 1951.

19. Masson, P.K. and Lundblad, A.: Mannosidosis: Detection of
     the disease and of heterozygotes using serum and leucocytes.
     Biochem. Biophys. Res. Comm. 56:296, 1974.

20. Norden, N., Lundblad, A., Svensson, S., Ockerman, P.A. and
     Autio, S.: A mannose-containing trisaccharide isolated from
     urines of three patients with mannosidosis. J. Biol. Chem.
     17:6210, 1973.

21. Norden, N.E., Ockerman, P.A. and Szabo, L.: Urinary mannose
     in mannosidosis. J. Pediat. 82:686, 1973.

22. Ockerman, P.A.: A generalized storage disorder resembling
     Hurler's syndrome. Lancet ii:239, 1967.

23. Ockerman, P.A.: Mannosidosis: Isolation of oligosaccharide storage material from brain. J. Pediat. 75:360, 1969.

24. Phillips, N.C., Robinson, D. and Winchester, B.G.: Mannosidosis in Angus cattle. The enzymic defect. Biochem. J. 137: 363, 1974.

25. Phillips, N.C., Robinson, D. and Winchester, B.G.: Human liver α-mannosidase activity. Clin. Chim. Acta 55:11, 1974.

26. Poenaru, L. and Dreyfus, J.C.: Electrophoretic heterogeneity of human α-mannosidase. Biochim. Biophys. Acta 303:171, 1973.

27. Robinson, D., Phillips, N.C. and Winchester, B.: Affinity chromatography of human liver α-D-mannosidase. FEBS Lett. 53:110, 1975.

28. Sharp, H.L. and Desnick, R.J.: Sandhoff's disease: Diagnosis and evaluation by percutaneous liver biopsy. Gastroenterology 60:752, 1971.

29. Snaith, S.M.: Characterization of jack-bean α-D-mannosidase as a zinc metalloenzyme. Biochem. J. 147:83, 1975.

30. Snaith, S.M., Hay, A.J. and Levvy, G.A.: Relation between the α-mannosidase activity and the zinc content of mammalian sex organs. J. Endocrinol. 50:659, 1971.

31. Taylor, H.D., Thomas, G.H., Aylsworth, A., Stevenson, R.E. and Reynolds, C.W.: Mannosidosis: Deficiency of a specific α-mannosidase component in cultured fibroblasts. Clin. Chim. Acta 59:93, 1975.

32. Tsay, G.C., Dawson, G. and Matalon, R.: Excretion of mannose-rich complex carbohydrates by a patient with α-mannosidase deficiency (mannosidosis). J. Pediat. 84:865, 1974.

33. Tsay, G., Dawson, G. and Matalon, R.: Glycopeptide storage in skin fibroblasts cultured from a patient with α-mannosidase deficiency. J. Clin. Invest. 56:711, 1975.

34. Woolen, J.W. and Walker, P.G.: The fluorimetric estimation of β-glucuronidase in blood plasma. Clin. Chim. Acta 12:659, 1965.

MANNOSIDOSIS

Storage Material, α-Mannosidase Specificity and Diagnostic Methods

Arne Lundblad, Parvesh Masson, Nils E. Nordén,
Sigfrid Svensson and Per-Arne Öckerman

Department of Clinical Chemistry, University Hospital
S-221 85 Lund, Sweden

The first case of mannosidosis was reported by Öckerman in
1967 (1). Since then several new patients have been found. Their
symptoms resemble to some extent those of Hurler´s syndrome (2).
Psychomotor retardation, slightly gargoyle-like facies, recurrent
infections, and vacuolized lymphocytes are some of the more prominent findings.

The activity of tissue α-mannosidase is substantially decreased
leading to the accumulation and urinary excretion of mannose-rich
oligosaccharides (3). An analogous disease has also been detected
in Angus cattle (4,5). Here, as in human mannosidosis, the lack of
α-mannosidase also results in tissue accumulation and urinary
excretion of mannose-rich oligosaccharides.

STORAGE MATERIAL

Studies performed on the mannose-rich material from human
mannosidosis brain tissue (3), bovine mannosidosis lymph nodes
(5) and brain tissue (6) all suggest that this material is mainly
composed of oligosaccharides containing $\underline{D}$-mannose and N-acetyl-
$\underline{D}$-glucosamine in different proportions. Due to shortage of material
no detailed structural analyses were carried out on these oligosaccharides.

Human and bovine mannosidosis urine contains increased
amounts of low molecular weight mannose-rich oligosaccharides
(7-9). These compounds can be fractionated by gel chromatography
(Sephadex G-25). A typical gel chromatogram of a urinary ultra-

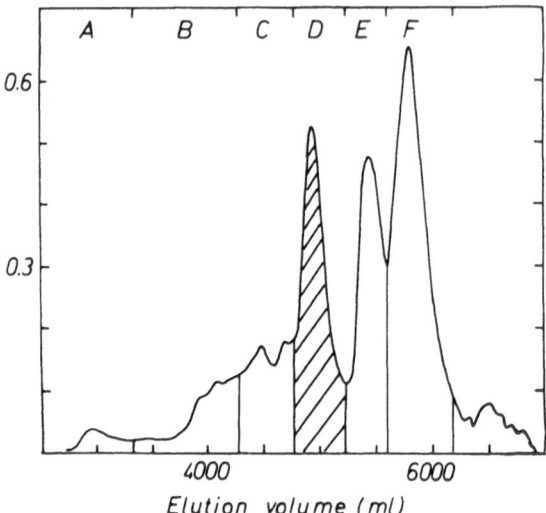

Fig. 1.   Gel chromatography on a column of Sephadex G-25, fine, (101 x 10 cm, void volume = 2950 ml) of a urinary ultrafiltrate from a patient with mannosidosis. Fractions (25 ml) were collected and assayed for hexose. (From ref. 7).

filtrate from a patient with mannosidosis is seen in Fig. 1. The material was pooled and concentrated as indicated. The material in fractions C and D was further purified by zone electrophoresis and paper chromatography yielding three pure oligosaccharides M_2G, M_3G, and M_4G (Table I). Their structures were established by sugar analysis, methylation analysis, and enzymatic degradation. M_2G was the most abundant compound.

Bovine mannosidosis urine proved to have different types of mannose-rich oligosaccharides as compared to human mannosidosis urine (9). The most abundant oligosaccharide, isolated by similar methods, was found to be a pentasaccharide (M_2G_3) (Table I).

The origin of these oligosaccharides is not known. Their structures do indicate, however, that they derive from the internal parts of different asparagine linked glycoprotein carbohydrate groups.

None of the human oligosaccharides was observed in the urine of calves with mannosidosis. This may indicate species differences in glycoprotein structure. The origin of the bovine mannosidosis pentasaccharide M_2G_3 is difficult to envisage since the unexpected chitotriose structure has so far not been demonstrated in any glycoprotein.

Table I. Structures of three oligosaccharides from human mannosidosis urine (M_2G, M_3G and M_4G) and one oligosaccharide from
bovine mannosidosis urine ($M_2G_3^4$)

Abb.	Compound
M_2G	a-$\underline{D}$-Manp-(1→3)-β-$\underline{D}$-Manp-(1→4)-$\underline{D}$-GlcNAc
M_3G	a-$\underline{D}$-Manp-(1→2)-a-$\underline{D}$-Manp-(1→3)-β-$\underline{D}$-Manp-(1→4)- -$\underline{D}$-GlcNAc
M_4G	a-$\underline{D}$-Manp-(1→2)-a-$\underline{D}$-Manp-(1→2)-a-$\underline{D}$-Manp-(1→3)- -β-$\underline{D}$-Manp-(1→4)-$\underline{D}$-GlcNAc
M_2G_3	a-$\underline{D}$-Manp-(1→6)-β-$\underline{D}$-Manp-(1→4)-β-$\underline{D}$-GlcNAcp- -(1→4)-β-$\underline{D}$-GlcNAcp-(1→4)-$\underline{D}$-GlcNAc

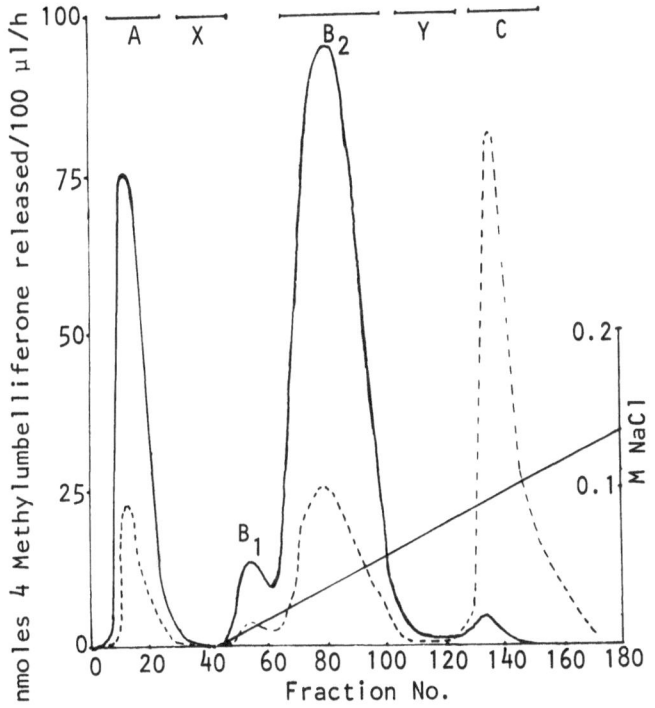

Fig. 2. Separation of a-mannosidase components on DEAE-cellulose
chromatography. ———, Activity of a-mannosidase at pH 4.0;
-----, activity of a-mannosidase at pH 6.0. The NaCl gradient is
indicated by the straight line. (From ref. 12).

A common feature to all the oligosaccharides isolated was a terminal non-reducing α-linked mannose residue giving further proof for the nature of the enzymatic defect.

α-MANNOSIDASE

Different Forms of α-Mannosidase

α-Mannosidase is present in several human tissues. Carroll et al. (10) resolved the activity of α-mannosidase from normal human liver into three components, A, B, and C, by chromatography on DEAE-cellulose. Forms A and B had acidic pH-optima and form C a neutral pH-optimum. Forms A and B were found to be absent in liver samples from patients with mannosidosis, whereas form C was unaffected. Similar results have also been observed in bovine mannosidosis (11).

A study of several different organs using DEAE-cellulose chromatography as before but with lower salt gradient resulted in a separation of the B-form of the liver enzyme into two forms (B_1 and B_2) (Fig. 2).

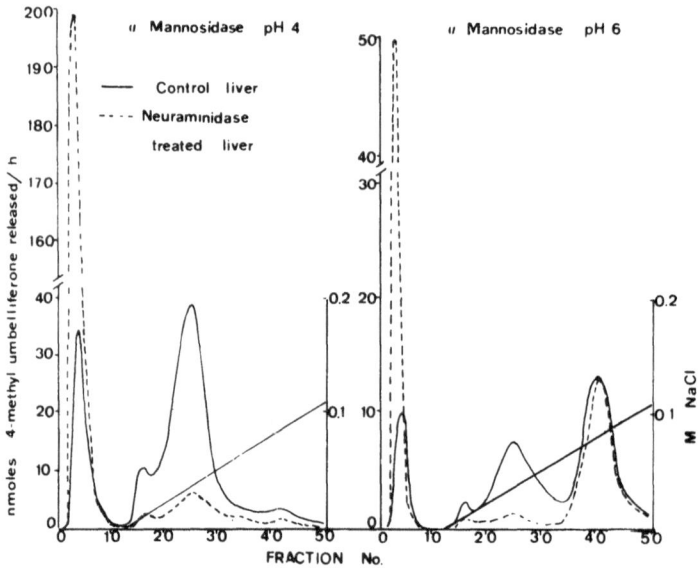

Fig. 3. DEAE-cellulose chromatography of liver supernatant before and after neuraminidase treatment. ——, NaCl gradient. (From ref. 12).

A more detailed investigation on the interrelationship of the different forms of a-mannosidase was performed (12). Treatment of tissue supernatant with neuraminidase followed by DEAE-cellulose chromatography indicated that the B-form lost sialic acid and was converted to an A-type of enzyme. Component C was unaffected by this treatment (Fig. 3). The individual forms (A, B_2) were isolated from liver by DEAE-cellulose chromatography, and treated separately with neuraminidase. Form A after re-chromatography on CM-cellulose appeared as a single less sialylated form, with no apparent loss of enzymic activity. CM-cellulose chromatography of neuraminidase-treated form B_2 indicated that the product was the less sialylated form of A. These results indicate that forms A and B are structurally interrelated, differing mainly in sialic acid content.

The close relationship between the A and B forms may explain that both are greatly reduced in mannosidosis, whereas form C which probably has a different origin is unaffected in the disease.

Specificity Studies on Different Forms

The specificities of a-mannosidases A, B_2, and C from human liver were tested towards the mannose-containing oligosaccharides M_2G, M_3G, M_4G, and M_2G_3. For the purpose of quantitation the products obtained after enzymic degradation of the substrates were reduced to their corresponding alditols with $[^3H]NaBH_4$, and separated by paper chromatography. The radioactivity in the separated alditols was measured (Table II) (13).

Forms A and B_2 had a pH-optimum of 4.5, and both hydrolysed all the natural substrates, irrespective of the fact that the terminal non-reducing mannose residue was linked by an $a(1\rightarrow3)$ linkage as in M_2G, an $a(1\rightarrow2)$ linkage as in M_3G and M_4G, and an $a(1\rightarrow6)$ linkage as in M_2G_3. However, a-mannosidase A was less active on the oligosaccharides than B_2, even though the K_m for each enzyme was similar with M_2G or M_4G. Similar results were obtained for the enzymes A and B_2 from bovine liver. In each case, the enzyme forms were most effective on the smallest of the oligosaccharides. Species differences between the human and the bovine enzymes may exist, since the enzymes from human liver were found to be more active towards substrates isolated from human than calf urine. None of the forms, either from human or bovine liver, hydrolysed the innermost mannosidic linkage, which is a β-linkage in all the substrates. This demonstrated that the "acidic" forms were non-specific towards positional isomers but were most likely specific for the a-linkage.

Human liver a-mannosidase C, which had a pH-optimum of 6.0 with the synthetic substrate, was inactive at this pH against the

Table II.   Specificity studies on human and bovine acidic α-mannosidases

Substrate	Human acidic α-mannosidases					Bovine acidic α-mannosidases				
	A % hydrolysis	B_2	K_m a) mM	$\dfrac{V_{max} B_2}{V_{max} A}$	$\dfrac{M\text{-ol}}{MG\text{-ol}}$ b)	A % hydrolysis	B_2	K_m a) mM	$\dfrac{V_{max} B_2}{V_{max} A}$	$\dfrac{M\text{-ol}}{MG\text{-ol}}$ b)
M_2G	55	95	5.5	1.7	1.0	37	64	5.2	1.7	1.0
M_3G	35	90	-	-	2.0	28	53	-	-	2.0
M_4G	27	90	5.5	3.4	3.0	20	37	4.9	1.7	3.0
M_2G_3	10	35	-	-	1.0 c)	-	-	-	-	-
4-MU-α-$\underline{\underline{D}}$-Man$\underline{p}$ d)	-	-	2.5	2.2	-	-	-	2.8	1.7	-

a)   The K_m values given are apparent K_m values calculated by the method of Lineweaver and Burk.

b)   M-ol = α-$\underline{D}$-mannitol;   MG-ol = β-$\underline{D}$-Man$\underline{p}$-(1→4)-N-acetyl-$\underline{D}$-glucosaminitol.

c)   The ratio expressed is that of M-ol to MG_3-ol (β-$\underline{D}$-Man$\underline{p}$-(1→4)-β-$\underline{D}$-GlcNAc$\underline{p}$-(1→4)-β-$\underline{D}$-GlcNAc$\underline{p}$-(1→4)-N-acetyl-$\underline{D}$-glucosaminitol.

d)   4-MU-α-$\underline{\underline{D}}$-Man$\underline{p}$ = 4-methylumbelliferyl-α-$\underline{\underline{D}}$-mannopyranoside.

natural substrates M_2G, M_3G, M_4G, and M_2G_3, but active at pH 4.5. Since neuraminidase had no effect on this enzymic form, but affected the adsorbed "acidic" activity (12), this property was utilised in order to separate the "residual neutral" activity from any contaminating "acidic" activity which may have co-eluted with it, and which may be responsible for the observed hydrolysis of the substrates. The resultant "residual neutral" activity obtained in this way was still capable of hydrolysing M_2G at pH 4.5 (13).

The results obtained with the studies using natural substrates added further support to the concept that the "acidic" forms of α-mannosidase were interrelated, and had a common genetic origin.

Effect of Metal Ions

Normal acidic α-mannosidase activity was activated slightly by Zn^{2+} and inhibited by Co^{2+}. Between 1 and 8 % of the normal acid activity was found in mannosidosis tissues. This residual acidic activity could be activated significantly by Zn^{2+} and Co^{2+} (Table III) (14) giving final activities which corresponded to between 15 and 40% of the activities found in normal tissues. The effect of Co^{2+} was interesting since this metal ion inhibited the acidic activity from normal tissues but was a better activator than Zn^{2+} on the residual acid α-mannosidase in mannosidosis tissues. The activated residual enzyme was also capable of hydrolysing more of the natural substrate M_2G. The results indicate that the residual "defective" enzyme has an altered capacity to bind metal ions. The demonstration that the enzyme can be activated in mannosidosis tissues may have an important bearing on the therapy of the disease.

Table III.   Effect of metal ions on the acidic activities of α-mannosidase in liver

Metal ion	mM	Normal	Mannosidosis
–	0	452	7.1
Zn^{2+}	2.5	493	50
Co^{2+}	2.5	390	66.3

The results are expressed as nmoles 4-methylumbelliferone released/g wet weight/min.

DIAGNOSIS OF MANNOSIDOSIS AND OF HETEROZYGOTES

One characteristic feature of mannosidosis is the accumulation and urinary excretion of mannose-rich oligosaccharides. The most abundant metabolite in human urine is M_2G (Table I). A diagnostic method employing gas liquid chromatography (GLC) and mass spectrometry (MS) was therefore developed for the direct quantitative determination of this compound in urine (15). Initially the trisaccharide was partially purified by gel chromatography (Fig. 1). The material in region D was pooled, an internal standard of maltotriose was added and the oligosaccharide mixture reduced, methylated, fractionated by GLC and quantitated. A typical gas chromatogram obtained from the Varian MAT 311A GLC-MS-computer system is seen in Fig. 4. The identification of M_2G is based on identical

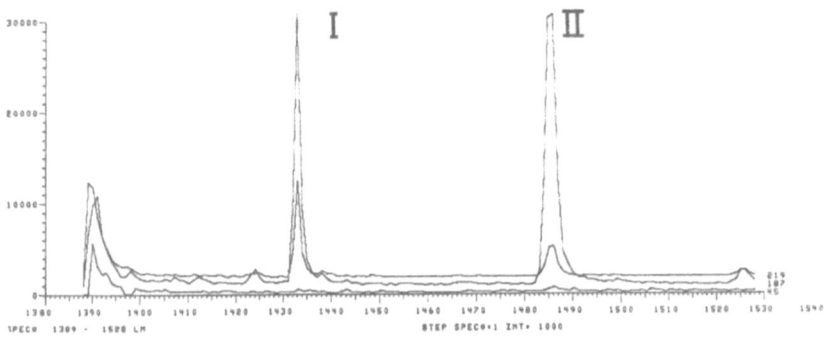

Fig. 4.   GLC-MS-computer analysis of M_2G, as its permethylated alditol derivative from a patient with mannosidosis. Peak I represents the internal standard (maltotriose) and peak II M_2G. The tracings represent some typical m/e values.

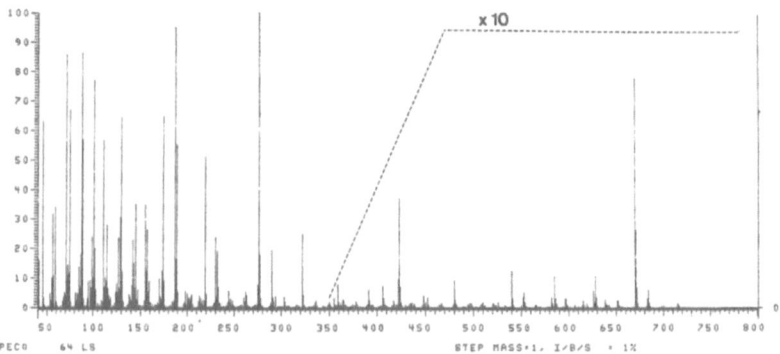

Fig. 5.   Mass spectrum of permethylated alditol derivative of the trisaccharide M_2G. (From ref. 15).

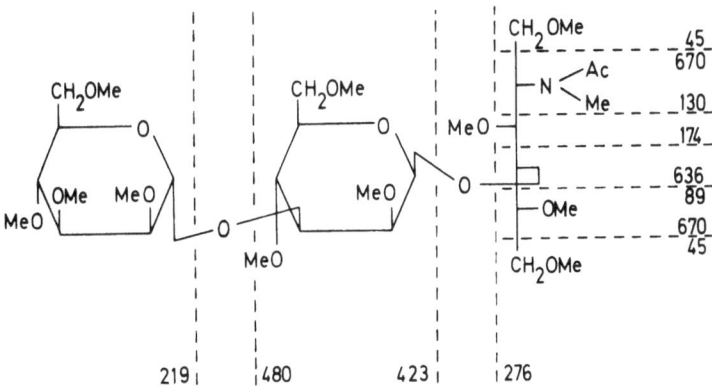

Fig. 6. The most characteristic primary fragmentations of the per-methylated alditol derivative of M_2G. (From ref. 15).

retention time and mass spectrum as compared to those of an authentic sample of the trisaccharide. The mass spectrum and main fragmentation routes of the permethylated alditol derivative of M_2G are seen in Figs. 5 and 6, respectively.

Four patients with mannosidosis were found to excrete between 123 and 469 mg of M_2G/l of urine (Table IV). It is interesting that the clinical symptoms of those patients who excreted less M_2G (cases 2 and 3) were milder than those for patients excreting more M_2G, suggesting that variants of mannosidosis may exist. The oligosaccharide was not detected in the urine of twenty normal individuals and two heterozygotes.

Table IV. Quantitative determinations of compound M_2G in urines

	M_2G	
	mg/l urine	mg/g creatinine
Case 2	234	264
Case 3	123	351
Case 4	469	832
Case 5	272	709
Heterozygote K.P.	n.d. [a]	n.d.
Heterozygote L.P.	n.d.	n.d.
Controls (n = 20)	n.d.	n.d.

[a] Not detectable.

For the purpose of heterozygote detection an enzymic method was developed using serum and leucocytes as the sources of the enzyme (Table V) (16). The activity of α-mannosidase at pH 4.4 was greatly diminished in both serum and leucocytes from patients with the disease. Although intermediate levels of α-mannosidase at pH 4.4 were found in heterozygotes, there was no clear-cut differentiation between this group and the normals. This difficulty was overcome when the activity of acidic α-mannosidase was related to another lysosomal enzyme, N-acetyl-β-glucosaminidase. This enzyme was chosen as the reference enzyme because its stability was similar to that of acidic α-mannosidase, and also because its total activity in leucocytes was unaffected in several pathological conditions even if it was altered in serum (17). The enzymatic method is the most rapid method for diagnosis and has the advantage that heterozygotes can be detected. α-Mannosidase is also present in amniotic fluid and cells which probably will enable prenatal diagnosis of mannosidosis.

Table V.   Ranges of α-mannosidase and hexosaminidase activities in serum and leucocytes

| | Serum | | Leucocytes | |
	Man 4.4[1]	$\dfrac{\text{Hex } 4.4^{[2]}}{\text{Man } 4.4}$	Man 4.4	$\dfrac{\text{Hex } 4.4}{\text{Man } 4.4}$
Controls				
Females (n=9)	4.9–7.7	10.7–18.3	28–142	5.7–9.4
Males (n=10)	4.5–8.0	10.0–19.2	30–92	5.8–9.2
Heterozygotes				
Female (S.S.)	6.8	33.6	33	14.8
Male (T.S.)	1.8	36.5	34	14.2
Female (R.K.)	2.0	26.0	28	15.3
Male (J.K.)	1.9	48.5	28	15.2
Female (P.N.)	6.0	24.4	–	–
Male (O.N.)	2.1	37.4	–	–
Mannosidosis				
Males (n=6)	0.3–0.5	185–620	3.3–8.0	67.0–75.2

(1) Man 4.4 = α-D-mannosidase activity at pH 4.4 (nmoles 4-methyl-umbelliferone released/ml/min).

(2) Hex 4.4 = Total N-acetyl-β-D-glucosaminidase activity at pH 4.4.

The GLC-MS method for direct determination of the main accumulated metabolite is a more tedious procedure and it also requires expensive and sophisticated instrumentation. The method can therefore not be adopted in any routine screening program but is a valuable tool for confirmation of the diagnosis of mannosidosis, since there is a potential risk for diagnostic errors when only enzymatic methods with artificial substrates are used (18).

REFERENCES

1. P.A. Öckerman (1967) Lancet 2, 239-241.
2. S. Autio, N.E. Nordén, P.A. Öckerman, P. Riekkinen, J. Rapola and T. Louhimo (1973) Acta Paediat. Scand. 62, 555-565.
3. P.A. Öckerman (1969) J. Pediat. 75, 360-365.
4. J.H. Whittem and D. Walker (1957) J. Pathol. Bacteriol. 74, 281-288.
5. J.D. Hocking, R.D. Jolly and R.D. Batt (1972) Biochem. J. 128, 69-78.
6. N.E. Nordén, A. Lundblad, S. Svensson, P.A. Öckerman and R.D. Jolly (1973) FEBS Letters 35, 209-212.
7. N.E. Nordén, A. Lundblad, S. Svensson, P.A. Öckerman and S. Autio (1973) J. Biol. Chem. 248, 6210-6215.
8. N.E. Nordén, A. Lundblad, S. Svensson and S. Autio (1974) Biochemistry 13, 871-874.
9. A. Lundblad, B. Nilsson, N.E. Nordén, S. Svensson, P.A. Öckerman and R.D. Jolly (1975) Europ. J. Biochem. In press.
10. N. Carroll, N. Dance, P.K. Masson, D. Robinson and B.G. Winchester (1972) Biochem. Biophys. Res. Commun. 49, 579-583.
11. N.C. Phillips, D. Robinson, B.G. Winchester and R.D. Jolly (1974) Biochem. J. 137, 363-371.
12. M.A. Chester, A. Lundblad and P.K. Masson (1975) Biochim. Biophys. Acta 391, 341-348.
13. B. Hultberg, A. Lundblad, P.K. Masson and P.A. Öckerman (1975) Biochim. Biophys. Acta. In press.
14. B. Hultberg and P.K. Masson (1975) In preparation.
15. A. Lundblad, P.K. Masson, N.E. Nordén, S. Svensson and P.A. Öckerman (1975) Biomedical Mass Spectrometry. In press.
16. P.K. Masson, A. Lundblad and S. Autio (1974) Biochem. Biophys. Res. Commun. 56, 296-303.
17. W.R. Den Tandt (1972) Clin. Chim. Acta 40, 199-204.
18. J.-C. Dreyfus, L. Poenaru and L. Svennerholm (1975) New Engl. J. Med. 292, 61-63.

HEXOSAMINIDASES: MULTIPLE COMPONENT ENZYMES

J.A.Lowden, J.W.Callahan, and F.N.Howard

Research Institute, The Hospital for Sick Children

Toronto, Ontario, Canada

In 1968 Robinson and Stirling (1) demonstrated that lysosomal N-acetylhexosaminidase could be separated into two species by starch gel electrophoresis. They noted that the more anodic form, A, was heat-labile and that it could be converted to the less anodic form, B, by the action of neuraminidase. In the intervening years, several groups have used various methods of purification of these two species and have compared the similarities and differences between them (2, 3,4). The two enzymes appear remarkably similar in amino acid composition, molecular weight, kinetic properties and, when highly purified have reported similar hydrolytic properties (4,5).

Because of the recognized association of hexosaminidase A defects and GM2 ganglioside storage (6,7,8) and because crude extracts of tissue can catabolize GM2 ganglioside more effectively than the isolated hexosaminidase A, attempts were made to find a loosely associated component or co-factor which may be lost during isolation. Li et al (9) found a heat-stable, small molecular weight (20,000 daltons) glycoprotein which stimulated the hydrolysis of several glycosphingloipids by partly purified lysosomal hydrolases. More recently, Hechtman and LeBlanc (10) have demonstrated a larger (49,000 daltons) protein, which is heat-labile and appears specific for hexosaminidase A and GM2 hydrolysis. They found this component of the system by noting that the GM2ase activity decreased when crude tissue extracts were chromatographed on DEAE Sephadex. By adding back aliquots of other fractions to the hexosaminidase A fraction they located the 'effector' in the material which did not bind to the ion exchanger. It could be readily separated from the hexosaminidase B activity on Sephadex G200. It did not confer GM2ase activity on hexosaminidase B. This work suggests that purified hexosaminidase A and B are not similar proteins but do differ in some significant fashion.

Immunochemical data indicate that the two enzymes have a common antigenic determinant but, in addition, hexosaminidase A also has a specific determinant (11). This difference could mean that A contains two peptide chains (α and β) or that the same primary sequence in the A enzyme has a different conformation in the B form. In the latter, one antigenic marker is occluded or unavailable. Hybridization studies indicate, however, that there are clearly two proteins in hexosaminidase A, one (β chain) encoded on chromosome 5 and the other (α chain) on chromosome 15 (12,13). Hexosaminidase B is encoded only on chromosome 5. Genetic complementation studies with Tay-Sachs and Sandhoff cell strains support this view (14).

Nevertheless for many years it was accepted dogma that hexosaminidase A could be converted to hexosaminidase B by the action of neuraminidase (1,15). Recent reports (16,17) have noted that the 'neuraminidase effect' described by Robinson and Stirling (1) was nonenzymatic and was caused by merthiolate in the neuraminidase preparations. Tallman et al (4) had claimed the two species of hexosaminidase were merely different conformations of the same protein. This type of conformational change could result from the action of merthiolate, perhaps, on disulfide bonds. We have therefore examined two questions. Are the two hexosaminidases identical in primary structure, and why does purified hexosaminidase A not catabolize GM_2 ganglioside more effectively than hexosaminidase B?

TABLE I

ISOLATION OF HEXOSAMINIDASE A FROM PLACENTA

	Units X 10^{-6}	Units /mg protein	Purification
Homogenate	75.5	958	–
NH_4SO_4 (30–65%)	49.1	8,913	9.3
Sephadex G_{200}	27.8	25,226	26.3
DEAE cellulose			
– A peak	7.9	70,057	73.9
– B peak	15.8	63,996	66.6
2nd DEAE cellulose	5.0	166,800	174
Sephadex G_{200}	2.3	615,900	642
Isoelectric focussing	0.717		
Sephadex G_{200}	0.497	1,656,800	1730

   The enzymes were isolated from human placenta by gel filtration
and ion exchange chromatography (Table I).The resultant hexosaminidase A was purified 1700-fold. It ran as a single peak on
Sephadex G200, DEAE cellulose and polyacrylamide gel electrophoresis.
The enzyme activity and protein peaks were coincident in each system.
Purified hexosaminidase A was then placed in a 0.1% solution of
merthiolate at 4°C for 16 hours. The enzyme solution was dialysed
to remove free merthiolate and spotted on a cellulose acetate strip
for electrophoresis (Fig.1). The hexosaminidase activity was now
distributed between 3 bands. One of these corresponded to the
original hexosaminidase A, a second to purified hexosaminidase B, and
the third migrated more anodically than hexosaminidase A. Mercapto-
ethanol and 8M urea did not disrupt the enzyme. The merthiolate-
treated enzyme solution was also applied to a DEAE cellulose column
prepared in citrate-phosphate buffer (0.04M, pH 6.0). After washing
with the starting buffer, the column was eluted with a NaCl gradient
(Fig.2). The three bands of hexosaminidase activity were clearly
separated by ion exchange chromatography. Comparison of the enzyme
activity and protein elution profiles show that the material which
did not bind to the cellulose ('new hex B') had remarkably high
specific activity. Furthermore, the protein elution peaks are no

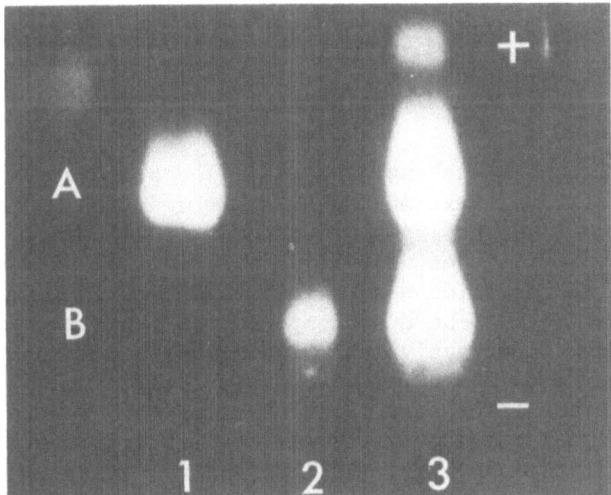

Fig.1 Cellulose acetate electrophoresis of hexosaminidases in
(citrate-phosphate buffer, 0.2M, pH 7.0 for 20 min at 6mA) enzymes
located by incubating strip between filter papers soaked in citrate
phosphate buffer (0.1M, pH 4.1) containing 1mM 4MU-GlcNAc. Band 1
hexosaminidase A. Band 2 hexosaminidase B. Band 3 mercapto-
ethanol-treated hexosaminidase A.

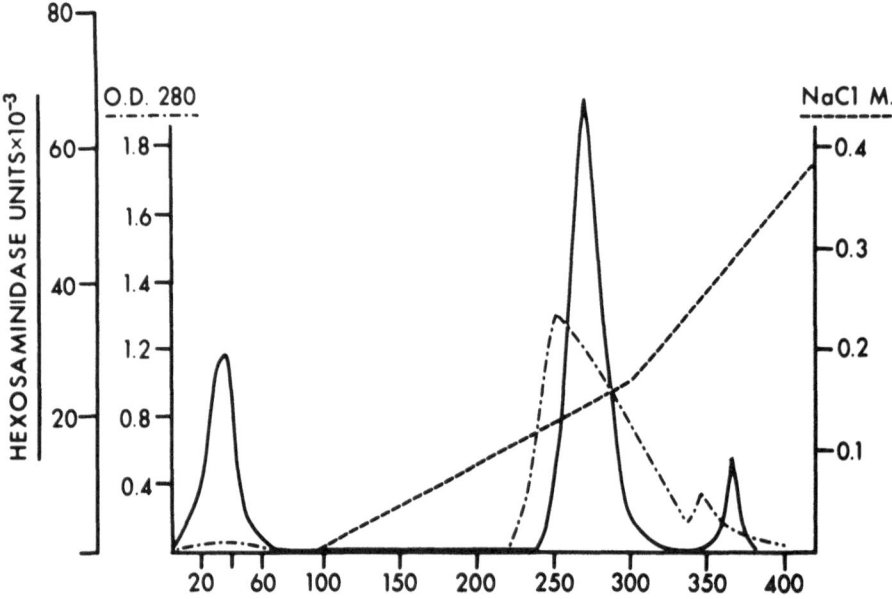

Fig.2   Elution chromatogram from DEAE cellulose column of residual protein and hexosaminidase activity of merthiolate-treated hexosaminidase A.   Column dimension (50 x 250 mm).

longer coincident with the enzyme peaks. The protein peak in the region of the residual hexosaminidase A preceeds the enzyme peak by several fractions, suggesting some conformational change. A clearly defined protein peak, independant of any enzyme activity is also seen after the hexosaminidase A activity has been eluted. We believe this material to be a subcomponent of hexosaminidase A which does not have enzymatic activity but which does confer some substrate specificity on the enzyme. Shortly after we made these observations in our laboratory, Beutler et al (16) published similar findings on polyacrylamide gel chromatography of merthiolate-treated hexosaminidase A. They believe the noncatalytic protein corresponds to their previously proposed α chain and the enzymatically-active protein to β chain.

We have compared some properties of the enzyme which did not bind to the DEAE cellulose with our purified hexosaminidase B and find them identical (Table II). We thus believe that hexosaminidase

A is composed of two subcomponents, one contains the active site
of the enzyme, and is identical to hexosaminidase B. In addition,
purified hexosaminidase A contains at least one other noncatalytic
component.

We then examined the interaction of the hexosaminidases with
4-methylumbelliferyl-β-D-N-acetylglucosaminide (4MU-GlcNAc) in the
presence of GM₂ ganglioside and some other hexosaminide-containing
materials. Our isolated hexosaminidases, like those of most others
(3,4,5) have little or no GM₂ase activity. GM₂ ganglioside,
however, inhibits the hydrolysis of 4MU-GlcNAc (Fig.3). The
inhibition is noncompetitive. On a Dixon plot one can see the Ki
for GM₂ with hexosaminidase A is twice that for hexosaminidase B.
Hydrolysis of 4MU-GlcNAc was not affected by glucose, glucosamine
or N-acetylglucosamine. Dermatan sulfate and mixed chondroitin
sulfates did inhibit the enzyme activity, however, in a competitive
fashion.

TABLE II

COMPARISON OF NATURAL HEXOSAMINIDASE B WITH ENZYME PREPARED

FROM HEXOSAMINIDASE A

	Natural Hex B	New Hex B
pH optimum	3.9	3.9
Km	0.59 mM	0.55 mM
MW (G_{200} filtration)	114,000	115,000
Heat stability (residual activity after heating)		
48° - 4 hr	94%	90%
60° - 5 min	62%	53%

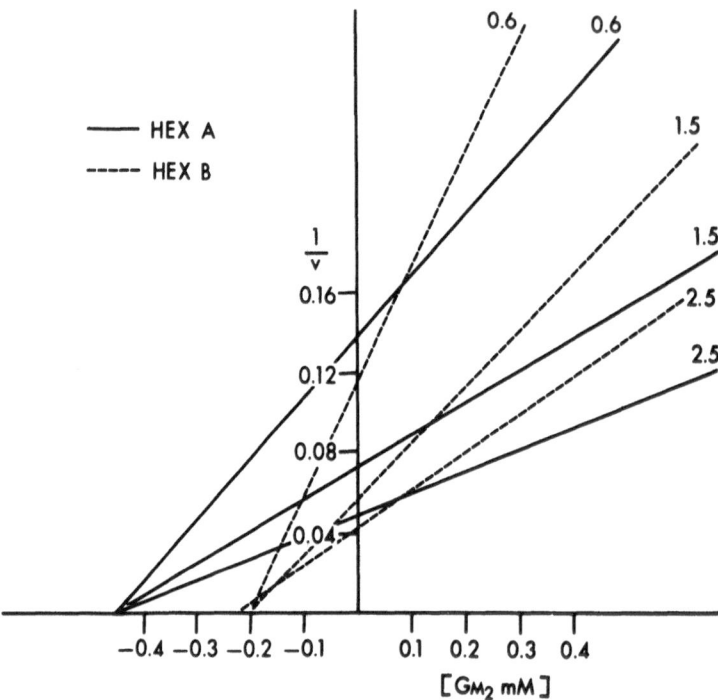

Fig. 3   Dixon plot to demonstrate inhibition of hexosaminidase activity by GM2 ganglioside.   Enzyme activity was measured as hydrolysis of 4MU-GlcNAc at pH 4.1 in 0.04M citrate-phosphate buffer (7).

These data suggest that the enzyme has not only an active centre on the hexosaminidase B component but another site which recognizes some other part of the ganglioside molecule. Furthermore, the noncatalytic component of hexosaminidase A probably also has another recognition site for GM2 ganglioside. Thus, hexosaminidase A has a greater affinity for GM2 than hexosaminidase B, but neither has the necessary component for GM2 hydrolysis. The theory is depicted in Figure 4 with GM2 ganglioside or GA2 glycolipid interacting with the enzyme. The N-acetylgalactosamine residue is inserted in the catalytic centre. Broken lines indicate other sites of interaction of substrate and enzyme or of the enzyme components. Present evidence suggests the natural enzymes are multiples of these components. Hexosaminidase A, for example, is probably $(\alpha\beta)_3$. Three forms of the enzyme are shown:

1. The complete enzyme consists of 3 components: the catalytic β chain, the noncatalytic α chain which provides a recognition site for GM2 ganglioside and for the third component,

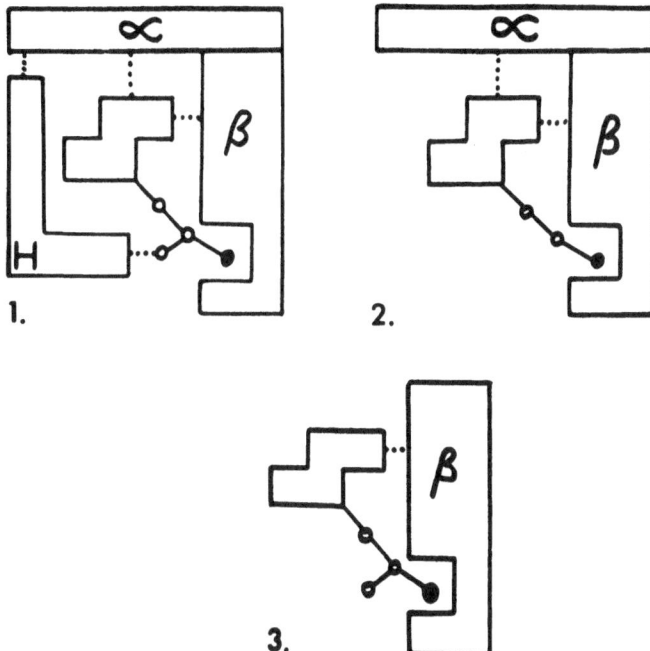

Fig. 4   Schematic representation of 3 forms of hexosaminidase.
         1. GM_2 gangliosidase   2. Hexosaminidase A
         3.   Hexosaminidase B (see Text for details).

Table III

GENETIC VARIANTS OF GM_2 GANGLIOSIDOSIS

		(References)
B Variant	Tay-Sachs	–
	Lebanese form	19
	Juvenile form	20
O Variant	Sandhoff's	–
	Nova Scotian form	21
	Juvenile form	22
AB Variant	Juvenile	23
	Infantile	24
	Juvenile – low A	25

the Hechtman effector (H). The effector recognizes both GM_2 ganglioside (perhaps through the sialic acid) and the α-chain.

2. During isolation, the loosely-associated Hechtman effector is separated from the enzyme. The two component enzyme is the functional unit usually named hexosaminidase A. It interacts with GM_2 or with GA_2 (as shown) but hydrolyses ganglioside at rates not differing from hexosaminidase B.

3. After treatment with merthiolate, the α-chain is lost. This enzyme is hexosaminidase B. It also can interact with GM_2 or GA_2 and slowly hydrolyses the N-acetylhexosaminyl bond.

Four years ago Konrad Sandhoff (18) proposed a nomenclature for the three recognized types of GM_2 gangliosidosis. Today, we can list nine phenotypic variants of this disorder (Table III). Sandhoff's nomenclature still holds but now each variant has several subspecies. If hexosaminidase A is a 3 component system, then the 3 variants described by Sandhoff can each result from a mutation in a different component. The B variants are due to α-chain mutations; the O variants to β-chain mutations, and the AB variants to defects in the Hechtman factor. Differences in subtypes are due to different point mutations on the specific protein.

Acknowledgement

This work was supported by grant MT 1602 from the Medical Research Council of Canada. J.W.C. is a Medical Research Council Scholar. We thank Dr. L.S.Wolfe, Montreal, Canada, for the generous gift of ^{3}H-GM_2 ganglioside.

REFERENCES

1. Robinson, D., and Stirling, J.L.   Biochem. J. 107: 321 (1968).

2. Verpoorte, J.A.   J.Biol.Chem. 247: 4787 (1972).

3. Srivastava, S.K., Awasthi, Y.G., Yoshida, A., and Beutler, E.
   J.Biol.Chem. 249: 2043 (1974).

4. Tallman, J.F., Brady, R.O., Quirk, J.M., Villalba, M., and Gal,
   A.E.   J.Biol.Chem. 249: 3489 (1974).

5. Bach, G., and Suzuki, K.   J.Biol.Chem. 250: 1328 (1975).

6. Kolodny, E.H., Brady, R.O., and Volk, B.W.   Biochem.Biophys.
   Res.Comm. 37: 526 (1969).

7. Okada, S., and O'Brien, J.S.   Science 165: 698 (1969).

8. Sandhoff, K.   FEBS Letters 4: 351 (1969).

9. Li, Y.T., Mazzota, M.Y., Wan, C.C., Orth, R., and Li, S.C.
   J.Biol.Chem. 248: 7512 (1973).

10. Hechtman, P., and LeBlanc, D.   Am.J.Hum.Genet. 27: 42A (1975).

11. Beutler, E., and Srivastava, S.K.   Isr.J.Med.Sci. 9: 1335 (1973).

12. Lalley, P.A., Ratazzi, M.C., and Shows, T.B.   Proc.Nat.Acad.
    Sci. 71: 1569 (1974).

13. Gilbert, F., Kucherlapati, R., Creagan, R.P., Murnane, M.J.,
    Darlington, G.J., and Ruddle, F.H.   Proc.Nat.Acad.Sci. 72: 263
    (1975).

14. Rattazzi, M.C., Brown, J.A., Davidson, R.C., and Shows, T.B.
    Am.J.Hum.Genet. 26: 71A (1974).

15. Swallow, D.M., Stokes, D.C., Corney, G., and Harris, H.   Ann.
    Hum.Genet. 37: 287 (1974).

16. Beutler, E., Villacorte, D., Kuhl, W., Guinto, E., and Srivastava,
    S.   J.Lab.Clin.Med. 86: 195 (1975).

17. Carmody, P.J., and Rattazzi, M.C.   Am.J.Hum.Genet. 25: 19A (1973).

18. Sandhoff, K., and Jatzkewitz, H.   *in* Sphingolipids,Sphingolipidose
    and Allied Disorders, B.W.Volk and S.M.Aronson, Eds. Plenum Press
    New York, 1972 p305.

19. Andermann, F., Andermann, E., Carpenter, S., Karpati, G. and Wolfe, L.S. Am.J.Hum.Genet. 26: 10A (1974).

20. Phillapart, M. Personal communication.

21. Spence, M.W. Ped.Res. 8: 628 (1974).

22. Wood, S., MacLeod, P.M., Applegarth, D.A., Jan, J.E., and Dolman, C.L. Proc.First International Congress of Child Neurology, Toronto, Canada, October 1975.

23. Gatt, S., and Rapport, M.M. Biochim.Biophys.Acta 113: 567 (1966).

24. Gordon, B.A., Pozsony, J., Geerling, S., Kaufmann, J.C.E., and Haust, M.D. Clin.Res. 22: 740A (1974).

25. Suzuki, Y., and Suzuki, K. Neurol. 20: 848 (1970).

PURIFICATION AND PARTIAL CHARACTERIZATION OF α-N-ACETYLGALACTOS-

AMINIDASE FROM PORCINE LIVER

Sun-Sang J. Sung and Charles C. Sweeley

Department of Biochemistry, Michigan State

University, East Lansing, Michigan 48824

INTRODUCTION

α-N-Acetylgalactosaminidase is an unusual lysosomal glycosidase in that no genetic abnormality involving this enzyme has been
discovered. It was discovered many years ago, when Freudenberg
and Eichel (1) found that extracts of the hepatopancreas from the
snail *Helix pomatia* inactivated blood group A substance with the
release of N-acetylhexosamine and galactose. Cell-free extracts
of the flagellate *Trichomonas foetus* were also observed to contain
activity that destroyed blood group A-active glycoprotein (2).
Subsequent studies with partially purified preparations from these
sources indicated that the loss of serological activity was accompanied by the concomitant liberation of terminal N-acetylgalactosamine (GalNAc) residues (3,4). Terminal GalNAc residues were also
released from desialized sheep submaxillary mucin by enzyme fractions from various animal sources (5-7) and *Clostridium perfrin-
gens* (8).

Stereochemical specificity for α-GalNAc residues was demonstrated with partially purified fractions from these organisms
using the artificial substrates, phenyl-α-GalNAc and phenyl-β-
GalNAc (9-11). Further specificity, for the conformation of the
hydroxyl group at C-4 of the hexosamine, is evident from the ease
with which α-N-acetylgalactosaminidase and α-N-acetylglucosamini-
dase activities have been separated (6,10,12,13).

Isoelectric focusing of α-N-acetylgalactosaminidase from pig
liver (6) suggests that there are multiple forms of the enzyme and
raises the question of whether these forms have different specific-

ities toward naturally occurring glycosphingolipids and glycoproteins with terminal α-GalNAc residues. There are at least ten
neutral glycosphingolipids, shown in Table I, that are eventual
substrates for lysosomal α-N-acetylgalactosaminidase; two of them
are Forssman haptens (14-16), four are blood group A-active glycolipids from human erythrocytes (17), and several are A-active fucolipids discovered in glandular epithelial tissues (18-21).

TABLE I

GLYCOSPHINGOLIPID SUBSTRATES FOR α-N-ACETYLGALACTOSAMINIDASE

1. Forssman glycolipids

    GalNAcα1→3GalNAcβ1→3Galα1→4Galβ1→4Glc→Cer

        (horse, dog, hamster, sheep)

    GalNAcα1→3GalNAcβ1→3Galα1→4Gal→Cer

        (hamster fibroblast NIL cells)

2. Blood group A-active glycolipids

    a. Type A[a]

    GalNAcα1→3Gal(2←1αFuc)β1→4GlcNAcβ1→3Galβ1→4Glc→Cer

        (human erythrocytes)

    b. Types A[b], A[c] and A[d] (incomplete structures)
        (human erythrocytes)

    c. Compounds from glandular epithelial tissues

    GalNAcα1→3Gal(2←1αFuc)β1→3GlcNAcβ1→3Galβ1→4Glc→Cer
    GalNAcα1→3Gal(2←1αFuc)β1→4GlcNAcβ1→3Galβ1→4Galβ1→4Glc→Cer
    GalNAcα1→3Gal(2←1αFuc)β1→4GlcNAc(3←1?Fuc)β1→3Galβ1→4Glc→Cer
    GalNAcα1→3Gal(2←1αFuc)β1→3Galβ1→4Galβ1→4Glc→Cer

        (hog gastric mucosa, dog intestine)

    The present study was undertaken to determine whether one or
more of the multiple forms of pig liver α-N-acetylgalactosaminidase
can hydrolyze dog intestinal Forssman pentaglycosylceramide,
2-acetamido-2-deoxygalactosyl(α1→3)-2-acetamido-2-deoxygalactosyl-
(β1→3)galactosyl(α1→4)galactosyl(β1→4)glucosylceramide (15).

MATERIALS AND METHODS

Isolation of Forssman Hapten

A crude preparation of Forssman pentaglycosylceramide was isolated from dog intestines by the method described by Saito and
Hakomori (22). Glycosphingolipids in the 1,2-dichloroethane-acetone
fraction from the Florisil column (Floridin Company, Tallahassee,
Fla.) were deacetylated with 0.5% sodium methoxide (22) and passed
through 100 gm of DEAE-cellulose to separate gangliosides from the
neutral glycosphingolipids (23). The glycolipids were further
fractionated on a 1.2 kg silicic acid (Unisil, Clarkson Chemical
Company, Williamsport, Pa.) column (7.5 x 100 cm) by gradient
elution with 4 1 of chloroform and 3 1 of methanol, starting with
the nonpolar solvent. Fractions from the column were monitored by
thin-layer chromatography on silica gel G plates (Analtech, Newark,
Del.) developed in chloroform/methanol/water (100:42:6, v/v). The
yield of Forssman pentaglycosylceramide was about 1.5 gm from 6 kg
of fresh dog intestines.

Preparation of $[6-^3H]$GalNAc-Labeled Forssman Hapten

The Forssman pentaglycosylceramide was labeled by the galactose
oxidase-sodium borotritiide method (24). The labeled glycolipid
was purified by extensive washing of a chloroform solution with
aqueous methanol followed by thin-layer chromatography on silica
gel G plates developed in chloroform/methanol/water (65:45:8, v/v).
About 41 mg of labeled lipid was recovered from 50 mg of starting
material; the specific activity was 240,000 cpm per mg.

Purification of Porcine Liver α-N-Acetylgalactosaminidase

ConA-Sepharose was prepared by coupling 440 mg of Concanavalin
A (Miles-Yeda, Kankakee, Ill.) with 45 ml of Sepharose 4B (Pharmacia, Piscataway, N.J.) as described by Lloyd (25). The product
contained about 29% of the added ConA at a concentration of 2.8 mg
per ml of gel, as determined by the protein procedure of Lowry *et
al.* (26). The gel (10 ml) was packed into a small glass column
(1 x 16 cm) and pre-equilibrated with 0.05 M citrate buffer, pH 6.0.

α-N-Acetylgalactosaminidase was purified by the procedure described by Weissmann and Hinrichsen (6), modified to incorporate
ConA-Sepharose affinity chromatography between the DEAE-cellulose
and Sephadex G-150 steps. Briefly, 1.46 kg of fresh ground pig
liver was homogenized with three volumes of distilled water containing 0.1 mM disodium EDTA. After centrifugation at 23,000 x g

the extract was adjusted to pH 3.7 with 1 M citric acid and stirred
overnight at 4°C. The mixture was then adjusted to pH 4.8 with 1 M
sodium citrate and centrifuged. Activity in the supernatant was
precipitated with ammonium sulfate, this step was repeated, and the
re-dissolved, dialyzed product was fractionated on 100 gm of DEAE-
cellulose suspended in 5 mM citrate buffer, pH 6.0. The column
was washed with the same buffer, then activity was recovered by
elution with 0.6 M sodium chloride in 5 mM citrate buffer.

Active fractions from the DEAE-cellulose column were adjusted
to pH 6.0 and the activity was precipitated with ammonium sulfate.
A dialyzed solution of the material was applied to the ConA-Sepharose column, unabsorbed proteins were washed through with 50 ml of
0.05 M citrate buffer, pH 6.0, and activity was then recovered with
50 ml of the same buffer containing 0.5 M α-methyl mannoside.

Active fractions were pooled, dialyzed and concentrated about
ten-fold with polyethylene glycol. The sample was further fractionated on a Sephadex G-150 column (1.1 x 60 cm) as described by
Weissmann and Hinrichsen (6).

Electrophoresis

Isoelectric focusing was performed using an established procedure (27). In each run 2.5 ml of an ampholine with pH range of
5 - 8 and 0.6 ml of an ampholine with pH range of 3 - 6 was used.
Electrophoretic separations were at 700 V for 60 hr.

Native polyacrylamide gel electrophoresis was carried out as
described by Gabriel (28), using a 7% gel and tris-glycine buffer
in the reservoir. Gels were stained for α-N-acetylgalactosaminidase activity by first shaking them at room temperature in 0.3 M
citrate buffer, pH 4.3, for 30 min, then transferring them to a
solution of 0.17 mM p-nitrophenyl-α-N-acetylgalactosaminide in
0.1 M citrate buffer, pH 4.3. After incubating the gels for 15 min
they were shaken in 0.6 M potassium borate buffer, pH 10.4, for
15 min and scanned immediately at 410 nm in a Gilford 2400 spectrophotometer with a linear transport assembly. Protein bands in the
gels were stained with Coomassie Brilliant Blue (29) and the bands
were determined by scanning at 550 nm in the Gilford spectrophotometer.

Assays

Forssman hapten hydrolase activity was determined by adding
50 μl of enzyme solution to 150 nmoles of labeled glycolipid (360
cpm per nmole), 0.6 mg of sodium taurocholate and 15 μmoles of sodium citrate, pH 4.3, in a final volume of 150 μl. After incubation

at 37°C for 30 min, the reaction was terminated with 4 ml of chloro-
form/methanol (2:1, v/v) and 0.85 ml of water was added. The upper
phase was washed with 2.5 ml of theoretical lower phase (31), dried,
and the residue was counted in 10 ml of a toluene-based cocktail in
a liquid scintillation spectrometer (24).

p-Nitrophenyl-α-N-acetylgalactosaminidase activity was assayed
by incubating 50 μl of enzyme solution in 100 μl of 5 mM p-nitrophenyl-α-N-acetylgalactosaminide and 50 μl of 0.3 M citrate buffer,
pH 4.3, at 37°C for 30 min. The reaction was terminated with 3 ml
of 0.6 M potassium borate buffer, pH 10.4, and absorbance was read
at 410 nm in a Gilford 2400 spectrophotometer.

Protein concentration was determined by a fluorescamine
method (30).

Radioactivity was monitored on thin-layer plates with a
Berthold LB 2723 Radio Scanner.

RESULTS

Products of Enzymatic Hydrolysis of Forssman Hapten

In a scaled-up reaction, 200 μg of labeled Forssman pentaglycosylceramide was hydrolyzed with α-N-acetylgalactosaminidase
recovered from the Sephadex G-150 column. The chloroform lower
phase contained about 15% of the added radioactivity and a major
glycolipid that corresponded to globotetraglycosylceramide (GL-4),
GalNAcβ1→3Galα1→4Galβ1→4Glc→Cer, on thin-layer chromatography, as
shown in Fig. 1. Approximately 81% of the radioactivity was recovered in the upper aqueous phase and was assumed to represent the
liberated GalNAc.

Purification of Forssman Hapten Hydrolase Activity

Glycosidase activity for the hydrolysis of Forssman pentaglycosylceramide paralleled α-N-acetylgalactosaminidase activity toward the artificial substrate through the acid precipitation step,
two batch treatments with ammonium sulfate and chromatography on
DEAE-cellulose, ConA-Sepharose and Sephadex G-150. As shown in
Tables II and III, Forssman hapten hydrolase activity was purified
about 26,000-fold whereas activity toward the artificial substrate
was purified about 8,000-fold. The Forssman hapten hydrolase was
recovered in an overall yield of about 34% with a final specific
activity of 32,000 nmoles GalNAc liberated per hr per mg protein.
The α-N-acetylgalactosaminidase for hydrolysis of artificial substrate had a final specific activity of 3,440 nmoles p-nitrophenol

TABLE II

PURIFICATION OF FORSSMAN HAPTEN HYDROLASE ACTIVITY

Fraction	Volume	Total Protein	Forssman Hapten Hydrolase Activity		Purification	Recovery
			Total	Specific	cation	ery
	ml	mg	$nmol/hr$	$nmol/hr/mg$	-fold	%
Crude extract	4030	424,563	515,116	1.2	1	100
Acid extract	4124	349,676	938,980	2.7	2	182
1st Amm. sulfate	240	52,920	1.3×10^6	24.5	20	252
2nd Amm. sulfate	65	12,368	857,252	69.3	57	166
DEAE-cellulose	24	349	600,950	1,723	1,424	117
ConA-Sepharose	0.5	⌐9	253,334	28,853	23,846	49
Sephadex G-150	0.3	⌐6	177,187	32,339	26,726	34

TABLE III

PURIFICATION OF α-N-ACETYLGALACTOSAMINIDASE ACTIVITY

Fraction	Volume	Total Protein	PNP-α-GalNAc Activity		Purification	Recovery
			Total	Specific	cation	ery
	ml	mg	$nmol/min$	$nmol/min/mg$	-fold	%
Crude extract	4030	424,563	182,782	0.43	1	100
Acid extract	4125	349,676	137,725	0.39	1	75
1st Amm. sulfate	240	52,920	66,516	1.26	3	36
2nd Amm. sulfate	65	12,368	41,349	3.34	8	23
DEAE-cellulose	24	349	61,222	175	408	33
ConA-Sepharose	0.5	⌐9	24,800	2,818	6,553	14
Sephadex G-150	0.3	⌐6	18,921	3,440	8,000	10

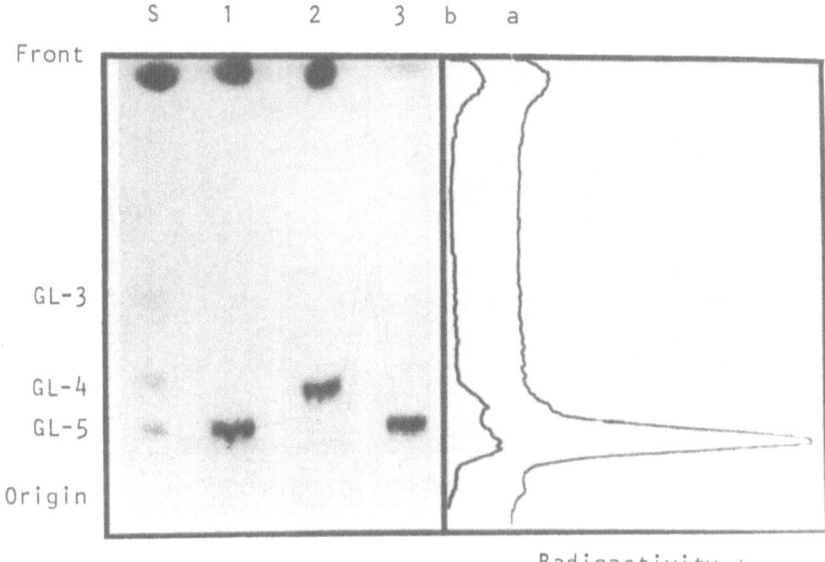

Figure 1. Thin-layer chromatography of the chloroform-soluble
fraction (lower phase) after hydrolysis of [6-^{3}H]GalNAc-labeled
Forssman hapten with α-N-acetylgalactosaminidase. Lane S, reference
Galα1→4Galβ1→4Glc→Cer (GL-3), GalNAcβ1→3Galα1→4Galβ1→4Glc→Cer (GL-4),
and Forssman hapten (GL-5); Lane 1, substrate plus boiled enzyme;
Lane 2, substrate plus enzyme; Lane 3, substrate alone. Lane a is
a radioactivity scan of Lane 1 and Lane b is a radioactivity scan
of Lane 2.

formed per min per mg protein; the recovery in terms of artificial
substrate activity was 10%. Activity toward β-N-acetylgalactos-
aminidase decreased from 3 x 10^8 nmoles per min in the total crude
extract to less than 1,500 nmoles per min in the fraction from the
Sephadex G-150 column. As observed previously by Weissmann and
Hinrichsen (6), activity toward α-GlcNAc artificial substrate was
negligible in the final product.

The ConA affinity chromatography step provided effective
additional purification (17-fold) as compared with the procedure
described by Weissmann and Hinrichsen (6) although slightly more
than half of the activity of the Forssman hapten hydrolase was lost
at this step. Fractions from this column were monitored with both
glycolipid and artificial substrate assays; the active fractions
for the artificial substrate (Fig. 2) were coincident with those
for glycolipid hydrolysis (not shown).

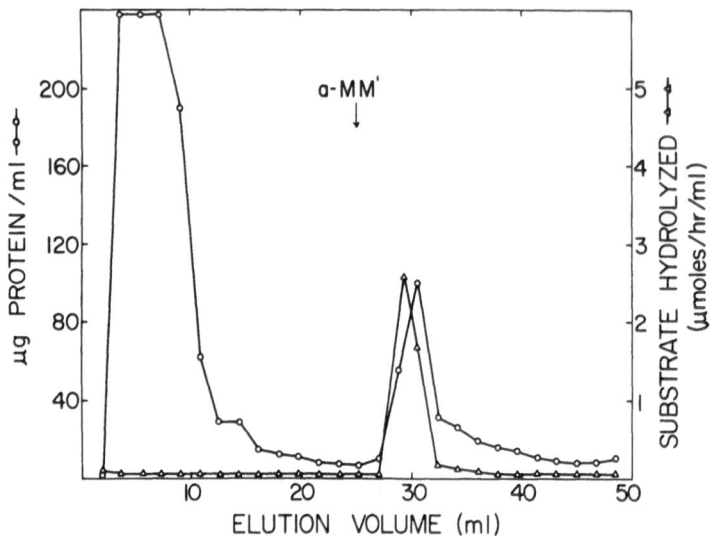

Figure 2. ConA-Sepharose affinity chromatography of partially purified pig liver α-N-acetylgalactosaminidase. The sample (9 mg protein) was loaded onto 2 ml of ConA-Sepharose gel pre-equilibrated with 0.05 M citrate buffer, pH 6.0. After washing with 25 ml of buffer the activity was eluted with 25 ml of 0.5 M α-methyl mannoside in buffer. Activity shown in the plot represents liberation of GalNAc from p-nitrophenyl-α-N-acetylgalactosaminide.

Kinetics of Forssman Hapten Hydrolase

The α-N-acetylgalactosaminidase fraction from the Sephadex G-150 column hydrolyzed Forssman pentaglycosylceramide linearly for at least 3.5 hr under standard assay conditions (Fig. 3) and the rate was also linear with respect to enzyme concentration when the enzyme was stabilized at low concentrations with bovine serum albumin (Fig. 4). The rate of GalNAc liberation from Forssman hapten was optimal at pH 3.9 when the activity was assayed in the presence of an optimal concentration (4 mg per ml) of sodium taurocholate. The apparent K_m under these conditions was 2.1×10^{-4} M.

Purity of the Porcine Liver α-N-Acetylgalactosaminidase

Polyacrylamide gel electrophoresis of the active fraction from the Sephadex G-150 column on 7% native gel indicated the presence

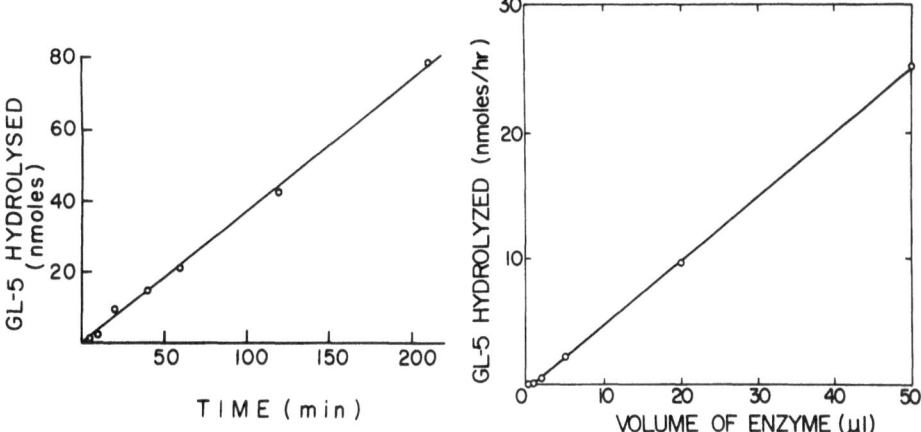

Figure 3 (left). Activity vs time plot of Forssman hapten (GL-5) hydrolase activity.

Figure 4 (right). Activity vs concentration of enzyme for Forssman hapten (GL-5) hydrolase activity.

of three major bands and some minor bands as well, all of which were located near the top of the gel (Fig. 5). The location of the yellow bands obtained when the gel was incubated with artificial substrate indicated that α-N-acetylgalactosaminidase was associated with the dark Coomassie-stained band nearest the top of the gel.

Isoelectric Focusing of the Purified Enzyme

Weissmann and Hinrichsen (6) found that a partially purified preparation of α-N-acetylgalactosaminidase from porcine liver could be separated by isoelectric focusing into eight bands, all of which were active toward phenyl-α-N-acetylgalactosaminide. Their isoelectric points varied from pH 5 to 6.5. Isoelectric focusing of the more highly purified enzyme obtained by our procedure showed the same general pattern of multiple peaks (Fig. 6). Forssman hapten hydrolase activity generally coincided with the peaks of activity toward artificial substrate, although the ratio of glycolipid to artificial substrate activity increased significantly with increasing pI of the multiple forms.

Individual peaks from the isoelectric focusing run were compared on native polyacrylamide gels. The peaks with the lowest isoelectric points contained a sharp band near the top of the gel that became weaker in intensity with increasing pI and was nearly absent from the peaks with the highest pI values. This is shown in

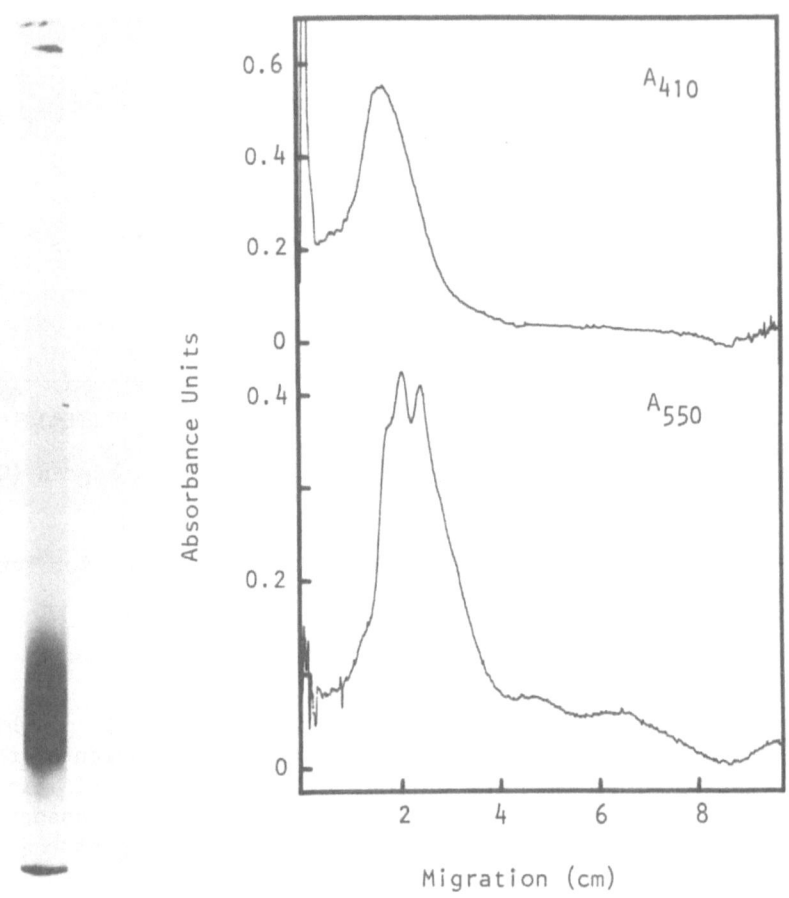

Figure 5.   Native polyacrylamide gel electrophoresis of α-N-acetylgalactosaminidase activity from Sephadex G-150 column. Coomassie
Blue stained gel (left) and scans of artificial substrate activity
(410 nm) and protein (550 nm) (right).

the comparison of Coomassie Blue bands of Peaks II (pI = 5.4) and
VI (pI = 6.4) in Fig. 7. All of the peaks from the isoelectric
focusing run contained a more diffuse band of greater mobility on
the gels; this band appeared to change somewhat with pI as well,
as shown in Fig. 7.

The activity of Peaks II and VI toward artificial substrate
is compared with Coomassie Blue stains of protein on native gels
in Fig. 8. Close inspection of the more diffuse band in these
graphs strengthens the view that it is not homogeneous and that its
composition varies with the isoelectric points of the Peaks I to

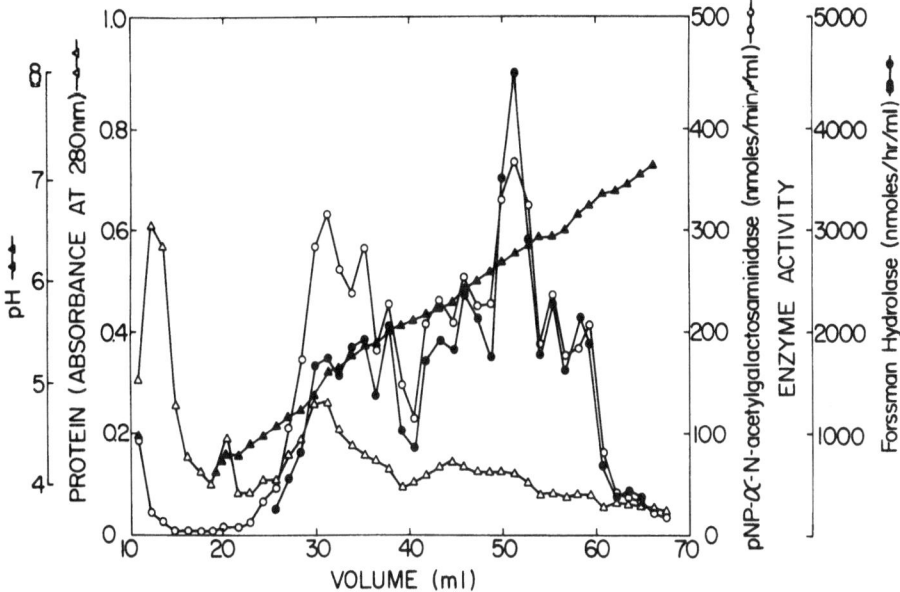

Figure 6.   Isoelectric focusing of α-N-acetylgalactosaminidase fraction from Sephadex G-150 column.   The peak at 30 ml elution volume is designated Peak I in the text; the remaining peaks are designated II to VIII with increasing elution volume and increasing isoelectric point.

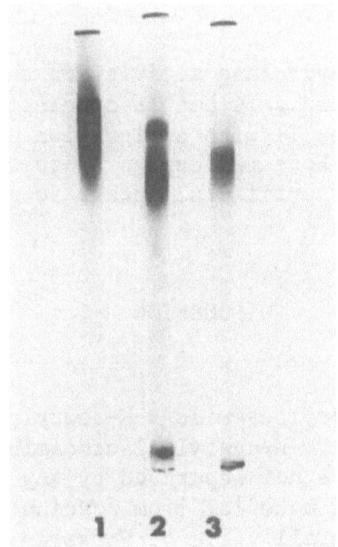

Figure 7.   Native polyacrylamide gel electrophoresis of α-N-acetyl-galactosaminidase from Sephadex G-150 column (Lane 1) and Peaks II (Lane 2) and VI (Lane 3) from isoelectric focusing separation of activity.   Gels are stained with Coomassie Blue.

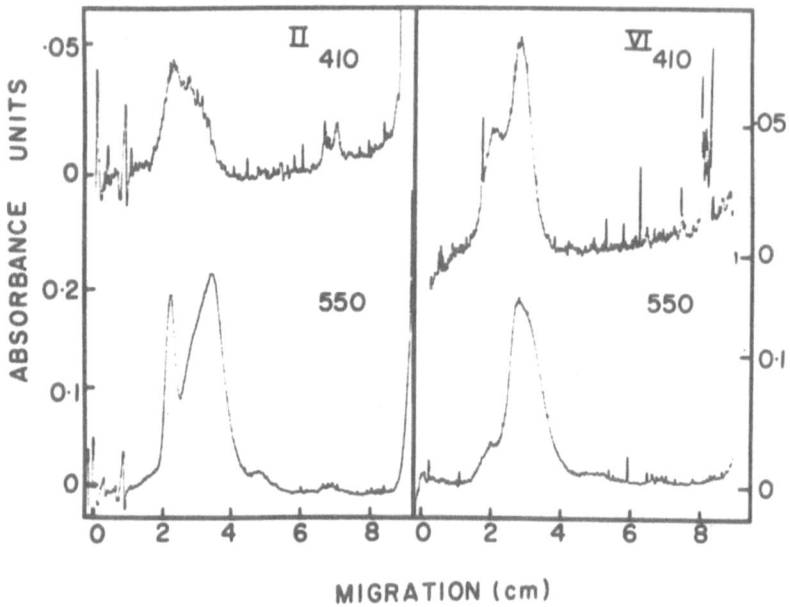

Figure 8. Native gel electrophoresis of Peaks II and VI from isoelectric focusing run. Scans of artificial substrate activity at
410 nm and protein at 550 nm.

VIII. Forssman hapten hydrolase activity in the separated bands
was not monitored on these gels but it appears possible that the
maximum at 550 nm in Peak II with a migration of about 3.5 cm may
represent primarily the Forssman hapten hydrolase as there is little
absorbance at 410 nm for artificial substrate activity at this
point.

DISCUSSION

        Forssman pentaglycosylceramide α-N-acetylgalactosaminidase
activity and nonspecific α-N-acetylgalactosaminidase activity toward
artificial substrate were not separated by any of the procedures
used in the isolation of material from porcine liver to near homogeneity. The higher overall yield of Forssman hapten hydrolase, as
compared with artificial substrate activity, can probably be
accounted for by the presence of inhibitory material in the crude
homogenate, since approximately two-fold increases in activity were
observed after the acid precipitation and ammonium sulfate precipi-

tation steps. ConA affinity chromatography was an effective means of increasing the purity of the α-N-acetylgalactosaminidase, compared with fractions obtained earlier (6). The loss of activity at this step was attributed to the instability of the enzyme at low protein concentrations rather than poor recovery from the column.

Forssman hapten hydrolase activity in rat brain and kidney was described previously, and conditions of the reaction were investigated (32). In the presence of optimal taurocholate (1.5 to 2.0 mg per ml) the apparent K_m of the rat brain and kidney enzymes was 1.0×10^{-4} M and 3.5×10^{-4} M, respectively. These values compare very well with that which we obtained with the porcine liver enzyme (2.1×10^{-4} M).

We observed almost the same behavior of the enzyme on isoelectric focusing that was reported by Weissmann and Hinrichsen (6). It is attractive to believe that this phenomenon reflects the presence of a complex of multiple forms of the enzyme in pig liver, much like that of α-fucosidase reported recently for human liver by Alhadeff *et al.* (33). There are alternative explanations that cannot be ruled out yet, however. The overnight treatment of the crude fraction at an acid pH may have resulted in variable changes in the degree of amidation of the enzyme. When sufficient amounts of each of the peaks from isoelectric focusing have been obtained, this possibility can be evaluated by direct ammonia determinations. Secondly, some proteolytic activity during the fractionation procedure may have produced several active but partially degraded proteins. The α-N-acetylgalactosaminidase needs to be purified in the presence of protease inhibitors to rule out this possibility. Finally, it is conceivable that the native enzyme is a multimer, and that subunits may be forming and randomly reassembling during one or more of the purification steps. Tests can be designed using purified peaks from isoelectric focusing to evaluate this possibility.

On careful inspection of the protein and artificial substrate scans of native gel electrophoresis runs of individual peaks from isoelectric focusing, it appears likely that Forssman hapten hydrolase and nonspecific α-N-acetylgalactosaminidase toward artificial substrate are not identical. A much more pronounced specificity pattern may have been observed in these experiments had we used actual substrates native for these enzymes. Forssman pentaglycosylceramide does not occur in pig tissues and, of course, neither does PNP-α-GalNAc. These substrates may, however, represent hydrophobic and hydrophilic substances that can be distinguished to some degree by the enzymes. It will be interesting to compare the specific activities of the various isoelectric focusing peaks with blood group A-active glycoprotein, desialized submaxillary mucin and several of the gastric mucosal and intestinal fucolipids.

Speculation about the absence of a defined clinical abnormality with deficiency of α-N-acetylgalactosaminidase is probably not warranted at this time. A variety of explanations, such as multiple genetic loci for the synthesis of the several forms of the enzyme or insufficient turnover of blood group A-specific and fucolipids to be clinically significant, are possible. Nevertheless, it may be fruitful to seek such a genetic disease in an animal with large amounts of a glycolipid with a terminal α-GalNAc residue, as it could be a useful model for the study of sphingolipidoses and evaluation of various approaches to enzyme replacement therapy. Forssman hapten and the dog appear to represent an attractive model in this respect.

ACKNOWLEDGMENT

This investigation has been supported in part by a research grant (AM 12434) from the U. S. Public Health Service.

REFERENCES

1. Freudenberg, K., and Eichel, H. (1935) *Ann.* 518, 97
2. Watkins, W. M. (1959) *Biochem. J.* 71, 261
3. Tuppy, H., and Staudenbauer, W. L. (1966) *Biochemistry* 5, 1742
4. Harrap, G. J., and Watkins, W. M. (1964) *Biochem. J.* 93, 9p
5. Schauer, H., and Gottschalk, A. (1968) *Biochim. Biophys. Acta* 156, 304
6. Weissmann, B., and Hinrichsen, D. F. (1969) *Biochemistry* 8, 2034
7. Bhargava, A. S., Buddecke, E., Werries, E., and Gottschalk, A. (1966) *Biochim. Biophys. Acta* 127, 457
8. McGuire, E. J., and Roseman, S. (1967) *J. Biol. Chem.* 242, 3745
9. Weissmann, B., and Friederici, D. (1966) *Biochim. Biophys. Acta* 117, 498
10. Muramatsu, T. (1968) *J. Biochem. (Tokyo)* 64, 521
11. Buddecke, E., Schauer, H., Werries, E., and Gottschalk, A. (1969) *Biochem. Biophys. Res. Commun.* 34, 517
12. Weissmann, B., Rowin, G., Marshall, J., and Friederici, D. (1967) *Biochemistry* 6, 207
13. Werries, E., Wollek, E., Gottschalk, A., and Buddecke, E. (1969) *Eur. J. Biochem.* 10, 445
14. Siddiqui, B., and Hakomori, S. (1971) *J. Biol. Chem.* 246, 5766
15. Sung, S. J., Esselman, W. J., and Sweeley, C. C. (1973) *J. Biol. Chem.* 248, 6528
16. Gahmberg, C. G., and Hakomori, S. (1975) *J. Biol. Chem.* 250, 2438
17. Hakomori, S., Stellner, K., and Watanabe, K. (1972) *Biochem. Biophys. Res. Commun.* 49, 1061

18. Smith, E. L., and McKibbin, J. M. (1972) *Anal. Biochem.* 45, 608

19. Slomiany, A., and Horowitz, M. I. (1973) *J. Biol. Chem.* 248, 6232

20. Slomiany, A., Slomiany, B. L., and Horowitz, M. I. (1974) *J. Biol. Chem.* 249, 1225

21. Slomiany, B. L., Slomiany, A., and Horowitz, M. I. (1975) *Eur. J. Biochem.* 56, 353

22. Saito, T., and Hakomori, S.-i. (1971) *J. Lipid Res.* 12, 257

23. Rouser, G., Kritchevsky, G., Yamamoto, A., Simon, G., Galli, C., and Bauman, A. J. (1969) in *Methods in Enzymology* (Lowenstein, J. M., ed) Vol. XIV, pp. 272, Academic Press, New York

24. Suzuki, Y., and Suzuki, K. (1972) *J. Lipid Res.* 13, 687

25. Lloyd, K. O. (1970) *Arch. Biochem. Biophys.* 137, 460

26. Lowry, O. H., Rosebrough, N. J., Farr, A. L., and Randall, R. J. (1951) *J. Biol. Chem.* 193, 265

27. Vesterberg, O. (1971) in *Methods in Enzymology* (Jakoby, W. B., ed) Vol. XXII, pp. 389, Academic Press, New York

28. Gabriel, O. (1971) in *Methods in Enzymology* (Jakoby, W. B., ed) Vol. XXII, pp. 565, Academic Press, New York

29. Malik, N., and Berrie, A. (1972) *Anal. Biochem.* 49, 173

30. Böhlen, P., Stein, S., Daireman, W., and Udenfriend, S. (1973) *Arch. Biochem. Biophys.* 155, 213

31. Folch, J., Lees, M., and Sloane-Stanley, G. H. (1957) *J. Biol. Chem.* 226, 497

32. Israel, M., Bach, G., Miyatake, T., Naiki, M., and Suzuki, K. (1974) *J. Neurochem.* 23, 803

33. Alhadeff, J. A., Miller, A. L., Wenaas, H., Vedvick, T., and O'Brien, J. S. (1975) *J. Biol. Chem.* 250, 7106

IDENTIFICATION OF TAY-SACHS GENOTYPES BY HEXOSAMINIDASE

ANALYSIS OF URINE AND TEAR SAMPLES

Abraham Saifer, June Amoroso and Guta Perle

Department of Biochemistry, Isaac Albert
Research Institute of the Kingsbrook Jewish
Medical Center, Brooklyn, N.Y. 11203

The absence of N-acetyl-β-D-hexosaminidase A
(Hex A, EC 3.2.1.52) activity in the body fluids and
tissues of patients with Tay-Sachs disease (TSD) (1,2)
results in the cerebral accumulation of the G_{M2}-ganglio-
side [N-acetylgalactosaminyl -(N-acetylneuraminyl)-
galactosylglucosyl-ceramide] (3) and is responsible
for all the clinical symptoms and pathological findings
in the disease (4,5). TSD is a prototype representative of many other hereditary disorders (6).

Three basic criteria must be satisfied in order to
prevent a genetic-recessive type of disease. First, is
a clearly defined ethnic group with a high gene frequency for the disease, e.g., 1:30 for TSD in the Ashkenazic Jewish population of a community (7). Second,
is the availability of a simple quantitative biochemical test, preferably based upon the automated analysis
of the activity of the deficient enzyme (8,9), which
will permit the detection of heterozygotes (carriers)
in the ethnic group. Third, is the potential for
diagnosis of the disease prenatally, by enzymatic analysis of the amniotic fluid or cultured cells obtained
from fetuses of carrier-couples (1,10) sufficiently
early in the pregnancy to give parents the choice of
terminating it safely. All three of these criteria
are ideally satisfied by TSD, so that more heterozygotes have been uncovered by mass-screening and more
high-risk pregnancies of carrier-couples monitored for
this disease than all other genetic disorders combined
(11).

Since 1970, this Institute has screened more than 18,000 persons, about 95% being of Ashkenazic Jewish ancestry, for carriers of the TSD gene. For this purpose, samples of venous blood were obtained from the individuals being tested and their sera analyzed for Hex A content by the automated pH inactivation procedure (9). With this method for Hex A, as well as with those based on heat denaturation (8), the sera of normal (non-carrier) pregnant women (12,13) and of persons with diabetes and other debilitating diseases (12,14) generally yield Hex A values which fall within the carrier range (15). Since many parents become concerned about giving birth to a genetically defective child only after conception has occurred, and since diabetes is not infrequently found among Jews, false positive serum Hex A results are not uncommon in community mass screening programs for TSD. In such cases, the test has to be repeated on a lysed leukocyte sample which reduces the incidence of such false values in pregnancy sera to less than 20 percent.

In a recent publication (16), we have described an automated DEAE cellulose microcolumn procedure for the automated differentiation and measurement of hexosaminidase isoenzymes in biological fluids similar to that published by Ellis et al (17). With this technique the serum isoenzyme patterns of normal pregnant women contained appreciable amounts of heat stable intermediate forms and were similar to those of TSD carriers (16). Application of this technique to fluids such as urine and tears showed the absence of appreciable amounts of heat stable intermediate peaks in samples obtained from normal pregnant women. These experimental data appeared to confirm the findings of Navon and Padeh (18) for urine and of Carmody et al (19) for tears as fluids, other than serum (12,20) and leukocytes (21,22), which are suitable for the detection of TSD heterozygotes. The use of such fluids instead of blood samples for identifying TSD carriers has advantages of being less costly in material and personnel required and of being more efficient in the collection and processing of large numbers of samples. In addition, the report of Carmody et al (19) that normal pregnancy did not interfere with tear Hex A values is contrary to that published by Singer et al (23).

We have, therefore, investigated urine and tear specimens, in comparison with serum and leukocyte samples from the same individuals, for the identification of TSD genotypes based on their Hex A content as determined with both the heat denaturation (12,24) and

the pH inactivation (20,24) procedures. Our results led
us to conclude that urine is not a useful fluid for this
purpose but that tears constitute an almost ideal fluid
for heterozygote detection in TSD.

MATERIAL AND METHODS

A. Automated Column Method of Hexosaminidase Analysis

The flow diagram of the manifold for the automated
system for the simultaneous separation of the hexosaminidase isoenzymes and the quantitative measurement of
their activities by means of fluorescent analysis is
illustrated in Figure 1. The equipment used is the
"Autoanalyzer II" system (Technicon Instruments Corp.,
Tarrytown, N.Y. 10591) for fluorometric analysis. It
consists of a Proportioning Pump III, a Fluornephelom-
eter with a flowcell (No. 126-B014-02), primary filter
(365 nm, No. 7-60) and secondary filter (460 nm, No. 48
plus 426 nm, No. 3-73) and a single- or double-pen Re-
corder modified for fluorometric measurements. The reagents pumped through the system and its calibration for
fluorometric analysis have been described in detail in
a previous publication (16). The DEAE-cellulose microcolumn is connected to the sample line on the proportioning pump and then equilibrated with phosphate buffer
for 15 min. A sample (e.g., serum, urine, tears, etc)
is either diluted with or dialyzed against phosphate
buffer (pH 6.0, 0.01 mol/liter) to an activity of about
40 nmol/ml. A 50 to 400 µl aliquot (usually 200 µl) is
aspirated onto the column with the aid of a phosphate
buffer wash and the buffer pumped through the column for
10 min. Then 40 ml of a 0 to 0.5 mol/liter NaCl gradient
in the phosphate buffer is passed through the column.

It requires about an hour to elute the sample from
the column and record the hexosaminidase isoenzyme
pattern. The area under each peak is measured by tri-
angulation and the activity of each component calculated
either as nanomoles per ml or as a percentage of the
total activity. Hexosaminidase isoenzyme patterns were
obtained by the automated microcolumn DEAE-cellulose
chromatographic system for serum (Figure 2), urine
(Figure 3) and tear (Figure 4) samples for TSD genotypes.

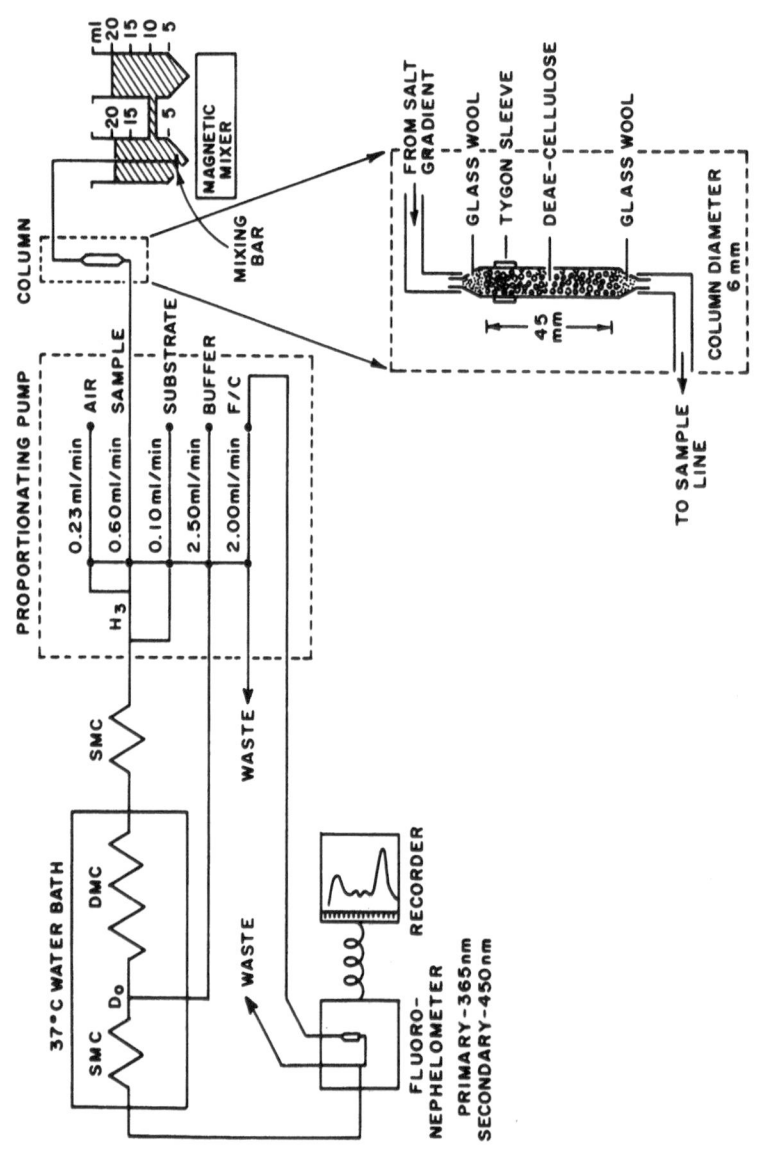

Figure 1. Flow diagram for measurement of N-acetyl-β-D-hexosaminidase B (Hex B) activity by pH inactivation (16). NOTE:- The same manifold is used for the total hexosaminidase method, except that the mixed buffer reagent is substituted for the pH 4.5 and pH 2.8 buffers.

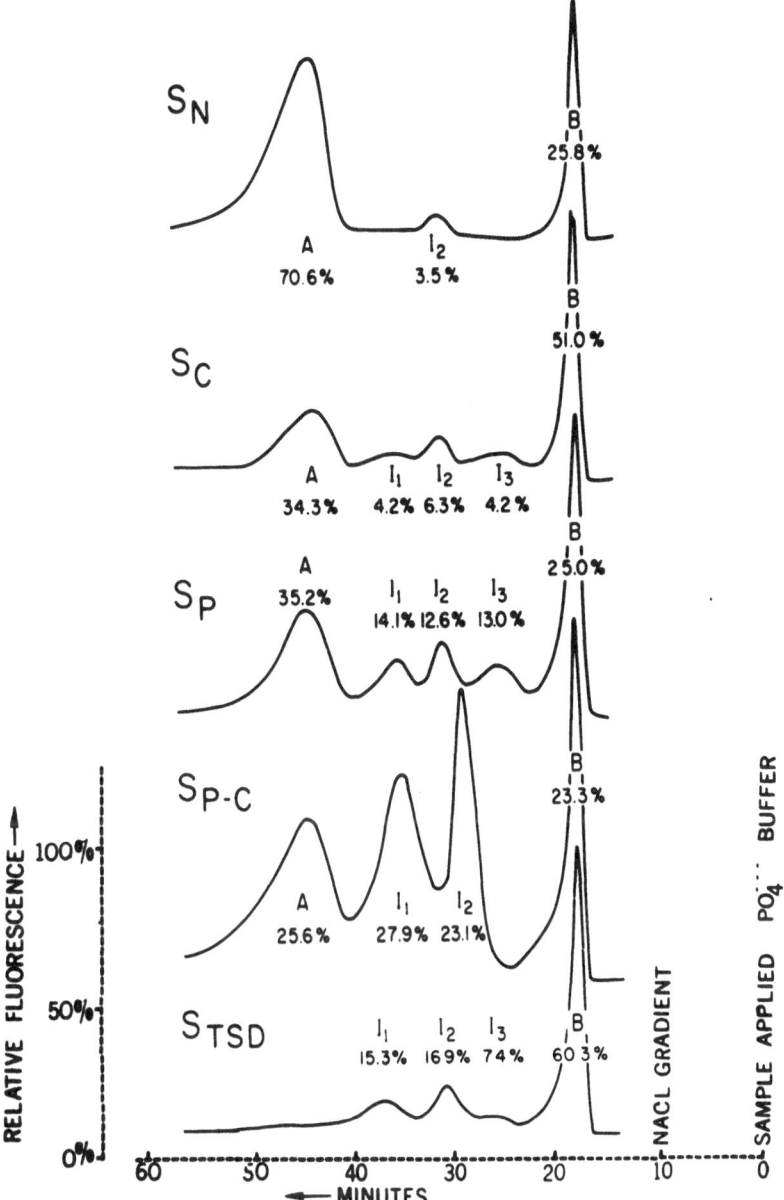

Figure 2. Serum hexosaminidase patterns obtained by automated DEAE-cellulose microcolumn chromatography. S_N=normal serum. S_C=carrier serum. S_P=pregnancy serum. S_{P-C}=pregnancy-carrier serum. S_{TSD}=Tay-Sachs disease patient's serum. A, I_1, I_2, I_3 and B refer to the various isoenzymes. The numbers are percentage of the total area under a given peak.

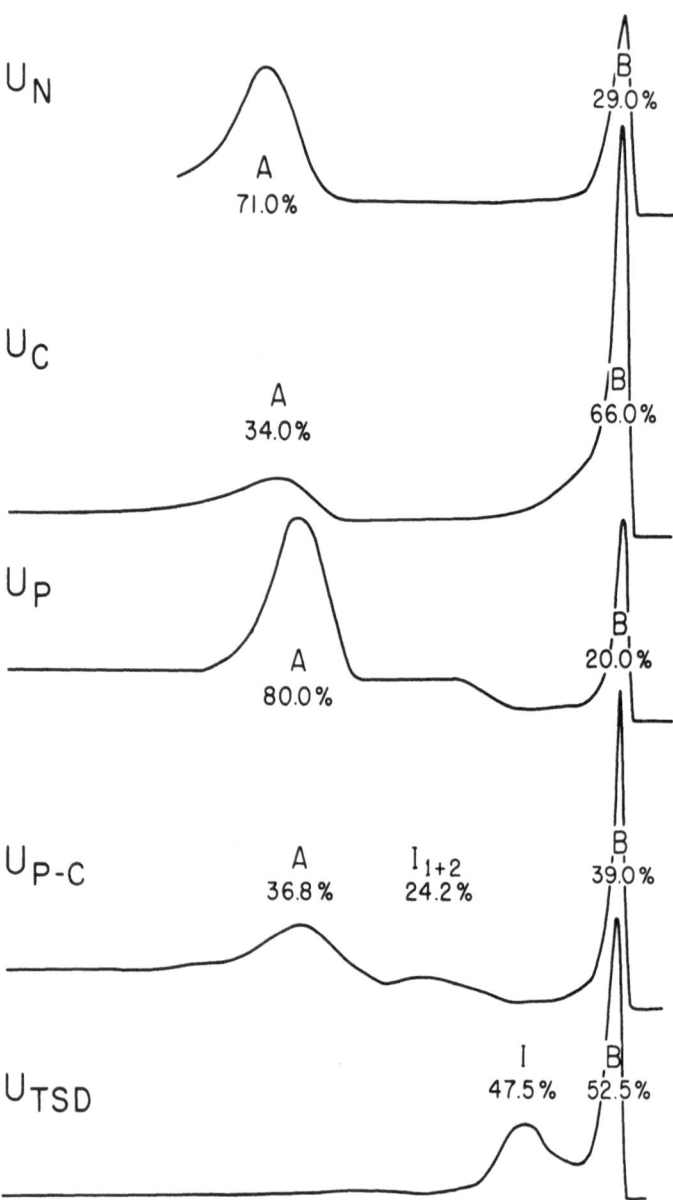

Figure 3. Urinary hexosaminidase patterns obtained by automated DEAE-cellulose chromatography. Nomenclature and time course are the same as in Figure 2.

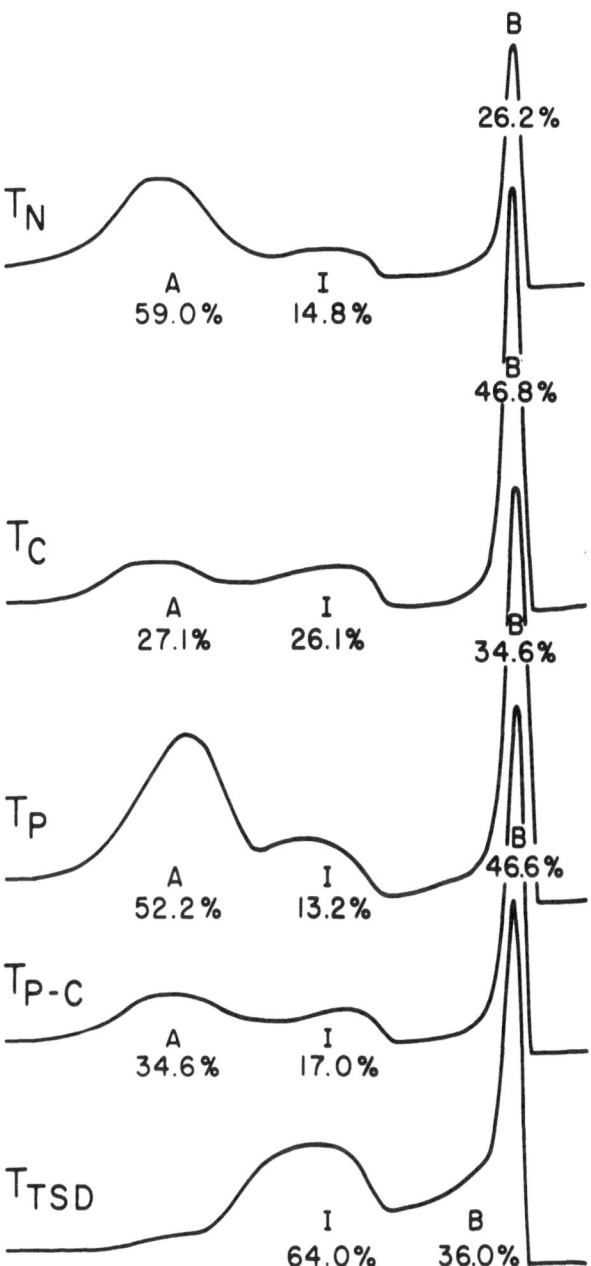

<u>Figure 4</u>.   Tear hexosaminidase patterns obtained by
automated DEAE-cellulose chromatography.   Nomenclature
and time course are the same as in Figure 2.

B. Urinary Hexosaminidase-pH Inactivation Procedure

1. Reagents. The reagents used in the analysis of
urinary total hexosaminidase activity and of Hex B by
pH inactivation are the same as those described previously
for serum (24) except that both the glycine hydrochloride
(pH 2.80, 0.50 moles/liter) and sodium citrate (pH 4.50,
0.10 moles/liter) buffers contained 1.0g/liter crystalline bovine serum albumin (Pentex, Kankakee, IL 60901).
The concentration of the termination buffer (pH 10.3)was
also increased from 0.02M to 0.06M 2-amino-2-methyl-
propanol.
2. Urinary Hexosaminidase B Analysis. For each
sample prewarm two tubes containing 300 μl of pH 2.80
glycine hydrochloride buffer to 37°C. At timed intervals (15-30 seconds) add 50 μl of urine to each tube
maintained at 37°C. After exactly 5 minutes of incubation, 100 μl of each mixture is pipeted into another set of tubes containing 350 μl of substrate
solution which has been prewarmed to 37°C. After exactly 20 minutes of incubation, the reaction is stopped
by the addition of 2.0 ml of termination buffer. Fluorescent readings are made as described below.
3. Urinary Total Hexosaminidase Analysis. For each
sample prewarm two tubes containing 300 μl of pH 4.50
sodium citrate buffer with 1.0g/liter albumin to 37°C.
The rest of the procedure is carried out exactly as described above for Hex B beginning with "At timed in-
tervals---etc".

The fluorescence of each sample is read in a
Beckman Ratio Fluorometer at an excitation wavelength
of 365 nm and an emission wavelength of 450 nm. The
termination buffer is set at 0% and the fluorescent
standard (1.3 x 10^{-6} moles/liter of 4-methylumbellifer-
one) is set at 100%.

C. Urinary Hexosaminidase-Heat Denaturation Procedure

1. Reagents. The reagents used in the analysis of
urinary total hexosaminidase activity and of Hex B by
heat fractionation are the same as those of Navon and
Padeh (18) except that 1.0g/liter of crystalline bovine
serum albumin was added to the pH 4.50 sodium citrate
incubation buffer rather than to the buffered substrate.
2. Urinary Total Hexosaminidase and Hexosaminidase
B Analysis. Dilute 0.5 ml of urine with 2.0 ml of 0.05M
sodium citrate (pH 4.5) buffer containing 1.0g/liter
bovine plasma albumin. Pipet 100 μl aliquots of this

mixture into 6 separate test tubes and cap the tubes.
Two tubes are frozen immediately for the total hexosaminidase assay and the remaining tubes are placed in a
50°C water bath for the Hex B assay. After 2 hours, two
tubes are removed from the 50°C bath and are frozen. The
two remaining tubes are removed from the bath and frozen
after 3 hours of incubation. All tubes are then thawed
and transferred to an ice bath. 0.2 ml of substrate is
then added to each tube. After 60 minutes of incubation
at 37°C, the tubes are returned to the ice bath and the
enzyme reaction is terminated by adding 2.0 ml of the 0.2
M glycine-NaOH buffer (pH 10.6). Fluorescence is read
in a Beckman Ratio Fluorometer against termination buffer
set at 0% and the fluorescent standard set at 100%. For
the Hex B value, the 2 and 3 hour readings are averaged.

D. Tear Hexosaminidase-pH Inactivation Procedure

1. <u>Tear Sample Collection</u>. The person being tested
is seated in an examining chair preferably with the head
resting against a headrest. The rounded wick end of the
standardized, sterile Schirmer tear strip (SMP Division,
Cooper Labs, San Germán, Puerto Rico 00753) is bent 90°
(angle) at the indentation before opening the sterile in-
side envelope. The envelope is then cut at the end opposite the wick and the strip is removed with a forceps
to prevent contamination. The subject is asked to look
up and the lower eyelid is drawn gently downward. The
rounded bent end of the sterile tear strip is then hooked
over the lower eyelid. A second strip may also be hooked
over the lower eyelid of the other eye. The subject may
continue normal blinking although some persons will prefer
to keep their eyes closed during the collection. The
strips are removed when they are moistened along their
full length and placed in properly labeled (13 x 100 mm)
test tubes. The tubes are stoppered tightly and refrig-
erated prior to analysis.
2. <u>Tear Total Hexosaminidase and Hexosaminidase B
Analysis</u>. 300 µl of 1.0g/liter of bovine serum albumin
per strip is added to each tube and the contents mixed
on a Vortex mixer to elute tears from the strips. For
the pH inactivation analysis, 50 µl aliquots of the tear
sample are processed in the same manner as is used to per-
form the serum Hex A analysis (24) except that the substrate incubation period at 37°C has been extended to
45 min.

E. Tear Hexosaminidase-Heat Denaturation Procedure

For the heat denaturation method, 300 µl of 1.0g/
liter of bovine serum albumin in 0.04 moles/liter
citrate-phosphate buffer, pH 4.45 is added to 100 µl of
the eluted tear fluid. 50 µl aliquots of this mixture
are then treated in the same manner as that previously
described for the serum Hex A analysis (24) except that
denaturation at 50°C is carried out for one and two hours.

RESULTS

Serum hexosaminidase was separated into as many as
five peaks of enzyme activity with the automated DEAE-
cellulose microcolumn chromatographic system (Figure 1).
The most representative pattern for each category, i.e.,
(a) normals (b) heterozygotes (c) pregnant-normals
(d) pregnant-carriers and (e) TSD children, is illustrated in Figure 2. These patterns show a clear-cut dis-
tinction between the normal, carrier and TSD groups but
almost identical patterns for the carrier and normal
pregnancy groups and are confirmatory of the statistical data previously obtained with the pH inactivation
and heat denaturation methods (9). While it would
appear likely that this technique would permit differentiation between the serum pattern of a pregnant-
carrier and that of a normal (non-carrier) pregnant
woman, the small number of cases of the former analyzed
thus far precludes any valid conclusion at this time.

Urinary hexosaminidase isoenzyme patterns, representative of the same categories as the above serum
samples, are shown in Figure 3. The urinary isoenzyme
patterns also indicate good differentiation between the
normal, carrier and TSD groups. However, the most
striking differences between the serum and urine hexosaminidase patterns are the absence of any intermediate
peaks for the latter fluid, except for samples from
pregnant-carriers and TSD children, and the similarity
of the normal and pregnancy urinary patterns. These
results, and the previously published conclusion of
Navon and Padeh (18) that the urinary hexosaminidase
assay is as dependable as that with leukocytes for the
identification of TSD genotypes, led to a more intensive
investigation of the use of this fluid for heterozygote
detection.

Since the ease of obtaining urine samples would make
this the method of choice for the mass screening of TSD
carriers, we proceeded to investigate about 200 urine

samples with the heat denaturation and pH inactivation Hex A procedures. The urinary Hex A values were compared with those determined for sera with the pH inactivation method (9,20) and for leukocytes with the heat denaturation method (24) for a large number of samples obtained simultaneously from the same subjects. Statistical data for Hex A values (as a percentage of total hexosaminidase activity) are given in Table 1 for 137 normal (non-carrier) sera and for 62 leukocyte samples obtained from this group. The mean and SD for normal sera with the pH inactivation method, listed in Table 1, are in good agreement with the value of 68.1 $\pm$ 5.2% reported for 170 normal sera in a previous publication (9). The Hex A results obtained for normal leukocytes with the heat denaturation procedure are also in close agreement with both the serum values in Table 1 (F = 1.6) and are higher by about 5% Hex A than previously reported values for normal leukocytes (22). The somewhat lower CV (5.8%) for the leukocyte Hex A values, as compared to those for normal sera (7.9%), is due in large part to the fact that the former were obtained by averaging four readings while the latter were run in duplicate.

The data in Table 1 show only a slight overlap of serum Hex A values between the normal and TSD carrier groups and almost complete differentiation between the two groups based on their leukocyte Hex A values. The segregation of individuals being tested into normal (or non-carrier), TSD carrier (heterozygote) and TSD patient (homozygote) groups was therefore based primarily on serum and leukocyte Hex A analysis (24).

In contrast to the leukocyte Hex A results, the urinary Hex A values with the pH inactivation method (Table 1) gave a large CV (17.8%), a wide normal range (43 to 91% Hex A) and a very large F number (8.4 as compared to an expected value of F = 1.4, if the sets of results differed only by chance) for the ratio of their variances. The least squares regression line for the two fluids was calculated as:- Urinary Hex A (%) = 0.88 Leukocyte Hex A (%) + 4.0 and the correlation coefficient (r) is 0.83.

Somewhat better, although still unsatisfactory, Hex A results were obtained with the heat denaturation method for normal urines in comparison with the leukocyte Hex A data analyzed with the same procedure. The CV is 11.7%, as compared to 5.8% for leukocytes, the normal range (55.6 to 89.6% Hex A) is considerably

TABLE 1

COMPARATIVE DATA OF URINARY, SERUM AND LEUKOCYTE HEX A VALUES (AS %) FOR NORMALS AND FOR TSD CARRIERS.

Sample (Subjects)	Controls(Hex A%) Mean ± SD (Range ± 2SD)	TSD Carriers (Hex A%) No.	Mean ± SD (Range ± 2SD)
Sera pH Inactivation) (137)	69.4 ± 5.5 (58.4-80.4)	(19)*	47.5 ± 6.0 35.5-59.5
Leukocytes (Heat Denaturation) (62)	70.9 ± 4.1 (62.7-79.1)	(14)	53.9 ± 4.2 (45.5-62.3)
Urines (pH Inactivation) (143)	67.0 ± 11.9 (43.2-90.8)	(23)	57.5 ± 7.4 (42.7-72.3)
Urines (Heat Denaturation) (150)	72.6 ± 8.5 (55.6-89.6)	(25)	57.4 ± 5.8 (46.8-69.0)

*Determined by heat denaturation

closer to the leukocyte normal range (Table 1) and
F = 4.3. The regression line equation for the two fluids
is:- Urinary Hex A (%) = 0.93 Leukocyte Hex A (%) + 6.3
and r = 0.85. When urine is the fluid being analyzed
for Hex A with the heat denaturation method, then all
the known TSD carriers also yield values in the carrier
range, i.e., 46.8 to 69.0% Hex A. However, about 30%
of the individuals, shown to be non-carriers by blood
analysis, will give urinary Hex A values in the carrier
range, i.e., less than 69% Hex A. These persons will
require retesting with leukocyte samples as compared to
5% of the original test group for serum Hex A analysis.
These data would preclude any practical use of urinary
Hex A analysis for distinguishing heterozygotes from
normal individuals among the Ashkenazic Jewish population of a community.

However, our urinary Hex A results for ten TSD
children show a clear-cut statistical differentiation
between heterozygote (Table 1) and homozygote values.
Low Hex A (%) values, i.e., below the statistical limits
of the carrier range, are obtained for homozygotes regardless of the fluid being analyzed or of the method
employed for the Hex A analysis. Because of the ease with
which a urine sample can be obtained from an infant, a
urinary value of less than 20% Hex A would confirm a
suspected clinical diagnosis of TSD.

Several investigators (19,23) had proposed the use
of tears as a suitable and readily obtainable fluid for
the determination of TSD genotypes. The tear hexosaminidase patterns for the various categories of individuals, previously investigated for serum and urine,
were determined with the automated DEAE-cellulose chromatographic system and the results are presented in Figure
4. The tear isoenzyme patterns obtained closely resemble those of urine with respect to the absence of
mutliple intermediate peaks and in the similarity of
their normal and the pregnancy patterns. These data
appeared to confirm the findings of Carmody et al (19)
that pregnancy did not interfere with TSD heterozygote
detection when tear samples were used for the Hex A
analysis.

Since previous investigators had utilized either heat
denaturation or cellulose acetate electrophoresis (1923)
for tear Hex A analysis, the optimal experimental factors
for the pH inactivation method for this fluid needed to
be established. Aliquots of a pooled tear sample were

treated in the same manner as described above for the
pH inactivation procedure under "Material and Methods"
except that the glycine hydrochloride buffer used was
adjusted to the pH listed in Figure 5. Each tear sample
was kept at the indicated pH for 5 minutes at 37°C. The
mixture was then adjusted to pH 6.0 with concentrated
phosphate buffer, i.e., 1.0 mole/liter, and the samples
were run with the automated DEAE-cellulose microcolumn
chromatographic technique. The tear isoenzyme patterns
obtained at the various pH's are illustrated in Figure
5 and show an almost complete disappearance of Hex A
at pH 2.9 and some slight destruction of Hex B at pH 2.6.
It was for this reason that pH 2.80 ± 0.05 was chosen as
the optional pH for the given temperature (37°C) and time
period (5 minutes). The 37°C temperature was chosen
mainly because it is a readily available laboratory temperature at which most enzymatic reactions are performed.
The time course, in minutes, of the inactivation of the
Hex A activity of an aliquot of a pooled tear sample is
shown in Figure 6. The tear sample was maintained at
pH 2.80 for the time period indicated by each point in
Figure 6. The residual enzyme activity for each time
interval was determined by the manual pH inactivation
procedure and is expressed as a percentage of the activity at zero time, i.e., the total hexosaminidase activity. These results demonstrate that a plateau level of
activity is reached between four and eights minutes
after which time there is a slow decline indicating
continuing destruction of Hex B.

In this Laboratory we have confirmed the findings
of earlier investigators (25) that biological fluids
with low protein content such as urine, leukocytes, tears,
etc, require the addition of protein e.g., albumin, to
the enzyme reaction mixture for enzyme stability and
accurate assays. In order to duplicate the conditions
used for the serum assay, we have preferred to add the
albumin during the heat denaturation or heat inactivation steps rather than to the substrate. Neither of
the two published heat denaturation procedures for the
assay of tear Hex A (19,23) utilized albumin in their
analyses. We, therefore, investigated the effect of the
time of incubation at 50°C on the change in Hex A and
Hex B activity of a tear sample in the absence and presence of 1.0g/liter of albumin. The amount of each isoenzyme present in the tear sample was measured with
automated DEAE-cellulose microcolumn chromatography at
the time intervals indicated in Figure 7. The results
of these experiments show that all of Hex A is denatured

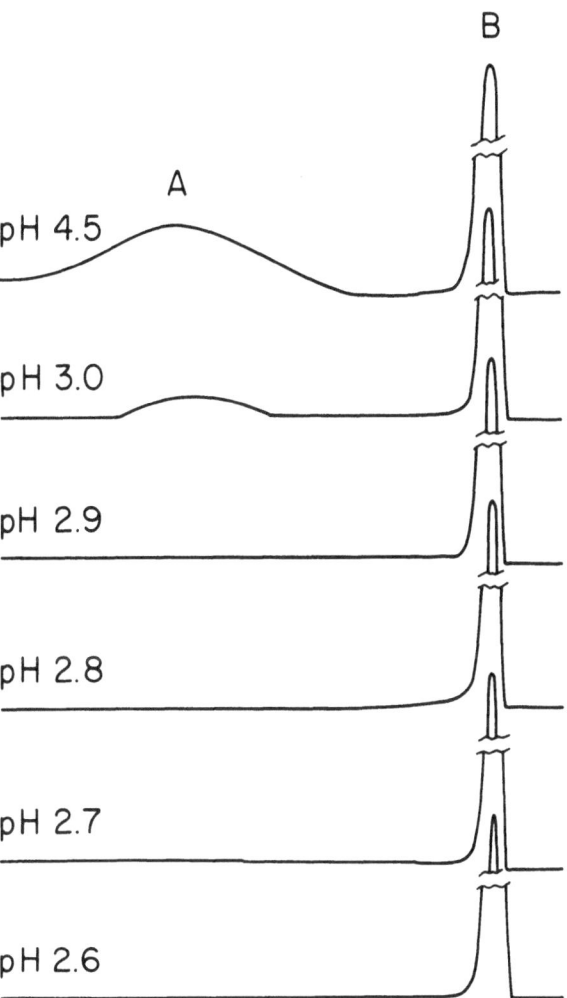

<u>Figure 5</u>. Tear hexosaminidase patterns obtained by automated DEAE-cellulose chromatography after tear samples were kept at the indicated pH for 5 min. at 37° and then brought to pH 6.0 with phosphate buffer.

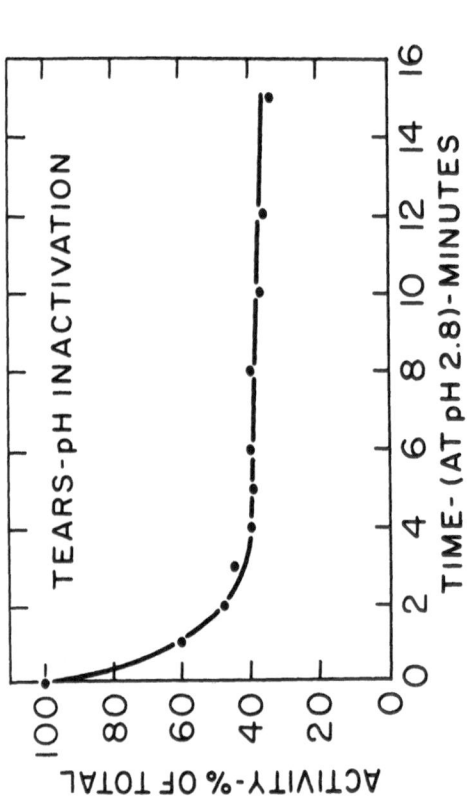

Figure 6. Time course (min.) of tear Hex A inactivation at pH 2.80 glycine-hydrochloride (0.5 moles/liter) buffer expressed as a percentage of the total activity.

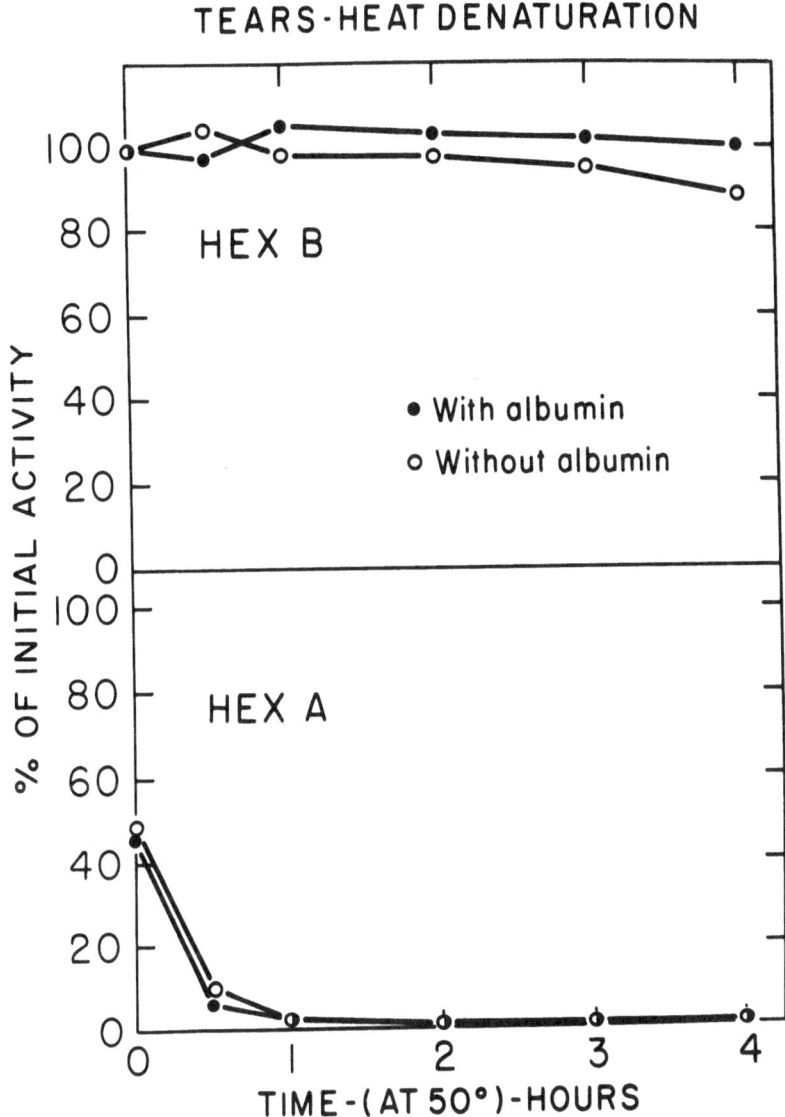

Figure 7. Effect of time (hr.) of incubation at 50°
on the activity of Hex B (top) and Hex A (bottom) of a
tear sample in the absence (-O-) and presence (-●-)
of albumin (1.0g/liter). The results are expressed as
a percentage of the initial activity of each isoenzyme
as measured with automated DEAE-cellulose chromatography.

after about one hour of incubation both in the absence
and presence of albumin but that there is less destruction of Hex B in the presence of albumin, than in
its absence, over a four hour time period. Based on
these data, the heat denaturation step for the analysis
of Hex B in tears was carried out for one and two hour
intervals in the presence of albumin and the Hex B values
obtained by the subsequent enzymatic assay were averaged.

Some 100 tear samples were divided into separate
categories based on the results obtained with serum and
leukocyte Hex A analysis (24). The tear samples were
then analyzed by the pH inactivation and heat denaturation methods described above. A correlation plot comparing the heat denaturation results with those obtained
with the pH inactivation method is presented in Figure 8.
The regression equation for the relationship is: y(pH
Inactivation) = 1.02 x (Heat Denaturation) - 1.50; the
correlation coefficient (r) is 0.92; which is significant at the 1% level.

Statistical analysis of the data obtained for tear
Hex A (as % of total hexosaminidase) is illustrated in
Figure 9 for the various groups of subjects tested with
the heat denaturation and pH inactivation methods. The
heat denaturation method provides clear-cut differentiation between the normal (non-Jewish) group, the
carrier (Tay-Sachs parents) group and the TSD children.
There is, however, a small overlap, i.e., less than 10%,
between the normal (non-carrier) pregnancy and the
carrier groups. The experimental data for tear Hex A
(%) with the pH inactivation method show considerably
greater degree of overlap between the normal and carrier
groups, i.e., about 20%, and about a 10% overlap between
the carrier and pregnancy groups. However, there is
complete statistical differentiation between homozygotes
and heterozygotes with this procedure. For the purpose
of TSD heterozygote detection by mass screening of the
Ashkenazic Jewish segment of a community, the manual
heat denaturation method appears to be preferable to
the manual pH inactivation procedure when tear samples
are used for the Hex A assay.

                            DISCUSSION

Because of the ease with which a urine sample can
be obtained, it would be the fluid of choice in any mass
screening program for heterozygote detection in a high
risk population with genetic disorders. Unfortunately,

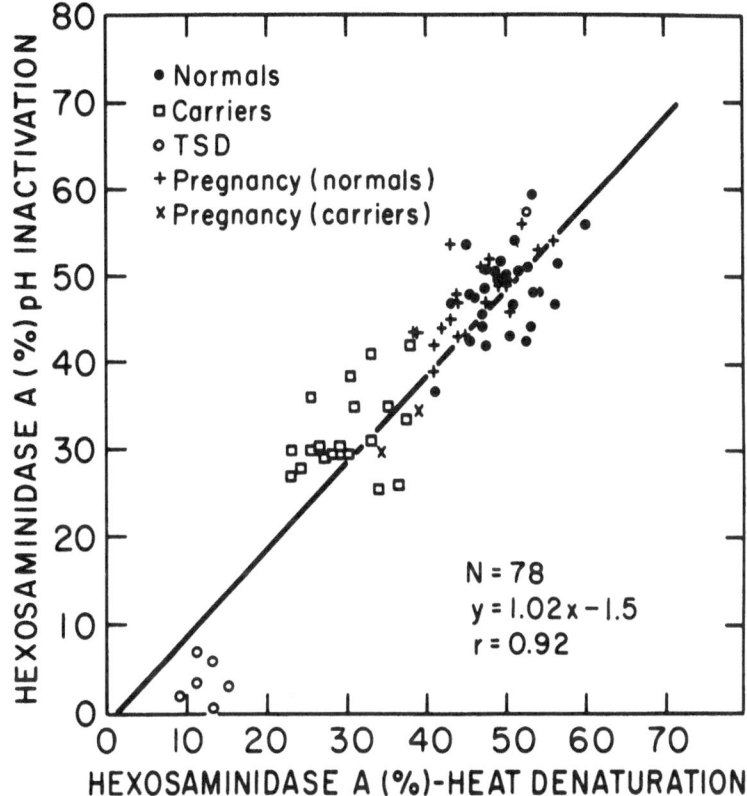

Figure 8. Comparison of data obtained for percentage of activity that is attributable to hexosaminidase A, as measured by the heat denaturation and pH inactivation methods, for tear samples from normal persons, TSD carriers, normal pregnant women, pregnant-carriers and children with TSD.

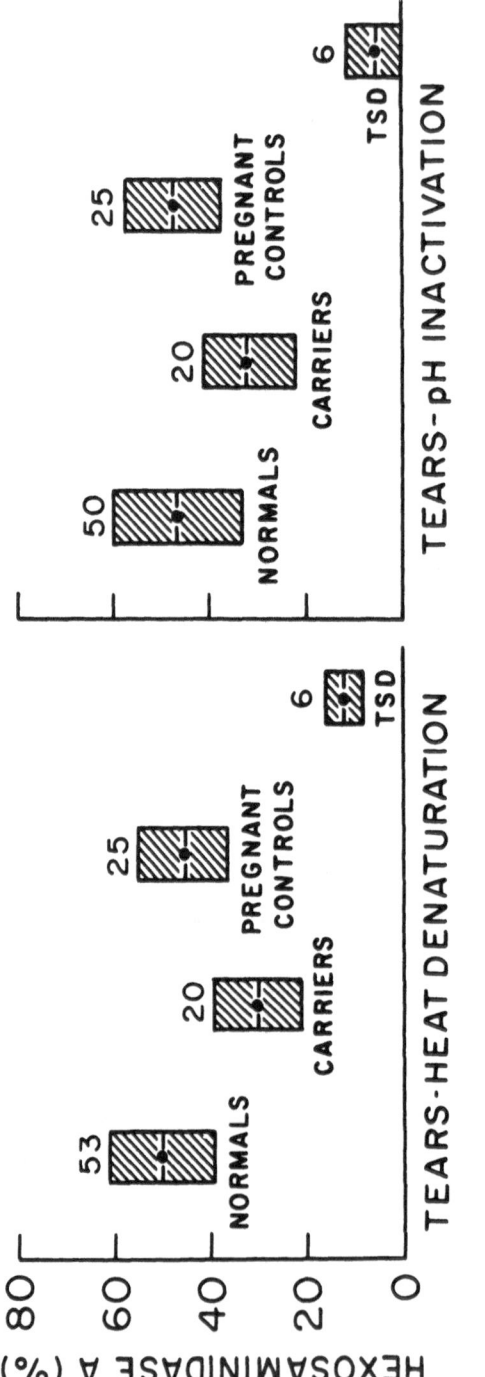

Figure 9. Statistical data (Mean (⊕) ± 2 SD) of tear hexosaminidase A levels obtained with the heat denaturation and pH inactivation methods for:- normal controls, TSD carriers, normal pregnancies, and TSD children. The number in parenthesis designates the number of subjects tested in each category.

our urinary Hex A statistical data for TSD genotypes does not substantiate the published conclusion of Navon and Padeh (18) that their results "demonstrate that the urine test is as dependable as that with leukocytes". Part of the reason for this discrepancy may lie in the small number of normal controls, i.e., 20 subjects, used by them in establishing their normal range. Also the total urinary hexosaminidase activity, and its iso-enzyme distribution,may represent an efflux from both intralysomal and non-lysosomal portions of the tubule cells as well as the action of neuraminidase on these enzymes (26). Not only would this situation result in a wide variation of normal urinary total hexosamin-idase and Hex B (1 to 30%) values but many persons with kidney disease would also give Hex A values similar to those obtained for TSD heterozygotes (18). The wide scatter of the data for urinary Hex A, in comparison with serum and leukocyte Hex A on the same individuals, and the statistical data in Table 1 preclude its use-fulness as a test for segregating TSD heterozygotes from non-carriers in the Ashkenazic Jewish population of a community. However, we are in agreement with other in-vestigators (18,27) that urine may be the preferable fluid to test for the absence of Hex A in an infant suspected clinically of having TSD as it eliminates the need for a blood sample.

The use of tear samples for the detection of TSD heterozygotes was proposed simultaneously by Carmody et al (19) and Singer et al (23). The many practical and economic advantages of the use of this fluid, in preference to serum or leukocyte samples, led Goldberg (28) to suggest its potential applicability for hetero-zygote detection and genetic counseling in other genetic disorders. In this connection, Johnson et al (29) found that tears provided an easily obtainable source of freshly excreted α-galactosidase for the diagnois of hemizygotes and heterozygotes with Fabry disease.

Our sampling technique for tear collection was similar to that of Singer et al (23) except that our filter paper strips consisted of the sterile, stand-ardized Schirmer tear test strips used by opthalmol-ogists to measure tear flow. The actual amount of sample collected on the tear strip is of little im-portance since the results of the analysis are ex-pressed as a ratio, i.e., % Hex A of the total hexos-aminidase activity. Except for the incorporation of albumin into the incubation buffer and modification

of the incubation time at $50^{\circ}C$, the heat denaturation
procedure for the tear Hex A analysis was similar to
that employed by previous investigators (19,23).

The statistical data in Figures 8 and 9 show widespread scatter and significant overlap of normal and
heterozygote ranges for the pH inactivation as compared
to the heat denaturation method. Part of the reason
for this discrepancy may lie in the fact that the pH
inactivation method is more subject to error as a
manual procedure because of the short incubation time,
i.e., 5 minutes, and because the samples were run in
duplicate instead of quadruplicate as for the heat denaturation method. As was the case for serum (9), conversion of the tear pH inactivation method from a manual
to an automated procedure may result in more accurate
Hex A ratio values and better differentiation between
normals and TSD heterozygotes. As with urine samples,
there is no difficulty in distinguishing TSD homozygotes
from all other categories by means of tear Hex A% values
regardless of which one of the two procedures is used for
the analysis.

In general, the Hex A% values obtained for tears with
the heat denaturation method are considerably below those
for serum or leukocytes for both normal and heterozygote
groups, c.f., Table 1. Our normal range for tear samples
obtained from 50 controls (39 to 61% Hex A) is close to
that of Singer et al (23) for 92 subjects; in that their
lower limit was 38% Hex A. The upper limit of our range
for 20 carriers (21 to 39% Hex A) is also in agreement
with theirs (39% Hex A) for 13 carriers. Our results
for tear samples (Figure 9) substantiate their conclusion that there is about a 3% overlap between tear
Hex A levels of "normals" and those of obligate heterozygotes. This is somewhat lower than the 5% overlap of
the Hex A% values in these groups found by O'Brien et
al (30) for serum, and higher than that reported for
leukocytes by Kaback and Zeiger (11). This means that
when tear samples are used for purposes of mass screening
for TSD Heterozygotes, about 5% of the test group may
require retesting with leukocyte samples with both acrylamide gel electrophoretic and heat denaturation methods
for Hex A (24). In line with the known carrier rate for
TSD in the Ashkenazic Jewish population, i.e., 1:30 (7),
3% of the original test group will be confirmed as carriers of the TSD gene. Of the remaining 2% in the "inclusive range", only 1 out of 10 individuals will prove
to be a TSD carrier and less than 1 in 1000 persons

tested will remain as "inconclusive" (11). This is not
a serious matter in regard to preventing the birth of
a Tay-Sachs child as it is unlikely that the spouse of
such an individual will be either a TSD carrier or will
also fall into the "inconclusive" category.

The problem of pregnancy is of great concern to
all genetic centers engaged in TSD carrier detection
of which there are now more than 50 such facilities in
the United States and Canada. Many parents become concerned about the possibility of having a genetically
defective child only after conception has occurred. It
has also become a routine practice for many obstetri-
cians with a Jewish clientele to send such pregnant
patients and their husbands to genetic centers to be
tested as potential carriers of the Tay-Sachs gene.
Since there is a complete overlap between serum Hex A%
values in normal pregnancy with those found in the
carrier range (9,11,15), the analysis has to be performed on lysed leukocyte preparations. This is both
a laborious and time-consuming operation which does not
yield entirely satisfactory results since we have found
about a 20% overlap between the normal pregnancy and
TSD carrier ranges for leukocyte Hex A% values with the
heat denaturation method (15). It is for these reasons
that we were most interested in the report of Carmody
et al (19) that the Hex A ratio in tears is not altered
during pregnancy. Shortly thereafter, we came across
the finding of Singer et al (23) that there is no significant difference between the tear and serum Hex A
ratio values of pregnant women, i.e., results for both
fluids fell within the TSD heterozygote range. Our
tear Hex A ratio values by heat denaturation for 25
women in various stages of pregnancy ranged from 36 to
55% Hex A and show less than a 10% overlap with the
carrier range. These results are contrary to those of
Singer et al (23) and lend support to the findings of
Carmody et al (19) that tear sample Hex A ratios are
considerably less influenced by pregnancy than are serum
Hex A% values. This finding constitutes still another
important reason why we believe that tear specimens will
eventually replace all other sampling techniques for
providing the concentrated enzymes needed to study and
prevent the many inborn errors of metabolism which
affect man (28).

SUMMARY

1. Two readily obtainable biological fluids, i.e.,
urine and tears, were investigated as possible sub-
stitutes for serum and leukocytes for the detection
of Tay-Sachs disease (TSD) heterozygotes based on
quantitative hexosaminidase A (Hex A) determinations.

2. Hexosaminidase isoenzyme patterns were determined,
by means of an automated DEAE-cellulose microcolumn
procedure, for serum, urine and tear samples from
normals, TSD carriers, normal pregnancies, carrier-
pregnancies and TSD children.

3. Normal pregnancy and TSD carrier sera gave almost
identical hexosaminidase patterns with multiple intermediate peaks. Whereas, urine and tear samples from
normal pregnant women showed hexosaminidase isoenzyme
patterns resembling those of normal controls. These
results suggested that use of these fluids might eliminate the effect of pregnancy on the Hex A ratio which
occurs when serum is used as the test fluid. In addition these fluids are more economical and simpler to
obtain than a blood sample.

4. About 200 urine samples, from the various categories
listed above, were analyzed for Hex A with both the heat
denaturation and pH inactivation methods and the results
compared with serum and leukocyte levels from many of
the same individuals. With either method, the wide
overlap between the urinary Hex A normal and heterozygote
ranges would require retesting with leukocytes of about
30% of the subjects. These results would preclude the
use of urines as a suitable fluid for the mass screening
of the Ashkenazic Jewish population for TSD heterozygotes.

5. The experimental parameters for tear Hex A analysis
by the pH inactivation and heat denaturation methods
were investigated.

6. Application of these procedures to the quantitative
analysis of the Hex A content of tear samples obtained
from the various groups listed above, indicated the
superiority of the manual heat denaturation procedure
over that of the pH inactivation method with respect to
separation of the normal and carrier ranges. Unlike
serum, where there is an almost complete statistical
overlap between the normal pregnancy and TSD carrier

Hex A% ranges, tear samples show less than a 10% over-lap for these groups.

7. Homozygotes (TSD children) show clear-cut statistical differentiation from all TSD genotypes regardless of the biological fluid, or the method used, for the Hex A analysis. However, either urine or tears are more easily obtainable than a blood sample for confirming a diagnosis of TSD based on the determination of their Hex A content.

8. Tear samples, absorbed on sterile, standardized (Schirmer) filter paper test strips, provide a practical, economical and readily obtainable source of concentrated enzymes, e.g., hexosaminidase, α-galactosidase, etc, suitable for heterozygote detection of inborn errors of metabolism by mass screening of the population at risk.

ACKNOWLEDGEMENTS

This study was aided by a grant from the National Tay-Sachs and Allied Diseases Association, New York, N.Y.

The authors wish to acknowledge the technical assistance of Mr. Ronald Silverman in obtaining some of the experimental data used in these studies and the aid of Mrs. Lillian Salowitz with the editing and typing of the manuscript.

REFERENCES

1. Okada,S., and O'Brien,J.S., Tay-Sachs disease. Generalized absence of a beta-D-N-acetylhexosaminidase component. Science 165, 698 (1969).

2. Sandhoff,K., Variation of β-N-acetylhexosaminidase-pattern in Tay-Sachs disease. FEBS Letters 4:351,1969.

3. Svennerholm,L., The chemical structure of normal human brain and Tay-Sachs gangliosides. Biochem. Biophys. Res. Commun. 9, 436 (1962).

4. Saifer,A., and Wishnow,D.E., Disturbances of lipid metabolism and their relationship to the lipidoses. In "Handbook of Clinical Neurology", Vol. 10, P.J.Vinken and G.W.Bruyn, Eds. North-Holland Publ. Co., Amsterdam, 1970, pp265-324.

5.   Volk,B.W., and Schneck,L., "The Gangliosidoses". Plenum Press, New York, N.Y., 1975.

6.   Stanbury,J.B., Wyngaarden,J.B., and Fredrickson, D.S., "The Metabolic Basis of Inherited Disease", 3rd ed., McGraw-Hill, New York, N.Y., 1972.

7.   Aronson,S.M., and Volk,B.W., Genetic and demographic considerations concerning Tay-Sachs' disease. In "Cerebral Sphingolipidoses", S.M.Aronson and B.W. Volk, Eds., Academic Press, New York, N.Y., 1962, pp375-394.

8.   Lowden,J.A., Skomorowski,M.A., Henderson,F., and Kaback,M., Automated assay of hexosaminidases in serum. Clin. Chem. 19, 1345 (1973).

9.   Saifer,A., and Perle,G., Automated determination of serum hexosaminidase A by pH inactivation for detection of Tay-Sachs disease heterozygotes. Clin. Chem. 20, 538 (1974).

10. Schneck,L., Friedland,J., Valenti,C., Adachi,M., Amsterdam,D., and Volk,B.W., Prenatal diagnosis of Tay-Sachs disease. Lancet 1, 582 (1970).

11. Kaback,M.M., and Zeiger,R.S., Heterozygote detection in Tay-Sachs disease:A prototype community screening program for the prevention of recessive disorders. In "Sphingolipids, Sphingolipidoses and Allied Disorders". B.W.Volk and S.M.Aronson, Eds., Plenum Press, New York, N.Y., 1972, pp613-632.

12. O'Brien,J.S., Okada,S., Chen,A., and Fillerup,D.L., Tay-Sachs disease: Detection of heterozygotes and homozygotes by serum hexosaminidase assay. New Engl. J. Med. 283, 15 (1970).

13. Stirling,J.L., Separation and characterization of N-acetyl-β-glucosaminidases A and P from meternal serum. Biochim. Biophys. Acta 271, 154 (1972).

14. Price,G., and Dance,N., The demonstration of multiple heat stable forms of N-acetyl-β-glucosaminidase in normal human serum. Biochim. Biophys.Acta 271,145 (1972).

15.   Saifer,A., Perle,G., Valenti,C., and Schneck,L.,
Pre- and postnatal detection of Tay-Sachs disease. A
comparative study of biochemical screening methods.
In "Sphingolipids, Sphingolipidoses and Allied Disorders".
B.W.Volk and S.M.Aronson, Eds. Plenum Press, New York,
N.Y., 1972, pp599-611.

16.   Saifer,A., Parkhurst,G.W., and Amoroso,J., Automated differentiation and measurement of hexosaminidase
isoenzymes in biological fluids and its application to
pre- and postnatal detection of Tay-Sachs disease. Clin.
Chem. 21, 334 (1975).

17.   Ellis,R.B., Ikonne,J.U., and Masson,P.K., DEAE-
cellulose microcolumn chromatography coupled with automated assay:Application to the resolution of N-acetyl-
β-D-hexosaminidase components. Anal. Biochem. 63, 5
(1975).

18.   Navon,R., and Padeh,B., Urinary test for identification of Tay-Sachs genotypes. J. Pediat. 80, 1026
(1972).

19.   Carmody, P.J., Rattazzi, M.C., and Davidson, R.G.,
Tay-Sachs disease-the use of tears for the detection of
heterozygotes. New Engl. J. Med. 289, 1072 (1973).

20.   Saifer,A., and Rosenthal,A.L., Rapid test for the
detection of Tay-Sachs disease heterozygotes and homozygotes by serum hexosaminidase assay. Clin.Chim. Acta
43, 417 (1973).

21.   Friedland,J., Schneck,L., Saifer,A., Pourfar,M.,
and Volk,B.W., Identification of Tay-Sachs disease
carriers by acrylamide gel electrophoresis. Clin.
Chim. Acta 28, 397 (1970).

22.   Padeh,B., and Navon,R., Diagnosis of Tay-Sachs
disease by hexosaminidase activity in leukocytes and
amniotic cells. Isr. J. Med. Sci. 7, 259 (1971).

23.   Singer,J.D., Cotlier,E., and Krimmer,R., Hexosaminidase A in tears and saliva for rapid identification of Tay-Sachs disease and its carriers. Lancet
2, 1116 (1973).

24.   Perle,G., and Saifer,A., Methods for pre- and
postnatal detection of Tay-Sachs disease heterozygotes
(carriers) and homozygotes (patients) by means of

hexosaminidase analysis of their fluids and tissues.
In "Amniotic Fluid". S. Natelson, A. Scommegna and M.B.
Epstein, Eds. J. Wiley & Sons, New York, N.Y., 1974,
pp373-381.

25.   Sandman,R., Margules,R.M., and Kountz,S.L., Urinary
liposomal glycosidases after renal allotransplantation:
correlation of enzyme excretion with allograft rejection
and ischemia. Clin. Chim. Acta 45, 349 (1973).

26.   Hultberg,B., Ockerman,P.A., Norden,N.E., Isoenzymes
of four acid hydrolases in human kidney and urine. Clin.
Chim. Acta 52, 239 (1974).

27.   Grebner,E.E., and Tucker,J., Human urinary N-acetyl-
β-hexosaminidases. Biochim. Biophys. Acta 321, 228(1973).

28.   Goldberg,M.F., The use of tears for heterozygote
detection and genetic counseling (An editorial). Invest.
Ophthal. 13, 159 (1974).

29.   Johnson, D.L., Del Monte, M.A., Cotlier,E., and
Desnick, R.J., Fabry disease: Diagnosis by α-galactosidase activities in tears. Clin.Chim.Acta 63, 81(1975).

30.   O'Brien,J.S., Ho,M.W., Okada,S., Zielke,K., Veath,
M.L., and Tennant,L., Sphingolipidoses: Detection of
heterozygotes and homozygotes. In "Sphingolipids,
Sphingolipidoses and Allied Disorders". B.W.Volk and
S.M.Aronson, Eds. Plenum Press, New York, N.Y., 1972,
pp581-597.

SPHINGOMYELINASES AND THE GENETIC DEFECTS IN NIEMANN-PICK DISEASE

John W. Callahan and Mary Khalil

The Hospital For Sick Children

555 University Avenue, Toronto, Ontario

The Niemann-Pick Diseases (N-P) are clinically and biochemically heterogeneous. The common name is derived from the early work of Albert Niemann and Ludwig Pick who described the classical form in the years 1914-1928 (1) The first documented variation of these classical characteristics was described by Videbaek in 1949 (2) The latter patient was remarkable since no neurological impairment was found whereas all previous patients did show severe neurological degeneration. Later, in 1958, Crocker and Farber (3) described 18 patients with variable clinical expression and developed a classification which remains in use today (4) The features of each type of disease are shown in Table 1.

The major storage product in the N-P diseases is sphingomyelin. Various theories were proposed to explain the storage of this phospholipid but it was not until 1966 that the genetic defect was recognized. Brady et al (5) showed for the first time that sphingomyelin was hydrolyzed by the lysosomal acid hydrolase, sphingomyelinase. The activity of this enzyme in tissues from the classical disease (now called Type A) was virtually undetectable. The genetic defect in this disease had thus been found. Schneider and Kennedy (6) confirmed the observations of Brady and coworkers and noted further a marked deficiency of sphingomyelinase in the non-neuronopathic form (Type B). Tissues from patients with the juvenile form (Type C) showed normal enzyme levels while in the so-called Nova Scotia variant (Type D) the activity was lower than normal.

Several major gaps in our understanding of these diseases exist. We have been impressed by the variations in nervous system involvement and the relatively minor storage of sphingomyelin in

TABLE 1

DIFFERENTIAL DIAGNOSIS OF NIEMANN-PICK DISEASE, TYPES A-E

CRITERION	TYPE A	TYPE B	TYPE C	TYPE D	TYPE E
Neurological Symptoms	onset within first year of life	Normal	onset after 1-2 years	early to middle childhood	often normal
Age at death	about 3 years	many live into adult-hood	variable, some live into adolescence	late teens, early 20's	20's--
Hepatosplenomegaly	Pronounced	Pronounced	Moderate	Moderate	Moderate
Foam cells in bone marrow	Yes	Yes	Yes	Yes	Yes
Sphingomyelin storage Brain Viscera	Yes Massive	No Massive	No Moderate	N.D. Moderate	N.D. Moderate
Sphingomyelinase Activity	virtually absent in all tissues	about 10% of normal in viscera brain levels unknown	near normal in all tissues	variable, often normal	Normal

the brain in Type A. Children with Type C clearly store sphingomyelin in their visceral organs yet show no obvious abnormality in
sphingomyelinase activity. In Type B, despite low levels of sphingomyelinase activity, there is no apparent neurological deficit. We
reasoned that multiple species of sphingomyelinase may exist and
that a deficiency in one or several species reflected the genetic
defect in each disorder. If so, then it would be possible to explain the variability in clinical and biochemical presentation.
The experiments we have performed attempt to determine the expression of the defects in several of the Niemann-Pick diseases.

As a necessary first step, we have measured sphingomyelinase
activity in crude extracts of several tissues obtained from controls
and patients with N-P disease. In liver, sphingomyelinase activity
is readily demonstrable (Table 2). Sphingomyelinase activity was
barely detectable in Type A (three cases) while in the single case
of Type B, the residual activity was substantially higher. Essentially normal levels of activity were found in all three cases of
Type C and a single case of Type D.

TABLE 2

LYSOSOMAL HYDROLASES IN HUMAN LIVER

Diagnosis		Specific Activities[+]		
		Sphingo-myelinase	β Hexo-saminidase	β-galactosidase
Normal (7)		12.0 ± 5.5 (5.5 - 21.0)	3.86 ± 2.16 (1.80 - 6.92)	92.5 ± 50.5 (25.2 - 160.0)
Niemann-Pick				
Type A	1.	1.3	2.20	59.1
	2.	0.4	3.39	20.5
	3.	0.1	5.43	45.5
Type B		3.4	4.68	90.0
Type C	1.	8.3	5.72	76.0
	2.	10.1	7.04	172.0
	3.	21.4	4.15	44.0
Type D		24.2	5.11	11.0

[+] Specific activities refer to the nanomoles (μmoles for β hexosaminidase) product formed per hour per mg protein. β-Hexosaminidase and β-galactosidase were assayed with the respective nitro-
phenylglycosides as described (7,8).

TABLE 3

SPHINGOMYELINASE IN NIEMANN-PICK TISSUES[+]

	BRAIN SM		LIVER SM		SPLEEN SM		KIDNEY SM	
	^{32}P	^{3}H	^{32}P	^{3}H	^{32}P	^{3}H	^{32}P	^{3}H
Normal	31.0	22.9	34.2	22.6	17.6	14.6	53.8	53.9
Niemann-Pick, A 1	6.3 / 8.3	0.3	0.0	1.3	0.4	0.2	0.4	0.8
2			0.3	0.4	1.6	0.1	0.7	1.1
3			0.2	0.1				
Niemann-Pick, C 1	26.1	11.8	7.5	5.0	25.9	14.2	28.8	19.8
2	28.2	22.3	3.9	3.7	11.5	10.4	42.6	29.0

+ Sphingomyelinase activity is the nanomoles sphingomyelin hydrolysed/hr/mg protein. Tissues were homogenized in 10 volumes 0.25 M sucrose. Sphingomyelinase activity with ^{32}P-labeled sphingomyelin was assayed according to Kanfer et al (11) while with ^{3}H-labeled sphingomyelin the method was that of Schneider and Kennedy (5).

The same pattern emerges when other tissues such as brain, spleen, kidney and cultured fibroblasts are tested. With ^{32}P-labeled sphingomyelin isolated from fibroblast cultures exposed to $H_3{}^{32}PO_4$ the results are the same as with ^{3}H-sphingomyelin (Table 3). The expression of the genetic defects in cultured fibroblasts confirms the findings in other tissues (Table 4). The cultured cells der- ived from a patient with Type B showed a residual sphingomyelinase activity of 3.5% of normal which is far less activity than detected in liver of another case while in Type A, the levels of residual activity were approximately the same in all tissues.

TABLE 4

LYSOSOMAL HYDROLASES IN CULTURED FIBROBLASTS

Cell Strain		Specific Activities		
		Sphingo-myelinase	β-Hexo-saminidase	β-Galacto-sidase
Normal	1.	25.8	1096	160
	2.	27.6	2250	275
	3.	21.5	7028	273
	4.	23.0	-	357
Pathological Cystic Fibrosis		58.9	3619	876
GM$_1$-gangliosidosis		62.3	15,525	20
GM$_2$-gangliosidosis		31.2	2930	324
Niemann-Pick Type A	1.	0.35	3125	400
	2.	0.40	6325	355
	3.	0.20	1830	-
Type B		0.83	2361	342
Type C	1.	17.0	1330	-
	2.	9.0	1700	-
	3.	17.6	3683	44
Type E		55.7	3866	461

* The cells were harvested by trypsinization, washed and lyophil- ized. The dried powder was weighed, homogenized in 1% glycine and centrifuged. The specific activities, determined in the super- natant fluids, refer to the nanomoles product formed per hour per mg protein. All numbers are averages of measurements taken at four protein concentrations. With Types A and C, the cell lines were derived from additional patients not referred to in Table 1.

There is virtually normal total activity in cultured cells
derived from Type C patients while the single example of Type E gave
a higher than normal result.

To test the hypothesis that multiple species of sphingomyelinase existed we chose to analyze tissue extracts by isoelectric
focusing. Our experience with other separation techniques such
as the ion-exchange celluloses and Sephadex columns suggested that
these methods were unsatisfactory for this purpose. Isoelectric
focusing was carried out in a Uniphor column electrophoresis
system according to standard methods (7-9). Liver sphingomyelinase
activity was resolved into five distinct peaks of activity, called
I-V according to their increasing isoelectric points (Figure 1).
Normal liver contains two major peaks I and II (pI 4.6 and 4.8)
which together constitute about 80% of the total activity recovered.
Similar profiles were obtained for spleen and placenta. Liver from
three cases of N-P disease, Type C showed only peak I while peak II
was absent (Figures 1 & 2). When the activity in this major peak
was recovered and re-focused under the same conditions, the enzyme
again focused to the same point (pI 4.6). Peaks II and III when
re-focused also concentrate at their respective isoelectric points
(4.8 and 5.0) (8). Recovery of enzyme activity was excellent (70-
90%) for the initial analysis and for the re-focused enzyme. Liver
from the case of Type B was also analyzed (Figure 3). All the major
peaks seen in normal liver could be discerned. Peaks I-IV were markedly reduced whereas peak V (pI 7.1) was found at or near the normal
level. The enzyme activity in the latter peak usually constitutes
about 5-10 of the total activity. Liver from a single case of
Type D had a normal isoelectric focusing pattern (10).

Brain sphingomyelinase was analyzed in the same manner but the
profile was different (Figure 4). The majority of the activity
focused in a wide zone (pI 4.4-4.7). On the shoulder of the major
peak a second peak was seen at pI 5.0. The latter is likely peak
II as seen in normal liver since in the two brain specimens from patients with Type C, the enzyme activity in this region of the gradient was greatly reduced. Small peaks of activity could also be seen
at pI 5.4 (comparable to peak IV in liver) and pI values near 7
(peak V).

Sphingomyelinase activity in cultured fibroblasts was resolved
into three peaks (I-III) whose isoelectric points (4.6, 4.8, 5.1)
were identical to those found in the liver (Figure 5). Peaks IV
and V have not been observed in extracts prepared in glycine (9).
In the two Type A cases, peak I was the major residual enzyme observed while trace activity in peaks II and III was detected. The
Type B pattern found was consistent to that obtained in liver; namely,
a marked reduction in all peaks but maintenance of a normal enzyme
distribution. We have analyzed one cell line from Type E and two
from Type C cases. The Type E fibroblasts showed a prominent peak

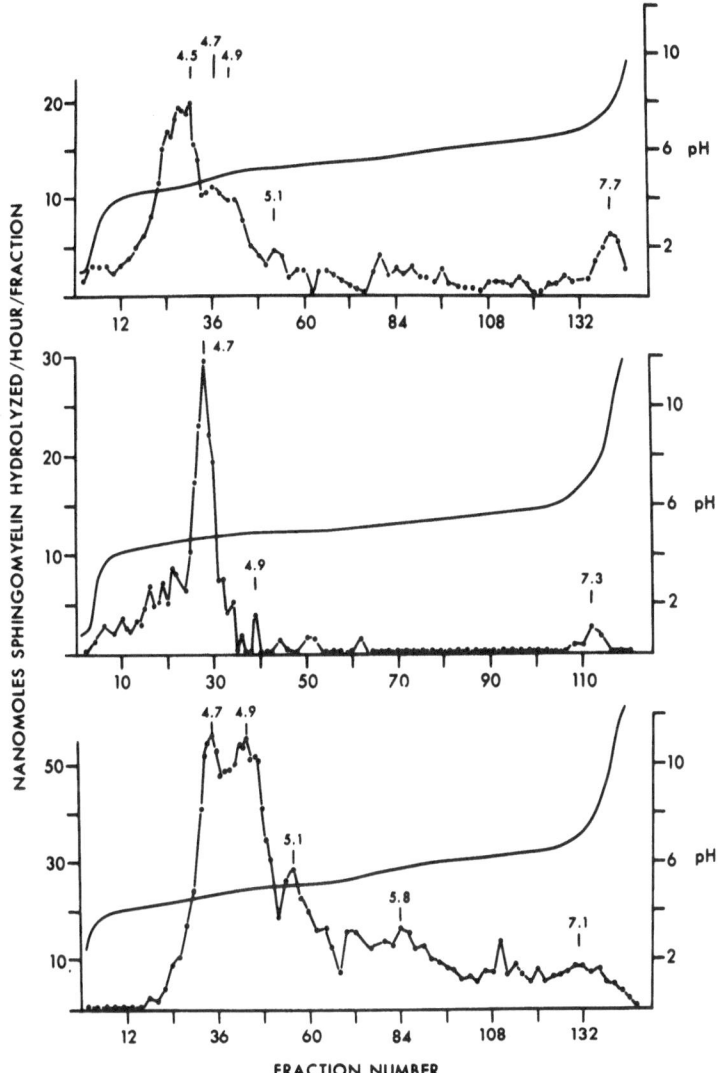

Figure 1

Sphingomyelinase activity in normal liver and in Niemann-Pick, Type C. The extracts were prepared from 1 g frozen liver and analyzed separately. Normal liver (lower panel) is compared with liver from Case I (upper panel) and from Case 2 (middle panel). The isoelectric points of the major peaks are indicated. Recovery was 85,65 and 78 per cent for the normal Cases I and 2 respectively. The pH gradient is the solid line.

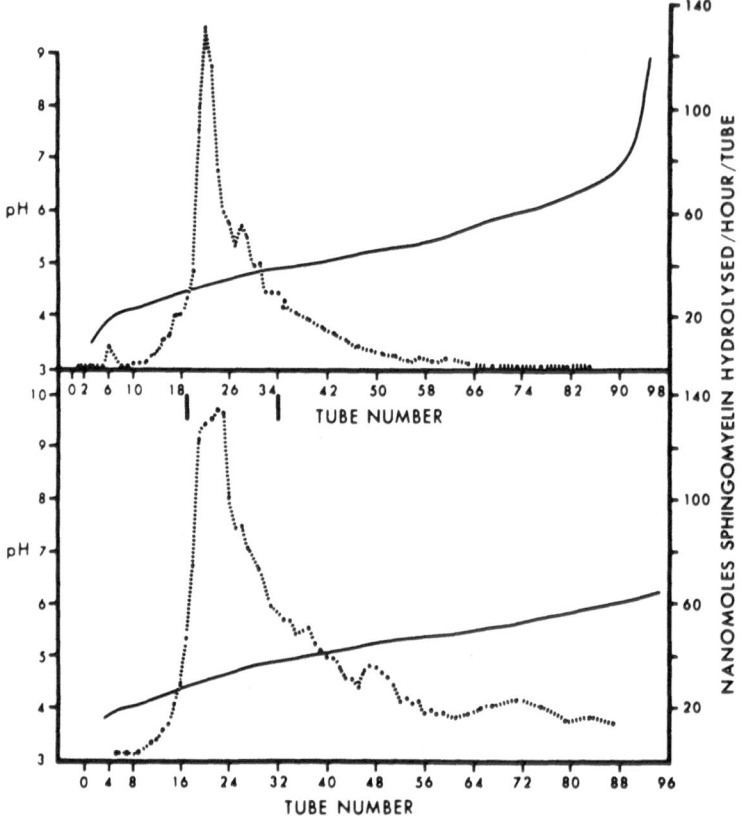

Figure 2

Isoelectric focusing of Niemann-Pick Type C liver. The extract
prepared from one gram of tissue (Case 3) contained 62 mg protein and 3,500 units of sphingomyelinase (Lower). The pH gradient measured at 4° C is shown as the solid line. Recovery of
enzyme was 79%. The enzyme in tubes 17-32 was pooled, centrifuged
and re-focused with a pI of 4.6 (Upper).

I, peak II was absent and peak III was normal (Figure 5). The
pattern in Type C was identical to that of Type E and confirmed a
specific loss of peak II in patients with this disease.

These data strongly suggest that multiple forms of sphingomyelinase exist in human tissues. The data on tissues from Types
A and B indicate a genetic and structural relationship between
all forms of the lysosomal sphingomyelinase. It is not clear
whether the multiple peaks of activity seen on isoelectric

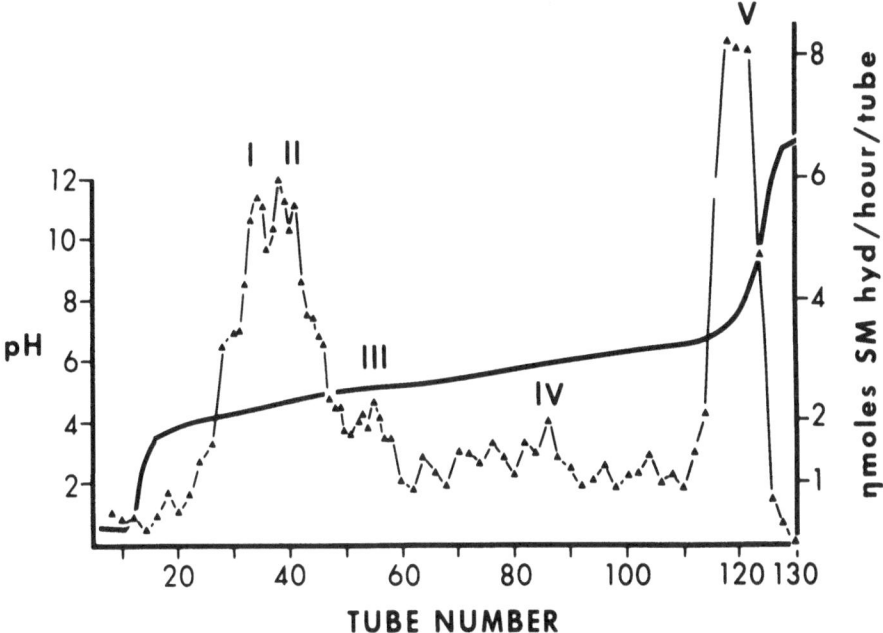

Figure 3

Sphingomyelinase profile in Niemann-Pick, Type B Liver. Liver
(1g) was processed in the usual manner (7-9). Five peaks of activity (I-IV) were found at the same isoelectric points as in the
normal. Not the reduced levels of peaks I-IV while peak V is
near normal. Recovery was 85%. The solid line is the pH gradient.

focusing reflect isoenzymes of sphingomyelinase since little is
known about their protein structure. It is conceivable that the
enzyme is a multimer with each species composed of one or more
different protein monomers. Further research is needed to clarify
this point.

    Recent data have indicated the existence of an additional
sphingomyelinase which acts at physiological pH in the brain (10).
This enzyme is highly unstable but shares properties similar to
those described by Schneider and Kennedy (6).

    It is likely that the properties of the brain sphingomyelinases
analyzed in this work coupled with the presence of a neutral brain
sphingomyelinase contribute to the diverse neurological and biochemical manifestations of the Niemann-Pick diseases in the central
nervous system.

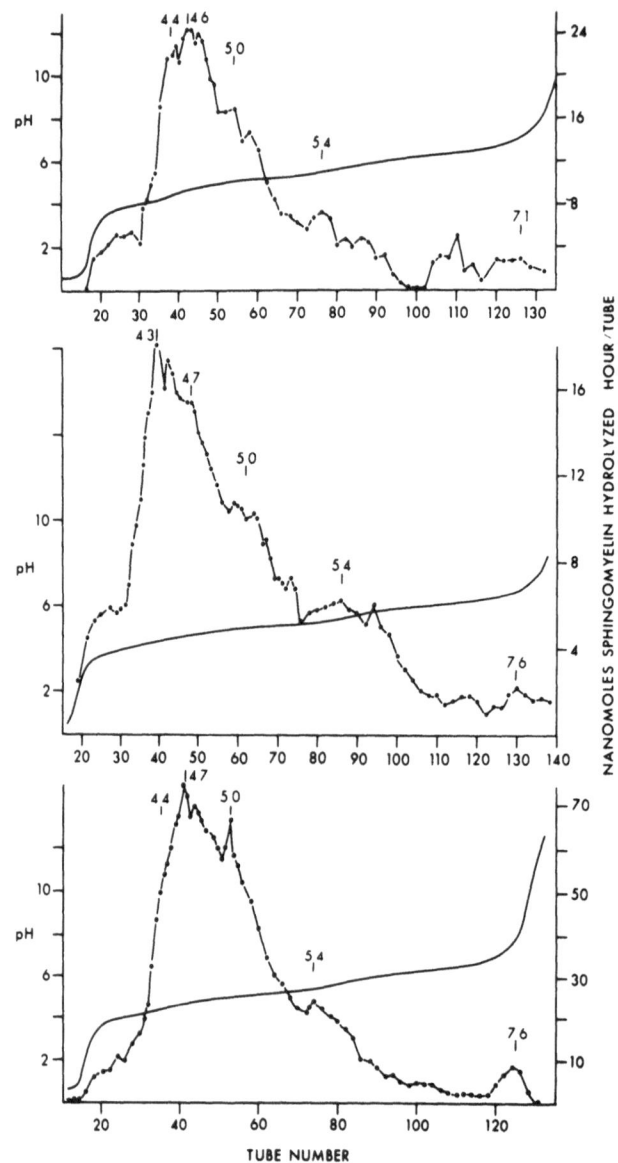

Figure 4

<u>Sphingomyelinase activity in human brain.</u> Brain samples (2 g)
from normal (lower panel), Case 1 (upper panel) and Case 2
(middle panel) were analyzed. Two major peaks of activity (pI
4.7 and 5.0) were found in the normal but were incompletely resolved. In the diseased brain, only the first major peak (pI
4.3 - 4.7) was prominent. Recovery of activity in all instances
was over 90 per cent. The solid line represents the pH graai-
ent.

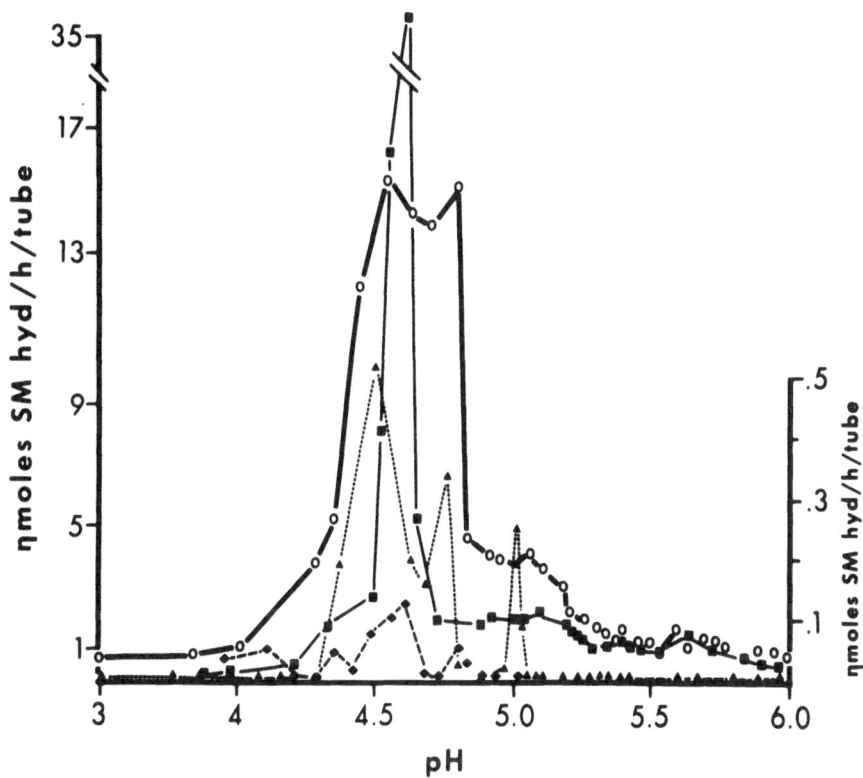

Figure 5

Sphingomyelinases in Fibroblasts from Patients with Niemann-Pick
Disease. All cells were lyophilized, weighed and homogenized in
cold 1% glycine. The left ordinate scale refers to cells from a
normal strain (O—O) and from Type E (■—■), while the right
ordinate refers to cells derived from patients with Type B (▲--▲)
and Type A (case 1,◆-◆). Little sphingomyelinase activity was
found above pH 6.0. Total protein applied to the column was 6.7,
3.2, 3.3 and 5.8 mg protein for the control and Niemann-Pick
Disease cells from Types E, A (Case 1) and B respectively. Electrofocusing of cells from Type A (Case 2) gave the same results as
shown for case 1. The pattern obtained for cells derived from
two cases of Type C was the same as for Type E.

It is our view that the genetic defects in Types A and B are different from one another and together are different from Types C and E. We have proposed that the genetic defect in Type C is the specific loss of sphingomyelinase II. This also seems to be true for cases with Type E.

ACKNOWLEDGEMENTS

This work was supported by province of Ontario Health Grant (PR 360 C) and by the Medical Research Council of Canada (MA-4873). J.W.C. is a MRC scholar.

REFERENCES

1. Fredrickson, D.S. and Sloan, H.R.: Sphingomyelin Lipidoses in The Metabolic Basis of Inherited Diseases J.B. Stanbury, J. B. Wyngaarden and D.S. Fredrickson (Eds) Chap. 35 McGraw Hill Publ. Co., New York, 1972 p. 783.

2. Videbaek, A. (1949) Acta Paediat. 37, 95.

3. Crocker, A.C. and Farber, S. (1958) Medicine 37, 1.

4. Crocker, A.C. (1961) J. Neurochem. 7, 69.

5. Brady, R.O., Kanfer, J.N., Mock, M.B. and Fredrickson, D.S. (1966) Proc. Natn. Acad. Sci. U.S.A., 55, 366.

6. Schneider, P.B. and Kennedy, E.P. (1967) J. Lipid Res. 8, 202.

7. Callahan, J.W., Khalil, M. and Philippart, M. (1975) Pediat. Res (in press).

8. Callahan, J.W., Khalil, M. and Gerrie, J. (1974) Biochem. Biophys. Res. Comm. 58, 384.

9. Callahan, J.W. and Khalil, M. (1975) Pediat. Res. (in press).

10 Rao, B. Ph.D. Thesis 1974. Dalhousie University, Halifax, N.S.

11. Kanfer, J.N., Young, O.M., Shapiro, D. and Brady, R.O. (1966) J. Biol. Chem. 241, 1081.

ADRENOLEUKODYSTROPHY:

A CLINICAL, PATHOLOGICAL AND BIOCHEMICAL STUDY

H.H. Schaumburg,[x] J. M. Powers,[xxx]   C. S. Raine,[xx]
A.B. Johnson,[xx] E.H. Kolodny,[xxxx] Y. Kishimoto,[xxxx]
M. Igarashi,[x] and K. Suzuki[x]

The Saul R. Korey Department of Neurology,[x] Department
of Pathology,[xx] and the Rose F. Kennedy Center for
Research in Mental Retardation and Human Development,[x,xx]
Albert Einstein College of Medicine, Bronx, N.Y. 10461;
Department of Pathology,[xxx] Medical University of South
Carolina, Charleston, South Carolina 29401; and the
Eunice Kennedy Shriver Center for Mental Retardation,[xxxx]
Waltham, Mass. 02154

HISTORICAL BACKGROUND

The association of diffuse cerebral demyelination and adrenal
disease was first adequately described by Siemerling and Creutzfeldt in 1923 (13). The report of Siemerling and Creutzfeldt
was followed by similar isolated case studies. Despite the start-
ling nature of these reports, the association of adrenal atrophy
and cerebral demyelination was considered coincidental, and these
cases were usually described as melanodermic leukodystrophy or
brown Schilder's disease. The studies of Gagnon and Leblanc in
1959 (4), Hoefnagel et al. in 1962 (5) and especially Fanconi et
al. in 1963 (3) established this combination of neurologic and endocrine abnormalities as a hereditary disease, probably with a
sex-linked recessive transmission. Since that time there have
been at least 40 well-documented cases. Blaw, in 1971, introduced
the term adrenoleukodystrophy (ALD) to describe this condition (1).
Our identification, in 1972 of specific light microscopic cytoplasmic changes in the adrenal cortical cells of nine males diagnosed as having Schilder's disease (10), and the subsequent ultrastructural characterization of the inclusions (7), led to the
recognition of similar abnormal inclusions in Schwann cells, testis,
and brain (8,11,12).

379

A recent review of case material relating to Schilder's disease collected at the Massachusetts General Hospital (MGH) and of the cases reported as Schilder's disease in the literature has determined that the overwhelming majority of the cases in males are instances of ALD (9). The cases occurring in females and in males with no adrenal atrophy most probably represent a variety of multiple sclerosis. Our experience supports Richardson's conclusion that Schilder's disease is no longer a justifiable designation.

This report describes some of the results of a five year mutlidisciplinary study of 41 autopsy proven cases of ALD, which has lead us to propose that it is a lipid storage disease, resulting in a striking variety of clinical and pathological findings in the adrenal gland, brain, peripheral nerve and testis.

CLINICAL STUDIES

A retrospective analysis of the clinical findings indicates that ·the development of abnormal behavior and disturbance of vision or gait in a young boy should suggest a diagnosis of ALD. If there is any demonstrable evidence of diminished adrenal cortical function, the diagnosis is virtually certain.

Central Nervous System

Central nervous system signs and symptoms have been consistently more prominent than signs of adrenal involvement. Behavioral changes were the most common initial finding and ranged from aggressive outbursts to withdrawal. Such behavior was generally accompanied by a gradually failing memory and poor school performance. Loss of vision was an early finding in some patients and was a prominent feature at some stage in almost every patient. The initial visual loss appeared as homonomous hemianopsia in some patients and was usually associated with intact pupillary reflexes. Optic atrophy was less common as an initial finding but eventually developed in all cases. Gait disturbance was also an early finding and usually was stiff-legged, unsteady and accompanied by hyperreflexia. Eventually, in every case, there was spastic quadraplegia and a variable degree of decorticate posturing. Hearing loss, dysarthria and dysphagia developed at about the same time as gait disturbance. Cerebellar and sensory ataxia were not prominent in any patient, and none had signs of lower motor neuron or peripheral nerve dysfunction. Seizures were present at the end stages in several patients.

The course of the CNS disease was that of relentless progression. The rate of progression of the CNS disorder varied

considerably. In two cases, whose illness began shortly after
severe head trauma, a transient improvement provided a diagnostic
dilemma. In all cases, the rate of CNS degeneration bore no relationship to the severity of adrenal cortical dysfunction and was
not affected by steroid therapy.

Adrenal Gland

The majority of the 41 patients in this series did not have
clinical stigmata of adrenal insufficiency at the time the CNS
illness became manifest. Five cases were addisonian for up to
10 years before any CNS findings developed. Adrenal insufficiency
in most of the other cases was detectable only as an impaired
response to ACTH infusion. With one exception, all cases displayed
some laboratory evidence of a diminished adrenal cortical reserve
at some point in the illness.

Laboratory Findings

The single most reliable test for ALD was an open adrenal
biopsy. This procedure was of enormous importance in establishing histological and biochemical abnormalities in ALD. However,
it is rarely necessary as a diagnostic maneuver since the ACTH
infusion test has proven to be a reliable indicator of a diminished adrenal cortical reserve in this illness. Peripheral nerve
and testis biopsy have rarely been diagnostic. Brain biopsy has
proven extremely misleading, and is clearly not indicated in ALD
because of the extreme rostro-caudal regional variation in the
pathological changes. We have, in fact, encountered two instances
where occipital biopsy resulted in an erroneous diagnosis of astro-
cytoma, resulting in radiotherapy, and other instances of negative
brain biopsies obtained from the uninvolved frontal white matter.
Other laboratory tests have been of limited use. The CAT scan
has shown early occipital lobe involvement in two cases, and the
EEG and conventional isotope brain scans have occasionally shown
similar findings. The CSF protein is usually elevated and the
gamma globulin has occasionally been elevated.

PATHOLOGICAL STUDIES

Central Nervous System

The severity of brain involvement in most cases bore little
relationship to the duration of the process, the age of the patient,
the family history, or the degree of adrenal insufficiency.

   The cerebral cortex was of normal thickness in all cases,
and the atrophic external appearance of some of the brains proved
to be secondary to loss of subcortical white matter. The subcortical arcuate fibers and the band of Gennari were, to a variable
extent, spared in every case. Moderate to severe ventricular
dilation was present in cases with extensive loss of white matter.
The cerebral lesion was consistently most severe in the parietal,
occipital and posterior temporal lobes with a highly variable
involvement of frontal white matter. Coronal sections showed that
the lesion in each cerebral hemisphere was confluent and that it
extended across the splenium of the corpus callosum to establish
continuity with the lesion in the opposite hemisphere. The fornix,
hippocampal commissure, and posterior cingulum and corpus callosum
were usually heavily involved. The posterior cerebral lesions
were usually widespread and symmetrical, while the cases with
frontal lobe involvement often showed a striking asymmetry. The
posterior limb of the internal capsules, lateral two thirds of
the cerebral peduncles, basis pontis, pyramids, and corticospinal
tracts were gray and shrunken. Lesions in the cerebellar white
matter were often visible grossly. The central portions of the
optic nerves and tracts were severely involved in every case
examined.

   Histopathological examination revealed that the ctyoarchi-
tecture of the cerebral cortex appeared generally normal except
for scattered neuronal loss and gliosis in layers five and six.
Cortical gliosis was most severe in posterior areas where the
white matter lesion occasionally did not spare the subcortical
arcuate fibers and was contiguous with the deep layers of the
cortex. In the white matter of the cerebral hemispheres, the
distribution of the microscopic lesions corresponded to the gross
changes; the nature of the histopathological chance varied greatly
from region to region, however. There appeared to be three histopathological zones in each lesion. The first zone, which contained
scattered PAS-postive and sudanophilic macrophages and destruction
of myelin with axonal sparing, was closely followed by a second
zone in which there were many lipid-laden macrophages, some
surviving myelinated axons, many preserved demyelinated axons, and
a vigorous perivascular mononuclear cell response. These two
zones were most prominent in the frontal edges of the lesion. The
third, and largest, zone consisted of a dense mesh of glial fibrils
and scattered astrocytes without any evidence of an active process.
The gliosis was both isomorphic and anismorphic in alternating
and sometimes concentric patterns. In well-defined pathways, e.g.
corpus callosum, the gliosis was consistently isomorphic. Oligodendroglia, axons, and myelin sheaths were absent in the third
zone; surrounding the vessels there were occasional PAS- and oil
red 0-positive macrophages, but few lymphocytes or plasma cells.
This pattern was most prominent in the center of the occipito-

parietal portion of the white matter lesion. Degeneration in the
brain stem and spinal cord was confined to the descending fiber
tracts and there were no small, independent foci of demyelination.
The corticospinal and corticobulbar tracts were involved in every
case. Electron microscopy revealed that many of the macrophages
contained distinctive cytoplasmic inclusions. These inclusions
were made up of paired electron-dense leaflets, each measuring
2.5 to 3.5 nm and separated by an electron-lucent space varying
from 4.0 to 10.0 nm in width. The length and configuration of
these profiles were highly variable, but the majority were curvilinear. By utilizing the tilting stage of the electron microscope,
continuity between the profiles and lipid droplets was established.
These inclusions were not found in oligodendroglia or astrocytes.

Peripheral Nervous System

In four cases, histologic examination of multiple, paraffin-
embedded sections of the peripheral nervous system including anterior root, posterior root, and dorsal root ganglia, disclosed no
abnormalities. Ultrastructural examination of a capsular nerve
found in an adrenal biopsy specimen from one case revealed abnormal cytoplasmic inclusions in Schwann cells consisting of paired,
electron-dense, 2.5 nm leaflets separated by a 3.0 to 4.0 nm
electron-lucent space. In a sural nerve biopsy specimen from
another case, many of these electron-dense, 2.5 nm leaflet profiles,
undetectable by light microscopy, were present in the Schwann cells
of some myelinated fibers and bands of Büngner, as well as in endo-
neurial macrophages. The dimensions and morphologic characteristics
of these inclusions were identical to those present in the Schwann
cells in the adrenal nerve from the other case. Ultrastructural
examination of the sural nerve biopsy specimens from three other
cases demonstrated no important abnormalities.

Adrenal Glands

The histologic changes in the adrenal glands from these cases
have largely been restricted to the ZFR of the cortex with only
slight involvement of the zona glomerulosa. The histologic feature
common to all the adrenals, and specific for this disease, is the
presence of ballooned cortical cells (ZFR), many of which have a
striated cytoplasm with macrovacuoles. With one exception, in
our 41 cases there have been no major accumulations of inflammatory cells. Ultrastructurally, the striations have consisted
of linear, or occasionally twisted, lamellar accumulations within
the adrenal cortical cell cytoplasm. An individual lamella has
demonstrated a trilaminar structure, consisting of paired, electron-
dense leaflets, each approximately 2.5 nm thick separated by an

electron-lucent space of 2.0 to 7.0 nm. There was usually a
perilamellar clear space around the trilaminar structures. The
abnormal lamellae did not appear to arise from cytoplasmic membranes
of adrenal cells.

Testis

In all cases, postmortem histologic examination of the testis
revealed it to be within normal limits for the stated age. Fully
developed Leydig cells were rarely present. In the testicular
biopsy specimen from one case and the postmortem specimen of testis
from another, there were sufficient numbers of interstitial cells
that fulfilled the ultrastructural criteria for presumptive Leydig
cells. In the postmortem specimen of testis these interstitial
cells contained many linear, clear clefts with electron-dense lamellar fragments. In the testicular biopsy specimen there were
lamellar profiles similar to those in the Schwann cells from the
sural nerve biopsy specimen of the same case. Inflammatory cells
were not present.

Other Organs

Histologic examination of the pituitary glands has shown a
mild proliferation of basophils in five cases. Ultrastructural examination of postmortem specimens of pituitary, spleen, liver, pancreas,
and kidneys from 3 cases circulating leucocytes from 2 cases and
cultured fibroblasts from one case have shown no significant abnormalities.

BIOCHEMICAL STUDIES

The biochemical studies on the inclusions in brain and adrenal gland from four cases of adrenoleukodystrophy were greatly
facilitated by the histochemical studies performed in Dr. A.B.
Johnson's laboratory. These studies were based on the earlier
observation that the inclusions display a brilliant birefringence
under polarized light (10). Utilizing the birefringence as a
marker, a series of experiments demonstrated that these abnormal
inclusions in both the adrenal and in brain macrophages were
insoluble in acetone, which extracts naturally-occurring cholesterol
esters and cholesterol. However, the inclusions could readily be
dissolved by the non-polar solvent, n-hexane. Thus the biochemical
studies began with a thin-layer chromatography analysis of the
n-hexane extract of the acetone-insoluble residue from ALD adrenals.
The hexane extract of an ALD adrenal yielded a distinct spot that
was not present in similarly treated controls. Analysis of this

spot in the hexane extract of the ALD adrenal revealed the presence of cholesterol esterified to saturated fatty acids of unusually long chain length. As an intact molecule, it behaved
essentially as esterified cholesterol in several systems of thin-
layer chromatography, including silver-impregnated TLC. The material showed characteristics of cholesterol when heated after spray-
ing with sulfuric acid, a procedure which differentiates various
sterols by their hues of colors as well as their fluorescence
under UV light. When subjected to alkaline hydrolysis procedure,
the material liberated a free sterol which could be identified as
cholesterol by similar criteria and also by gas-liquid chromatography (GLC). The material also liberated a series of compounds
which could be tentatively identified by GLC as saturated fatty
acids with chain-length longer than 23. These findings prompted
a systematic analysis of fatty acids in brain and adrenal cholesterol esters from ALD patients (6). Four ALD and four control
adrenals, and five ALD and two normal brains were studied. In
addition, brains from patients with G_{M1}-gangliosidosis and with
cerebral infarct were included as pathological controls. In the
control brain, almost all the fatty acids were shorter than C_{22}.
On the other hand, the cholesterol esters from an ALD brain contained a series of very long chain fatty acids, longer than C_{22}.
They were almost completely saturated, and they always showed
a smooth bell-shaped distribution with C_{25} or C_{26} at the peak.
The identity of these fatty acids was definitively established
by GLC-mass spectrometry, kindly carried out by Drs. Klaus Bie-
mann and Catherine Costello at the Massachusetts Institute of
Technology.

All the adrenals and brains from ALD patients showed the
same abnormality in fatty acid composition of cholesterol esters.
To determine if this unusual fatty acid abnormality is limited to
cholesterol esters, fatty acid composition of other lipids from
ALD patients was also analyzed. In general, fatty acids of
sphingolipids showed a qualitatively similar but quantitatively
lesser abnormality of increased saturated long-chain fatty acids.
However, no fatty acid abnormality was found for any of the
glycerophospholipids, and, in the adrenal, for the free fatty
acid pool or triglyceride. Furthermore, serum cholesterol esters
did not show the type of fatty acid abnormality found in brain
and adrenal cholesterol esters.

The fatty acid abnormality we have identified appears to be
present consistently in ALD tissues. To our knowledge, it has
not been found in any other pathological conditions. Cholesterol
esters with this abnormal fatty acid composition appears to represent the histologically characteristic cytoplasmic inclusions
in ALD tissues. Therefore, it is not unreasonable to formulate
a working hypothesis that this abnormality reflects the fundamental

genetic metabolic abnormality of ALD, although one cannot explain all of the known characteristics of the disease on this basis at the present time. The immediate question is whether the abnormality represents defective metabolism of cholesterol esters or fatty acids. It seems most likely that there is an abnormality of fatty acid metabolism because of the presence of similar abnormalities in sphingolipids. However, abnormal cholesterol ester metabolism, as suggested by Burton and Nadler cannot yet be rigorously excluded (2).

Acknowledgements

This work was supported by research grants, NS-10885, NS-00356, HD-01799, HD-05515, NS-08952 from the United States Public Health Service, by R.D.-982-A-4, R.D.-721-B-4 from the National Multiple Sclerosis Society and a grant from the ALD Foundation.

References

1. Blaw, M.E.: Melanodermic type leukodystrophy (adreno-leuko-dystrophy) in Vinken, P.G., Bruyn, G.W. Handbook of Clinical Neurology, New York, American Elsevier, 1970, Vol. 10, pp 128-133.

2. Burton, B.K. and Nadler, H.L.: X-Linked Schilder's disease: A generalized disorder of cholesterol metabolism? Pediatr. Res. 8:170, 1974.

3. Fanconi, V.A., Prader, A., Iser, W., Luthy, F. and Siebenmann, R.: Morbus Addison mit Hirnsklevose in Kindesalter Ein heritares Syndrom mit x-chronosomaler Verebung? Helv. Pediatr. Acta 13:480, 1963.

4. Gagnon, J. and Leblanc, R.: Sclerose cerebrale diffuse avec melanodermie et atrophy surrenale. Un Med. Can. 88:391,1959.

5. Hoefnagel, D., VandenNoort, S., and Ingbar, S.H.: Diffuse cerebral sclerosis with endocrine abnormalities in young males. Brain 85:553, 1962.

6. Igarashi, M., Schaumburg, H.H., Powers, J.M., Kishimoto, Y., Kolodny, E.H. and Suzuki, K.: Fatty acid abnormality in adrenoleukodystrophy. J. Neurochem., in press.

7. Powers, J.M. and Schaumburg, H.H.: Adrenoleukodystrophy: Similar ultrastructural changes in adrenal cortical cells and Schwann cells. Arch. Neurol. 30:406, 1974.

8. Powers, J.M. and Schaumburg, H.H.: Adrenoleukodystrophy (sex-linked Schilder's disease): A pathogenetic hypothesis based on ultrastructural lesions in adrenal cortex, peripheral nerve and testis. Am. J. Path. 76:481, 1974.

9. Richardson, E.P.: Schilder's disease: What is it? J. Neuropath. Exp. Neurol., in press.

10. Schaumburg, H.H., Richardson, E.P., Johnson, P.C., Raine, C.S., and Powers, J.M.: Schilder's disease: Sex-linked transmission with specific adrenal changes. Arch. Neurol. 27:458, 1972.

11. Schaumburg, H.H., Powers, J.M., Suzuki, K. and Raine, C.S.: Adrenoleukodystrophy: Ultrastructural demonstration of specific cytoplasmic inclusions in the central nervous system. Arch. Neurol. 31:210, 1974.

12. Schaumburg, H.H., Powers, J.M., Raine, C.S., Suzuki, K. and Richardson, E.P.: Adrenoleukodystrophy: A clinical and pathological study of 17 cases. Arch. Neurol. 32:577,1975.

13. Siemerling, E. and Creuzfeldt, H.G.: Bronzen-Krankenheit und skerosierende Encephalomyelitis. Arch. Psychiatr. Nervenkr. 68:217, 1923.

POLYUNSATURATED FATTY ACID LIPIDOSIS: A NEW NOSOLOGICAL ENTITY

Lars Svennerholm

Department of Neurochemistry, Psychiatric Research Centre

University of Göteborg, Göteborg, Sweden

INTRODUCTION

In 1963 Dr Bengt Hagberg saw in the Pediatric Service, University Hospital, Uppsala, a 2-year-old girl who was severely retarded, had no speech or grasping ability, could sit but not stand by herself and had pronounced truncal ataxia. Her reflexes were normal. She had no optic atrophy, but her vision was impaired, and she did not react in a normal manner to optic stimuli. Her EEG showed severe and diffusely spread abnormalities with an irregular delta activity and bilateral synchronous sharp waves of a low amplitude. She then rapidly deteriorated and half a year later she could no longer sit or utter any sound. Soon afterwards she lost the ability even to turn round, and her eye movements became irregular. Fits increased in frequency and intensity. When 2 years 9 months old she was soporous and in a neonatal motoric state with a flexion pattern, no head control and general floppiness. She then remained in a soporous state, quite flaccid and was unable to make any purposeful movements for more than three years and died at the age of 6 years.

The clinical picture suggested a previously unknown disorder for which reason brain biopsy was performed. The child was then 2 years 8 months old. The biopsy specimen revealed severe loss of neurons and marked cellular gliosis. The remaining cells and many of the glial cells were swollen and contained large amounts of material that reacted strongly positively with the PAS technique. At post mortem examination the brain was strikingly small and weighed only 305 g. There was total derangement of the cortical cytoarchitecture, severe degeneration of white matter and both the grey and the white matter contained deposits of granular material with histochemical properties of characterizing unsaturated polymerized and oxidized fatty acids.

389

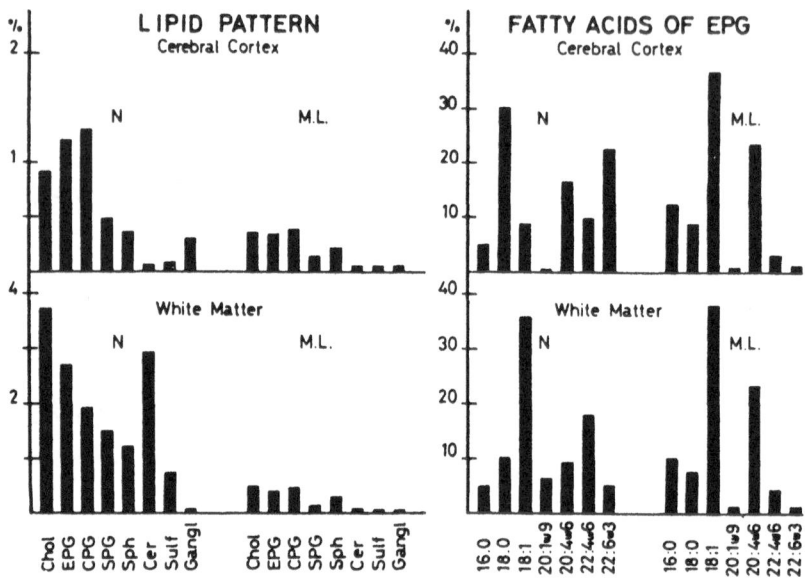

Figure 1. The lipid pattern and the fatty acid composition of ethanolamine
          phosphoglycerides (EPG) of cerebral cortex and white matter in
          a case of PFAL (M.L.) and in an age-matched control.

The chemical investigation revealed a drastic reduction of all lipids,
especially of the gangliosides of grey matter and the cerebrosides of white
matter (Fig. 1). The fatty acid composition of the phosphoglycerides revealed
several characteristic features: a large increase of monoenoic fatty acids in
cerebral cortex and a reduction of docosatetraenoic and particular of dokosahexaenoic acids. We therefore thought it warranted to conclude that the
clinical, the histological and the chemical examinations had all shown that
we had detected a previously unknown disorder (4).

I have given this rather long introduction because this first case of the
new disease showed the characteristic features, which have since been found
in all the cases afterwards detected in Finland.

MATERIAL AND METHODS

PFAL

Clinical Course. The total number of cases so far known in Finland and
Sweden is 70. The largest number of cases have been examined by dr Pirkko
Santavuori at the Children's Hospital, University of Helsinki. In her last

Table 1.   Symptoms and signs appearing between the ages
             of 12 and 24 months in 46 INCL patients.

Mental retardation	46
Visual failure	46
Myoclonic jerks	45
Microcephaly	42
Ataxia	39
Muscular hypotonia	28
"Knitting" hyperkinesia	28
Squint	17
Convulsion	9
Rigidity	6

From: Santavuori, P., Haltia, M, and Rapola, J.;
Infantile Type of So-called Neuronal Ceroidlipo-
fuscinosis; Develop. Med. and Child. Neurol.,
16, 644-653, 1974.

publication (7) she reported the clinical features of 46 patients from 38 families. The main symptoms and signs are given in Table 1. In all her patients
the disease reached a quiescent stage during the third year, but they survived
for further several years. The mean age at death was 6 1/2 years (range 3
years 8 months to 10 years 3 months).

At the first examination 90 % of all the patients had shown signs of
visual deterioration. The electroretinogram was extinguished in all patients.
In none of the patients was the electroencephalogram (EEG) normal. The first
signs were loss of the usual rhythmic components and an increase in slow
waves. By the age of 3 years all children had an isoelectric EEG.

Pathology. The brains were exceedingly small and weighed between
305 and 420 g. The cerebrum and cerebellum were severely affected, but the
brain stem, and particularly the spinal cord, were relatively spared. In the
final stage, the cortex was entirely depleted of nerve cells and consisted of
a spongy network of fibrillary astrocytes and capillaries with a small number
of macrophages. The ultrastructure of the stored material remained constant
through all these stages: membrane-bound spherical globules with a homogenous finely granular content. The material occurred not only in the cytoplasm of nerve cells and macrophages, but also in other neuroectodermal cells
and in many extraneural organs.

Chemical examination. In all, 8 cases have been examined. Six of them are from Finnish families living in Sweden, and the last two are from Finland. In 5 of the 8 cases autopsy material was analysed. The age at death varied between 5.2 and 10.3 years, but there was no significant difference with age in the biochemical changes. The results obtained in the 5 autopsy cases were pooled and only the mean values are given. In the remaining 3 cases only small tissue fragments of biopsy material of frontal lobe were available. A strictly quantitative determination was not possible and the results are only provisional and are therefore not included in the tables.

Juvenile amaurotic idiocy (JAI)

In the extensive review of neuronal ceroidlipofuscinoses Zeman and co-workers (1970) considered our first case of PFAL to be a case of Batten-Vogt syndrom. Therefore, 8 cases of the juvenile form of familial amaurotic idiocy (Spielmeyer-Sjögren-Vogt) have been included. The neuropathological exa-mination of all the cases has been performed by Dr Patrick Sourander (5). The ages of the cases have varied between 16 and 24 years. The analyses of this brain material were performed between 1963 and 1970.

Control material

In all together 20 cases who had died in accidents or from diseases with no primary involvement of the CNS, were examined.

Methods

The quantitative methods used for the lipid analyses are the same as those used since 1961 (9-11).

RESULTS AND DISCUSSION

Lipid Composition

In the terminal stage of PFAL the cerebral cortex was very poor in lipids and the concentration of phosphoglycerides (Fig. 2) was only 40% of that in age-matched controls. The phospholipid pattern showed a significant decrease in ethanolamine phosphoglycerides and a significant increase in sphingomyelin. In the white matter the concentration of phospholipids was the same as in the

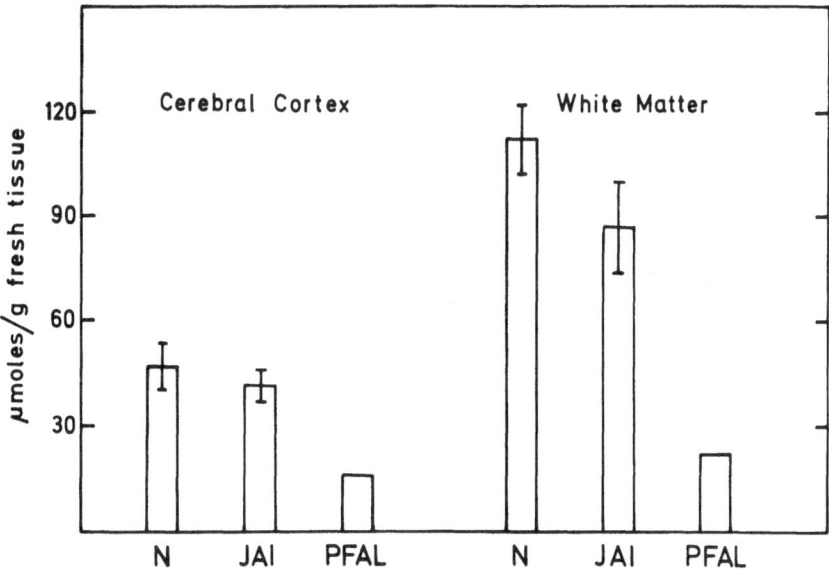

Figure 2. The concentration of phospholipids in cerebral cortex and white matter of controls, cases of juvenile familial amaurotic idiocy (JAI) and cases of polyunsaturated fatty acid lipidosis (PFAL).

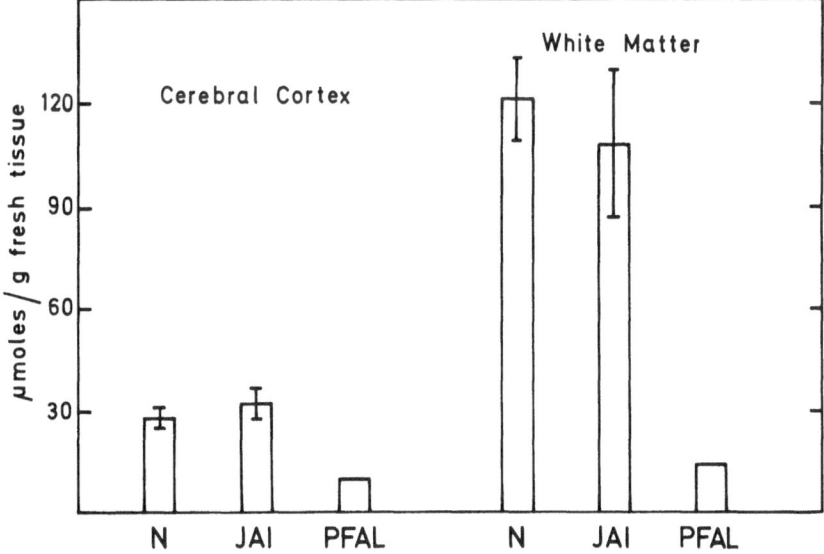

Figure 3. The concentration of cholesterol in cerebral cortex and white matter.

cerebral cortex and less than 20 % of the control value. The pattern was identical with that in the cerebral cortex. In JAI the phospholipid concentration and the proportion of individual phospholipids were the same as in the controls. In the white matter the concentration was slightly, but significantly, reduced.

The cholesterol concentration of the cerebral cortex in PFAL was also only 40 % of the control value, but in JAI it was slightly higher than in the controls (Fig. 3). In the white matter the cholesterol concentration was 15 % of the control value in PFAL white matter, while it was not significantly reduced in JAI.

In PFAL the cerebroside concentration was extremely low and the concentration was only 2 % of the control value (Fig. 4). In JAI the cerebroside concentration was slightly, but significantly, reduced, which suggests a myelin deficiency of white matter in JAI, which was rather mild in some cases, but more pronounced in others. The cerebroside changes in JAI did not show any correlation with the patients' ages at death.

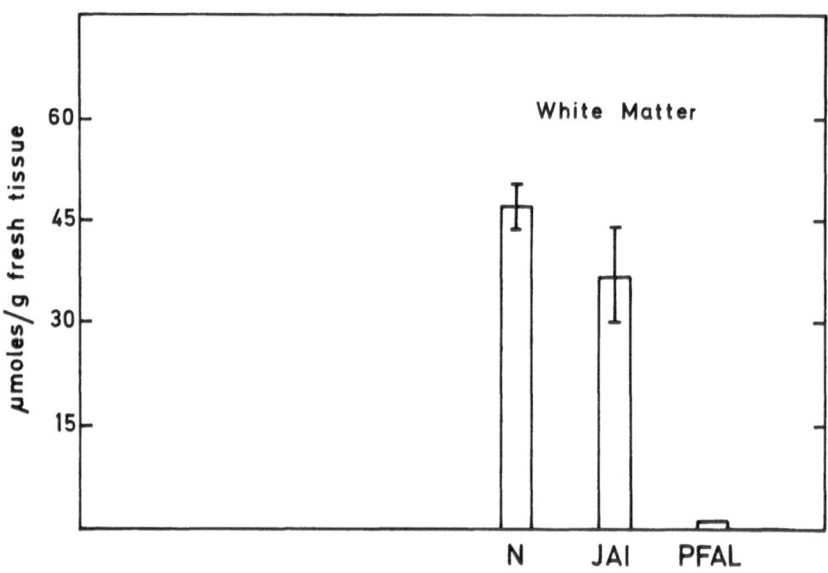

Figure 4. The concentration of cerebrosides in cerebral white matter.

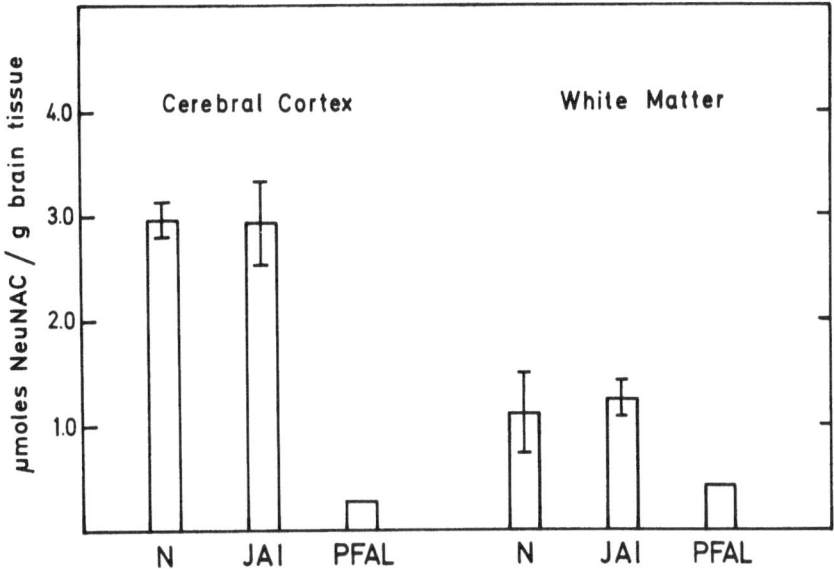

Figure 5. The concentration of gangliosides, expressed as lipid-NeuNAc
in cerebral cortex and white matter.

Ganglioside Concentration and Pattern

In PFAL the ganglioside concentration, expressed as lipid-NeuNAc,
was extremely low and was the same in the cerebral cortex as in white matter
(Fig. 5). In the cerebral cortex of the PFAL cases the ganglioside concentration was only 10 % of the control value. In JAI the ganglioside concentration
of cerebral cortex was the same as in the controls, but the standard deviation
was slightly larger, and in the white matter it was slightly higher than in the
controls. The ganglioside pattern of cerebral cortex in JAI was the same as in
the controls, but in the white matter the gangliosides GM3 and GD3 were increased. There was also a small increase of GD2.

The ganglioside pattern in PFAL was the same in cerebral cortex as in
white matter and showed the same features: the gangliosides GD1a and GM1,
which are normally the largest two ganglioside fractions had diminished to
such an extent as to be barely detectable (Fig. 6). On the other hand the
other two major brain gangliosides GD1b and GT1 were much less reduced.
The concentrations of the minor gangliosides were only slightly reduced and
that of GD3 was increased, so that this ganglioside was the largest fraction
in both cerebral cortex and white matter at the final stage.

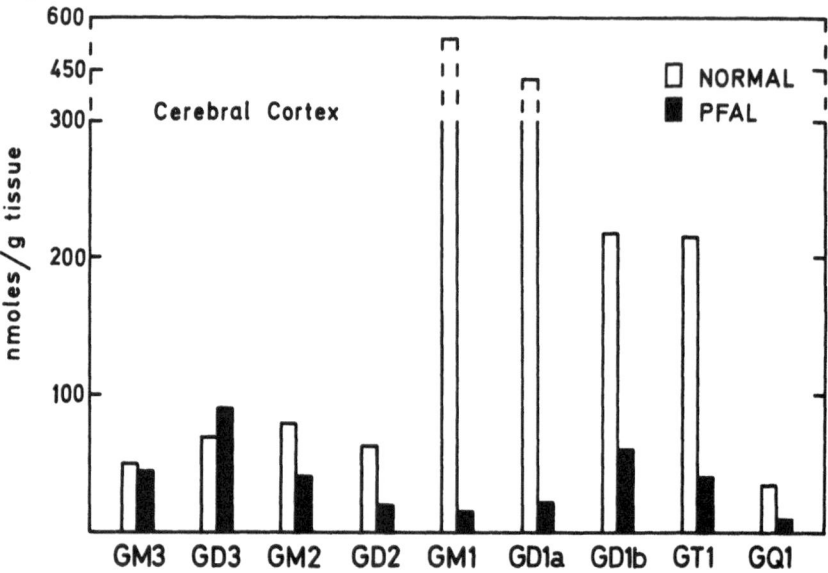

Figure 6. The pattern of individual gangliosides in controls and cases with
polyunsaturated fatty acid lipidosis (PFAL).

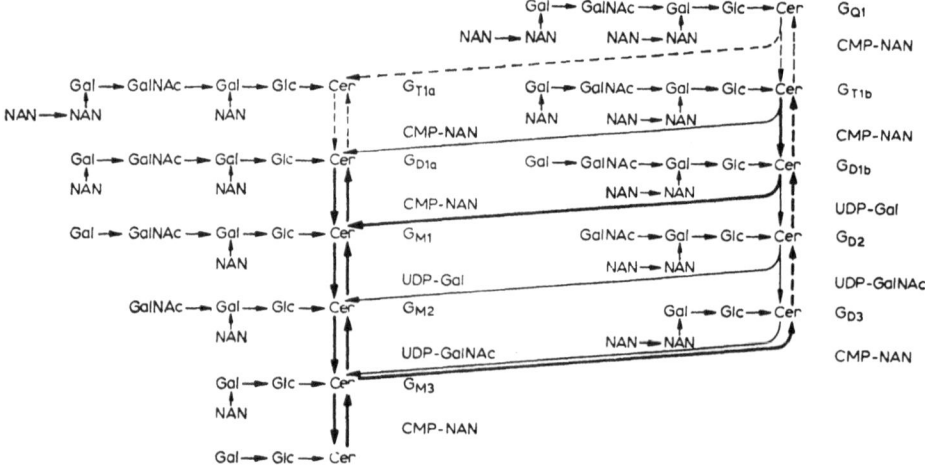

Figure 7. Metabolism of brain gangliosides. Thick line = major pathway,
thin line = minor pathway, unbroken line = demonstrated
pathway, dashed line = assumed pathway.

The diminution of gangliosides in PFAL was very striking and we have never found such a low concentration of brain gangliosides in any other condition except in a case described under the name of congenital amaurotic idiocy (3). Also in that case ganglioside GD3 was a major fraction and the cerebral hemispheres showed no cells recognizable as neurons, but only spherical granular masses. We are therefore inclined to ascribe the serious diminution of gangliosides in PFAL to the extensive loss of cortical nerve cells and particularly their synaptic connections.

The higher gangliosides can be synthesized by two routes (Fig. 7). The very low concentrations of gangliosides GM1 and GD1a suggest that this route is seriously impaired, and the formation will occur mostly via GD3 and GD2 to GD1b and GT1. In other connections I have assumed that the two routes for the formation of gangliosides will occur in different compartments. This assumption was based on the finding that there was a different ceramide composition of GD1b and GT1 than of GM1 and GD1a in normal brain (Svennerholm, in preparation) and in Krabbe brain (14).

The present study has provided results which suggest that GM1 and GD1a are confined mainly to the neurons and particularly to their nerve endings.

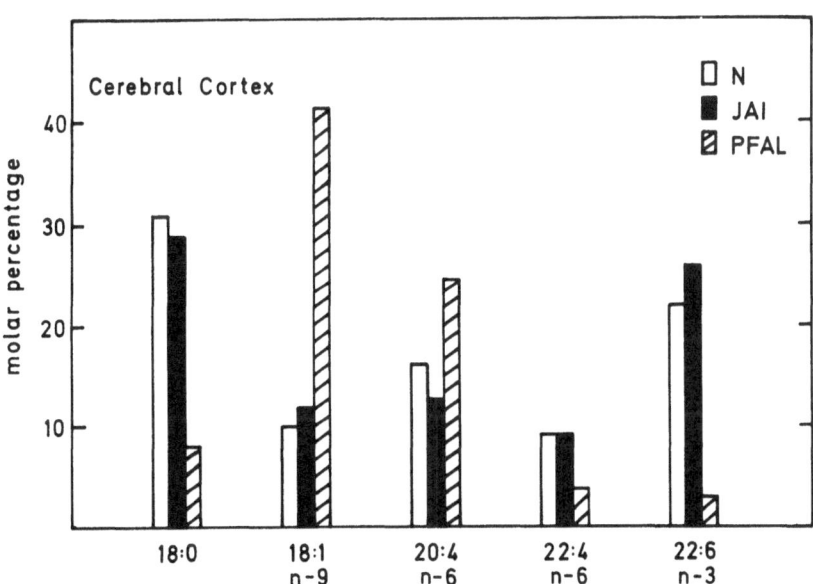

Figure 8. Fatty acid composition of ethanolamine phosphoglycerides in cerebral cortex.

Fatty Acid Composition of Phosphoglycerides and Sphingolipids

All the cases of juvenile JAI had the same or essentially the same fatty acid patterns as the control cases. In contrast the PFAL cases showed very large deviations from the normal patterns. The most striking findings were the very close similarities in fatty acid composition of all lipids in cerebral cortex and white matter, and the strong diminution of fatty acids of the linolenic acid series, particularly pronounced in the serine and ethanolamine phosphoglycerides of cerebral cortex. In cerebral cortex (Fig. 8) the proportions of the monoenoic acids were strongly decreased, while stearic acid was the only saturated fatty acid that was diminished. The proportion of dokosahexaenoic acid 22:6 (n-3), the major metabolite of linolenic acid, was reduced to less than 1 % in serine phosphoglycerides and to 2-5 % in ethanolamine phosphoglycerides. The proportion of fatty acids of the linoleic acid series was the same in the patients as in the controls, but the range of variation of the levels of the individual fatty acids was wide. Arachidonic acid 20:4 (n-6) was significantly increased in ethanolamine and serine phosphoglycerides, while 22:4 (n-6) was markedly decreased. In biopsy samples from less advanced cases the concentration of 22:6 (n-3) was normal or only slightly reduced, but all the other fatty acids showed the same trend as in the chronic cases – the proportion of monoenoic acids was increased, and those of 22:4 (n-6) and 22:5 (n-6) decreased (Fig. 9). In the white matter the phosphoglyceride changes

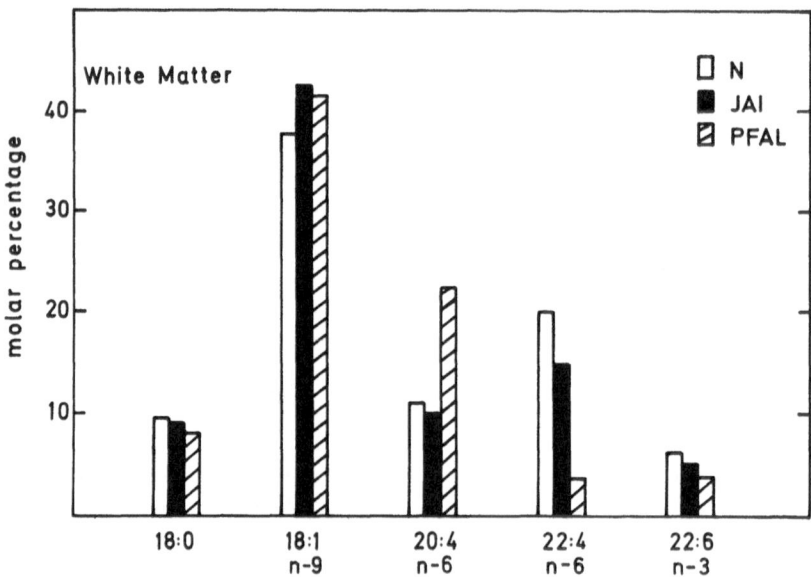

Figure 9. Fatty acid composition of ethanolamine phosphoglycerides in cerebral white matter.

were less striking since the white matter normally has a much higher concentration of monoenoic acids than the cerebral cortex and a lower concentration of polyenoic acids of the linolenic acid series (10). The proportions of 22:6 (n-3) and 22:4 (n-6) were diminished, while that of 20:4 (n-6) was increased in all the three phosphoglycerides. The increase of 20:4 was most striking in ethanolamine phosphoglyceride, which normally has a much larger proportion of this acid than choline and serine phosphoglycerides. The diminution of stearic acid was particularly pronounced in choline phosphoglycerides.

Sphingolipid Fatty Acids

The gangliosides had a higher proportion of long chain fatty acids than normally, while C_{20}-sphingosine was diminished. The fatty acid patterns were the same in grey and white matter. The fatty acid patterns of cerebrosides and sulfatides were difficult to determine and the values cannot be considered completely valid. The proportions of 16:0, 18:0 and 22:0 were increased, while that of the long-chain fatty acids were reduced. The sphingomyelin showed an extraneural pattern with increased proportions of 16:0 and 22:0.

Phosphoglyceride Fatty Acids in Liver and Serum

The fatty acid patterns of plasma choline phosphoglycerides have shown the same changes in all our Swedish cases in an early stage of the disease. The choline phosphoglycerides showed a reduction of linoleic acid and an increase of arachidonic acid, but with a normal proportion of oleic acid. In many disorders with a deficiency of dietary linoleic acid, there occurs a decrease of the proportion of linoleic acid and an increase of arachidonic acid, but the proportion of oleic acid is then always increased (1). The fatty acid changes of lecithin are the same in the liver as in serum – a reduction of linoleic acid and an increase of arachidonic acid. In the early biopsy cases of PFAL, the proportion of arachidonic acid was increased also in the brain phosphoglycerides when the proportion of dokosahexaenoic acid still was quite normal. This might be interpreted to suggest that the primary lesion in PFAL is a disturbance of the further metabolism of arachidonic acid, which will lead to an increased proportion in tissue phosphoglycerides of this fatty acid. The formation of malondialdehyde which will condense and react with aminogroups, will proceed at a high rate, and ceroid will accumulate in the neuronal bodies.

Protein of Cerebrospinal Fluid

Another common feature of the disease is the rapid disappearance of the so-called tau-fraction of cerebrospinal fluid. It is formed by the release of two moles of sialic acid from transferrin by the action of sialidase. This enzymic hydrolysis by sialidase will normally occur during the passage of the fluid from brain to lumbar region. When fresh normal lumbar cerebrospinal fluid is analysed, the absolute amount of tau is fairly constant, and it is increased in conditions in which there are signs of tissue nervous damage. In PFAL there is a true diminution of the tau-fraction, and this diminution will continue rapidly until no tau-fraction can be seen in the final stage. Sialidase activity could not be demonstrated with ganglioside GD1a as substrate in cerebrospinal fluid or in brain tissue of PFAL patients.

Biochemical Parameters of the Nerve Endings

Previous studies have shown the highest ganglioside concentration in the synaptic membranes (2). In the same structure there is an enrichment of sialidase (6, 13) and a high proportion of dokosahexaenoic acid in ethanolamine and serine phosphoglycerides. In the final stages of PFAL there is an almost complete disappearance of the synapses, and also an almost complete disappearance of some characteristic brain substances. It is therefore tempting to speculate that these three substances, ganglioside GD1a, sialidase and phosphoglycerides with dokosahexaenoic acid, are confined to the synapses. These three substances decrease continously as the disease proceeds. I do not believe that these changes are the primary ones in the disease, but only secondary to the destruction of the neuron. This suggests that the stored granular material is cytotoxic in PFAL, but not in JAI in which no similar changes are observed.

ABSTRACT

Lipid analyses in the terminal stage of the disease polyunsaturated fatty acid lipidosis (PFAL), showed a brain very poor in lipids. The concentration of sphingolipids was particularly low: gangliosides of cerebral cortex was only 10 % of the control value, and cerebrosides of white matter only 2 %. Of the gangliosides, GM1 and GD1a were reduced more than any other ganglioside fraction. The fatty acid compositions of the phosphoglycerides were the same in cerebral cortex and white matter. Compared with what was found in the controls, ethanolamine phosphoglycerides had much higher proportions of 18:1 and 20:4 (n-6) and much lower proportions of 22:4 (n-6) and 22:6 (n-3) in the cerebral cortex. Similar changes in the fatty acid patterns were found in the

other phosphoglycerides. It is assumed that in PFAL there is a primary disturbance in the metabolism of arachidonic acid, which leads to a series of
secondary changes. The results suggested that the gangliosides GM1 and GD1a,
sialidase and phosphoglycerides with dokosahexaenoic acid are confined to
the nerve endings.

ACKNOWLEDGEMENT

This work has been supported by grants from the Swedish Medical Research
Council (Project No 3X-627).

REFERENCES

1 Alling, C., Dencker, S.J., Svennerholm, L. and Tichý, J. Serum fatty
   acid pattern in chronic alcoholics after acute abuse. Acta Med. Scand.
   185, 99-105, 1969.

2 Breckenridge, W.C., Gombos, G. and Morgan, I.G. The lipid composition of adult rat brain synaptosomal plasma membranes. Biochim. Biophys.
   Acta 266, 695-707, 1972.

3 Hagberg, B., Hultquist, G., Öhman, R. and Svennerholm, L. Congenital
   amaurotic Idiocy. Acta Paediat. Scand. 54, 116-130, 1965.

4 Hagberg, B., Sourander, P. and Svennerholm, L. Late infantile progressive encephalopathy with disturbed polyunsaturated metabolism. Acta
   Paediat. Scand. 57, 495-499, 1968.

5 Kristensson, K. and Sourander, P. Occurrence of lipofuscin in inherited
   metabolic disorders affecting the nervous system. J. Neurol. Neurosurg.
   Psychiat. 29, 113-118, 1966.

6 Öhman, R. Subcellular fractionation of ganglioside sialidase from human
   brain. J. Neurochem. 18, 89-95, 1971.

7 Santavuori, P., Haltia, M. and Rapola, J. Infantile type of so-called
   neuronal ceroid lipifuscinosis. Developm. Med. Child. Neurol. 16,
   644-653, 1974.

8   Svennerholm, L. Ganglioside metabolism. In M. Florkin and E.M.
    Stotz (eds): Comprehensive Biochemistry, vol. 18, Lipid Metabolism.
    Amsterdam, Elsevier, 1970, 201-227.

9   Svennerholm, L. and Vanier, M.T. The distribution of lipids in the
    human nervous system. II Lipid composition of human fetal and infant
    brain. Brain Res. 47, 457-468, 1972.

10 Svennerholm, L. and Vanier, M.T. The distribution of lipids in the
    human nervous system. III Fatty acid composition of phosphoglycerides
    of human fetal and infant brain. Brain Res. 50, 341-351, 1973.

11 Svennerholm, L. and Vanier, M.T. The distribution of lipids in the
    human nervous system. IV Fatty acid composition of major sphingo-
    lipids of human infant brain. Brain Res. 55, 413-423, 1973.

12 Svennerholm, L. and Vanier, M.T. Brain ganglioside in Krabbe disease.
    In B. W. Volk and S. M. Aronson (eds): Sphingolipids, Spingolipidoses
    and Allied Disorders, New York, Plenum Press. Adv. Exp. Med. Biol.
    19, 499-514, 1972.

13 Tettamanti, G., Morgan, I.G., Gombos, G., Vincendon, G. and
    Mandel, P. Sub-synaptosomal localization of brain particulate
    neuraminidase. Brain Res. 47, 515-518, 1972.

14 Vanier, M.T. and Svennerholm, L. Chemical Pathology of Krabbe
    Disease. III Ceramide-hexosides and gangliosides of brain. Acta
    Paediat. Scand. 64, 641-648, 1975.

15 Zeman, W., Donahue, S., Dyken, P. and Green, J. The neuronal
    ceroid-lipofuscinosis. (Batten-Vogt syndrome). In P. J. Vinken and
    G.W. Bruyn (eds). Handbook of Clinical Neurology vol. 10.
    Amsterdam, North-Holland Publ. Co, 1970, 588-679.

THE BIOCHEMICAL DEFECT IN FARBER'S DISEASE

John Dulaney(a), Hugo W. Moser(a), James Sidbury(b),
and Aubrey Milunsky(a)
(a) Eunice Kennedy Shriver Center at the Walter E. Fernald
    State School, 200 Trapelo Road, Waltham, Massachusetts;
    Massachusetts General Hospital, Boston, Massachusetts
(b) National Institute of Child Health and Human
    Development, Bethesda, Maryland

In 1967 Prensky et al. reported the accumulation of ceramide
in the postmortem tissues of a patient with Farber's disease (1),
and in 1971 Samuelsson and Zetterström reported such an accumulation in a second case (2). In 1972 Sugita, Dulaney and Moser
demonstrated the deficient activity of an acid ceramidase in the
tissues of the case reported by Prensky et al. (3). Since this
same enzymatic defect has now been demonstrated in three additional
unrelated patients, it appears likely that the deficient activity
of acid ceramidase represents the basic defect in this disease,
and makes it appropriate to appraise our current knowledge about
this striking rare disorder.

The clinical and pathological features of Farber's disease
were very well described in the original report of three cases by
Farber, Cohen and Uzman (4), and in the review by Crocker, Cohen
and Farber which formed part of a previous symposium held at this
Institute (5). The characteristic feature is a granulomatous
lesion which contains a varying number of foam cells. The granu-
lomas involve the joints, subcutaneous tissues (usually at points
subject to pressure), the larynx, the lungs, often the kidney, and
less commonly the heart, liver and spleen. The changes in the
joints and subcutaneous nodules lead to striking deformities and
those in the larynx to hoarseness and aphonia. These features
make the diagnosis in classical cases unmistakeable. The main
abnormality in the nervous system is the accumulation of storage
material in the neuronal ytoplasm. This material is PAS positive
and for the most part extractable with lipid solvents (6, 7),
although some histochemical studies also suggested that there was
polysaccharide accumulation (8). Neuronal storage is most

403

prominent in the anterior horn cells of the spinal cord, the large
nerve cells of the brain stem nuclei, in the posterior root cells,
and the autonomic ganglia. Cortical neurones also show storage,
but less so than in other parts of the nervous system. While few
ultrastructural studies have been performed, their results suggest
that there is intralysosomal accumulation of lipids and possibly
polysaccharides (9, 10, 11).

Farber's disease usually is rapidly progressive; of the 14
reported cases 10 died before age 2 years (4, 6, 8, 9, 12, 13, 14,
15). One patient who was already severely involved during his
first year survived until age 16 years (2, 16). A one year old
child, who is now severely disabled, is at present being followed
by one of us (Sidbury). In addition, two patients have been
reported who are more mildly disabled; one is a French girl who
was 13 years old when she was reported in 1973 (10), and the other
a boy of Portuguese extraction, reported by Crocker, Cohen and
Farber at the previous symposium here (5). This boy, now 12 years
old, is doing well in school and is only very mildly disabled by
joint changes. While the clinical and pathological features in
the mild and severe cases suggest strongly that they represent
the same disease process, the biochemical studies to be reported
here have been carried out only in the severely involved cases.
Genetic data about Farber's disease are very limited; among the
14 reported cases 9 were females and five males. There is only
one instance in which a pair of sibs were affected. There were a
total of 19 unaffected sibs. In one instance parents were first
cousins; in eleven instances parents were reported not to be
related to each other. No cases have been described in previous
generations. Thus, while the limited genetic data are compatible
with an autosomal recessive mode of inheritance, this is far from
proven.

Changes in Levels of Tissue Components

The late Lahut Uzman reported the presence in Farber's
disease tissues of an abnormal "lipoglycoprotein" complex, which
accounted for 8 to 30% of total lipids (4). This material was not
fully characterized. Increases in neutral glycolipid or in ganglioside levels were reported by Clausen and Rampini (17) and by
Moser et al. (6). In one case there was a considerable increase
in the level of tissue mucopolysaccharides and a moderate increase
in urinary polysaccharides (12), but this has not been found in
other cases (2, 5, 6, 13). The most striking abnormality has been
the accumulation of ceramide. It should be noted that ceramides
are normally only present in small quantity ranging from 0.05% of
total lipid in plasma to 1% in brain. Quantitation of ceramide
levels often is not attempted when tissue components are analyzed,
and had not been performed in the Farber's disease cases studied

prior to 1967. So far, tissue ceramide levels have been tested in four cases. The greatest accumulation has been demonstrated in the subcutaneous nodules of three cases where ceramides accounted for 12 to 20% of total lipids (6, 9), or for 1.2% of fresh weight (2).

Eight to ten fold elevations of ceramide levels were found in the kidneys of the two cases which have so far been tested (2, 6). In one case (6) ceramides were also elevated 10 to 60 fold in the liver and spleen, and 2 to 6 fold in brain, but in the older patient studied by Samuelsson and Zetterström (2) ceramide accumulation was confined to the subcutaneous nodule and the kidney, and ceramide levels in the brain, liver, spleen and lung were not significantly altered. In one additional case (14), the ceramide level in the spinal cord was estimated by thin layer chromatography and reported not to be increased. Plasma ceramide levels are normal. However, in one case urinary ceramide levels were increased markedly, a finding which may prove to be of diagnostic value (18).

Unlike the normal, the ceramides in Farber's disease patients may contain a significant proportion of 2-hydroxy fatty acids: 43% in the kidney (2), 39% in cerebellum (19) and 10% in the liver (6). The 2-hydroxy acids consisted mainly of cerebronic acid, with lesser amounts of C_{22}, C_{20} and C_{18} 2-hydroxy acids, a pattern which resembles that seen normally in galactocerebrosides and sulfatides. In other respects the composition of fatty acids and long-chain bases in Farber's disease ceramide resembled that found in the control tissues. No hydroxy fatty acids were demonstrable in the ceramides isolated from Farber's disease subcutaneous nodules (2).

Table 1 summarizes the enzymatic studies performed in the postmortem tissues or cultured skin fibroblasts of four patients with Farber's disease. In each of these cases the activity of acid ceramidase (acylsphingosine deacylase E.C.3.5.1.23) was reduced to less than 5% of control, while the activities of a variety of other lysosomal enzymes were normal. Experimental details and additional results are given elsewhere (3, 21). The fact that the same enzymatic deficiency has now been demonstrated in four unrelated patients indicates that the finding is genuine, and when taken together with the observation that tissue levels of ceramide are elevated, reinforces the suggestion that it represents the basic biochemical defect in this disease. The enzyme defect would readily account for the accumulation of ceramide and probably also for the more variable accumulations of more complex sphingo-lipids. The ceramidase which appears to be deficient in Farber's disease has a pH optimum of 4 to 4.5, and is most active in lysoso-mal cell fractions (22, 23). This, together with the previously cited observation that there is lysosomal lipid storage in Farber's

Table 1

Farber's Disease: Activities of Acid Ceramidase and β-N-Acetylhexosaminidase

(nmole substrate cleaved per mg protein per hour)

	Ceramidase	β-Hexosaminidase	Acid Phosphatase	Arylsulfatase A
Postmortem Kidney				
Case 1	<0.01	8000	1340	
Case 2	<0.01	3160	930	
Controls (N=7)	2.55±0.48	4440±1510	1160±290	
Postmortem Cerebellum				
Case 1	<0.001	770	450	
Controls (N=5)	0.706±0.35	818±309	624±86	
Cultured Skin Fibroblasts				
Case 3	0.073	2542		350
Controls (N=2)	1.28-1.52	3024-3908		263±136
Case 4	0.036	4640		
Controls (N=4)	0.65±0.10	3439±538		

Table 1. Case 1 is that of Prensky and Moser (1, 6), Case 2 has been reported by Zetterström and by Samuelsson (2, 16), Case 3 is a case of Farber's disease now being followed by one of us (Sidbury), and Case 4 has been reported by Dustin et al. (9). Fibroblast cultures from Case 4 had previously been examined by Philippart et al. (20), and the fibroblast cultures of this case were obtained from The Human Genetic Mutant Cell Repository at the Institute for Medical Research, Camden, New Jersey (donated by Dr. M. Philippart). Synthetic N-(1-14C)oleoylsphingosine was used as substrate. The reaction was carried out at pH 4.0, in the presence of the detergents Tween, Triton X-100 and sodium cholate. See Ref. (3) for details for the studies with postmortem tissues and Ref. (21) for the studies with cultured skin fibroblasts.

disease (9, 10, 11), suggests that this disorder should be considered as one of the lysosomal storage diseases and sphingolipidoses.
It thus appears that Farber's disease represents an inborn error of
metabolism, a conclusion, which as noted before, could not have
been made on the basis of the sparse genetic data which are available at this time. Farber et al. in their original publication (4)
had also emphasized that this disorder appeared to represent a
bridge between the non-hereditary reticuloendothelioses, such as
Hand-Schueller-Christian disease or eosinophilic granuloma, and
the inherited sphingolipidoses. Again, the demonstration of the
enzymatic defect suggests (as Farber et al. had predicted), that
the disorder differs fundamentally from the reticuloendothelioses.

The description of the enzymatic defect in Farber's disease
also may lead to some points of general biological interest. Gatt
and Yavin in their studies of ceramidase reported that the enzyme
was also capable of catalyzing the reverse reaction: i.e. the
synthesis of ceramide from sphingosine and free fatty acids (22,
23). They found that the capacities to catalyze the reactions in
both directions remained inseparable and proportional, during all
stages of enzyme purification, and they concluded that one enzyme
was responsible for both: (Reaction 1)

$$\text{Sphingosine + Free Fatty Acid} \underset{\substack{\text{Acylsphingosine}\\\text{Deacylase}}}{\overset{}{\rightleftarrows}} \text{Ceramide} \qquad (1)$$

It is of interest, and in keeping with Gatt and Yavin's findings,
that in Farber's disease the degradative and synthetic activities
of ceramidase are impaired to the same extent (3). This provides
additional support for the supposition that the enzyme catalyzes
both directions of this reaction; the physiological significance
of the synthetic aspect of the reaction remains undetermined.

Sribney (24) has demonstrated another pathway of ceramide
synthesis, which utilizes Coenzyme A derivatives of fatty acid:
(Reaction 2)

$$\text{Sphingosine + Fatty Acid CoA} \xrightarrow{\substack{\text{Sphingosine}\\\text{N-acyltransferase}}} \text{Ceramide + CoA} \quad (2)$$

This reaction is catalyzed by the enzyme sphingosine N-acyltransferase (E.C.2.3.1.24). It has a pH optimum of 7.5, and is carried
out mainly in the microsomal fractions. We have been unable to
determine directly the status of this reaction in Farber's disease,
since in the frozen postmortem tissues available to us, it could
not be demonstrated in either the control or Farber's disease
tissues. We have not yet assessed this reaction in cultured skin

fibroblasts. However, in view of the "one gene, one enzyme" concept it is our speculation that this reaction will be found to be unimpaired in Farber's disease. As already noted the levels of ceramides and of more complex sphingolipids are increased in Farber's disease. This finding suggests that the main physiological role of ceramidase is concerned with ceramide degradation, and that ceramide synthesis is catalyzed mainly by other enzymes, presumably by sphingosine N-acyltransferase.

In considering the pathogenesis of Farber's disease one of the points that requires explanation is the variability of involvement of different tissues. Tissues such as bone marrow and spleen, which presumably have an active sphingolipid metabolism, are relatively uninvolved. Furthermore, even in the few cases studied so far, the degree of ceramide accumulation has been found to vary. Thus the subcutaneous nodule and the kidney appear more consistently involved than the liver or brain. A possible explanation for this difference is our recent demonstration of an alkaline ceramidase (pH optimum 9.0), which appears to be normally present in some but not in all tissues, and the activity of which appears normal in Farber's disease (25). The alkaline ceramidase was found to be present in the cerebellum, in white blood cells and in cultured skin fibroblasts, but not in the kidney, which normally appears to contain only the acid ceramidase. Nilsson had previously demonstrated possibly yet another ceramidase with a pH 7.6 optimum in the brush border of the small intestine (26). Possibly the degree of involvement of specific tissues of Farber's disease may be a function of the normal distribution and relative activities of the acid and alkaline ceramidases, keeping in mind that only the acid ceramidase activity appears to be deficient in the disease. To establish this point, more systematic studies are required of the normal distribution and function of these various ceramidases.

We have shown recently that cultured amniotic fluid cells have acid ceramidase activity (21), thus making it likely that the disorder can be diagnosed prenatally. Normal leukocytes also have acid ceramidase activity, and we are presently evaluating the activity of this enzyme in white blood cells of patients with Farber's disease.

ACKNOWLEDGEMENTS

Supported in part by Project 906 of the Maternal and Child Health Service and Grants HD05515, HD04147 and NS10473 from the U. S. Public Health Service. We wish to thank Drs. Ralph Zetterström and Karen Samuelsson for the postmortem tissues of their Farber's disease patient, and Dr. Michael Philippart for access to the cultured skin fibroblasts of case 4.

REFERENCES

1. Prensky, A. L., Ferreira, G., Carr, S. and Moser, H. W. Ceramide and ganglioside accumulation in Farber's lipogranulomatosis. Proc. Soc. Exp. Biol. Med. 126:725-728, 1967

2. Samuelsson, K. and Zetterström, R. Ceramides in a patient with lipogranulomatosis (Farber's disease) with chronic course. Scand. J. Clin. Lab. Invest. 27:393-405, 1971

3. Sugita, M., Dulaney, J. T. and Moser, H. W. Ceramidase deficiency in Farber's disease (lipogranulomatosis). Science 178:1100-1102, 1972

4. Farber, S., Cohen, J. and Uzman, L. L. Lipogranulomatosis. A new lipoglyco-protein "storage" disease. J. Mt. Sinai Hosp. 24:816-837, 1957

5. Crocker, A. C., Cohen, J. and Farber, S. The "Lipogranulomatosis" syndrome; Review, with report of patient showing milder involvement. In: Inborn Disorders of Sphingolipid Metabolism. Edited by S. M. Aronson and B. W. Volk. Pergamon Press, Ltd., Oxford, 1967, pp. 485-503

6. Moser, H. W., Prensky, A. L., Wolfe, H. J. and Rosman, N. P. with the technical assistance of S. Carr and G. Ferreira. Farber's lipogranulomatosis. Report of a case and demonstration of an excess of free ceramide and ganglioside. Amer. J. Med. 47:869-890, 1969

7. Cogan, D. G., Kuwabara, T., Moser, H. and Hazard, G. W. Retinopathy in a case of Farber's lipogranulomatosis. Arch. Ophthal. 75:752-757, 1966

8. Abul-Haj, S. K., Martz, D. G., Douglas, W. F. and Geppert, L. J. Farber's disease. Report of a case with observations on its histogenesis and notes on the nature of the stored material. J. Pediat. 61:221-232, 1962

9. Dustin, P., Tondeur, M., Jonniaux, G., Vamos-Hurwitz, E. and Pelc, S. La maladie de Farber. Etude anatomo-clinique et ultrastructurale. Bull. Acad. Med. Belg. 128:733-762, 1973

10. Barriere, H. and Gillot, F. La lipogranulomatose de Farber. Nouv. Presse med. 2:767-770, 1973

11. Van Hoof, F. and Hers, H. G. Farber's disease. In: Lysosomes and Storage Diseases. Edited by H. G. Hers and F. Van Hoof. Academic Press, Inc. N. Y., 1973, pp. 559-563

12. Bierman, S. M., Edgington, T., Newcomer, V. D. and Pearson,
    C. M. Farber's disease: A disorder of mucopolysaccharide
    metabolism with articular, respiratory, and neurologic
    manifestations. Arthritis & Rheumat. 9:620-630, 1966

13. Rampini, S. and Clausen, J. Farbersche Krankheit
    (disseminierte Lipogranulomatose) Klinisches Bild und
    Zusammenfassung der chemischen Befunde. Helvetica
    Paediatrica Acta 22:500-515, 1967

14. Battin, P. J., Vital, C. L. and Azanza, X. Une neuro-
    lipidose rare avec lesions nodulaires sous-cutanees et
    articulaires: La lipogranulomatose disseminee de Farber.
    Annales de Dermatologie et de Syphiligraphie, Paris,
    97:241-248, 1970

15. Schönenberg, H. and Lindenfelser, R. Farber-Syndrom
    (Disseminierte lipogranulomatose). Mschr. Kinderheilk
    122:153-159, 1974

16. Zetterström, R. Disseminated lipogranulomatosis (Farber's
    disease). Acta Paediatr. 47:501-510, 1958

17. Clausen, J. and Rampini, S. Chemical studies of Farber's
    disease. Acta Neurol. Scandinav. 46:313-322, 1970

18. Iwamori, M. and Moser, H. W. Above-normal urinary excretion
    of urinary ceramides in Farber's disease, and characteriza-
    tion of their components by high-performance liquid chromato-
    graphy. Clin. Chem. 21:725-729, 1975

19. Sugita, M., Connolly, P., Dulaney, J. T. and Moser, H. W.
    Fatty acid composition of free ceramides of kidney and
    cerebellum from a patient with Farber's disease. Lipids
    8:401-406, 1973

20. Philippart, M., Nakatani, S., Zeilstra, K., Tondeur, M.,
    Vamos-Hurwitz, E. and Pelc, S. Farber's disease: Ceramide
    accumulation in cultured skin fibroblasts. Trans. Amer. Soc.
    Neurochem. 6:152, 1975

21. Dulaney, J. T., Milunsky, A., Moser, H. W. Diagnosis of
    Farber's disease by use of cultured fibroblasts. Submitted
    for publication, 1975

22. Gatt, S., Enzymatic hydrolysis of sphingolipids. I. Hydro-
    lysis and synthesis of ceramides by an enzyme from rat brain.
    J. Biol. Chem. 241:3724-3730, 1966

23. Yavin, E. and Gatt, S. Enzymatic hydrolysis of sphingolipids.
     VIII. Further purification and properties of rat brain
     ceramidase. Biochemistry 8:1692-1698, 1969

24. Sribney, M. Enzymatic synthesis of ceramide. Biochim.
     Biophys. Acta. 125:542-547, 1966

25. Sugita, M., Williams, M., Dulaney, J. T. and Moser, H. W.
     Ceramidase and ceramide synthesis in human kidney and
     cerebellum. Description of a new alkaline ceramidase.
     Biochim. Biophys. Acta. 398:125-131, 1975

26. Nilsson, A. The presence of sphingomyelin- and ceramide-
     cleaving enzymes in the small intestinal tract. Biochim.
     Biophys. Acta 176:339-347, 1969

ULTRASTRUCTURE AND PEROXIDASE OF LEUCOCYTES IN FIVE PATIENTS WITH JUVENILE FORM OF CEROID LIPOFUSCINOSES*

M. Daria Haust, Bruce A. Gordon, and George G. Hinton

The Departments of Pathology, Biochemistry and Pediatrics
CPRI and The University of Western Ontario
London, Ontario, Canada

In the past decade several advances have been made regarding the nature of diseases formerly known as amaurotic familial idiocies (AFI). This group was characterized clinically by cerebro-retinal degenerations and morphologically by the accumulation of heterogeneous substances, all believed to have some lipid component.

The identification of various gangliosides among these accumulating substances in some patients and the subsequent demonstration of reduced levels of the specific enzymatic activity at the corresponding catabolic steps of gangliosides, allowed for the separation of a gangliosidic group from the original AFI. In the belief that various proportions of ceroid and lipofuscin accumulate in the remaining patients, the term: neuronal ceroid-lipofuscinoses (NCLF) was coined for the second group of the AFI (13).

Both the gangliosidic and non-gangliosidic groups of the AFI have been further subdivided. The subgrouping of the NCLF is based largely on the age of onset of signs and symptoms. In each of the four groups the infantile (10), late infantile, juvenile and the adult group (14) there is a different natural history, and thus prognostic value.

It has been widely accepted that ultrastructurally characteristic cytoplasmic "inclusions" that are present in many cells, not only neurons, typify each subgroup (5), and recently Armstrong and

---
*Supported by grants-in-aid of research No. 214-69C and No. 413 from The Ontario Mental Health Foundation, Toronto, Canada.

his associates have reported (1,2) that a specific peroxidase activity was deficient in the peripheral leucocytes in the late
infantile, juvenile and adult forms.

    The above advances in the area of NCLF were hardly made when
uncertainties and discrepancies emerged again on several fronts
including the question of the place of the specific peroxidase activity in the NCLF and their diagnosis, as well as the matter of
the ultrastructural specificity for each of the subgroups.

    In an attempt at clarifying some of the above problems a study
was undertaken with the aim at correlating the ultrastructural
appearance and the assayed values for the specific peroxidase activity of peripheral leucocytes in a group of patients with NCLF.
To avoid uncertainties or possible errors in previously made diagnoses only five of the eleven patients in this group were selected
for examination as their clinical histories and studies were documented in detail. All five patients belonged to the juvenile type
of the NCLF.

    The purpose of this communication is to report the results of
the above study and to discuss their possible relevance to the im-
plied significance of the specific peroxidase in the pathogenesis
of this group of diseases.

                          CLINICAL DATA

    All five patients were Caucasian girls. The clinical histo-
ries were typical of the juvenile type of NCLF (synonym: the
Spielmeyer-Vogt disease). The respective pregnancies and deliver-
ies were uneventful and the term infants developed normally in the
early period of life.

    Data pertinent to the disease under consideration are summar-
ized in Table I. Visual problems were the first manifestations of
the disease at the age of six, seven or eight years, with the exception of one patient (J.Z., Table I), whose visual acuity became
impaired at the age of 18 months, i.e., six months following an
acute episode of measles. Her vision deteriorated gradually and at
the age of eight years the child was only able to recognize bright
lights. At the time of measles the then one-year-old patient had
febrile convulsions and experienced similar convulsive episodes with
high fever in the following years. These febrile convulsions ceased
to occur at the age of five years.

    The impairment of vision progressed in all patients, in some to
almost complete blindness, over a period of three to four years.
At that stage the funduscopic examination was recorded as bilateral
retinitis pigmentosa with or without optic atrophy.

Incidental to the changes in vision, the children were observed to show evidence of mental deterioration, but neither the rate nor the severity of the mental retardation was uniform in the group. Some still function at only mildly retarded level (M.P.; C.V.; Table I) six or eight years following the first signs of regression, whereas one patient deteriorated severely in the short span of three years (L.M.; Table I).

Grand mal seizures developed six months, three years and as late as seven years following the onset of visual impairment (L.M.; Table I), and their frequency also varied considerably. Seizures were never experienced by one patient whose visual loss began at the age of eight years and who at present is fourteen years old. In view of experience with the one patient mentioned above, it is quite conceivable that this girl will yet develop seizures.

The tonus and power of muscles was normal in three patients, whereas increasing weakness and fatigability caused confinement of one patient to a wheelchair since the age of ten years; the fifth patient has preferred using a wheelchair since the age of twelve years.

At present the youngest of the patients is twelve and the oldest 18 years of age; the latter shows the most severe deterioration of the group.

ASSAYS OF LEUCOCYTIC PEROXIDASE

The leucocytes of each patient were harvested from 8 ml of venous blood mixed with 2 ml of a solution of heparin-dextran-saline (6), and washed with ammonium chloride solution and phosphate buffered saline. The peroxidase activity was assayed (with p-phenylene-diamine as the co-substrate) according to the procedure outlined by Patel and associates (8). The peroxidase activity of leucocytes obtained from 16 normal subjects and assayed under identical conditions served as control values.

The cumulative peroxidase activity in leucocyte preparations carried out on two different occasions for each patient was compared with the normal control levels. This activity was considerably lower in three patients (Fig. 1; M.P.; C.V.; L.M.) than that of the control subjects, but was within normal range in the two other patients (Fig. 1: J.Z.; C.M.).

ULTRASTRUCTURE OF LYMPHOCYTES

A 10-ml venous blood sample was obtained from each patient at the same time as the blood drawn for the enzymatic assay. The

Table 1. SUMMARY OF OCULAR, CEREBRAL AND MOTOR STATUS

Pat.	Age	Visual Status	Funduscopic Findings	Mental Status	Seizures	Motor Status
JZ	12	Impaired visual acuity since 1¼ (6 mo. after measles) progressive to age 8 then able to recognize only bright light.	Bilateral retinal pigmentation.	Functioning at borderline normal level; no consistent evidence of deterioration.	Convulsion with measles at age 1. Subsequent febrile convulsions but none since age 5.	From age 10 increasing weakness and fatigability; now confined to wheelchair.
MP	13	Visual problems age 7; slowly progressive: at 10 only able to recognize bright light.	Bilateral optic atrophy with peripheral retinal pigmentation.	At age 7 lost learned ability to write name.	Since age 7½ 1 grand mal seizure/month.	Muscle power and tone normal.
CM	14	Visual loss progressive since age 8.	Bilateral retinitis pigmentosa.	School difficulties from kindergarten on; now moderately retarded.	No seizures.	Muscle power and tone normal.
CV	14	Visual loss progressive since age 6.	Bilateral optic atrophy with scattered retinal pigmentation.	In grade I at age 6, regarded as slow learner; now moderately retarded.	First grand mal seizure at age 9 with 1 or 2 per year since.	Shuffling gait for 2 years. Walks only with support. Prefers wheelchair.
LM	18	Failing eyesight since age 7; progressive slowly.	Bilateral optic atrophy with retinitis pigmentosa.	Began to deteriorate at about age 10; now severely retarded.	Grand mal seizures since age 14, 1 or 2 per month.	Muscle power and tone normal.

N.B. Unless specified otherwise, numbers referring to ages indicate years.

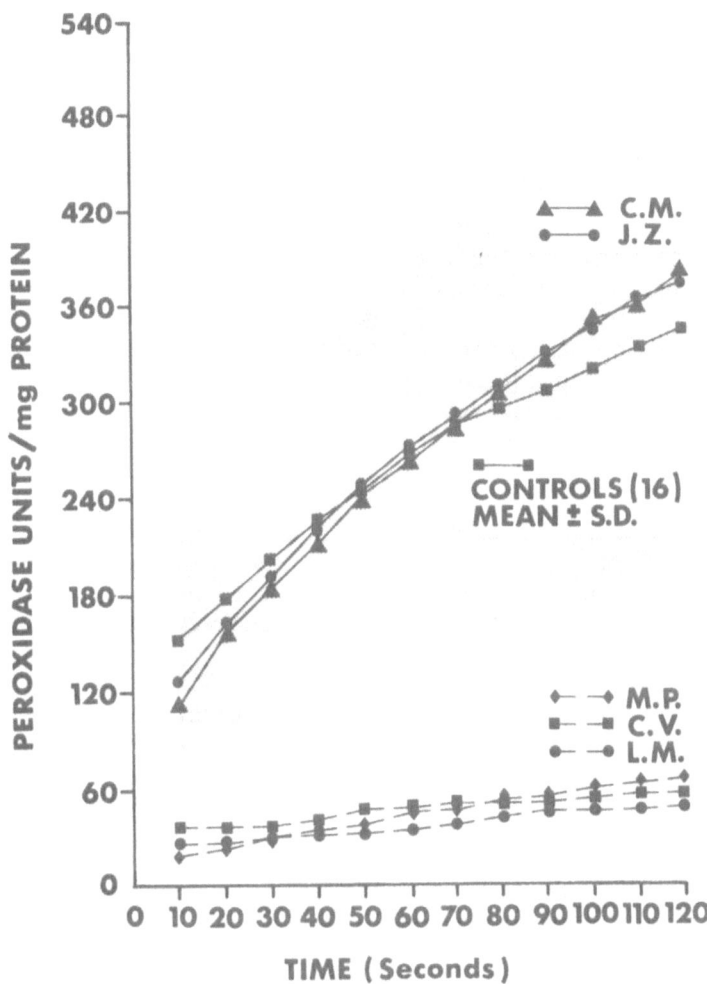

Fig. 1 Peroxidase activity in peripheral leucocytes from patients,
C.M., J.Z., M.P., C.V., and L.M., with juvenile neuronal
ceroid-lipofuscinosis. The shaded area represents ± 1 SD
from the control mean. Absorbance measurements were converted to units of peroxidase activity by comparison with a
standard curve; one unit gave an optical density equivalent
to that produced by 1 μg of horseradish peroxidase (Sigma
Type VI) in 1 minute.

leucocytic layer was processed for electron microscopic examination by the well established methods; the pellet of cells was
embedded in Epon-812 and thin sections were stained with uranyl
acetate and lead citrate. Identically processed lymphocytes available from two normal subjects served as controls.

The ultrastructural appearance of lymphocytes was similar in
all five patients and therefore will be described with no reference to the individual patients.

Numerous small and large size lymphocytes contained partly or
entirely empty vacuoles (or sacs) which varied in number and size
in the same patient and from one patient to another. In some lymphocytes the vacuoles were numerous (Fig. 2), whereas in other cells
only a few were present (Fig. 3). The size of these vacuoles varied
from those smaller to considerably larger than the average-sized
mitochondria. All vacuoles were limited by a trilaminar unit membrane.

Some of the vacuoles contained structured and unstructured
osmiophilic bodies. The structured vacuolar inclusions consisted
of parallel arrays of alternating electron-dense and electron-
lucent bands. These had either a straight course (Fig. 4), or were
slightly curved and concentric (Fig. 2), and were thus reminiscent
of finger-print images.

Similar arrays of stacked membranous structures were present
at times free in the hyaloplasm (Fig. 5); here they usually assumed
somewhat complex configurations with angular, highly irregular bor-
ders and often abutted upon, or were in continuity with the limiting
membranes of empty or distorted vacuolar remnants (Fig. 6). Often
these "free" bodies blended imperceptibly with the hyaloplasm (Figs.
5 and 6) and their constituent membranes were intertwined and con-
glomerated (as if condensed).

In suitably cut sections, presumably in a plane perpendicular
to the long axis of the membranous stacks, a distinct tubular nature,
or lattice-like arrangement of these parallel structures could be

---

Fig. 2 (See opposite). The large peripheral lymphocyte contains
        several vacuoles limited by a trilaminar membrane. Distinct
        tubulo-membranous arrays, some with fingerprint images, are
        seen in four of these; in others, nondescript and variably
        osmiophilic substances are present; nonspecific membranous
        remnants are seen in the vacuole on the extreme upper right
        side of the photograph. In the plane immediately above the
        nucleus, note a prominent Golgi on the left and on the right
        a multi-vesicular body (arrow).
        Magnification = x 26,000.

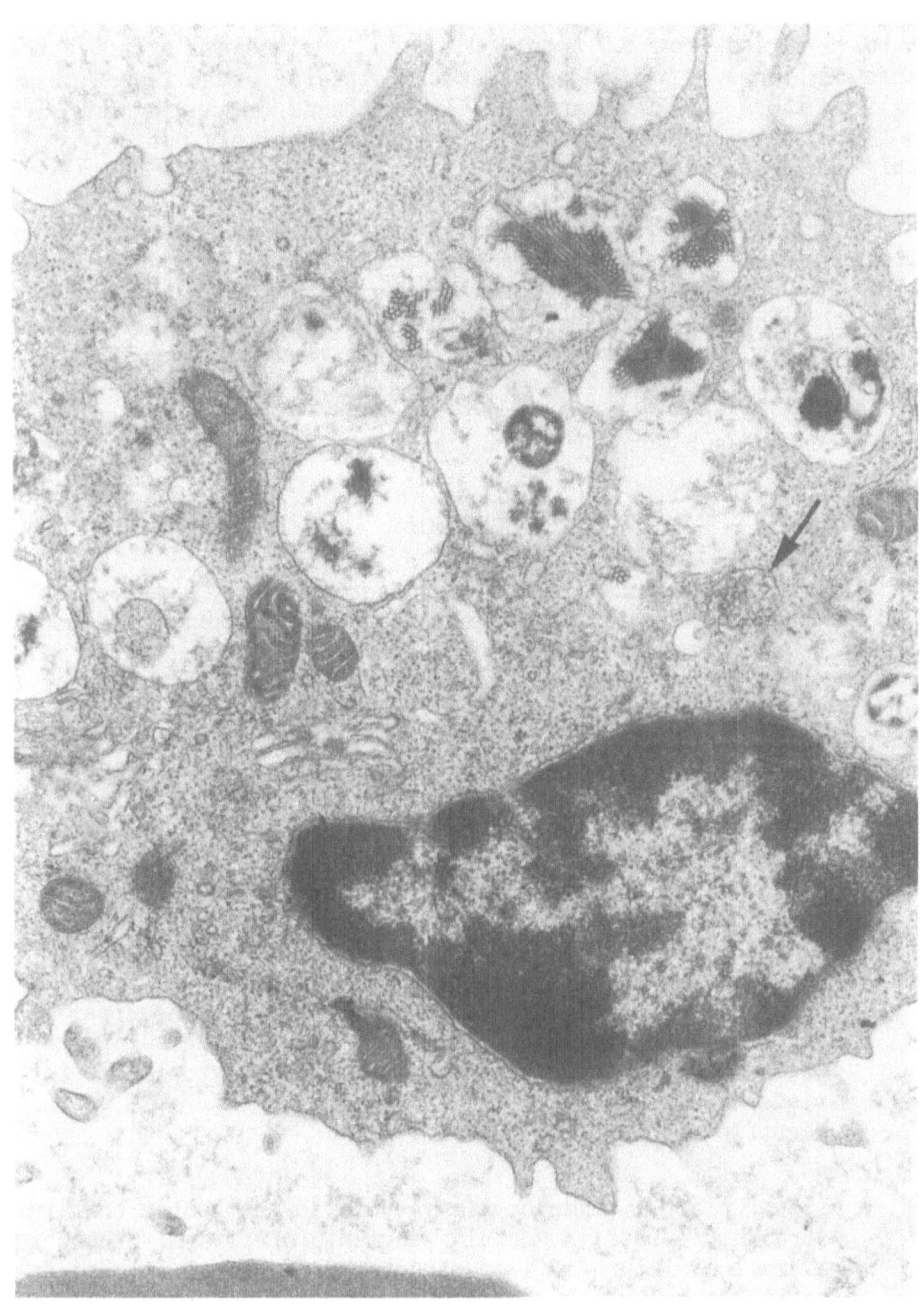

visualized (Figs. 2, 3, 6 and 7). In the cross sections the lumen appeared to be entirely electron-lucent measuring from 160 Å to 180 Å in diameter; the surrounding electron-dense membrane measured from 70 Å to 90 Å in thickness. Thus, the outer diameter of a "tubule" varied from 300 Å to 360 Å. In longitudinal sections the dense membranes of two adjacent stacks appeared often fused (measuring from 140 Å to 180 Å) and the "light" bands (measuring from 160 Å to 180 Å) between the dark bands were never entirely but only moderately electron-lucent (Fig. 7).

In addition to the above inclusions, structureless, extremely electron-dense material was present either alone in cytoplasmic vacuoles (Fig. 3), or intermingled with the above structured inclusions (Fig. 2). When in vacuoles, the dense structureless substance often was associated with membranous unorganized remnants (Fig. 2).

The described alterations were not observed in lymphocytes of normal control subjects.

DISCUSSION

The membrano-tubular inclusions observed in the lymphocytes of all five patients are similar to the organelles reported in the literature as cytosomes with "fingerprint" profiles (10). These were at first regarded as being pathognomonic of the juvenile form of the neuronal ceroid lipofuscinoses (NCLF) and were observed in various tissues (4,10) including the peripheral lymphocytes (11). Subsequently, however, similar profiles were found also in patients with

---

Fig. 3 (Upper plate). There are only a few vacuoles of small and medium size (compare with the size of the mitochondria) in this lymphocyte. Some vacuoles do not have a well defined limiting membrane and their contents merge with those of the hyaloplasm. A few straight, slightly curved and tubular arrays are present in the vacuolar spaces at the upper right segment of the cell; a nondescript osmiophilic substance is present in the vacuole at the lower right cytoplasmic portion.
Magnification = x 17,000.

Fig. 4 (Lower plate). Lymphocytic vacuole in the center contains straight, curved and tubular segments of arrays. There is a small admixture of less structured (? granular or degenerating tubular) osmiophilic substance. The content of the other vacuoles is of nondescript nature.
Magnification = x 41,000.

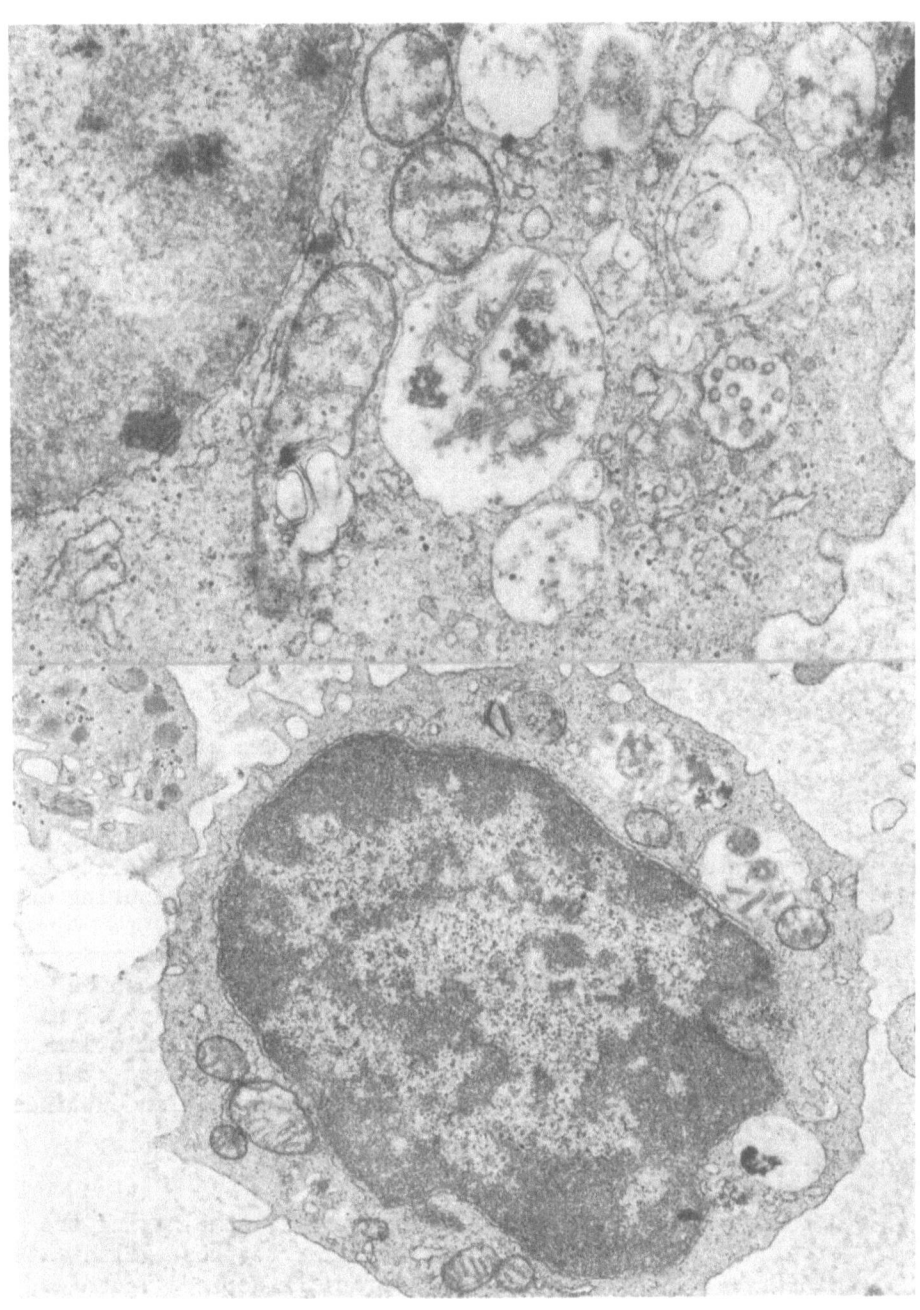

a clinical history and course typical of the late infantile form of
NCLF. Conversely, the cytosomes with the so-called curvilinear profiles, once thought to be characteristic of the late infantile form,
were observed also in the juvenile type of this disease group (4).
Nevertheless, assuming that similar or identical inclusions do not
occur also in other diseases, one may state that the presence of the
structures with the fingerprint images, indicates that all five patients belong to the group of NCLF.

At variance with these morphological observations are the results obtained for the assay of leucocyte peroxidase activity (Fig.
1) reported to be specifically low in patients with NCLF (2). Of
the five patients studied only three showed a value lower than that
for the sixteen normal controls, and the remaining two had levels
not different from those of the controls.

The discrepancy between the results of morphological observations and peroxidase activity may be interpreted in one of several
ways. It may imply that the ultrastructural features, the cytosomes with fingerprint images, lack specificity not only for one of
the subgroups, i.e., the juvenile form, but for the entire group of
NCLF. Conceivably, these cytosomes may occur in a wide variety of
diseases and have either an identical or slightly altered appearance
and measurements. Indeed, parallel tubular inclusions reminiscent
of those reported in the present study, were observed in peripheral
lymphocytes from patients with various hematological disorders (3).
Whereas the measurements of the internal structure of the cytosomes
observed in this study were provided above, these are being viewed
with some scepticism as representing true values. It has become
evident to the present authors as well as many other morphologists
that measurements in the range expressed above are in reality extremely unreliable and subject not only to errors in measuring and

Fig. 5 (Upper plate). This lymphocyte contains two cytosomes
        consisting of intertwining membrano-tubular arrays of no
        definite arrangement; these are "free" in the hyaloplasm.
        The elements of these merge imperceptibly with the hyalo-
        plasm and the structures have angulated irregular outlines.
        Magnification = x 52,000.

Fig. 6 (Lower plate). Membrano-tubular arrays, some having the
        typical fingerprint appearance similar to those illustrated
        in Figs. 2-5, are present either in ill-defined vacuoles,
        or "free" in the hyaloplasm. Some of the latter abut on
        or fuse with the nearby vacuolar remnants.
        Magnification = x 21,000.

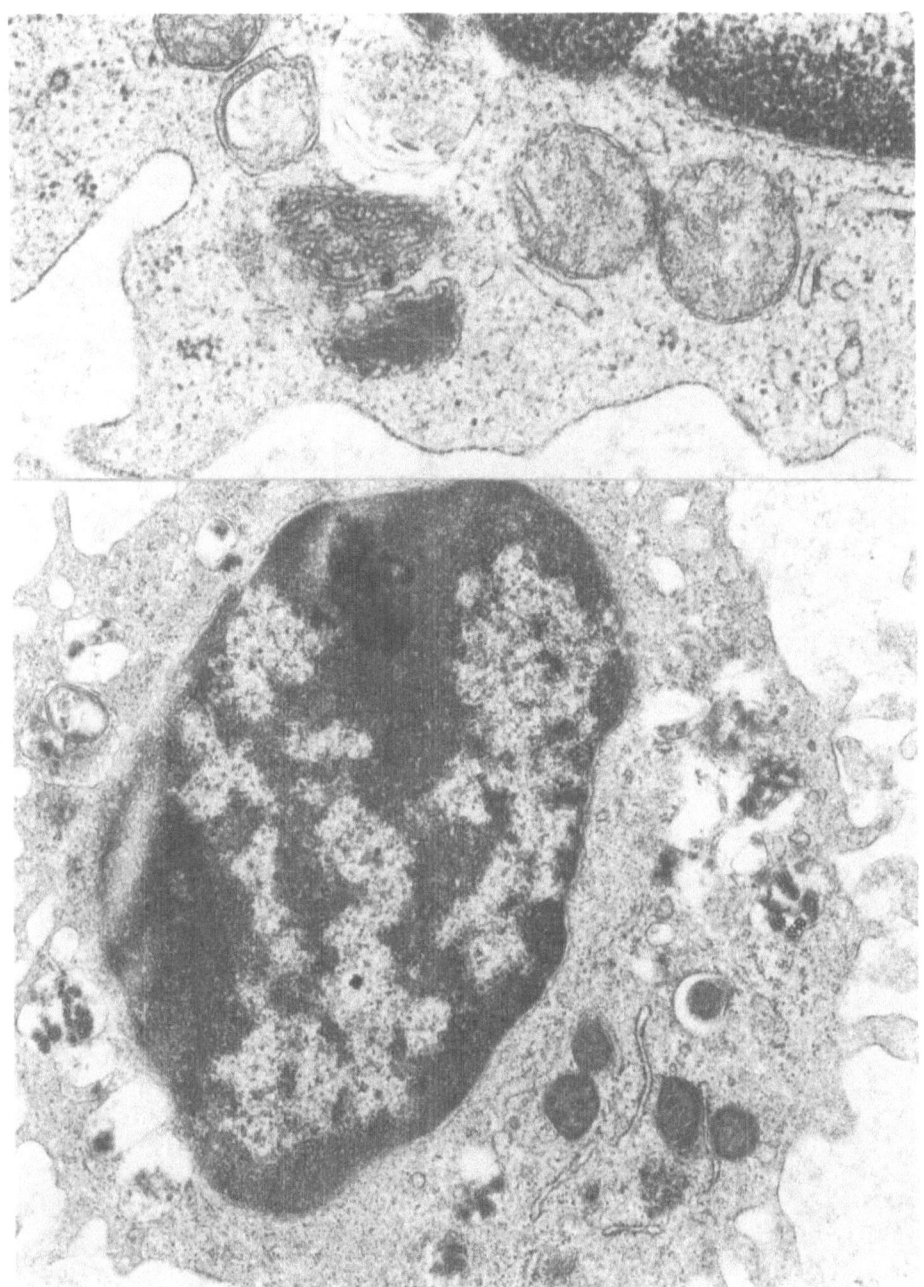

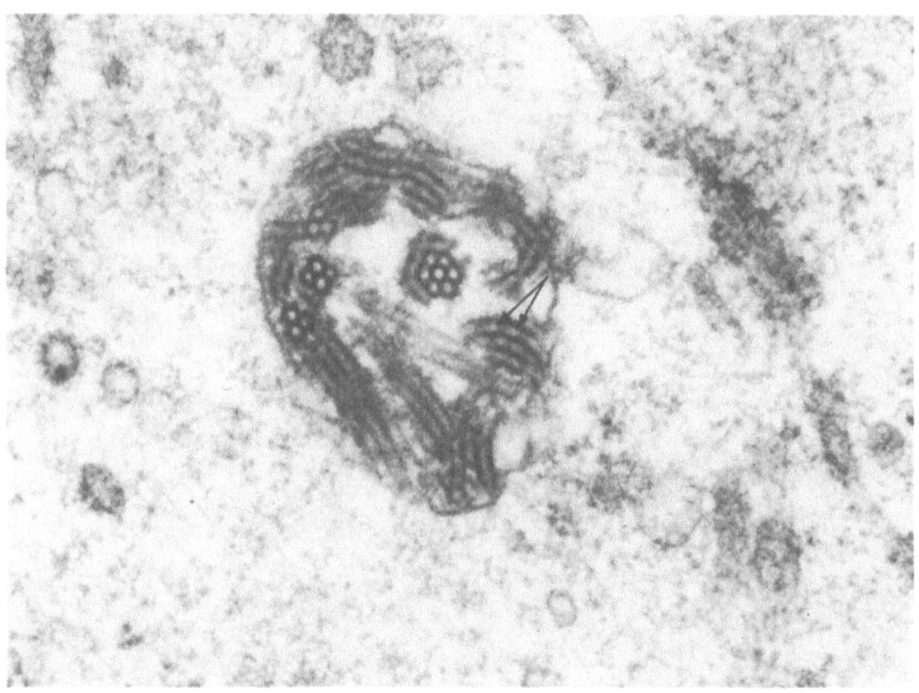

Fig. 7.   Higher magnification of the membrano-tubular arrays of a
          section, presumably cut in a plane perpendicular to the
          long axis of the membranous stacks. Note the lattice-
          like arrangements of the tubular structures. The lumen
          of a tubule is entirely electron-lucent and measures from
          160 Å to 180 Å in diameter. The surrounding electron-
          dense membrane measures from 70 Å to 90 Å in thickness.
          The dense membranes of two adjacent stacks appear to be
          fused (measuring from 140 Å to 180 Å). The "light" bands
          (measuring from 160 Å to 180 Å) between the dark bands
          are not entirely electron-lucent; there is a suggestion
          of circular areas of greater electron-lucency of an ap-
          proximate size of the tubular lumen (arrows).
          Magnification = x 80,000.

calibration of the electron microscope, but subject to the many unpredictable and variable steps in tissue processing. In summary, whereas the lymphocytes of all patients examined showed the presence of similar cytosomes that were not observed in normal controls, it is still not known whether these are indeed pathognomonic for the NCLF. Moreover, a recently reported case of a juvenile cerebro-macular degeneration indicates that in some instances the inclusions may be largely of a granular type (5).

The second explanation for the above discrepancy between the morphological and enzymatic results could be considered from the point of assaying the peroxidase. It is possible that the method employed to determine the peroxidase is either not sufficiently sensitive to measure the defective enzyme in all cases of this disease, or alternatively, the reported activity of the peroxidase tested is only a secondary and a rather variable phenomenon in a chain of processes "operating" in the pathogenesis of the NCLF. If the latter were true the concept as proposed for the pathogenesis of the NCLF would be no longer tenable (12). From our own experience it may be of interest to cite an example in support of the latter possibility. A teenage girl with a history of progressive mental deterioration had leukocyte peroxidase activity levels as low as those in 3 of our 5 patients with NCLF, and proved subsequently to have metachromatic leucodystrophy (7).

The presence of the characteristic cytosomes in the peripheral lymphocytes emphasizes again the fact that the term NCLF is somewhat inaccurate at least on the account of the first word, i.e. "neuronal" in this terminology. It has been known for quite a while now that many tissues and organs rather than only the nervous system, are involved in the accumulation of the substances characterizing this group of diseases (4). Recently, the advisability of continuing the usage of this terminology was questioned for another reason (5).

It is apparent from all data emerging lately that despite numerous advances in recent years in the field of the so-called NCLF much more work is still necessary for the understanding of the basic nature of these diseases.

SUMMARY

Peripheral leucocytes obtained from five patients with clinical histories and funduscopic findings typical of the juvenile form of the so-called neuronal ceroid lipofuscinosis (NCLF) (synonym: Spielmeyer-Vogt disease) were assayed for peroxidase activity and examined by electron microscopy. The peroxidase levels were considerably lower in three but normal in two patients. Ultrastructurally, the lymphocytes of all five patients showed the presence of tubulo-

membranous cytosomes many displaying the fingerprint images at
present regarded as being typical for the NCLF.

The possible implications of the discrepancy between the morphological observations and the enzymatic findings are discussed.

ACKNOWLEDGEMENTS

The authors wish to thank Mr. Roger Dewar and Mrs. Vera Feleki
for skillful technical assistance and Mrs. Phyllis Cloghesy for efficient typing of the manuscript.

REFERENCES

1. Armstrong, D., Dimmitt, S., Boehme, D.H., Leonberg, S.C., Jr.
   and Vogel, W. Leukocyte peroxidase deficiency in a family
   with a dominant form of Kuf's disease. Science 186:155, 1974.

2. Armstrong, D., Dimmitt, S. and Van Wormer, D.E. Studies in
   Batten disease. I. Peroxidase deficiency in granulocytes.
   Arch. Neurol. 30:144, 1974.

3. Brunning, R.D. and Parkins, J. Ultrastructural studies of
   parallel tubular arrays in human lymphocytes. Am. J. Pathol.
   78:59, 1975.

4. Carpenter, S., Karpati, G. and Anderman, F. Specific involvement of muscle, nerve and skin in late-infantile and juvenile
   amaurotic idiocy. Neurol. 22:170, 1972.

5. Carpenter, S., Karpati, G., Wolfe, L.S. and Anderman, F. A
   type of cerebromacular degeneration characterized by granular
   osmiophilic deposits. J. Neurol. Sci. 18:68, 1973.

6. Kampine, J.P., Brady, R.O., Kanfer, J.N., Feld, M. and
   Shapiro, D. Diagnosis of Gaucher's disease and Neimann-Pick
   disease with small samples of venous blood. Science 155:86,
   1966.

7. Lowden, J.A. Personal communication.

8. Patel, V., Koppang, N., Patel, B. and Zeman, W. p-Phenylene-
   diamine-mediated peroxidase deficiency in English setters with
   neuronal ceroid-lipofuscinosis. Lab. Invest. 30:366, 1974.

9. Santavuori, P., Haltia, M. and Papola, J. Infantile type of
   so-called neuronal ceroid-lipofuscinosis. Develop. Med. Child.
   Neurol. 16:644, 1974.

10. Suzuki, K., Johnson, A.B., Marquet, E. and Suzuki, K. A case
     of juvenile lipidosis: Electron microscopic, histochemical
     and biochemical studies. Acta neuropath. (Berl.) 11:122, 1968.

11. Witzleben, C.L., Smith, K., Nelson, J.S., Monteleone, P.L.
     and Livingston, D.J. Ultrastructural studies in late-onset
     amaurotic idiocy: Lymphocyte inclusion as a diagnostic marker.
     J. Ped. 79:285, 1971.

12. Zeman, W. Studies in the neuronal ceroid-lipofuscinoses. J.
     Neuropath. Exp. Neurol. 33:1, 1974.

13. Zeman, W. and Dyken, P. Neuronal ceroid-lipofuscinosis
     (Batten's disease) relationship to amaurotic family idiocy.
     Pediat. 44:570, 1969.

14. Zeman, W. and Siakotos, A.N. The neuronal ceroid-lipofuscinoses
     in lysosomes and storage diseases. Hers, H.G. and Van Hoof, T.,
     (eds.), New York, Academic Press, 1973, p. 519.

ULTRASTRUCTURE AND BIOCHEMICAL STUDIES OF RAT CNS
AND VISCERA AFTER SUBCUTANEOUS INJECTION
OF CHLORPHENTERMINE*

Masazumi Adachi, Chhin-Yang Tsai,
Mark Greenbaum, Barbara Mask and Bruno W. Volk

Isaac Albert Research Institute of the
Kingsbrook Jewish Medical Center
Brooklyn, New York

Chlorphentermine, known as an anoretic drug, has been
reported by Franken and associates to induce the formation of foamy cells in the lungs of rats (1). Subsequently, several investigators have described cytoplasmic
inclusion bodies in the viscera (2-9) which are considered to be the experimental counterpart of human lipidosis.

Since suitable experimental models of sphingolipidoses are difficult to obtain, the present study was
carried out to investigate whether or not chlorphentermine induces true lipidosis in rats.

MATERIAL AND METHODS

The animals were divided into three groups (Table 1).

The first group consisted of 30 young adult Sprague-
Dawley rats of either sex weighing 170 gm. which were
injected with a single subcutaneous daily dose of 40 mg./
kg. body weight of chlorphentermine hydrochloride. In a
control group of 16 rats, each animal received a single
subcutaneous daily dose of saline solution.

The 20 surviving experimental rats as well as the
control animals were sacrificed at intervals varying from

* This work was supported by a grant from the National
Tay-Sachs and Allied Diseases Association, Inc.

TABLE 1

SYNOPSIS OF EXPERIMENTAL GROUPS INDICATING INJECTED DOSES, NUMBER OF RATS AND SACRIFICE SCHEDULE OF EACH GROUP

GROUP	STATE	INJECTED SOLUTION (DOSES)	NO. OF RATS	SACRIFICE SCHEDULE DAY 1	WEEKS 1	2	3	4	6	8	10	12
1	Experimental	Chlorphentermine (40 mg./kg. b.w.)	20	—	5	5	5	—	—	—	—	—
1	Control	Physiologic Saline Solution	16	—	4	4	4	—	—	—	—	—
2 *)a)	Experimental	Chlorphentermine (40 mg./kg. b.w.)	6	6	—	—	—	—	—	—	—	—
2 *)a)	Control	Physiologic Saline Solution	3	3	—	—	—	—	—	—	—	—
3 *)b)	Experimental	Chlorphentermine (10 mg./kg. b.w.)	40	—	5	5	5	5	5	5	5	5
3 *)b)	Control	Physiologic Saline Solution	32	—	4	4	4	4	4	4	4	4

*) In groups 2 and 3 injections were administered to pregnant rats.
a) In group 2, the offspring were sacrificed on the first day of life.
b) In group 3, the newborn animals were sacrificed at the weeks indicated in the above table.

one to four weeks after the first injection. Portions of brain, liver, lungs and pancreas were directly immersed in 3% glutaraldehyde solution without perfusion so that fresh frozen tissues could be used for biochemical studies. Samples of the CNS tissue were taken from the frontal cortex and white matter, the basal ganglia, the cerebellar cortex and white matter and spinal cord.

The second group consisted of 12 pregnant rats at 10 days gestation weighing 300 gm. which were injected with a single subcutaneous daily dose of 40 mg./kg. of body weight of chlorphentermine hydrochloride. In the control group, three pregnant rats received a single subcutaneous daily dose of saline solution. Since the majority of the litters died within two days after delivery, six newborn rats and three control animals had to be sacrificed at one day after birth. The selection of tissue was similar to that in the first group.

In the third group, 30 pregnant rats received a single subcutaneous daily injection of 10 mg./kg. of body weight of chlorphentermine. In order to get a continuous effect on the babies, the same dose was given to the nursing mothers until three weeks after delivery. Three weeks after birth the young rats received the same injection schedule. In a control study, five pregnant rats and 32 delivered babies received the same dose of saline solution. The 40 surviving animals and the 32 control baby rats were sacrificed at intervals from one to 12 weeks. The tissue samples were similar to those used in the first group.

Ultrastructural and biochemical studies on the specimens were carried out according to previously described standard techniques (10,11).

RESULTS

In the first group, the animals contained a moderate number of cytoplasmic inclusion bodies in the lungs and liver during the first week. In the alveolar cells, the inclusion bodies consisted of loosely arranged concentric lamellae which were surrounded by a limiting membrane (Fig. 1). In the liver, the cytoplasmic bodies in the hepatocytes were composed of aggregates of concentric, but more compact, membranous structures (Fig. 2). The Kupffer cells showed similar inclusions.

During the first three weeks after the first injection

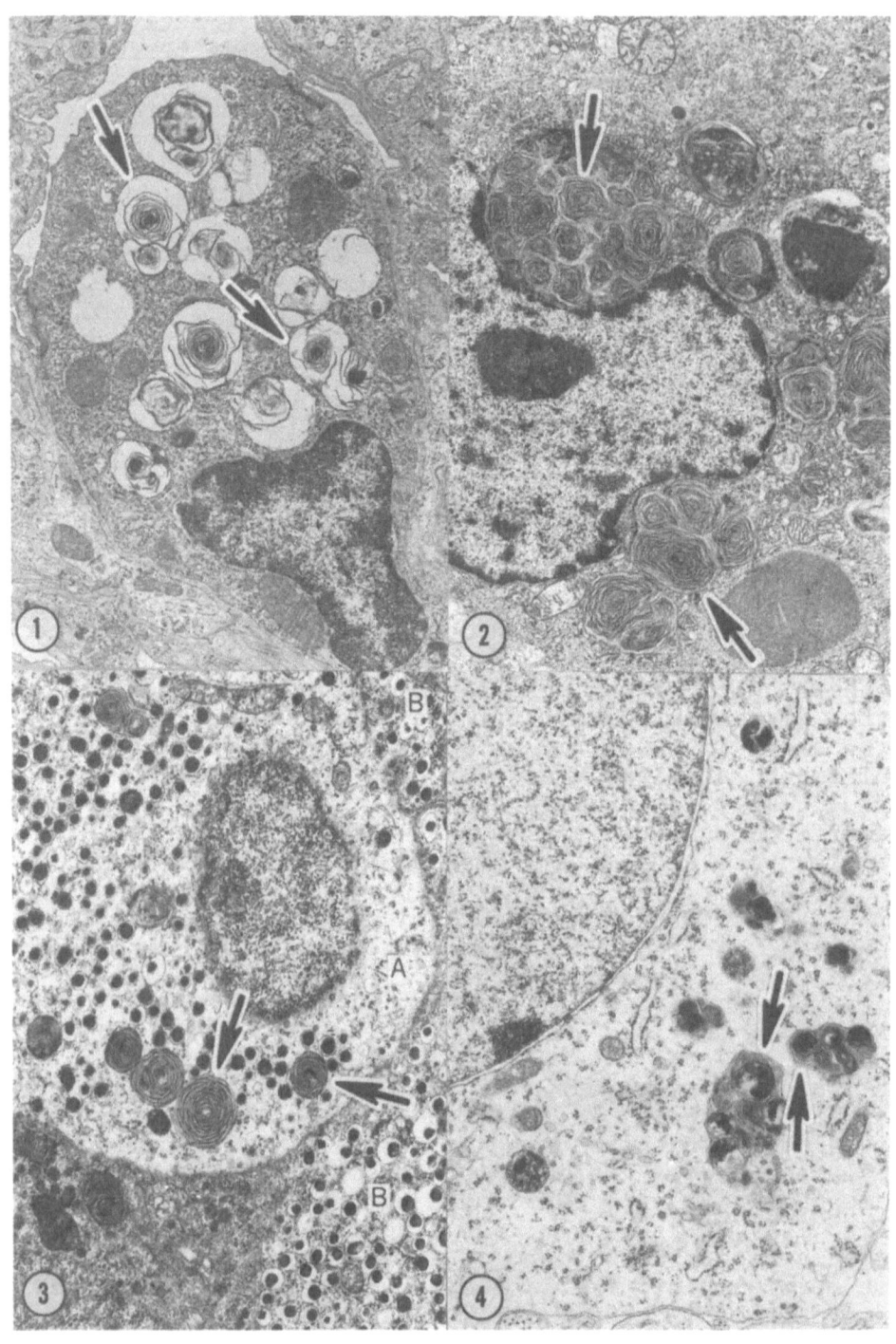

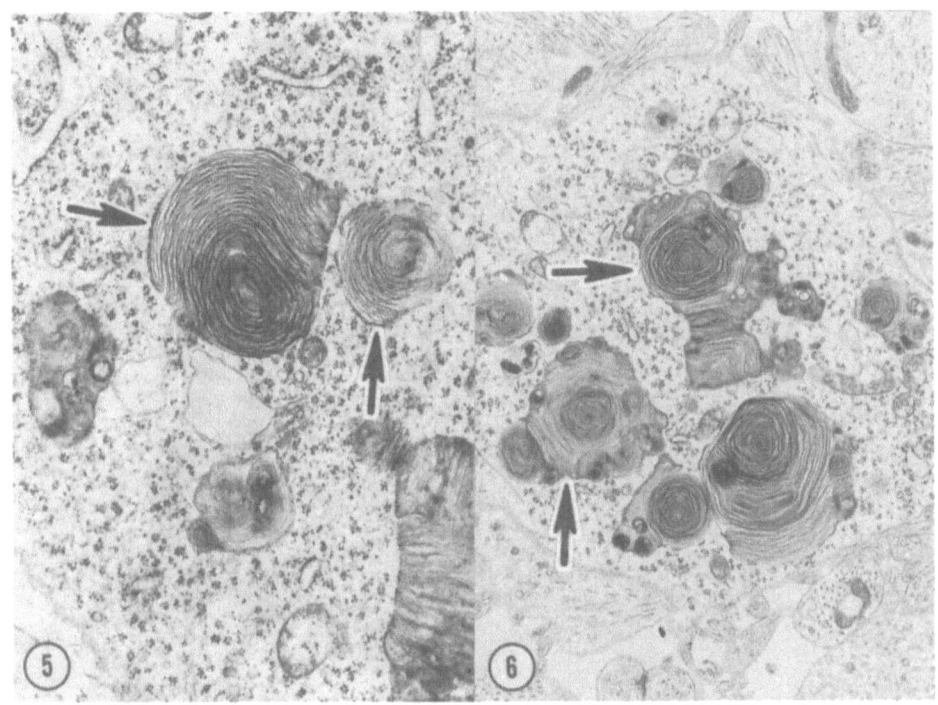

FIGURE 1: Portion of alveolar cell of animal of group 1, sacrificed during the first week showing cytoplasmic inclusion bodies which are composed of loosely arranged membranous structures surrounded by a single limiting membrane (arrows). X 10,500.

FIGURE 2: Portion of hepatocyte of rat (group 1) sacrificed during the first week showing cytoplasmic inclusion bodies which are composed of aggregates of concentric and compact membranous structures (arrows). X 10,500.

FIGURE 3: Portion of islet of Langerhans of animal of group 1 sacrificed during the fourth week showing a few membranous bodies (arrows) in A(A) and B(B) cells. X 11,700.

FIGURE 4: Portion of neuron of animal of group 1 sacrificed during the fourth week showing irregularly shaped dense bodies which are surrounded by laminated structures (arrows). X 15,200.

FIGURE 5: In another neuron of the same animal as shown in Fig. 4, there are well developed concentrically arranged membranes (arrows). X 18,700.

FIGURE 6: Frequently the cytosomes form congeries of laminated bodies which are surrounded by a limiting membrane (arrows). X 11,700.

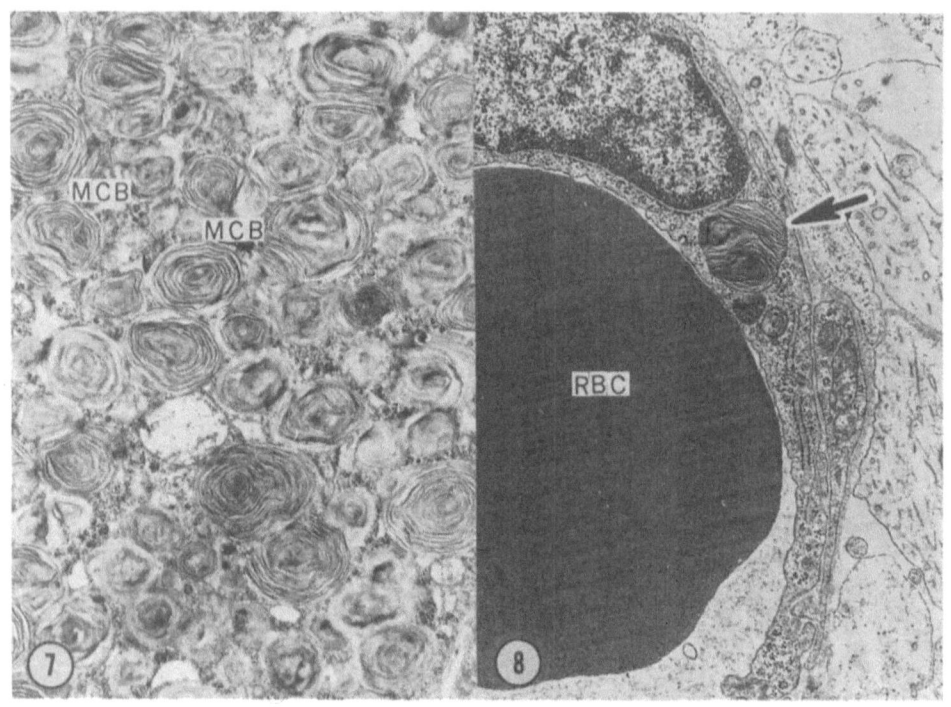

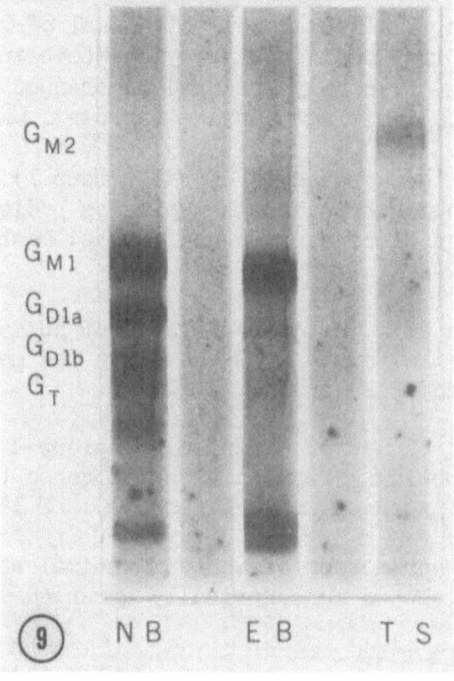

TABLE 2

LIPID BOUND SIALIC ACID*

Brain		Liver	
Exper.	Control	**Exper.**	Control
0.078	0.076	0.0056	0.0058

* Expressed as percent dry weight

TABLE 3

CEREBRAL GANGLIOSIDE PATTERNS*

Data	Normal Brain	Exper. Brain
G_{M1}	44.0	90.9
G_{D1a}	33.1	6.64
G_{D1b}	9.9	0.97
G_T	9.9	1.27
G_O	3.1	0.22

* Expressed as percent of total
N-acetyl neuraminic acid

FIGURE 7: Some of the neurons are densely filled with membranous cytoplasmic bodies (MCB's). X 14,000.

FIGURE 8: Portion of capillary endothelial cells also showing occasional inclusion bodies (arrow). RBC-Red Blood Cell. X 15,200.

FIGURE 9: Thin layer chromatograms of the brain of an animal (group 1) sacrificed during the fourth week (EB). The major ganglioside fraction has an Rf value which is similar to that of G_{M1}-ganglioside. NB-Control Rat Brain; TS-Brain of Patient With Tay-Sachs Disease.

TABLE 4

PHOSPHOLIPID ANALYSIS OF BRAIN AND LIVER

Data	Brain Exper.	Control	Liver Exper.	Control
Total Phospholipids*	10.5	10.4	4.8	4.7
Phosphatidyl Ethanolamine[+]	36.0	32.81	23.8	23.5
Phosphatidyl Choline[+]	38.0	38.28	45.6	48.0
Sphingomyelin[+]	6.75	7.14	4.3	3.8
Phosphatidyl Inositol[+]	5.13	4.67	8.7	6.3
Phosphatidyl Serine[+]	11.4	13.67	10.1	12.2
Diphosphotidyl Glycerol[+]	3.72	3.52	-	-
Origin Unknown[+]	-	-	7.0	5.9

* Expressed as percent dry weight

+ Expressed as percent of total phospholipids

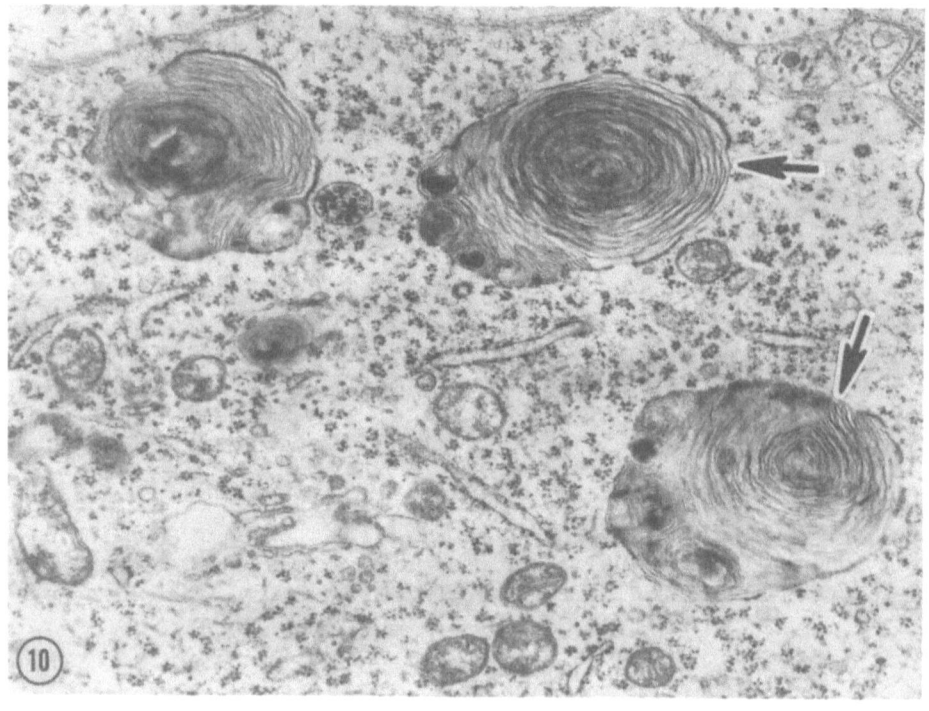

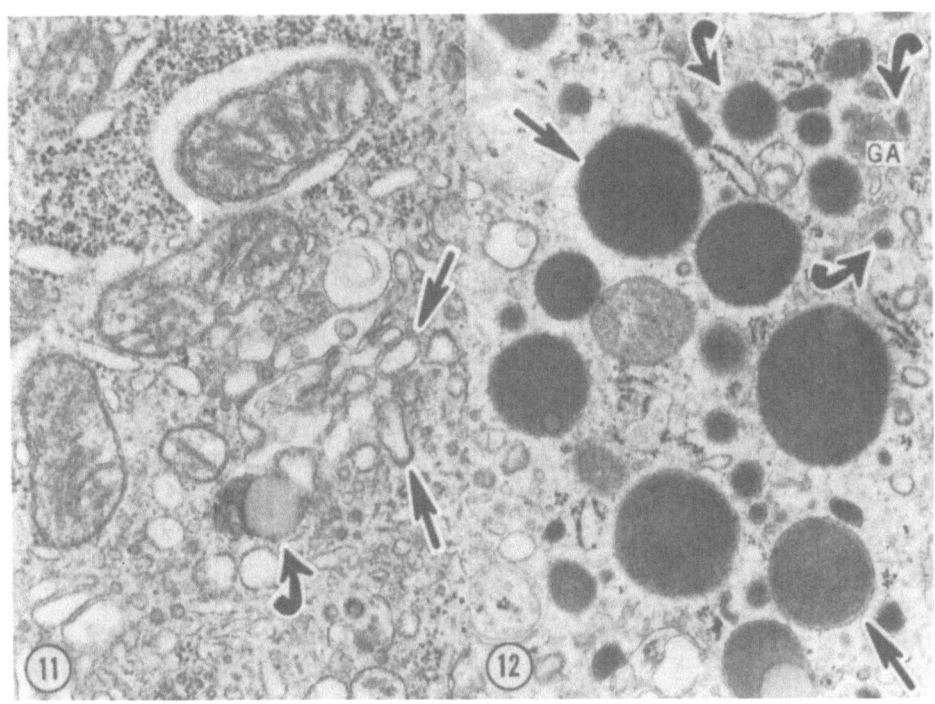

FIGURE 10: Portion of cortical neuron of a one day old rat (group
2) showing well formed concentric membranes (arrows). X 21,000.

FIGURE 11: Portion of neuron of animal (group 3) sacrificed during
the first week showing dilatation of the cisternae of the Golgi
complex (arrows) some of which contain a moderately electron-dense
homogeneous material (curved arrow). X 32,300.

FIGURE 12: During the second week the neurons of animals of group
3 show an increased number of lysosomes (arrows), the origin of
which can be traced (curved arrows) to the cisternae of the Golgi
apparatus (GA). X 23,300.

no ultrastructural changes were observed in the pancreas
and the CNS. During the fourth week, the pancreas contained a few membranous bodies in A cells and occasionally also in B cells of the islets of Langerhans (Fig.
3). The exocrine portion also showed abnormal membranous
inclusions within the acinar cells. Despite the changes
of the islet cells, the blood sugar levels remained within normal limits.

The brain showed various alterations in the neurons
at four weeks, some of which displayed irregular dense
bodies surrounded by laminated structures (Fig. 4). In
other areas, there were well-developed concentrically
arranged membranes (Fig. 5). The latter were more often
aggregated to form pleomorphic structures (Fig. 6). Only
occasionally, the neuronal cytoplasm was densely filled
with membranous cytoplasmic bodies (MCB's) during the
fourth week (Fig. 7), which were similar to those seen
in cases of Tay-Sachs disease and G_{M1}-gangliosidosis in
man (12,13). There was no neuro-anatomical predilection
of the cytoplasmic inclusion bodies in the CNS. The
endothelial cells in the brain also showed occasional
abnormal cytoplasmic inclusions (Fig. 8), while the
glial cells appeared unchanged.

In the control animals of the first experimental
group, no cytoplasmic changes were observed in either
the CNS nor in the viscera.

In biochemical studies of the first group, the brain
and liver at four weeks after the first injection showed
normal amounts of total sialic acid (Table 2). In thin
layer chromatograms of the brains obtained at four weeks,
the major ganglioside fraction had an Rf value which was
similar to that of G_{M1}-ganglioside (Fig. 9). In an
analysis of the total N-acetyl neuraminic acid, the brains
in the experimental group contained 90.9% G_{M1}-ganglioside
as compared with 44% in the control brains (Table 3).
The viscera in this group showed a normal ganglioside
pattern. The total phospholipids and the fractions
thereof were within normal limits during the fourth week
(Table 4).

In order to study further details of the subcellular
alterations during the process of lipid accumulation, the
second study was carried out during the fetal state. The
CNS and the viscera showed abnormal cytoplasmic inclusions
which consisted of well-formed concentric membranes in
the one day old rats (Fig. 10). In the control group,
these changes were absent.

In the third group in which the pregnant rats received a smaller dose of the drug, the brain showed
significant alterations of neuronal organelles. During
the first week of life, there was dilatation of the
cisternae of the Golgi complex, some of which contained
a moderately electron-dense homogeneous material (Fig.
11). During the second and third weeks of age, the
neuronal cytoplasm contained an increased number of
lysosomes (Fig. 12), the origin of which could be traced
to the cisternae of the Golgi apparatus. During the
fourth to sixth weeks, a membranous material appeared
within the lysosomal structures (Fig. 13). At eight to
ten weeks, a variety of membranous structures was observed in the neuronal cytoplasm (Fig. 14). The number
and shape of the inclusions varied from cell to cell.
At 12 weeks, there was a significant increase in the
number of membranous bodies within the neurons some of
which were pleomorphic (Fig. 15). At this stage, similar cytoplasmic inclusion bodies could be seen in the
astrocytes. In histochemical studies these pleomorphic
inclusion bodies displayed reaction granules in acid
phosphatase preparations (Fig. 15, inset).

At 12 weeks, the hepatocytes also contained inclusion
bodies which consisted of concentric or parallel loosely
arranged membranes (Fig. 17A) surrounded by a limiting
membrane (Fig. 16). The matrix of several lysosomes was
partially replaced by membranous structures (Fig. 17B)
which were similar to those previously described (Figs.
13 and 14).

None of the control animals showed these changes.

Biochemically, the brain and liver of the 12 week
old rats showed a slight increase of total sialic acid
as compared with the controls (Table 5). Thin layer
chromatograms of the brains obtained at 12 weeks showed
normal major ganglioside fractions (Fig. 18). In an
analysis of the total N-acetyl neuraminic acid, the brain
at 12 weeks displayed about a 14% increase of G_{M1}-ganglio-
side when compared with the controls. G_{D1b}-ganglioside
was also slightly increased (Table 6). The total phospholipids and fractions thereof in the brains of 12 weeks
old rats were within normal limits except for a moderate
increase of phosphatidic acid (Table 7).

Enzyme studies showed normal beta-galactosidase
activities in the experimental brain and liver.

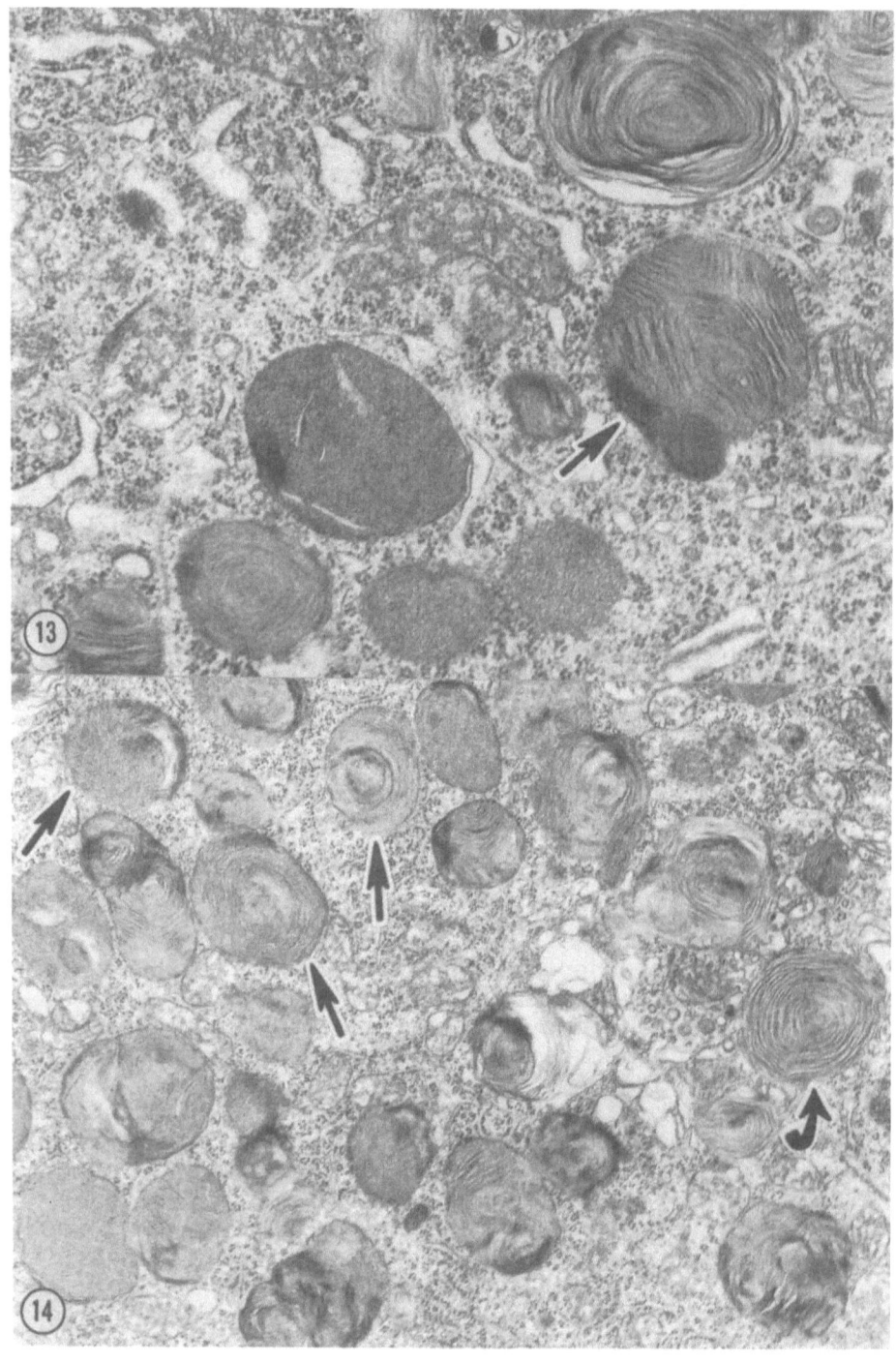

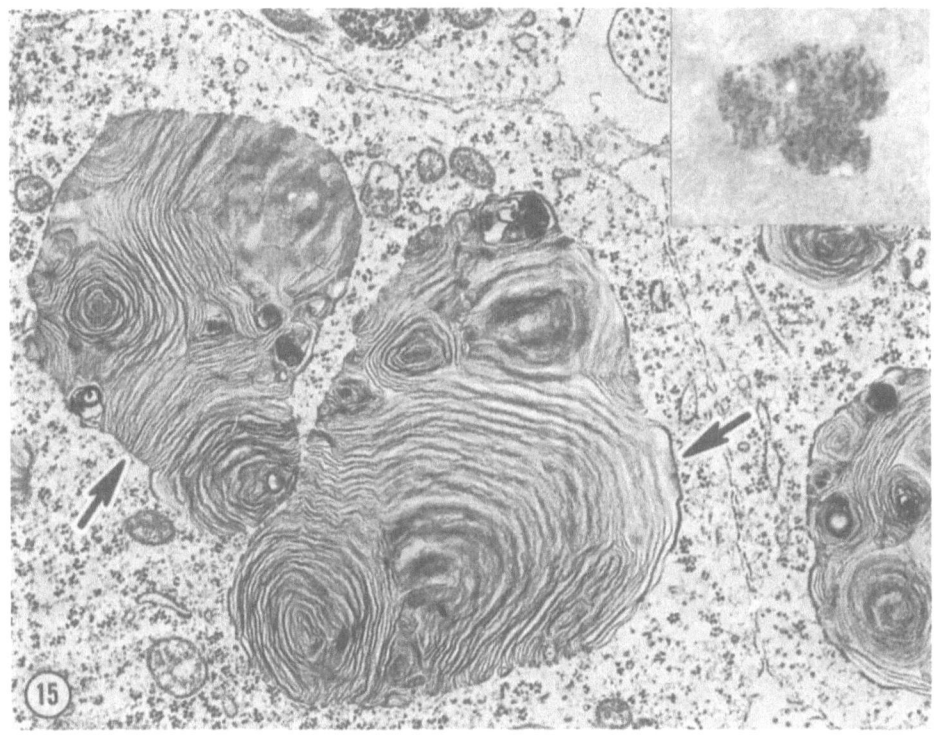

FIGURE 13: At four weeks the neurons of animals of group 3 show
membranous structures within lysosomes. A portion of the electron-
dense lysosomal matrix (arrow) is still visible. X 32,300.

FIGURE 14: At eight weeks the cerebral neurons of animals of group
3 display various stages of membrane formation (arrows) within
lysosomes, some of which have evolved to form concentric lamellar
bodies (curved arrow) similar to MCB's. X 18,700.

FIGURE 15: Portion of neuron of animal of group 3 sacrificed at
12 weeks exhibiting pleomorphic inclusion bodies (arrows) which contain irregularly arranged membranous structures. X 23,350. Inset:
With acid phosphatase preparations one of the inclusion bodies
shows reaction granules. X 23,350.

TABLE 5

LIPID BOUND SIALIC ACID*

Brain		Liver	
Exper.	Control	Exper.	Control
0.105	0.072	0.012	0.008

* Expressed as percent dry weight

TABLE 6

CEREBRAL GANGLIOSIDE PATTERN*

Data	Exper. Brain	Normal Brain
G_{M1}	18.3	14.4
G_{D1a}	33.4	32.4
G_{D1b}	23.7	17.9
G_T	18.9	24.7
G_O	5.7	10.6

* Expressed as percent of total
N-acetyl neuraminic acid.

TABLE 7

PHOSPHOLIPID ANALYSIS OF BRAIN

Data	Exper.	Control
Total Phospholipids*	7.1	7.2
Phosphatidyl Ethanolamine[+]	15.8	18.3
Phosphatidyl Choline[+]	49.0	49.0
Sphingomyelin[+]	9.3	7.4
Phosphatidyl Serine[+]	5.4	6.3
Phosphatidyl Inositol[+]	6.0	10.5
Phosphatidic acid[+]	14.5	8.5

* Expressed as present dry weight
+ Expressed as percent of total phospholipids

DISCUSSION

Chlorphentermine is a compound which contains a highly hydrophobic moiety, due to a chlorinated benzene ring, and a strongly hydrophilic side chain, containing ionized nitrogen (3) which can be bound to biological substances of amphipathic structures such as cell membranes.

In 1970, Franken and associates described the light microscopic features of huge foamy cells in the alveolar spaces in rat lungs treated by chlorphentermine (1). Ultrastructurally, these foamy cells contained numerous lamellar inclusion bodies (2), which developed from alveolar macrophages (3). Since the ultrastructural features of the lamellar inclusion bodies were similar to those seen in cases of lipidoses, the rat lung changes induced by chlorphentermine were believed to represent an experimental lipidosis, the mechanism of which was thought to be either inhibition of certain enzymes or formation of undigestable substrates by biochemical and pharmacological interactions by the drug (3).

Histochemical studies showed increased phospholipids in the inclusion bodies in the lungs which also displayed positive histochemical reactions in acid phosphatase pre-parations and, therefore, were considered to be residual bodies or secondary lysosomes (3). The activity of acid phosphatase in cytosomes in various lipidoses was demon-strated for the first time by the authors (14-17). Since acid phosphatase is a marker for lysosomes (18), these inclusion bodies, therefore, were interpreted to repre-sent secondary lysosomes of the residual type (14-17).

Further studies disclosed ubiquitous pathological findings in the animals exhibiting cytoplasmic inclusion bodies in the pancreas, liver, kidney, adrenal gland, heart and lymphatic tissue (4-9). Similar cellular changes were also demonstrated in guinea pigs, mice and rabbits (6,7,19,20).

The neuropathological features of these animals have been reported by several investigators (7,19-22), who noted various cytoplasmic alterations which vary from active degenerative changes to lamellar inclusion bodies in the CNS as well as in the peripheral nervous system. The inclusion bodies in the neuronal cytoplasm showed a periodicity of 40 Å to 50 Å in some of the lamellar structures (3) which were similar to those of the MCB's in cases of Tay-Sachs disease that varied from 50 Å to 60 Å (12).

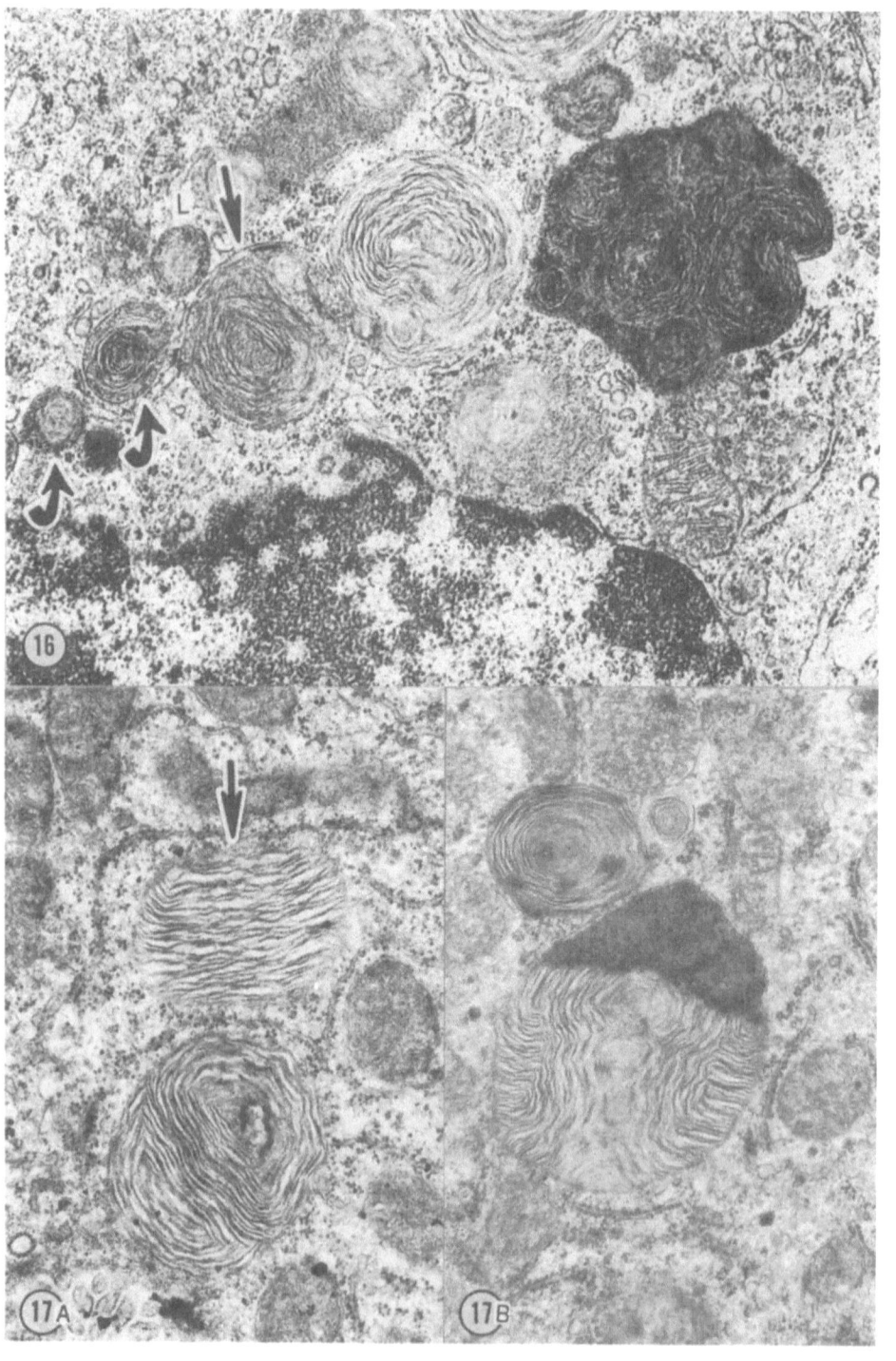

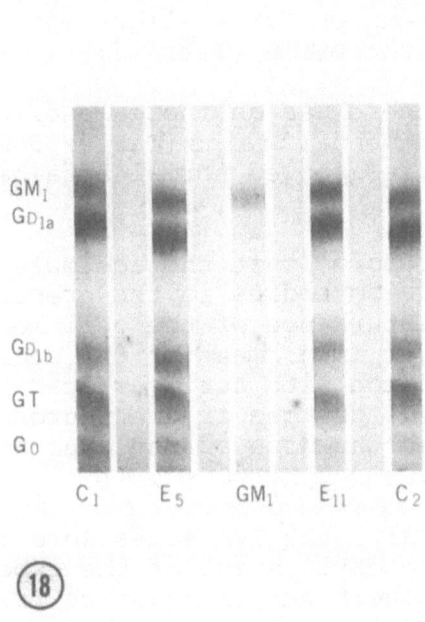

FIGURE 16: Portion of hepatocyte of animal of group 3 sacrificed at 12 weeks showing abnormal inclusion bodies which consist of concentric and loosely arranged membranes. They are surrounded by a limiting membrane (arrow) and some are located within the lysosomal matrix (curved arrows). L-Lysosome. X 25,900.

FIGURE 17: Hepatocytes of the same animal as in Fig. 16 showing a variety of inclusion bodies, some of which consist of parallel membranes (arrow)(Fig. 17A). Occasionally the inclusions seem to develop within the matrix of a lysosome (Fig. 17B). 17A) X 23,350; 17B) X 32,300.

FIGURE 18: Thin layer chromatograms of brains of animals of group 3 sacrificed at 12 weeks (E_5 and E_{11}) showing normal major ganglioside fractions. Cl and C2-Normal Control Brains. G_{M1}-Chromatogram of Brain of Patient With G_{M1}-gangliosidosis.

Biochemical details of the brain have, to the best of our knowledge, so far not been described. Although the lungs showed increased phospholipids in the experimental rats (23), the present studies revealed no increase of total or fractions of phospholipids in the brain and liver, except for a slight increase of phosphatidic acid in the brain (Table 7).

Furthermore, there was an increase of G_{M1}-ganglioside in the experimental brains (Tables 3 and 6). However, enzyme studies showed normal beta-galactosidase activity.

It seems, therefore, that the accumulation of the cytoplasmic inclusion bodies in the present study is due to a metabolic disturbance of the cell membranes rather than resulting from impairment of the degrading enzyme. This is in accordance with our previous studies in which active degenerative changes of the neurons in the CNS were observed when the dose of the drug administered was increased (7).

Ultrastructurally, the lysosomes were markedly increased during the early stage of the experimental studies (Fig. 12). Their origin could be traced to the cisternae of the Golgi complex which indicates that they are primary lysosomes. This impression was seemingly substantiated by the observation that, during the advanced stage, the animals showed membranous inclusion bodies which developed within the primary lysosomes (Fig. 14). In contrast to these experimental observations, in Tay-Sachs disease and other types of lipidoses, the cytoplasmic bodies are considered to be secondary or residual types of lysosomes (14-17).

The hypothesis that the lysosomes in the present experiment are of the primary type, has been proven by additional studies which demonstrated that the membranous structures in the primary lysosomes are reversible when in the third group the administration of the drug was withheld for two weeks from the animals. The brain and viscera of these rats displayed a reduction in the number of membranous bodies, the remainder of which showed an increased density of the lysosomal matrix obscuring the membranous structures at one week (Fig. 19A). During the

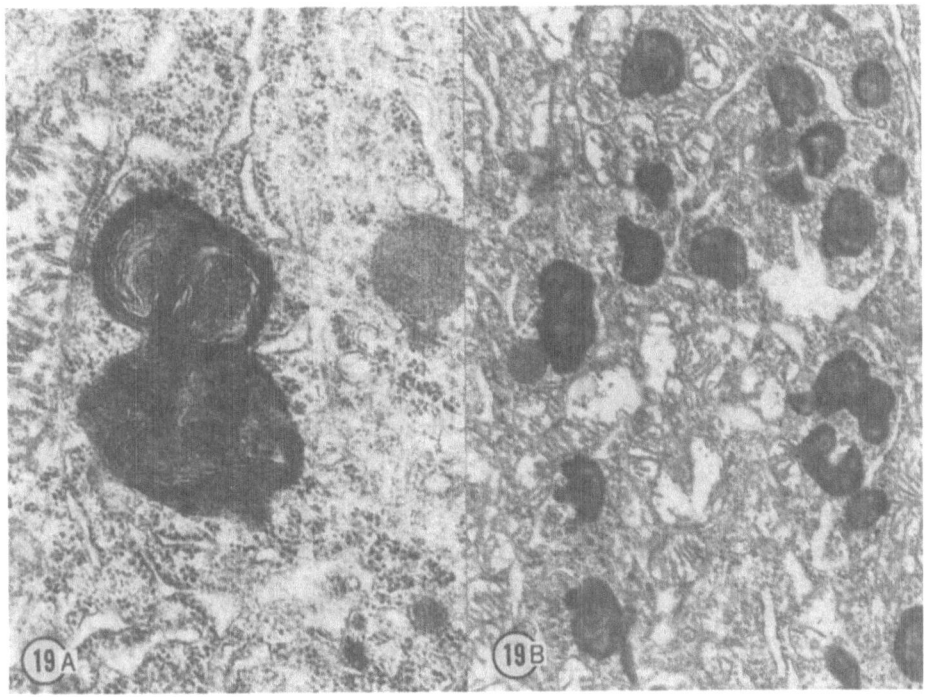

FIGURES 19A and B: Portion of neurons of animals of group 3 kept
without administration of the drug for one to two weeks. The cytoplasmic inclusion bodies display increased density of the matrix
and the obscured membranous structures at one week (A). During
the second week the lamellae disappear within the lysosomes, although pleomorphism and moderately increased numbers of organelles
are still observed. 19A) X 36,200; 19B) X 16,300.

second week, the membranous structures disappeared within the lysosomal matrix, although pleomorphic structures
and a moderately increased number of organelles were
still observed (Fig. 19B).

SUMMARY

     Ultrastructural and biochemical studies were carried
out on three groups of experimental models which were induced by a single subcutaneous daily dose of 10 to 40 mg./
kg. body weight of chlorphentermine hydrochloride. The
first group consisted of 20 young adult rats which were
sacrificed at intervals of from one to four weeks. The
liver and lungs showed concentrically arranged membranous
bodies in the hepatocytes and alveolar cells during the
first week after the first injection, while the CNS and
pancreas showed no ultrastructural alterations. During
the fourth week, the pancreas displayed abnormal cytoplasmic inclusion bodies in the A and B cells of the
islets of Langerhans as well as in the exocrine portion.
The brain showed various neuronal alterations at four
weeks which consisted of irregular dense bodies to well-
developed membranous structures which were similar to
those of Tay-Sachs disease. Biochemically, thin layer
chromatograms showed that the major ganglioside fraction
in the brains at four weeks had an Rf value similar to
that of G_{M1}-ganglioside. In an analysis of the total N-
acetyl neuraminic acid the brains in the experimental
group contained 90.9% G_{M1}-ganglioside as compared with
44% in the controls. The total and fractions of phospholipids in the brains and livers of the experimental
animals were within normal limits.

     In the second group, 12 pregnant rats received also
a single subcutaneous daily injection of 40 mg. of the
drug. Since most of the newborn animals died within two
days, six of them were sacrificed on the first day after
birth. The CNS and viscera showed abnormal cytoplasmic
bodies containing well-formed concentric membranes.

     In the third group, 30 pregnant rats received a re-
duced dose of 10 mg./kg. body weight of the drug subcutaneously. Forty of the baby rats were sacrificed at
intervals of from one to 12 weeks. During the first to
third week, dilatation of the cisternae of Golgi complex
and an increased number of lysosomes were observed in
the neuronal cytoplasm. During the fourth to 12th week,
formation of membranous structures was noted within
the lysosomal matrix.   At 12 weeks, the neurons often

displayed more pleomorphic membranous bodies which exhibited reaction granules in acid phosphatase preparations. Biochemically, the brains at 12 weeks showed a 14% increase of G_{M1}-ganglioside as compared with the controls. However, enzyme studies showed normal beta-galactosidase activity in the experimental brains and livers.

Additional studies demonstrated that the membranous structures within the cytosomes were also lysosomes of the primary type, since the lamellar material was reversible or digestible in the animals of the third group when the drug was withheld for two weeks.

ACKNOWLEDGEMENTS

The authors wish to acknowledge the technical assistance of Mrs. Bernice Franklin and Mr. Fritz Joseph; the photographic preparations of Mr. Herbert Fischler, and the assistance of Mrs. Renee Brenner in editing and typing the manuscript.

REFERENCES

1. Franken, G., Lüllmann, H. and Siegfriedt, A.: The occurrence of huge cells in pulmonary alveoli of rats treated by an anorexic drug. Arzneimittel-Forsch., 20:417, 1970.

2. Kiesel, I.: Grosse Zellen in der Rattenlunge nach Anwendung von Chlorphentermin. Quot. in Ref. 3.

3. Lüllmann-Rauch, R., Reil, G.H., Rossen, E., and Seiler, K.U.: The ultrastructure of rat lung changes induced by an anorectic drug (chlorphentermine). Virchows Arch. B Zellpath., 11:167, 1972.

4. Lüllmann, H., Lüllmann-Rauch, R. and Reil, G.H.: A comparative ultrastructural study of the effects of chlorphentermine and triparanol in rat lung and adrenal gland. Virchows Arch. B Zellpath., 12:91, 1973.

5. Lüllmann-Rauch, R.: Chlorphentermine-induced ultrastructural alterations in foetal tissues. Virchows Arch. B Zellpath., 12:295, 1973.

6. Lüllmann-Rauch, R. and Reil, G.H.: Chlorphenter-
    mine-induced ultrastructural changes in liver tissues
    of four animal species. Virchows Arch. B Zellpath.,
    13:307, 1973.

7. Adachi, M., Tsai, C.-Y., Wellmann, K.F. and Volk,
    B.W.: Ultrastructural alterations of liver, lung,
    pancreas and CNS of mice induced by chlorphenter-
    mine. Fed. Proc., 33:607, 1974.

8. Lüllmann-Rauch, R., and Pietschmann, N.: Lipidosis-
    like cellular alterations in lymphatic tissues of
    chlorphentermine-treated animals. Virchows Arch.
    B Zellpath., 15:295, 1974.

9. Lüllmann-Rauch, R.: Lipidosis-like renal changes
    in rats treated with chlorphentermine or with tri-
    cyclic antidepressants. Virchows Arch. B Cell Path.,
    18:51, 1975.

10. Adachi, M., Torii, J., Schneck, L. and Volk, B.W.:
    The fine structure of fetal Tay-Sachs disease. Arch.
    Path., 91:48, 1971.

11. Schneck, L., Adachi, M. and Volk, B.W.: The Fetal
    aspects of Tay-Sachs disease. Pediatrics, 49:342,
    1972.

12. Terry, R.D. and Weiss, M.: Studies on Tay-Sachs
    disease: II. Ultrastructure of the cerebellum.
    J. Neuropath. Exp. Neurol., 22:18, 1963.

13. Gonatas, N., and Gonatas, J.: Ultrastructural and
    biochemical observations on a case of systemic late
    infantile lipidosis and its relationship to Tay-
    Sachs disease and gargoylism. J. Neuropath. Exp.
    Neurol., 24:318, 1965.

14. Wallace, B.J., Volk, B.W. and Lazarus, S.S.: Fine
    structural localization of acid phosphatase activi-
    ty in neurons of Tay-Sachs disease. J. Neuropath.
    Exp. Neurol., 23:676, 1964.

15. Wallace, B.J., Volk, B.W., Schneck, L. and Kaplan,
    H.: Fine structural localization of two hydrolytic
    enzymes in the cerebellum of children with lipidoses.
    J. Neuropath. Exp. Neurol., 25:76, 1966.

16. Volk, B.W. and Wallace, B.J.: The liver in lipidosis. An electron microscopic and histochemical study. Am. J. Path., 49:203, 1966.

17. Wallace, B.J., Lazarus, S.S. and Volk, B.W.: Electron microscopic and histochemical studies of viscera in lipidoses. In: Inborn Disorders of Sphingolipid Metabolism. Aronson, S.M. and Volk, B.W. (Eds.). New York, Pergamon Press, 1967, P.107.

18. De Duve, C.: Lysosomes, a new group of cytoplasmic particles. In: Subcellular Particles. Hayashi, T. (Ed.). New York, Ronald Press, 1959, p. 128.

19. Anzil, A.P., Herrlinger, H. and Blinzinger, K.: Lipidose des Nervensystems nach Chlorphentermin-Applikation. Naturwissenschaften, 61:35, 1974.

20. Blinzinger, K., Anzil, A.P. and Herrlinger, H.: Intravitale Tellur-Markierung lysosomaler Speicherorganellen bei exogener Lipidose. Naturwissenschaften, 61:83, 1974.

21. Lüllmann-Rauch, R.: Retinal lesions in rat after treatment with chlorphentermine or with tricyclic antidepressants. Virchows Arch. B Zellpath., 15: 309, 1974.

22. Lüllmann-Rauch, R.: Lipidosis-like alterations in spinal cord and cerebellar cortex of rats treated with chlorphentermine or tricyclic antidepressants. Acta Neuropath., 29:237, 1974.

23. Schmien, R., Seiler, K.U. and Wassermann, O.: Drug-induced phospholipidosis. I. Lipid composition and chlorphentermine content of rat lung tissue and alveolar macrophages after chronic treatment. Naunyn-Schmiedberg's Arch. Pharmacol., 283:331, 1974.

CHEMICAL MODELS AND CHEMOTHERAPY IN THE SPHINGOLIPIDOSES

Norman S. Radin

Mental Health Research Institute and
Department of Biological Chemistry
University of Michigan
Ann Arbor, Michigan 48104

As I left the previous Sphingolipid Symposium that was held here in 1971, I decided to attempt intervening in glucocerebroside metabolism by synthesizing suitable enzyme inhibitors. It seemed possible to help the victims of Gaucher's disease, and possibly other sphingolipidoses, by slowing down the synthesis of the sphingolipid that accumulates. When you look at the hydrolase activities reported for the tissues from homozygous individuals suffering from sphingolipidoses, and compare the data with the activities in related, heterozygous individuals, the interesting point emerges: there is really not a great difference in specific activities. Where a sick person might exhibit an activity that is 10% of normal, the apparently healthy relative is getting along fine with an activity that may be 25% of normal. It is apparent that, at least in some organs, many victims of sphingolipidoses are hydrolyzing quite a bit of lipid each day. Their problem seems to be that they are making just a bit too much of the lipid each day and the overload is gradually producing a serious accumulation.

In the case of Gaucher's disease, this approach calls for a slowing of the synthesis of glucocerebroside (GL1a). Unfortunately such an action might affect a multitude of phenomena, some of which are suggested in the following reaction equations:

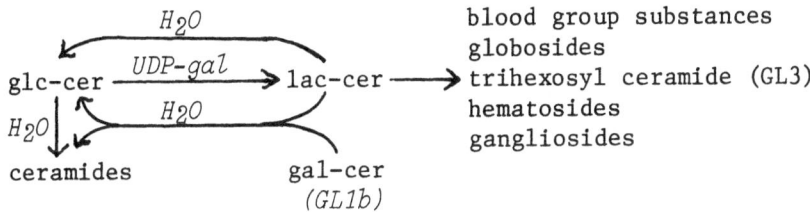

blood group substances
globosides
trihexosyl ceramide (GL3)
hematosides
gangliosides

Reducing the availability of GL1a might slow the synthesis of GL2 (lactoside), GL3, gangliosides, and a variety of nonacidic oligo-saccharide derivatives, virtually all of which are derived from GL1a. All these lipids occur in membranes and the functioning of these membranes might be adversely affected. There is still some reason to believe that the glycosphingolipids play an important role in cell function.

Not only might the concentrations of the various lipids be changed, but their specific hydrolases might adapt to the new situ-ation and produce secondary changes. Kampine et al. (18) seem to have produced such an adaptation by injecting red cell stroma into rats. The spleen level of glucocerebrosidase became somewhat ele-vated, presumably as the result of loading the spleen with extra stroma glycolipids. Moreover several laboratories have observed that patients with lysosomal diseases can exhibit markedly elevated levels of activity in several hydrolases, presumably the result of adaptation to changed membrane turnover and composition. Thus a change in one lipid could affect the levels of other lipids and their hydrolases.

The arrows pointing to the left in the above equations bring out a newly discovered complication in cerebroside metabolism, the dual role of the galactosidase (shown at the bottom) that attacks both lactoside and GL1a (34,35). GL2 is hydrolyzed to GL1a by two different enzymes which differ in their localization and aging dynamics. Thus a change in the level of GL1a could produce a change in the level of GL2, with a consequent change in the level of the hydrolase that attacks galactocerebroside. In such a way GL1a con-centration might control the concentration of GL1b, a glycolipid generally considered to be on a different plane of functional rele-vance.

Not shown in the above equations is an additional complication in sphingolipid metabolic interrelationships. There are now known to be several cofactor proteins which stimulate or activate sphingo-lipid hydrolases (13,17,21). Some or all of these are glycoproteins (like the hydrolases themselves) and their roles are yet to be elu-cidated. Perhaps they play a typical cofactor role by accepting the moiety that is cleaved off and then acting, themselves, as sub-strates. Perhaps they simply alter the structure of the hydrolase to make it more efficient. The relevance of this topic here is that Ho and O'Brien (12) found that the level of the glucosidase cofactor is markedly elevated in the spleen of a patient with Gaucher's dis-ease. Whether this marked elevation plays a role in the toxicity of the disease is an interesting question. No doubt the levels of such proteins are factors to be reckoned with in any tampering with sphingolipid levels.

Another set of considerations is shown in the equations below, which list some metabolic interrelationships at an earlier stage.

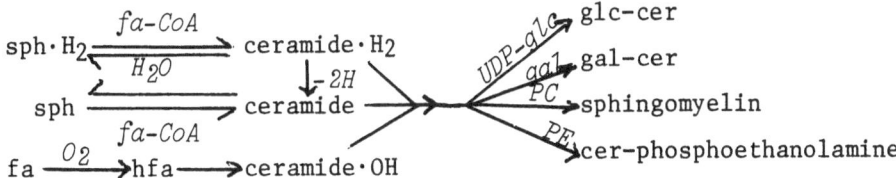

Ceramides lie at the center of sphingolipid metabolism, producing all of the more complex sphingolipids. The two sugars are transferred via uridine nucleotides. An unexpected feature of the transferases is that the galactosyltransferase shows great preference for ceramides containing hydroxy fatty acids (1,24), while the glucose transferase utilizes hydroxy and nonhydroxy ceramides approximately equally well (4, 28). Despite the former specificity, the brain accumulates both types of GL1b almost equally well; despite the latter lack of specificity, the brain's glucocerebroside derivatives contain no hydroxy acids at all.

The above equations show some recent findings in the biosynthesis of the phosphosphingolipids: the phosphoethanolamine and phosphocholine moieties are apparently derived from the corresponding glycerolipids by some kind of transfer reaction (5,9,31). Perhaps the phosphoethanolamine derivative is methylated to form sphingomyelin. Also listed above is the conversion of acyl dihydrosphingosine to acyl sphingosine, a dehydrogenation uncovered by in vivo isotope work (25). Not shown are the complications arising from the differences due to fatty acid chain length and hydroxylation of some of the fatty acids. The hydroxylase shows strong chain length preferences (14), at least four different acyltransferases handle the formation of ceramides (30), and the acyltransferases do not treat sphingosine and dihydrosphingosine equally (23). It is likely that many enzymes in sphingolipid metabolism are actually multiple, differing in substrate preferences.

The next set of enzyme reactions lists some alternative processes that have received some experimental support, as well as support from writers of textbooks.

$$\text{sph} \cdot \text{H}_2 \xrightarrow{FAD} \text{sph} \xrightarrow{UDP\text{-}glc} \text{glc-sph} \xrightarrow{fa\text{-}CoA} \text{glc-cer}$$
$$\xrightarrow{UDP\text{-}gal} \text{gal-sph} \xrightarrow{fa\text{-}CoA} \text{gal-cer}$$
$$\xrightarrow{CDP\text{-}chol} \text{sph-phosphocholine} \xrightarrow{fa\text{-}CoA} \text{SM}$$

$$\text{ceramide} \xrightarrow{CDP\text{-}choline} \text{SM} \; (sphingomyelin)$$

Perhaps some of these reactions occur only in certain tissues or
certain species. Perhaps they are relatively slow reactions that
become more prominent when one of the major pathways is interrupted
for genetic or other reasons. One of the problems in intermediary
metabolism is trying to decide whether a reaction that can be demonstrated in vitro truly operates in vivo, or whether it is simply
an accident of partial nonspecificity on the part of some enzyme.
Some reactions go so slowly in vitro that one must wonder if there
is not some other reaction yet to be discovered that goes at a more
reasonable speed.

The purpose of showing the above enzyme reactions is to indicate the dangers of slowing a single reaction, such as the glucosy-
lation of ceramide. This might result in diversion of unused ceramide for the formation of excessive amounts of the other sphingolipids or shifts in the proportion of sphingosine and dihydrosphingosine.

The scheme below illustrates some higher order complexities
that become visible when we think of cellular and intracellular
relationships.

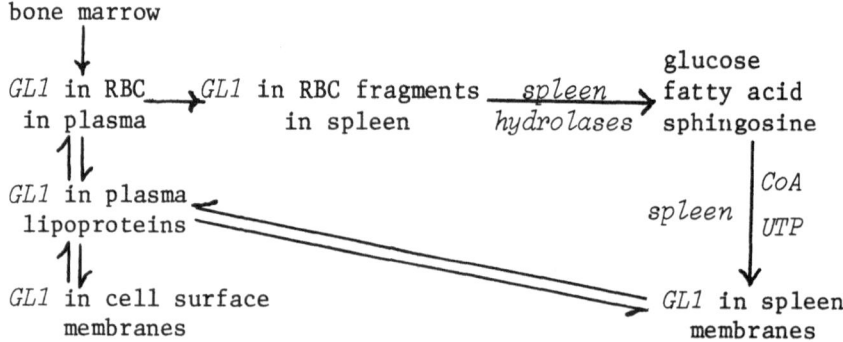

Circulating red blood cells contain GL1a and derived glucolipids,
presumably synthesized in the bone marrow together with the other
RBC constituents. We know from the work of Dawson and Sweeley (8)
that RBC exchange GL1a with plasma GL1a (like cholesterol) and it
is quite reasonable to assume that the plasma GL1a is exchanging
with the GL1a in all cells, via the intercellular fluid. In
support of the latter idea is the finding in several laboratories
that cultured cells readily absorb glycolipids from the medium
(e.g. 7). A recent report on Gaucher patients tells us (3) that
their RBC have a considerably elevated level of GL1a, so each
membrane's position in these equilibria can evidently be shifted.
(Incidentally, this observation raises the possibility that the
anemia seen in some Gaucher patients is due to a decreased RBC
life span, rather than to simple hyperactivity of the enlarged
spleen.)

Red cells ultimately reach a stage which somehow activates their capture and hydrolysis by the spleen. At this point the glucolipids are split, sugar by sugar, to GL1a and then to ceramide and glucose. This is the point that rubs the adult victim of Gaucher's disease so hard. Aggravating the problem is the fact that the spleen also makes GL1a (29), presumably for its own membranes, and the glucosidase there must bear the burden of two disposal problems, external and internal. Of course the white cells from the blood also contribute their glucolipids to the spleen and probably undergo similar exchange reactions with the plasma. It is interesting to question why the spleen bothers to make its own GL1a when so much is available from the blood cells. Probably the answer lies in the lysosomes, which must grasp cell fragments and hydrolyze them all the way down the road to sphingosine, fatty acids, and sugars. The spleen endoplasmic reticulum probably sees only the raw materials.

If we administer a drug which slows GL1a synthesis, we might expect to find membranes formed which are deficient in the glucolipids. Shifts in some of the related enzymes, lipids, and binding proteins will also occur. Whether such depleted, modified membranes can function satisfactorily is something we must discover. If glucolipid production rates in the bone marrow are important, we may find not so much a shift in composition as a reduction in cell release, that is, anemia and leukopenia. However, the exchangeability of GL1a between cells and plasma may act to transfer needed lipid from membranes carrying a surplus to the cells in the bone marrow. Another possibility is that the rate-limiting enzyme step in forming the higher glucolipids is the galactosylation of GL1a to form GL2. Judging by in vitro assays of this transferase (11), the reaction is quite slow and a shortage of GL1a might have little effect on the ceramide oligosaccharides.

A complexity that worries all workers designing drugs is the possibility that the enzyme inhibitor may not really be completely specific. It might inhibit another, innocent enzyme as well as the desired enzyme and produce a new disease while curing the genetic disease. Most of the compounds we have synthesized so far have been analogs of ceramide and it is possible that this centrally located lipid should not be tampered with.

One final factor to worry about: sphingolipids seem to have two roles. One is a position in membranes, acting as a structural component or protein-modifying component. The other is as an intermediate in the synthesis and breakdown of other sphingolipids. The former role raises the possibility that an enzyme inhibitor could produce membranes in which the lipid analog has usurped the rightful place of the related sphingolipid. The latter role raises the possibility that the enzyme inhibitor could be converted to an unnatural "sphingolipid" that also ends up in a membrane.

The above grim listing of possible complications is a useful "thought experiment" that warns us of measurements that we ought to make. After an enzyme inhibitor is administered to an animal, one should look for changes in a variety of sphingolipid concentrations. The life span of the animal's red cells and white cells should be checked. The inhibitor should be made radioactive to allow determination of its possible incorporation into membranes, either unchanged or as a metabolic derivative. The compound should be tested with several enzymes against which it might act. The animal's growth rate and level of physical activity should be checked, as elementary tests of toxicity.

Let's look at the optimistic side now. The field of chemotherapy is a flourishing one that faces many of the problems described above. Sick people and biochemists have both benefited enormously from the discovery of naturally occurring enzyme inhibitors or the synthesis of novel inhibitors. The reasons for this lucky situation are many. First is the differences in inhibition constants exhibited by a drug that acts on several enzymes; with proper design the drug will act most strongly on the target enzyme and the therapeutic dose is adjusted to reach the desired K_i and no higher. Second there is the matter of differential access by drugs; drugs don't go equally well to every organ, or every cell within an organ, or every membrane in the cell. Third is the differential metabolism of drugs, which leads to differing rates of inactivation in different body or cell areas. A drug that has only a transient existence in one site may not do lasting damage there. Fourth is the fact that for many disorders only a temporary administration of the inhibitor is needed. In the case of the chronic sphingolipidoses, such as adult Gaucher's disease, there is probably no need for continual inhibition of sphingolipid synthesis. These forms of the disorders progress so slowly that only intermittent treatment would be needed.

A sixth factor that can make chemotherapy successful, even when an inhibitor hinders more than one enzyme, is the fact that not every enzyme is equally important or that some occur in excess capacity. Some enzyme pathways simply operate at a slow rate, perhaps present primarily as relics of incomplete evolutionary elimination, or perhaps present for special emergency situations that rarely arise. Other enzymes may simply offer alternate pathways, a form of redundancy that is useful in the event of a failure in the primary pathway but of no value in an otherwise normal person.

There is, furthermore, the possibility that a toxic inhibitor, with unavoidable bad side effects, can still be useful when reduced in dose and combined with another form of therapy. Modern cancer chemotherapy is coming to use several different drugs at a time, as well as X-radiation. In the case of the sphingolipidoses, inhibitor therapy could be supplemented by administration of the missing enzyme at intervals. I should think that the two approaches would be mutually helpful.

IN VITRO EXPERIMENTS

Let us look now at the status of the project in my laboratory. In aiming at our organic syntheses, we chose the two easiest approaches. One was the synthesis of compounds derived from naturally occurring sphingolipids, the other was the synthesis of aromatic analogs of ceramide. The former approach is limited by the difficulty of isolating sphingolipids from natural sources. The latter approach is limited by the difficulty of synthesizing aromatic analogs, but we were unexpectedly the lucky recipients of a very kind donation of the total stock of a group of compounds from Drs. Mildred Rebstock and H. M. Crooks, Jr. of Parke, Davis & Company. The structural formulas below illustrate some of our starting materials:

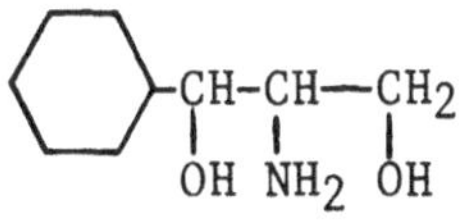

D-erythro-PAPD
($p$henyl$a$mino$p$ropane$d$iol)

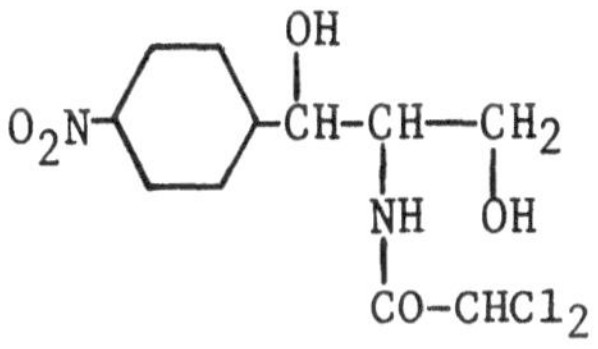

Chloramphenicol (N-dichloroacetyl-
    D-threo-p-nitro-PAPD)

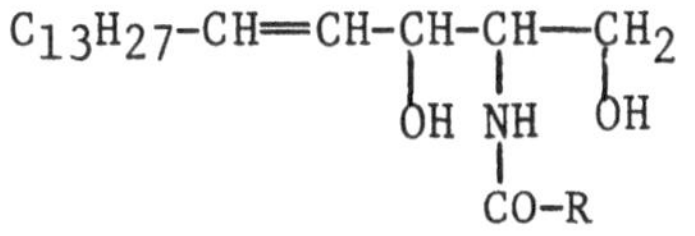

Ceramide (N-acyl sphingosine)

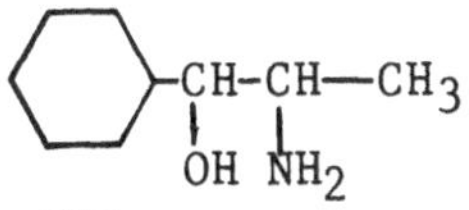

Norephedrine
    ("deoxy-D-erythro-PAPD")

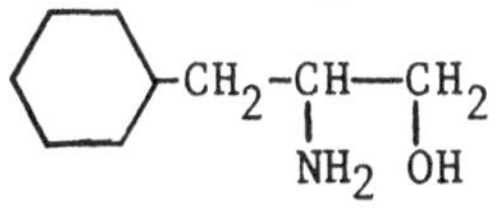

D-Phenylalaninol

We also had available the threo isomers of PAPD (in which the OH near the benzene ring is inverted). The second structure represents a naturally occurring useful drug that has been good to Parke, Davis. The benzene ring corresponds to the alkyl chain of

sphingosine and the dichloroacetyl group corresponds to the fatty
acid of ceramide. Note the difference in chiral structures:
sphingosine has the D-erythro configuration and chloramphenicol has
the D-threo form. Unfortunately we could not obtain erythro-PAPD
in the D and L forms and it has been too scarce to attempt resolution of the DL compound.

Our ceramide analogs have been tested in vitro with various
enzyme preparations. Galactocerebrosidase was assayed in a partially purified preparation from rat brain. Glucocerebrosidase was
assayed in partially purified preparations from human placenta and
rat spleen. The two sugar transferases that make GL1a and GL1b were
assayed in lyophilized rat brainhomogenates, or lyophilized brain
microsomes, which were coated with benzene solutions of ceramide
or ceramide plus putative inhibitor. In the case of the galactosyl
transferase, the ceramide substrate was prepared by degrading the
brain cerebrosides containing 2-hydroxy acids; in the case of the
glucosyltransferase the substrate was made from cerebrosides containing nonhydroxy fatty acids. (Thus the two enzymes are like
Jack Sprat and his wife, who between them licked the platter clean.)

Recently Dr. Kenneth Warren in my lab decided to check out the
chain length preferences of the two sugar transferases and synthesized a large number of fatty acid amides of sphingosine (32). The
findings with ceramides made from various D-hydroxy fatty acids
were surprising (Fig. 1). Galactosyltransferase worked much better
with the very short hydroxy acid ceramides and hydroxystearate was
the poorest galactose acceptor. The enzyme activities are plotted
on a logarithmic scale and the precision with which the points fall
on two different straight lines is striking, but not yet explainable.
Perhaps we are seeing data from two enzymes, one preferring the very
short acids, the other, the very long ones. The unnatural, L-
isomers of the hydroxy acids were somewhat less effective than the
D-isomers.

Glucosyltransferase, on the other hand, showed little preference with respect to chain length. In fact, this enzyme paid little
attention to the presence of a hydroxyl group on the fatty acid; for
example D-hydroxystearate yielded about 10% more GL1a than stearate.
However the L-hydroxystearate was only 2/3 as active as the D-isomer,
so the enzyme does see something there.

Chain length effects often showed up in our inhibitors and we
eventually made most of our comparisons with compounds bearing side
chains with 6, 10, and 14 carbon atoms. Unfortunately not all of
the compounds we made have been tested with all four enzymes. In
some cases the test with the 10-carbon homolog proved so disappointing that we didn't try the shorter and longer homologs. In other
cases, the compound was synthesized after a series of assays with

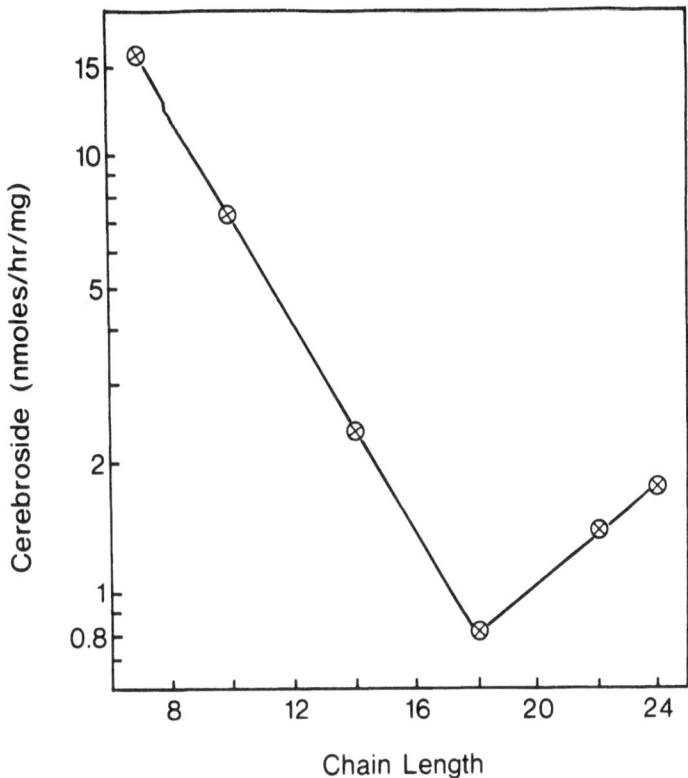

Fig. 1. Rate of synthesis of galactocerebroside from UDP-gal and various D-hydroxyacyl sphingosines. Each incubation tube contained 0.1 mg of lyophilized rat brain microsomes, washed with acetone, 0.2 mg ceramide, 0.1 M Tris pH 7.4, 15mM $MgCl_2$, 2 mM EDTA, 1 mM dithioerythritol, and 0.16 mM labeled UDP-gal in 0.2 ml water. The blank activity (without added ceramide) was 0.1 nmoles/hr/mg.

one enzyme was completed, and the final test data simply are not yet available. The data presented here are taken from studies in my laboratory by Drs. R. C. Arora, J. S. Erickson, J. C. Hyun, Y.-N. Lin, R. S. Misra, R. R. Vunnam, and K. R. Warren. Each compound was tested initially at a concentration of 0.3 mM, since that seems to be a reasonably stringent test of usefulness. Some therapeutic drugs are used at about that concentration (plasma level).

Table 1 shows some test findings with amides made from isomers of PAPD and related compounds. The first compound on the list, which most closely resembles natural ceramide containing a nonhydroxy acid, showed good inhibition of galactosidase but a stimulatory effect on glucosyltransferase. An examination of the radio-

Table 1. Inhibition of cerebroside enzymes by 0.3 mM amides of 1-phenyl-2-amino-1,3-propanediol and its desoxy derivatives. Data are percent of normal activity (a + signifies stimulation, not inhibition).

Fatty acid/Amino alcohol	Hydrolase Gal	Hydrolase Glc	Synthetase Gal	Synthetase Glc
1. 10:0 DL-e-PAPD	48	+ 6	5	+39
2. 10:0 L-t-PAPD	17	+14	10	44
3. 10:0 D-t-PAPD	15	+ 4	6	32
4. h10:0 DL-e-PAPD	67			
5. h10:0 L-t-PAPD	26			
6. h14:0 DL-e-PAPD	60		+73	+59
7. 10:0 L-phenylalaninol	18	23	25	42
8. 10:1 "			30	56
9. h10:0 "	3	18	8	20
10. 10:0 norephedrine			12	69
11. 10:1 "			8	44

10:0 is decanoic acid, 10:1 is 2-decenoic acid, h10:0 is 2-hydroxydecanoic acid (DL), e = erythro, t = threo.

active products of transferase action by thin-layer chromatography showed the presence in the stimulated system of a novel radioactive material. No doubt this is the glucoside formed from decanoyl PAPD. When the normal substrate was omitted, even more of the abnormal product was formed, evidently because the two lipids compete for the same binding site on the transferase. The abnormal product ran more slowly on the plate than the natural glucocerebroside, which is to be expected from the presence of the shorter fatty acid and the truncated amino alcohol moiety. Evidently an animal that is given the aromatic ceramide analog can be expected to exhibit slow degradation of GL1b and accumulation of an unnatural glucocerebroside. Possibly the aromatic "cerebroside" would enter the higher derivatives of GL1a, such as gangliosides.

The second and third compounds in Table 1 differ primarily in the configuration of the benzylic hydroxyl group. They are poor inhibitors of galactosidase but fairly good inhibitors of GL1a synthesis. Evidently the glucosyltransferase can bind but not utilize the threo isomers, even though it is the primary alcohol group that reacts with the glucose.

The small stimulation seen in glucosidase with compound #2 is a real effect, since a higher concentration of the amide (1.2 mM) produced a 47% enhancement of GL1a hydrolysis. This raises the possibility of another kind of chemotherapy, in which the defective or lacking glucosidases of the Gaucher patient might be stimulated.

As I pointed out earlier, the margin between sickness and health is small and a 50% stimulation might prove rather beneficial, especially if coupled with some inhibition of GL1a synthesis. Another compound that looks promising is methyl β-glucoside, which stimulated glucosidase 18% at 0.3 mM (16). We plan to test related compounds to see if a greater stimulation can be obtained, then try the best ones with the glucosidase in Gaucher tissues. The mechanism of the stimulation is still unknown; perhaps the compounds act like the Ho-O'Brien glucosidase stimulating protein.

The fourth compound on the list, made from DL-2-hydroxydecanoic acid instead of decanoic acid, may be compared with the first one. The extra OH group definitely enhanced the inhibition of the galactosidase. This is especially interesting because of the marked effect of the fatty acid OH group in natural ceramide when utilized as a galactose acceptor in GL1b synthesis. Perhaps this signifies that the hydrolase also shows a marked preference for hydroxy cerebrosides.

The longer hydroxy acid (hydroxymyristic, line 6) was found not only to block galactosidase well but also to greatly stimulate the two sugar transferases. Examination of the TLC plates produced a result like the above-mentioned effect of compound 1: apparently both transferases are able to utilize the hydroxy ceramide analog to form the unnatural galactoside and glucoside. The glucosyltransferase acted because it cannot discriminate against the OH group on the fatty acid, while the galactosyltransferase acted because it acts preferentially on ceramides containing a hydroxy acid. (Actually, we found a little of the abnormal galactoside formed with compound #1 too.)

The last five compounds in Table 1 show what happens when one of the hydroxyls is omitted from PAPD. The compounds seem to have only minor activity against the hydrolases, some promise against GL1b synthesis, and good activity against GL1a synthesis. In the case of the amides made from phenylalaninol, insertion of a trans double bond in the 2,3-position of the decanoic acid (compound 8) enhanced the inhibition. On the other hand, the double bond in the norephedrine amides (#10 vs #11) diminished the effect. The OH group in decanoic acid markedly weakened the inhibition of GL1a synthesis. Not shown in the table is a compound that we made recently, a derivative of compound 7 containing a ketone group next to the benzene ring: this produced 74% inhibition of glucosyltransferase and is our best inhibitor of that enzyme to date. We are hoping that the carbonyl group forms a Schiff base with the enzyme.

Also not shown in the table is the oxirane derivative of compound #11, made by epoxidation of the double bond. This too was rather inert toward galactosyltransferase, and inhibited GL1a synthesis 54%. Perhaps the oxirane ring reacts with a sensitive group in the enzyme.

Table 2 lists the findings with some similar compounds which were n-alkyl amines rather than N-acyl amides. These compounds have a + charge under the assay conditions, especially at the low pH used for the hydrolase assays. The most striking result is the observation that all the secondary amines had some blocking action against glucosidase; compound #1 gave substantially complete inhibition. There was also some blocking of glucosyltransferase, especially with N-decyl norephedrine (#5), which was almost as effective as the related amide. From this it would appear that the sugar transferase cannot distinguish between the diamine and amide structures, despite the difference in charge. However compound 1 in this table, made from DL-erythro-PAPD, was an inhibitor of GL1a synthesis while the corresponding amide had been found to be a substrate for the enzyme. Evidently the transferase can tell the difference between an amine and an amide in certain structures.

Not shown in this table is the high effectiveness against glucosidase by the somewhat unnatural isomer of N-decyl PAPD, DL-erythro-1-phenyl-1-decylamino-2,3-propanediol (89% inhibition). In this isomer the two hydroxyl groups are adjacent instead of 1,3. This compound was the result of attempting to make PAPD by a new method, the reaction of an amine with epoxy cinnamyl alcohol. Equally good (87%) was an amino analog of N-decyl PAPD: DL-erythro-1-phenyl-2-decylamino-3-amino-1-propanol.

Table 2. Inhibition of cerebroside enzymes by 0.3 mM secondary amines formed from alkyl groups and PAPD or desoxy PAPD. Legend as in Table 1.

Alkyl group/Amino alcohol	Glucosidase	Synthetases	
		Gal	Glc
1. 10:0 DL-e-PAPD	98	+12	38
2. 10:0 L-t-PAPD	59	+16	35
3. 10:0 D-t-PAPD	39	+16	26
4. h10:0 L-t-PAPD	78	+11	25
5. 10:0 norephedrine	34	+19	61
6. h10:0 "		20	
7. h10:0 p-nitro-D-t-PAPD	49	9	25

10:0 is the n-decyl group, attached by alkylation with n-decyl bromide. h10:0 is 2-DL-hydroxydecyl, attached by alkylation with 1,2-epoxydecane.

Table 3. Inhibition of cerebroside hydrolases by 6 µM decyl amine derivatives. Data are percent inhibition.

Alkylated amino alcohol	Glucosidase	Galactosidase
DL-e-PAPD	28	7
p-Nitro-DL-e-PAPD	66	5
p-Amino-DL-e-PAPD	50	2
p-Decanoylamido-DL-t-PAPD	68	5

Some of the most active compounds were reexamined at 1/50th the previous concentration with the two hydrolases (Table 3). It is evident that this family of amino analogs of ceramide constitutes a highly effective group, with negligible effects on GLlb hydrolysis. The para substituents augment the effect, particularly the bulkier groups, possibly because they increase the similarity of the benzene ring to the long alkyl chain in sphingosine.

Tests of some of the secondary amines with whole rat tissues showed that they were effective against rat glucocerebrosidase too (16). When p-nitrophenyl glucoside was used as substrate the amines proved quite effective too. Although there is evidence that this unnatural substrate gives activity data derived from at least two different glucosidases, it should be remembered that Gaucher patients exhibit low activities with both the natural and unnatural substrates. Perhaps the two glucosidases possess the same protein backbone but different carbohydrate side chains and the genetic error lies in the protein segment. Whatever the explanation, we were pleased to see that our inhibitors acted on both enzymes. This opened the way to inducing a model form of Gaucher's disease in animals or in isolated cells, allowing us to study the development of the disease symptoms in detail.

Table 4. Inhibition of rat spleen glucocerebrosidase by 6 µM N-alkyl derivatives of glucopsychosine (1-0-glucosyl sphingosine).

n-Alkyl group	Percent inhibition
18:0	56
10:0	74
8:0	79
6:0	85
4:0	42
3:0	21

In our earliest search for glucocerebrosidase inhibitors (10) we investigated derivatives of the substrate in which the amide group was reduced to a secondary alkyl amine (Table 4). All the compounds were excellent inhibitors at the 6 µM level; alkyl chains longer than four carbon atoms were the best. Hexyl psychosine was better than the two best aromatic analogs (Table 3). No doubt the glucose moiety enhances the attraction of the inhibitor for the active site of the enzyme. A test with the glucocerebrosidase from human placenta also revealed the N-hexyl glucosyl sphingosine (HGS) to be very effective (92% at 6 µM) while the analogous hexyl galactosyl sphingosine was almost ineffectual.

A study of plant α- and β-glucosidases by Legler (2,20) has shown that these enzymes possess a vital carboxyl group near the active site, which may take part in the hydrolytic reaction by forming a glycoside ester. He was able to synthesize an epoxy derivative of a cyclohexane related to inositol, which inhibited glucosidases by reacting covalently with the active COOH. The oxirane ring formed an ester, allowing Legler to isolate a peptide segment around the active COOH. There is thus little doubt that our inhibiting amines act because of their ionic attraction to the active COOH of mammalian glucocerebrosidase and because of their structural resemblance to the substrate lipid and sugar moieties.

While Legler's compounds, and glucose derivatives like glucono-lactone act against both α- and β-glucosidases, our derivatives presumably act only against the enzymes that attack the β-gluco-sides. However we have not yet tested our inhibitors with an α-glucosidase. Nonspecific inhibitors might not be useful in inducing a model form of Gaucher's disease because animals possess at least one α-glucosidase.

Presumably all glycosidases act like the glucosidases, through a COOH group at the enzyme's active site. When we tested galacto-cerebrosidase with N-hexyl galactosyl sphingosine (or with HGS) at a concentration of 6 µM, virtually no inhibition was seen (16). Either this enzyme uses a different hydrolytic mechanism, or the COOH group is located too far from the compound's amino group. We will have to prepare similar compounds but with the amino group at some other position.

IN VIVO STUDIES

I use the term "in vivo", not only for intact organisms, but also for cultured cells, which should more precisely be considered "in plastico." So far we have done four such studies, three of them in collaboration with other laboratories.

One was an evaluation of some effects of our best glucosidase inhibitor, HGS, on human skin fibroblasts. This was carried out by Kenneth Warren, Irwin Schaefer, Julia Sullivan, Mary Petrelli and myself (*33*). The first question was: is the inhibitor taken up from the culture medium by the cells? Experiments with different HGS concentrations in the medium showed that 1 μg/ml (1.8 μM) produced no visually discernible abnormalities in the cells, but concentrations above 4.5 μM produced morphological changes and death within a week. We don't know yet whether this toxicity is a sign that total inhibition of glucosidase is very toxic or whether HGS, in higher concentrations, acts to block other enzymes or processes.

Another test was made by growing the fibroblasts in the presence of HGS for various periods of time, then assaying them for several hydrolase activities with artificial substrates. In each case, aryl glucosidase was found to be almost absent. Since the enzyme assay involved a considerable dilution of the cells with buffer, any HGS that was stored within the cells must have been diluted considerably if it was free to dissociate. Previous tests had shown that the inhibitor acted competitively against the substrates (lipoidal and aryl), so that observation probably means that much of the inhibitor added with each change of medium had been absorbed and stored by the cells.

The most intriguing finding from this experiment was that the specific activities of the other hydrolases were generally elevated. This includes α-glucosidase, phosphatase, β-galactosidase, and β-hexosaminidase. The effect was not consistent from batch to batch, and the magnitude of the stimulation was also variable, but the effect seems quite real. Fibroblasts that had been grown with an equal concentration of N-hexyl <u>galactosyl</u> sphingosine showed little change. Since other investigators have noted similar (and similarly variable) increases in activity of lysosomal enzymes in patients with sphingolipidoses, it would appear that we have mimicked this aspect too in our model form of Gaucher's disease.

Analytical data are given for one set of fibroblasts grown for 28 days in the presence of HGS (Table 5). The HGS concentration in the medium was initially 0.5 μg/ml, then it was raised to 1 μg/ml. The yield of dry cells seemed to be consistently enhanced by the inhibitor, which seems to be a mimicking of the great enlargement seen in Gaucher spleen and liver. It will be interesting to elucidate the nature of the stimulation: was it due to an increase in the number of cells or was it simply an enlargement of cells? I don't think that this question has been investigated in cases of the human disease.

As expected, the HGS-treated cells showed an accumulation of glucocerebroside. The increase was only 2- to 3-fold (in this and other experiments), a disappointing ratio. Perhaps we had been overoptimistic, since skin (the source of the fibroblasts) is not

Table 5. Effects of hexyl glucosyl sphingosine on fibroblasts
          grown 28 days with a total of 95 µg/plate of HGS.

	-HGS	+HGS
Cell yield *(mg dry wt/plate)*	4.9	5.6
Cerebroside *(mg/g of dry cells)*	0.29	0.85
Trihexosyl ceramide "	1.8	2.7
Cholesterol "	20	21
Total lipids "	152	166
Total protein "	590	570

noted for being a great storage site for cerebroside in Gaucher's
disease. Moreover, the rate of accumulation even in spleen of
Gaucher adults is not great. Future studies of this sort should
include cerebroside in the culture medium, which might accentuate
the HGS effects.

The other change of interest in the above table was in the
concentration of ceramide trihexoside, which rose 17% in one experiment and 46% in another. Several studies of Gaucher spleens have
also reported elevated levels of GL3 (19,26), although other studies
have not found elevated values (6, 22). This effect might be due
to inhibition by GL1a of the enzymes that hydrolyze GL3, or simply
to increased synthesis of GL3 from its precursor, GL1a. One might
postulate a "damming up" effect when a metabolite cannot be hydrolyzed. The mechanism of such an effect might be a product-caused
inhibition of hydrolase activities by each accumulating intermediate in the degradative chain. However there is little evidence in
the literature for product-inhibition in the sphingolipid hydrolases
or for accumulation of GL2a in Gaucher tissues. Because of the low
concentration of GL2 in fibroblasts we were unable to look for
accumulation in this study.

I have one more explanation for the elevated GL3 values: this
lipid is a relatively plentiful component of liver lysosomes (15)
and it is likely that our fibroblast lysosomes accumulated together
with the cerebroside and miscellaneous lysosomal enzymes. It
could be shown by electron microscopy that organized particles
accumulated in our HGS-treated fibroblasts, although they didn't
look like the particles seen in Gaucher cells. Perhaps these particles are the site of GL3, as well as GL1a, deposition; the particles may also contain glucosidase, HGS, and the cohydrolase glycoprotein. Unfortunately the small amount of material that one gets
in tissue culture makes characterization of the particles difficult.

In an effort to study these phenomena on a larger scale, we
injected HGS intraperitoneally into young rats (27). Injection of

5 mg/rat proved fatal to 60% of the rats and the survivors showed slow growth. At a dosage level of 2 mg/rat, growth was normal and analysis of the spleens revealed no increase in weight but a 65% increase in GL1a concentration.

Based on this preliminary finding, we treated a larger group of weanling rats at the dosage ratio of 16 mg/kilo, which would yield an average body concentration of 38 μM if uniformly distributed in the body water. The HGS was injected every 4 or 5 days for a total of 28 days, after which the rats were analyzed. The livers appeared abnormally dark and lumpy, but electron microscopy showed no abnormalities. The spleens were 19% larger than the controls but the chemical differences were quite small, with only a slight elevation in GL1a concentration.

In a prior experiment we had followed the metabolic fate of injected HGS, labeled in the hexyl group. The spleen and liver were major sites of uptake, which was promising, and the spleen concentration of HGS decreased with a half-life of about 1.5 days. This rate of removal did not seem too serious since the concentration of HGS remained above 2 μM for about 5 days. In other words, one could expect to find HGS at strongly inhibiting levels for 5 days after each injection. Perhaps the rats injected for 28 days adapted to the drug and increased their rate of removal to the point where it lost its effectiveness. The moral of this unsatisfactory experiment is that we should check drug turnovers in both naive and chronically treated rats.

We are presently trying other ways of bringing glucosidase inhibitors to the spleen. One method that looks very promising is the use of red blood cells filled with inhibitor. Since the cells contain no glucocerebrosidase, it is possible that the inhibitor will not interfere with normal RBC function. As the assorted, loaded RBC reach the ends of their life spans, they should deliver a constant infusion to the spleen.

It is evident that this project has a long way to go yet. We are still synthesizing new compounds which may be more specific or more resistant to metabolic removal from the body. The search for better stimulators of glucosidase is also continuing. Hopefully a side benefit to our project will be the development of inhibitors suitable for other sphingolipidoses, such as Niemann-Pick disease.

This research has been supported in part by grants from the National Institutes of Health (NS 03192 and HD 07406) and the National Science Foundation (GB 36735).

REFERENCES

1. Basu, S., Schultz, A. M., Basu. M., and Roseman, S. Enzymatic synthesis of galactocerebroside by a galactosyltransferase from embryonic chicken brain. J. Biol. Chem. 246, 4272 (1971).

2. Bause, E. and Legler, G. Isolation and amino acid sequence of a hexadecapeptide from the active site of α-glucosidase A3 from *Aspergillus wentii*. Z. Physiol. Chem. 355, 438 (1974).

3. Brady, R. O., Pentchev, P. G., Gal, A. E., Hibbert, S. R., and Dekaban, A. S. Replacement therapy with purified glucocerebrosidase in Gaucher's disease. New Engl. J. Med. 291, 989 (1974).

4. Brenkert, A. and Radin, N. S. Synthesis of galactosyl ceramide and glucosyl ceramide by rat brain: assay procedures and changes with age. Brain Res. 36, 183 (1972).

5. Broad, T. E. and Dawson, R. M. C. Formation of ceramide phosphorylethanolamine from phosphatidylethanolamine in the rumen protozoon *Entodinium caudatum*. Biochem. J. 134, 659 (1973).

6. Dawson, G. Glycosphingolipid levels in an unusual neurovisceral storage disease characterized by lactosylceramide galactosyl hydrolase deficiency: lactosylceramidosis. J. Lipid Res. 13, 207 (1972).

7. Dawson, G., Stoolmiller, A. C., and Radin, N. S. Inhibition of β-glucosidase by N-(n-hexyl)-O-glucosyl sphingosine in cell strains of neurological origin. J. Biol. Chem. 249, 4634 (1974).

8. Dawson, G. and Sweeley, C. C. In vivo studies on glycosphingolipid metabolism in porcine blood. J. Biol. Chem. 245, 410 (1970).

9. Diringer, H. and Koch, M. A. Biosynthesis of sphingomyelin. Transfer of phosphoryl choline from phosphatidylcholine to erythro-ceramide in a cell-free system. Z. Physiol. Chem. 354, 1661 (1973).

10. Erickson, J. S. and Radin, N. S. N-Hexyl-O-glucosyl sphingosine, an inhibitor of glucosyl ceramide β-glucosidase. J. Lipid Res. 14, 133 (1973).

11. Hildebrand, J., Stoffyn, P., and Hauser, G. Biosynthesis of lactosylceramide by rat brain preparations and comparison with the formation of ganglioside G_{M1} and psychosine during development. J. Neurochem. 17, 403 (1970).

12. Ho, M. W. and O'Brien, J. S. Gaucher's disease: deficiency of

"acid" β-glucosidase and reconstitution of enzyme activity in vitro. Proc. Nat. Acad. Sci. USA 68, 2810 (1971).

13. Ho, M. W., O'Brien, J. S., Radin, N. S., and Erickson, J. S. Glucocerebrosidase: reconstitution of activity from macromolecular components. Biochem. J. 131, 173 (1973).

14. Hoshi, M. and Kishimoto, Y. Synthesis of cerebronic acid from lignoceric acid by rat brain preparation. J. Biol. Chem. 248, 4123 (1973).

15. Huterer, S. and Wherrett, J. R. Enrichment of lysosomes in glycosphingolipid content. Trans. Am. Soc. Neurochem. 5, 68 (1974).

16. Hyun, J. C., Misra, R. S., Greenblatt, D., and Radin, N. S. Synthetic inhibitors of glucocerebroside β-glucosidase. Arch. Biochem. Biophys. 166, 382 (1975).

17. Jatzkewitz, H. and Stinshoff, K. An activator of cerebroside sulfatase in human normal liver and in cases of congenital metachromatic leukodystrophy. FEBS Lett. 32, 129 (1973).

18. Kampine, J. P., Kanfer, J. N., Gal, A. E., Bradley, R. M., and Brady, R. O. Response of sphingolipid hydrolases in spleen and liver to increased erythrocytorhexis. Biochem. Biophys. Acta 137, 135 (1967).

19. Kuske, T. T. and Rosenberg, A. Quantity and fatty acyl composition of the glycosphingolipids of Gaucher spleen. J. Lab. Clin. Med. 80, 523 (1972).

20. Legler, G. Labeling the active center of β-glucosidases A and B of almond emulsin with [^{3}H]6-bromo-6-deoxy-conduritol B epoxide. Z. Physiol. Chem. 351, 25 (1970).

21. Li, Y.-T., Mazotta, M. Y., Wan, C.-C., Orth, R., and Li, S.-C. Hydrolysis of Tay-Sachs ganglioside by β-hexosaminidase A of human liver and urine. J. Biol. Chem. 248, 7512 (1973).

22. Makita, A., Suzuki, C., and Yosizawa, Z. Glycolipids isolated from the spleen of Gaucher's disease. J. Exptl. Med. (Tohoku) 88, 277 (1966).

23. Morell, P. and Radin, N. S. Specificity in ceramide biosynthesis from long chain bases and various fatty acyl Coenzyme A's by brain microsomes. J. Biol. Chem. 245, 342 (1970).

24. Morell, P. and Radin, N. S. Synthesis of cerebroside by brain from uridine diphosphate galactose and ceramide containing hy-

droxy fatty acid. Biochem. 8, 506 (1969).

25. Ong, D. E. and Brady, R. N. In vivo studies on the introduction of the 4-t double bond on the sphingenine-3-moiety of rat brain ceramides. J. Biol. Chem. 248, 3884 (1973).

26. Philippart, M. Glycolipid, mucopolysaccharide and carbohydrate distribution in tissues, plasma and urine from glycolipidoses and other disorders. In *Advances in Experimental Medicine and Biology*, V. Zambotti, G. Tallamanti, and M. Arrigone, eds. Plenum Press, New York, vol. 25, p. 231 (1972).

27. Radin, N. S., Warren, K. R., Arora, R. C., Hyun, J. C., and Misra, R. S. In *Modification of Lipid Metabolism*, E. G. Perkins and L. A. Witting, eds., Academic Press, New York, 1975, 87-104.

28. Shah, S. N. Glycosyl transferases of microsomal fractions from brain: synthesis of glucosyl ceramide and galactosyl ceramide during development and the distribution of glucose and galactose transferase in white and grey matter. J. Neurochem. 18, 395 (1971).

29. Trams, E. G. and Brady, R. O. J. Clin. Invest. 39, 1546 (1960).

30. Ullman, M. D. and Radin, N. S. Enzymatic formation of hydroxy ceramides and comparison with enzymes forming nonhydroxy ceramides. Arch. Biochem. Biophys. 152, 767 (1972).

31. Ullman, M. D. and Radin, N. S. The enzymatic formation of sphingomyelin from ceramide and lecithin in mouse liver. J. Biol. Chem. 249, 1506 (1974).

32. Warren, K. R., Misra, R. S., Arora, R. C., and Radin, N. S. Glycosyltransferases of rat brain that make cerebrosides: substrate specificity, inhibitors, and abnormal products. J. Neurochem. *in press*.

33. Warren, K. R., Schafer, I. A., Sullivan, J. C., Petrelli, M., and Radin, N. S. The effects of N-hexyl-O-glucosyl sphingosine on normal cultured human fibroblasts: a chemical model for Gaucher's disease. J. Lipid Res. *in press*.

34. Wenger, D. A. Studies on galactosyl ceramide and lactosyl ceramide β-galactosidase. Chem. Phys. Lipids 13, 327 (1974).

35. Tanaka, H. and Suzuki, K. Lactosylceramide β-galactosidase in human sphingolipidoses. J. Biol. Chem. 250, 2324 (1975).

CHEMICAL INDUCTION OF LYSOSOMAL STORAGE

Michel Philippart and Elsa Kamensky

Mental Retardation Center
University of California
Los Angeles, California

Primary lysosomal storage disorders involve the accumulation of lipids, mucopolysaccharides or saccharides following a genetic mutation of the corresponding lysosomal hydrolases. Aside from these conditions it is becoming apparent that there are other types of storage disorders which do not result from a specific hydrolase deficiency but reflect a more generalized impairment of the lysosomal digestion. We have proposed to call such disorders secondary lysosomal storage disorders (1).

A number of different mechanisms may be at play. There may be chemical denaturation or binding of the natural substrates or enzymes by peroxides in the ceroid-lipofuscinoses (2) or by drugs such as AC 3579 (3) or chlorphentermine (4). Another type of secondary lysosomal storage disorders may result from an impairment (5) of the proton pump suspected to generate the acid pH (6) which allows optimal hydrolysis of the lysosomal contents. A third type may reflect an impairment of the natural activator(s) (7) which probably contributes to proper substrate dispersion and hydrolase interaction with water-insoluble molecules such as lipids. The Tay-Sachs AB variant in which there is accumulation of GM_2 ganglioside in presence of normal hexosaminidase activity against water-soluble artificial substrates may represent an example of such a mechanism. Still another type of deficiency may result from either an abnormal "tagging" of the lysosomal enzymes which prevents their normal packaging into the primary lysosomes (8) or from abnormalities in the fusion between primary lysosomes and pinocytotic or autophagic vacuoles. These by no means inclusive possibilities emphasize that lysosomal function reflects much more than a normal complement of functional acid hydrolases.

The present study was undertaken to investigate the lysosomal function in normal cultured skin fibroblasts exposed to chemicals (chloroquine, and AC 3579) or excess amounts of natural biological molecules (retinol, sphingomyelin and N-acetylneuraminic acid). Comparisons with genetic diseases were attempted.

Retinol and Lysosome Function

Fell (9) in the early fifties started pioneering work on the biological action of vitamin A on cultured bone explants. The addition of retinol (10 IU/ml) to the culture medium stimulated lactic acid formation and the synthesis and excretion (up to 7 times more than controls) of the acid protease cathepsin D. In other experiments with radioactive sulfate retinol was shown to stimulate the liberation of polymeric chondroitin sulfate from the cartilage matrix of cultured bone rudiments. The secretion of lysosomal enzymes into the environment was thought to reflect a specific physical alteration of the lysosomal membrane, promoting its fusion with the plasma membrane. While the release of lysosomal enzymes into the cytoplasm has often been considered as a significant factor of lysosomal pathology, Fell did not believe that cytoplasmic release took place, except possibly with very toxic doses of retinol.

Chloroquine Toxicity

Retinopathy (10) neuromyopathy (11) and corneal opacities have long been associated with the side effects of chloroquine therapy in man. A cerebrospinal lipodystrophy could be induced in swine, giving rise to cellular inclusions which were compared to those of Tay-Sachs disease (12). Actually the toxicity was expressed in many types of cells by the accumulation of membranous and granular cytoplasmic inclusions suggesting impairment of the lysosomal digestion (13).

Since inclusions also occur in cells not known to engage in phagocytosis such as muscle (14), myelocytes and lymphocytes (15), these inclusions might result from increased autophagy. Pino-cytosis was briefly stimulated in cultured macrophages exposed to chloroquine but this was not accompanied by synthesis of large amounts of hydrolases by the cells (16). Inhibitors of pinocytosis in macrophages did not block the development of vacuoles in the chloroquine-treated cells (17). In L-strain fibroblasts, Golgi and smooth endoplasmic reticulum vesicles and cisternae partici-pated in the formation of the autophagic vacuoles, possibly reflecting fusion of membranes altered by chloroquine (17).

Mucopolysaccharide degradation was inhibited by chloroquine in normal human fibroblasts which showed an ultrastructural pattern resembling a lysosomal storage disease. This might reflect an accumulation rather than an increased production of vacuoles, resulting from inhibition of the normal process of autophagy (18).

Inhibition of Phospholipid Catabolism by AC 3579

In the rat the administration of the diazafluoranthen derivative AC 3579 induced an hypertrophy of the smooth endoplasmic reticulum and an accumulation of membranous inclusions in the liver (19). While phospholipid synthesis remained within normal limits, their catabolism was significantly impaired, leading to a phospholipid storage disorder (20).

Direct enzyme inhibition did not seem to be involved, as phospholipid degradation by endogenous phospholipases was not impaired when either AC 3579 or liver homogenate from treated rats was added to the assay mixture. An exogenous phospholipase A_2, however, had less activity in the treated rats than in controls. This was attributed to the in vivo formation of a complex between AC 3579 and membrane phospholipids which made them relatively resistant to hydrolysis, thereby causing an hypertrophy of the endoplasmic membranes and their secondary accumulation into lysosomes (3).

The Concept of Drug-Induced Lysosomal Storage Disorders

Lullman et al. (4) reviewed a number of drugs including anorectics, inhibitors of cholesterol synthesis, antihistaminics and psychotropic drugs which have been associated with the development of phospholipid storage disorders. They pointed out that all these compounds are amphiphilic and possess a cationic side-chain which might interact with the phosphate side-chain of the phospholipid. A strong interaction between chlorphentermine and phospholipid could be demonstrated by NMR spectroscopy. It was also shown by Sephadex gel filtration that chlorphentermine forms a stable complex with phosphatidyl-choline. The aromatic ring of the drugs might also interact with the hydrophobic moiety of the phospholipid molecules. The phospholipid-drug complex cannot be degraded by the lysosomal hydrolases and therefore accumulates within the lysosomes.

This type of drug-lipid interaction might also act at other cellular sites, for example, altering membrane properties such

as fusion. Interaction with proteins by these or other drugs
could be conceived too. Chloroquine induced morphologic abnormalities of the eosinophil granules (15) which contain mostly
peroxidase and are not associated with the lysosomal system (21).

MATERIAL AND METHODS

Norman human skin fibroblasts obtained from two adults
(#1 and #2) and one child (#3) were cultured as described
previously (22). Cells had undergone four to eight passages
prior to the experiments. Only confluent layers were used. One
T-250 flask was adequate for phospholipid (23) or hydrolase
determination (24). Six replicate T-30 flasks were used for
turnover studies (24). The selected drug concentration and time
of exposure did not cause excessive rate of cell death or
detachment of the monolayers.

Ultrastructural studies were conducted as reported
elsewhere (22).

RESULTS

Phospholipid Concentration and Distribution

At the 10 ug/ml level, AC 3579 elicited a doubling of
phospholipid concentration per flask after 12 days, following
which there was no further increase up to the 24th day (Table I).
Protein increased more slowly up to the 24th day. At the 20 ug
level, the phospholipid concentration per flask was normal while
the protein concentration increased significantly. The latter
effect was also observed with retinol (10 ug/ml). Chloroquine
(10 ug/ml) first caused increased protein concentration at day 6.
Longer exposure resulted in a further increase which was matched
by a parallel phospholipid accumulation. Sphingomyelin had no
significant effect at 0.1 mg/ml level. Phospholipid concentration per mg protein doubled at the 5.0 mg/ml level.

Of the major phospholipids, only sphingomyelin was significantly affected in these experiments (Table I). When expressed
as percent of total lipid phosphorus, sphingomyelin was only
half of the lowest normal concentration in all AC 3579
experiments. A similar but less pronounced effect was also seen
with retinol and chloroquine which caused sphingomyelin to fall
to or under the low normal range. As might be expected, the
most significant deviation from the normal phospholipid distribution resulted from exposure to excess sphingomyelin. Under
these conditions sphingomyelin concentration reached 22.8% at
the 0.1 mg/ml level and 79.1% at the 5.0 mg/ml level.

TABLE I

EFFECT OF VARIOUS CHEMICALS ON NORMAL HUMAN FIBROBLASTS

EXPERIMENT	PHOSPHOLIPID *	PROTEIN *	RATIO +	SPHINGOMYELIN #	PHOSPHATIDIC ACID #	LYSOBIS-PHOSPHATIDIC ACID #
Control mean (n = 7)	0.26	1.18	0.22	13.0	0.5	0.9
X range	0.2-0.47	0.8-1.45	0.19-0.28	11.0-15.3	0.4-0.7	0.6-1.1
AC 3579(10 ug)(12 days)	0.79	1.82	0.43	5.0	1.9	2.1
AC 3579(10 ug)(24 days)	0.82	2.48	0.33	6.0	1.3	1.2
AC 3579(20 ug)(12 days)	0.39	2.1	0.18	5.6	3.1	3.2
Retinol(10 ug)(14 days)	0.38	2.2	0.17	10.5	ND	3.3
Chloroquine(10 ug)(6 days)	0.28	2.68	0.1	11.0	ND	1.0
Chloroquine(10 ug)(24 days)	2.71	12.1	0.22	7.5	0.1	1.0
Sphingomyelin(0.1 mg)(24 days)	0.23	1.2	0.19	22.8	ND	ND
Sphingomyelin(5.0 mg)(15 days)	0.34	0.8	0.43	79.1	ND	ND

X Concentration per ml of culture medium

* mg per T-250 flask

+ mg phospholipids per mg protein

percent total lipid phosphorus

ND not determined

Among the minor phospholipids, phosphatidic acid and
lysobisphosphatidic acid were increased in the AC 3579
experiments. The latter lipid was also increased in retinol
experiments.

Hydrolase Activities

Protein concentration per T-250 flask increased 1.7- and
5.9-fold in two lines exposed to 10 ug/ml AC 3579 but dropped
to 48% of the control value at the 20 ug/ml level (Table II).
Specific activities of alpha-galactosidase, beta-hexosaminidase
and alpha-glucosidase were slightly decreased (40 to 76% of
control) in the lines exposed to 10 ug/ml. Sphingomyelinase
activity was significantly depressed to about 30% of control.
Acid phosphatase, beta-glucuronidase and alpha-mannosidase
specific activities were increased 2- to 3-fold. These results
suggested that the overall increase in protein concentration
tended to exceed a lesser increase in lysosomal hydrolases
resulting in reduced specific activities. At the 20 ug/ml level
considering the significant decrease in protein concentration
there seemed to be a general inhibition of hydrolase activities
with the exception of beta-glucosidase and acid phosphatase.

Retinol (10 ug/ml) caused a 3-fold increase in protein
concentration per T-250 flask (Table II). This resulted in
a corresponding dilution of alpha-galactosidase, beta-
hexosaminidase and arylsulfatase A activities, an inhibition
of beta-glucosidase, sphingomyelinase, alpha-fucosidase, and
beta-galactosidase activities, and some stimulation of
beta-glucuronidase activity.

Two adult lines exposed to chloroquine (10 ug/ml) also
had increased protein concentration per T-250 flask (Table II).
Most specific hydrolase activities were less reduced than would
be expected from simple dilution. Acid phosphatase, beta-
glucosidase and in one line only, beta-galactosidase had
significantly increased specific activities.

Sphingomyelin exposure (0.1 and 5.0 mg/ml) did not induce
changes in protein concentration (Table I). Most hydrolase
activities were significantly reduced and the reduction was
more severe at the 5.0 mg/ml level. Only acid phosphatase
activity remained within normal limits.

TABLE II

HYDROLASE ACTIVITIES IN NORMAL FIBROBLASTS EXPOSED TO VARIOUS CHEMICALS
(percent of control values)

HYDROLASES	AC 3579 10 ug #1	AC 3579 10 ug #3	AC 3579 20 ug #3	RETINOL 10 ug #3	CHLOROQUINE 10 ug #1	CHLOROQUINE 10 ug #2	SPHINGOMYELIN 0.1 mg #1	SPHINGOMYELIN 5.0 mg #3	N-ACETYLNEURAMINIC ACID 0.1 mg #3
α-galactosidase	73	67	25	38	33	37	41	21	142
β-galactosidase	83	228	13	15	49	788	39	18	393
β-glucosidase	251	100	100	8	200	883	80	46	100
β-glucosaminidase	76	40	20	48	36	93	63	11	117
sphingomyelinase	28	33		6	22		27	5	112
α-fucosidase	44	11	70	18	52		40	5	92
acid phosphatase	268		188		165		104	85	238
arylsulfatase A		127		38					
α-glucosidase	66	62	34	61	75	125			
α-mannosidase	214	29	18		61	115	263		
β-glucuronidase	74	100	47	154	52		59	48	786
protein	174	590	48	309	387	258	101	95	144

Exposure to N-acetylneuraminic acid (0.1 mg/ml) induced no change in protein concentration or in most hydrolase activities, while beta-galactosidase, acid phosphatase, and most strikingly beta-glucuronidase had significantly increased activities (Table II).

Various hydrolase activities were detectable in the cell culture medium. They tended to be low and often exhibited poor kinetics. As found in human serum, the highest activity by far was that of beta-hexosaminidase which could be reliably assayed (Table III). While the activity was similar to controls in the retinol experiments, it was doubled in medium from cells exposed to chloroquine and quadrupled in that from I-cells, confirming the original observation on which was based the hypothesis of lysosomal leakage (26).

$1-^{14}C$-Acetate Incorporation into Cultured Skin Fibroblasts

Following a 2-day pulse with $1-^{14}C$-acetate, fibroblasts were extracted into three major fractions: water-soluble, lipid-soluble and water- and lipid-insoluble residue (25). Exposure to retinol (10 ug/ml) for six days resulted in a slight decrease of incorporation into the water-soluble fraction (Table IV). Exposure to chloroquine (10 ug/ml) for seven days caused a significantly decreased incorporation into all three fractions.

TABLE III

BETA-HEXOSAMINIDASE RELEASED INTO THE CULTURE
MEDIUM OF HUMAN FIBROBLASTS

EXPERIMENT	MEAN	RANGE
Controls (6)[+]	1277[*]	1089 - 1462
Retinol (10 ug/ml)(9)	1216	981 - 1364
Chloroquine (10 ug/ml)(3)	2317	2133 - 2578
I-cell (5)	4715	4430 - 5102

+ number of experiments

* nmoles / hr / ml medium

1-^{14}C-Acetate Turnover in Fibroblasts Exposed to Chloroquine or Retinol.

Normal human fibroblasts were pulse-labelled for two days and then exposed to a medium containing chloroquine (10 ug/ml) for six weeks. Replicate flasks were extracted and fractionated at regular intervals. Half-lives of the different fractions could be estimated by plotting the logarithm of the corresponding counts per minute (CPM) against time. Under these conditions a fast, linear decay of the radioactivity of the three major fractions was observed for one week (Fig. 1).

Thereafter, a second, slower component became apparent in all fractions but the water-soluble one. In controls the plot remained linear throughout the experiment (Table V).

The lipid fraction was subdivided into neutral lipids, glycolipids, and phopholipids by 2-dimensional thin-layer chromatography (27) using known carrier lipids. After an

TABLE IV

1-^{14}C-ACETATE INCORPORATION INTO SUBFRACTIONS
FROM HUMAN FIBROBLASTS

EXPERIMENT	WATER	LIPID	INSOLUBLE
Control	14.6[+]	21	2.2
Retinol[X]	10.6	20.6	2.7
Control	11.5	20	7.7
Chloroquine[*]	4.2	7.2	0.7

+ CPM X 10^{-4}

X 10 ug/ml for 6 days

* 10 ug/ml for 7 days

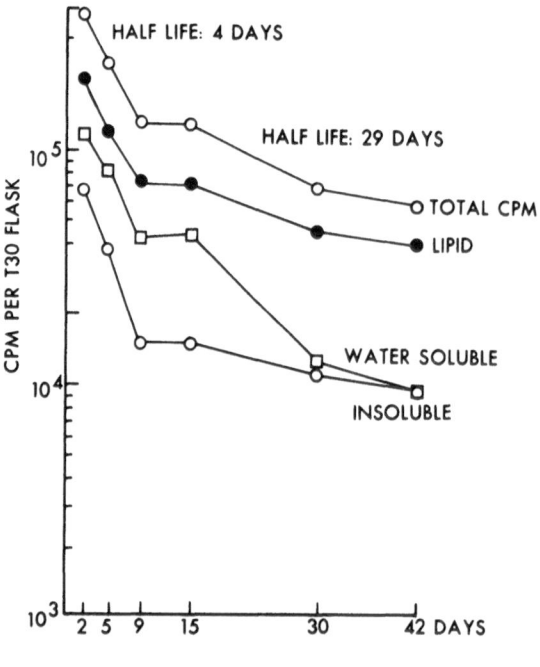

RADIOACTIVITY IN FIBROBLASTS EXPOSED TO
CHLOROQUINE FOLLOWING A ^{14}C-ACETATE PULSE

Fig. 1

Impaired turnover of lipid and water-and-lipid insoluble
label.

TABLE V

1-^{14}C-ACETATE TURNOVER IN SKIN FIBROBLASTS

EXPERIMENT	HALF-LIFE (days)			
	Total CPM	LIPID	WATER	INSOLUBLE
Control adults (n=6)	12(4-24)*	10(4-21)	13(2-25)	8(5-46)
Chloroquine (10ug/ml)				
2d to 9th day	4	4	4	4
9th to 42nd day	29	29	13	29
Control children (n=7)	10(8-11)	9(6-13)	9(6-11)	13(5-19)
Retinol (10ug/ml)				
2d to 15th day	4	5	3	4^X
15th to 45th day	41	13	18	∞

* mean and range

X not linear

initial decrease of phospholipid and neutral lipid CPM at the benefit of the glycolipid CPM for the first two weeks, the proportion of the different lipid classes remained constant for the rest of the experiment (phospholipids 65 percent, neutral lipids 20 percent and glycolipids 15 percent) which was within normal limits. The proportion of phosphatidyl choline (about 35 percent of total phospholipids) and sphingomyelin (about 15 percent of total phospholipids) remained essentially constant during the last four weeks of the experiment (Fig. 2), while under normal conditions the proportion of labelled sphingomyelin tended to increase and eventually exceeded that of labelled phosphatidyl choline which decreased. This type of abnormal phospholipid turnover was also observed in I-cell fibroblasts (Fig. 3).

When 1-^{14}C-acetate turnover was similarly studied in presence of retinol (10 ug/ml), lipid CPM as percent of total CPM remained significantly lower than normal controls at all times. There was a corresponding increase in the proportion

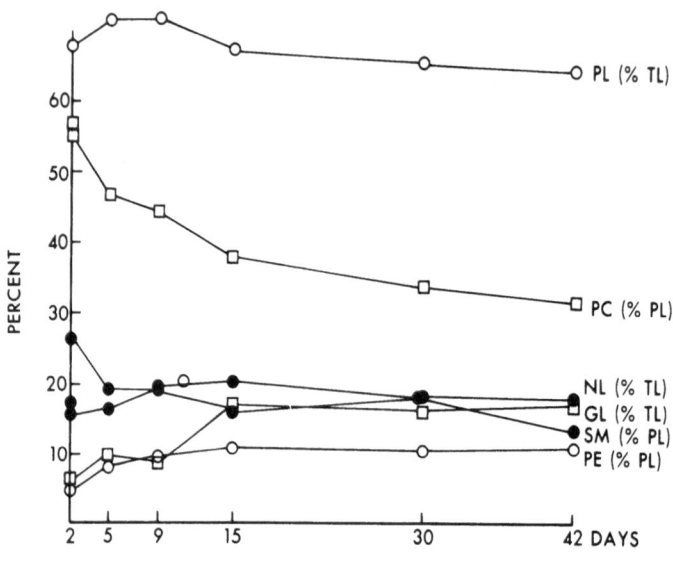

Fig. 2

Label distribution in the major lipid classes and phospholipids following a two-day pulse with 1-¹⁴C-acetate (neutral lipids = NL, phospholipids = PL, glycolipids = GL, as percent of total lipid CPM = TL; phosphatidylcholine = PC, sphingomyelin = SM and phosphatidylethanolamine = PE, as percent of total phospholipids = PL)

of insoluble CPM which was above the normal range at all times, reaching almost twice the upper normal limit at 42 days (Fig. 4). As in the chloroquine experiments, two components could be distinguished in the decay plot of the three major fractions. The fast component with a half-life of four days between day 2 and 15 lasted longer than in the chloroquine experiment. The slow component of the water-soluble fraction had an abnormal half-life. There was a gradual increase of the insoluble CPM.

Lipid classes had an abnormal distribution, neutral lipid CPM being increased at all times at the expense of phospholipid CPM (Table VI).

Ultrastructural Studies

We have previously shown (22) that a number of lysosomal storage disorders can be recognized by the development of characteristic lysosomal inclusions in cultured skin fibroblasts.

LIPID LABEL IN I-CELL FIBROBLASTS FOLLOWING A ^{14}C-ACETATE PULSE

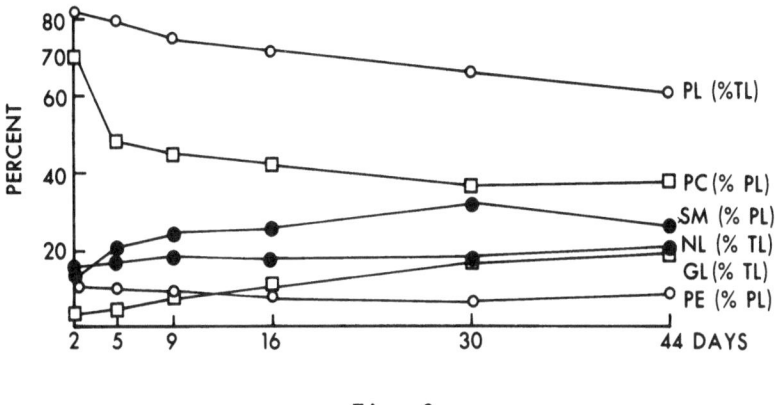

Fig. 3

Label distribution in the major lipid classes and phospholipids (same abbreviations as in Fig. 2).

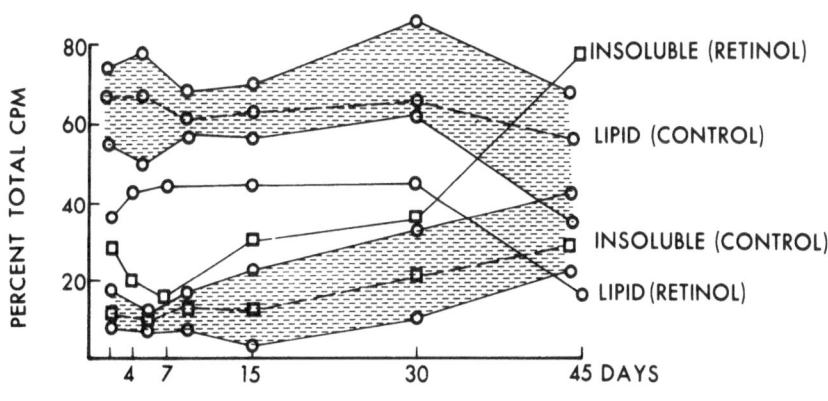

Fig. 4

Distribution of lipid and water-and lipid-insoluble label
following a 2-day pulse with 1-^{14}C-acetate.

TABLE VI

LIPID RADIOACTIVITY IN HUMAN FIBROBLASTS EXPOSED TO RETINOL
FOLLOWING A 2-DAY PULSE WITH 1-^{14}C-ACETATE

TIME (DAYS)	NEUTRAL LIPIDS CONTROL	NEUTRAL LIPIDS RETINOL	PHOSPHOLIPIDS CONTROL	PHOSPHOLIPIDS RETINOL
2	44^X	44	55	50
4		29		64
5	27		65	
7		34		56
9	20		67	
15	18	33	65	53
30	25	37	63	48
45	28	43	63	42

X percent of total lipid CPM

        Exposure to excess sphingomyelin (5mg/ml of culture medium)
produced inclusions rather different from those observed in
Niemann-Pick disease, type A. Aside from lamellar and poly-
morphous inclusions, tightly packed, unusual curved tubules
were seen. These were similar to inclusions found in Farber's
disease (28). A sizeable amount of ceramides could be demonstrated in these cultures, corroborating the ultrastructural
clue to the nature of these inclusions.

        Chloroquine exposure gave rise to the development through-
out the cytoplasm of numerous granular inclusions containing
polycyclic, dense lamellar rings with a granular core.

        Inclusions elicited by retinol exposure had the same
basic morphology as the chloroquine inclusions, but their
distribution was more strictly perinuclear and the lamellar
formations were much denser. The lamellae seemed to originate
within the granular matrix and occasionally resembled fingerprint bodies.

N-acetylneuraminic acid appeared to stimulate extensive plasma membrane infoldings. They were a few large membrane-bound inclusions containing stacks of needle-like crystals often in a fan-shaped arrangement.

DISCUSSION

These experiments illustrate what seemed to be a rather indiscriminate uptake by cultured skin fibroblasts of a large variety of substances which may turn out to be difficult or impossible to catabolize or to return to the outside environment. Many substances taken up are lysosomotropic (29), that is to say they will find their way into lysosomes where they may have beneficial pharmacologic properties. This is the rationale for enzyme replacement in cases of hydrolase deficiency (30). Lysosomal accumulation of substances susceptible to interfere with the lysosomal function is another aspect of lysosomotropism which may have wider-ranging consequences in the field of pharmacology than heretofore realized (31).

The physical properties of the lysosomal contents make them an efficient trap for weak bases, such as chloroquine, which are protonated within the acid environment and presumably become unable to pass across the lysosomal membrane (32). Complex formation with phospholipid would further prevent their disposition. Drug storage is not necessarily irreversible, disappearance of myeloid bodies and exocytosis were documented in some tissues (14,33). Detectable amounts of chloroquine could be found in body fluids from patients for as long as five years after the last ingestion (34). While interference with lysosomal function may be the crucial factor of chloroquine toxicity, other sites of action are clearly involved. For example, in cultured fibroblasts decreased rate of mitosis and cell migration were reported along with morphologic alterations which were time and dose dependent (35). Ultra-structural studies revealed the appearance of large electron-lucent vacuoles within 15 minutes of exposure (16) possibly reflecting water uptake by osmosis (32). Membranous and granular inclusions were more commonly described (10,13,14,18, 33,36). Although most reported biological effects were inhibitory, stimulation of protein synthesis was shown in the rat liver (37). In our fibroblast experiments, the increase in protein preceded that in phospholipid concentration (Table I). Labelled acetate incorporation, however, was uniformly decreased after one-week exposure to chloroquine (Table IV) while acetate turnover was initially accelerated in cells exposed to the drug following a 2-day pulse (Table V). Most hydrolase activities were decreased in the treated cells (Table II). This may have represented dilution by non-lysosomal proteins rather than actual inhibition,

since when the results were calculated as activities per flask
instead of per mg protein, they were equal or slightly superior
to the controls while β-glucosidase was significantly increased.
Losses into the medium (Table III) likely contributed to the
decrease in hydrolase activities. Actually the values obtained
in line #1 were almost identical to those of the milder variant
of I-cell disease, the so-called mucolipidosis III (24). A
marked impairment of cellular turnover is characteristic of
I-cell disease (38,39). Impaired mucopolysaccharide turnover
was previously reported in fibroblasts exposed to chloroquine
(18). In fibroblasts pulse-labelled with 1-^{14}C-acetate, chloroquine first induced an acceleration of the turnover for one
week (Fig. 1), then lipid and insoluble CPM half-lives became
significantly increased (Table V). The faster turnover component
which was never observed in I-cell strains, might be secondary
to an initial stimulation of hydrolase synthesis. No such
stimulation and no hydrolase release into the medium was apparent
in macrophages exposed to chloroquine for 24 hours (16). The
remarkably invariable lipid distribution during the last four
weeks of the chloroquine experiment (Fig. 2) was also observed
in I-cell fibroblasts (Fig. 3). This may reflect stoichiometric
physical interaction between undegraded molecules (40). Despite
striking resemblances in fibroblast studies the chloroquine model
does not perfectly mimick the pathology of I-cell disease. The
severe lesions produced by chloroquine intoxication in the liver
and brain (13) were not observed in the genetic disorder (41)

Retinol is highly surface active. Lecithin was primarily
concerned in the penetration of lipid films by retinol (42).
Excess retinol (33 ug/ml of medium) after a few hours altered
cell membranes, elicited the formation of numerous myelin bodies,
and affected the functions of the mitochondria and endoplasmic
reticulum in rat fibroblasts (42,43). Retinol concentration
within lysosomes was demonstrated by fluorescent microscopy (44).
In vitro, high amounts of retinol (200 ug/ml) stimulated
arylsulfatase A while it inhibited β-glucuronidase activity (45).

In our experiments, retinol induced an increase in protein
and to a lesser extent in phospholipid concentration (Table I).
Most hydrolase activities were decreased with the exception of
β-glucuronidase (Table II). No loss of acid hydrolases into
the medium was detected (Table III). The decreased activities
seemed to result in part from dilution by non-lysosomal proteins,
and in part from actual inhibition. Incorporation of acetate
into fibroblasts, previously incubated for six days in presence
of retinol, was decreased in the water-soluble fraction only
(Table IV). Acetate turnover was less uniformly impaired than
in the chloroquine experiments. The progressive increase of
the insoluble radioactivity suggested denaturation or trapping

of components originating from the water-soluble and lipid
fractions. Retinol is a fusogenic lipid (46) which by combination with phospholipids may influence membrane fusion (47), and,
as suggested by in vitro experiments (48), the formation of
lamellar bodies. The abnormal distribution of the label between
neutral lipids and phospholipids was a further indication of
the abnormal lipid metabolism.

As shown in the N-acetylneuraminic acid experiment, some
hydrolase activities could be independently stimulated.

The sphingomyelin experiments illustrated the limited
capacity of fibroblasts to protect themselves from being
invaded by excess substances in their environment either by
adjusting the rate of pinocytosis or hydrolase synthesis.
Induced sphingomyelin storage was actually much more marked than
in fibroblasts genetically deficient in sphingomyelinase
activity. Further experiments will be necessary to determine if
other phospholipids would generate a comparable situation.
Although sphingomyelinase activity was most depressed in the
chloroquine, retinol and AC 3579 experiments, there was
proportionally less accumulation of sphingomyelin in comparison
to other phospholipids and no indication of an abnormal sphingomyelin turnover, suggesting that sphingomyelin catabolism
remained adequate.

All the substances used had some common effects. Numerous
lysosomal inclusions were generated in all cases, with the
exception of the N-acetylneuraminic acid experiment in which
inclusions were sparse and metabolic changes discreet. A
significant accumulation of inclusions was generally accompanied
by a decrease in many hydrolase activities which became more
severe when the time of exposure or the concentration of the
toxic substance was increased. There was not always a parallel
increase in protein and phospholipid concentration as illustrated
in Table I. In phenobarbital-treated rats, the phospholipid/
protein ratio of the smooth endoplasmic reticulum membranes may
also change independently (49). By calculating the concentration
per single cell as well as the absolute amount per organ, one
may be able to detect abnormalities not apparent when concentrations are expressed as protein or weight ratios.

ACKNOWLEDGMENTS

We wish to thank Dr. Pasquale A. Cancilla for his help in
carrying ultrastructural studies, and Mrs. Angie Chapple, Mr.
Stephen Frommes, Mr. Elton Lassila, Mr. Seiji Nakatani, Ms.
Helen Roberson, and Ms. Klaske Zeilstra for expert technical
assistance. This study was supported in part by USPHS Research
Grant HD-05615.

REFERENCES

1. Philippart, M. Diagnosis and treatment of inborn errors of
    lipid metabolism. In: Modification of lipid metabolism.
    Ed. by E.G. Perkins and L.A. Witting. pp. 57-84, Acad. Press
    New York, 1975.
2. Chio, K.S., Reiss, U., Fletcher, B. and Tappel, A.L. Perox-
    idation of subcellular organelles: formation of lipofuscin-
    like fluorescent pigments. Science, 166, 1535-1536, 1969.
3. Laurent, G., Hildebrand, J., and Thys, O. Alterations of
    rat liver lysosomes and smooth endoplasmic reticulum
    induced by the diazafluoranthen derivative AC-3579. Lab.
    Invest., 32, 580-584, 1975.
4. Lullmann, H., Lullmann-Rauch, R. and Wassermann, O. Drug-
    induced phospholipidosis. Germ. Med., 3, 128-135, 1975.
5. Lie, S.O., McKusick, V.A. and Neufeld, E.F. Simulation of
    genetic mucopolysaccharidoses in normal human fibroblasts
    by alteration of pH of the medium. Proc. Nat. Acad. Sci.
    USA, 69, 2361-2363, 1972.
6. Mego, J.L., Farb, R.M. and Barnes, J. An adenosine triphos-
    phate-dependent stabilization of proteolytic activity in
    heterolysosomes. Biochem. J., 128, 763-769, 1972.
7. Li, S-C., Wan, C-C., Mazzotta, M.Y. and Li, Y-T. Requirement
    of an activator for the hydrolysis of sphingoglycolipids by
    glycosidases of human liver. Carbohydr. Res., 34, 189-193,
    1974.
8. Hickman, S., Shapiro, L.J. and Neufeld, E.F. A recognition
    marker required for uptake of a lysosomal enzyme by cultured
    fibroblasts. Biochem. Biophys. Res. Commun., 57, 55-61, 1974.
9. Fell, H.B. The direct action of vitamin A on skeletal tissue
    in vitro. In: The Fat Soluble Vitamins. Ed. by H.F. De
    Luca and J.W. Suttie, pp. 187-202, Univ. Wisconsin Press,
    Madison, 1970.
10. Hobbs, H.E., Sorsby, A. and Freedman, A. Retinopathy follow-
    ing chloroquine therapy. Lancet, 2, 478-480, 1959.
11. Whisnant, J.P., Espinosa, R.R., Kierland, R.A., and Lambert,
    E.H. Chloroquine neuromyopathy. Mayo Clin. Proc., 38,
    502-513, 1963.
12. Gleiser, C.A., Bay, W.W., Dukes, T.W., Brown, R.S., Read,
    W.K. and Pierce, K.R. Study of chloroquine toxicity and a
    drug-induced cerebrospinal lipodystrophy in swine. J. Am.
    Pathol., 53, 27-46, 1968.
13. Read, W.K., and Bay, W.W. Basic cellular lesion in chloro-
    quine toxicity. Lab. Invest., 24, 246-259, 1971.
14. Gerard, J.M. Stoupel, N., Collier, A. and Flament-Durant, J.
    Morphologic study of a neuromyopathy caused by prolonged
    chloroquine treatment. Eur. Neurol., 9, 363-379, 1973.
15. Fedorko, M. Effect of chloroquine on morphology of cytoplas-
    mic granules in maturing human leukocytes - an ultrastruct-
    ural study. J. Clin. Invest., 46, 1932-1942, 1967.

16. Fedorko, M.E., Hirsch, J.G. and Cohn, Z.A. Autophagic vac-
    uoles produced in vitro. I. Studies on cultured macrophages
    exposed to chloroquine. J. Cell Biol., 38, 377-391, 1968.
17. Fedorko, M.E., Hirsch, J.G. and Cohn, Z.A. Autophagic vacuoles
    produced in vitro. II. Studies on the mechanism of formation
    of autophagic vacuoles produced by chloroquine. J. Cell.
    Biol., 38, 392-402, 1968.
18. Lie, S.O. and Schofield, B. Inactivation of lysosomal
    function in normal cultured human fibroblasts by chloroquine.
    Biochem. Pharmacol., 22, 3109-3114, 1973.
19. Thys, O., Hildebrand, J., Gerin, Y. and Jacques, P.J. Alter-
    ations of rat liver lysosomes and smooth endoplasmic reticulum
    induced by the diazafluoranthen derivative AC-3579. I.
    Morphologic and biochemical lesions. Lab. Invest., 28,
    70-82, 1973.
20. Hildebrand, J., Thys, O. and Gerin, Y. Alterations of rat
    liver lysosomes and smooth endoplasmic reticulum induced
    by the diazafluoranthen derivative AC-3579. II. Effects
    of the drug on phospholipid metabolism. Lab. Invest.,
    28, 83-86, 1973.
21. Miller, F., De Harven, E. and Palade, G.E. The structure
    of eosinophil leukocyte granules in rodents and in man.
    J. Cell Biol., 31, 349-362, 1966.
22. Kamensky, E., Philippart, M., Cancilla, P. and Frommes, S.P.
    Cultured skin fibroblasts in storage disorders. An analysis
    of ultrastructural features. Am. J. Pathol., 73, 59-72, 1973.
23. Rouser, G., Fleisher, S. and Yamamoto, A. Two-dimensional
    thin-layer chromatographic separation of polar lipids and
    determination of phospholipids by phosphorus analysis of
    spots. Lipids, 5, 494-496, 1970.
24. Den Tandt, W.R., Lassila, E. and Philippart, M. Leroy's
    I-cell disease: Markedly increased activity of plasma acid
    hydrolases. J. Lab. Clin. Med., 83, 403-408, 1974.
25. Philippart, M. (^{14}C) incorporation into brain explants from
    lipofuscinosis and sulfatidosis. Third International Meeting
    of the International Society for Neurochemistry, Budapest,
    p 343, 1971.
26. Wiesmann, U.N., Lightbody, J., Vassella, F. and Herschkowitz,
    N.N. Multiple lysosomal enzyme deficiency due to enzyme
    leakage? N. Engl. J. Med., 284, 109-110, 1971.
27. Rouser, G., Kritchevsky, G., Yamamoto, A., Knudson, A. and
    Simon, G. Accumulation of a glycerophospholipid in classical
    Niemann-Pick disease. Lipids, 3, 287-293, 1968.
28. Van Hoof, F., Hers, H.G. Other lysosomal storage disorders.
    In: Lysosomes and storage diseases. Ed. by H.G. Hers &
    F. Van Hoof, pp 553-573, Acad. Press, New York, 1973.
29. De Duve, C., De Barsy, T., Poole, B., Trouet, A., Tulkens, P.,
    and Van Hoof, F. Lysosomotropic agents. Biochem. Pharmacol.,
    23, 2495-2531, 1974.

30. De Duve, C. From cytases to lysosomes. Fed. Proc., 23, 1045-1049, 1964.

31. Allison, A. The role of lysosomes in the action of drugs and hormones. Adv. Chemotherapy, 3, 253-302, 1968.

32. Wibo, M. and Poole, B. Protein degradation in cultured cells. II. The uptake of chloroquine by rat fibroblasts and the inhibition of cellular protein degradation and cathepsin B_1. J. Cell. Biol. 63, 430-440, 1974.

33. Abraham, R. and Hendy, R. Effects of chronic chloroquine treatment on lysosomes of rat liver cells. Exp. Mol. Pathol., 12, 148-159, 1970.

34. Rubin, M., Bernstein, H.N. and Zvaifler, N.J. Studies on the pharmacology of chloroquine. Arch. Ophthalmol., 70, 474-481, 1963

35. Gaddoni, G., Carraro, P.R. and Capitani, G. Azione della clorochina sui fibroblasti coltivati in vitro. Nota III - Effetti sulla morfologia cellulare. Arch. Ital. Dermat. Vener. Sess., 33, 397-414, 1964.

36. Abraham, R., Hendy, R. and Grasso, P. Formation of myeloid bodies in rat liver lysosomes after chloroquine administration. Exp. Mol. Pathol., 9, 212-229, 1968.

37. Delpino, A. and Ferrini, U. Protein synthesis stimulation in rat liver by chloroquine. Experientia, 28, 1061-1062, 1972.

38. Philippart, M., Nakatani, S., Kamensky, E., and Zeilstra, K. Impaired turnover of lipid, protein and mucopolysaccharide in Leroy's Inclusion-cell disease. Pediatr. Res., 7, 392, 1973.

39. Philippart, M., Zeilstra, K. and Kamensky, E. Impaired sulfate turnover in cultured skin fibroblasts and amniotic cells from patients with mucopolysaccharidosis. Pediatr. Res., 7, 348, 1973.

40. Samuels, S., and Aleu, F. The formation of membrane aggregates. In: Inborn Disorders of Sphingolipid Metabolism. Ed. by S.M. Aronson and B.W. Volk, pp 317-324, Pergamon Press Oxford, 1967.

41. Tondeur, M., Vamos-Hurwitz, E., Mockel-Pohl, S., Dereume, J.P., Cremer, N., and Leob, H. Clinical biochemical, and ultrastructural studies in a case of chondrodystrophy presenting the I-cell phenotype in tissue culture. J. Pediatr., 79, 366-378, 1971.

42. Dingle, J.T. and Lucy, J.A. Vitamin A, carotenoids and cell function. Biol. Rev., 40, 422-461, 1965.

43. Daniel, M.R., Dingle, J.T., Glauert, A.M. and Lucy, J.A. The action of excess of vitamin A alcohol on the fine structure of rat dermal fibroblasts. J. Cell Biol., 30, 465-475, 1966.

44. Allison, A.C. and Young, M.R. Uptake of dyes and drugs by living cells in culture. Life Sci., 3, 1407-1414, 1964.

45. Hsu, L. and Tappel, A.L. Effect of vitamin A on the activity of arylsulfatase and β-glucuronidase of rat tissues. Biochem. Biophys. Acta, 101, 113-120, 1965.

46. Ahkong, Q.F., Fisher, D., Tampion, W. and Lucy, J.A. The fusion of erythrocytes by fatty acids, esters, retinol and α-tocopherol. Biochem. J., 136, 147-155, 1973.

47. Lucy, J.A. The fusion of biological membranes. Nature, 227, 814-817, 1970.

48. Howell, J.I., Fisher, D., Goodall, A.H., Verrinder, M., and Lucy, J.A. Interactions of membrane phospholipids with fusogenic lipids. Biochem. Biophys. Acta, 332, 1-10, 1973.

49. Higgins, J.A. Studies on the biogenesis of smooth endoplasmic reticulum membranes in hepatocytes of phenobarbital-treated rats. II. The site of phospholipid synthesis in the initial phase of membrane proliferation. J. Cell Biol., 62, 635-646, 1974.

Glycolipids in Cultured Fetal Tay-Sachs Disease Cerebellar Cells

Larry Schneck, Linda M. Hoffman, Daniel Amsterdam,
Steven Brooks and Betty Pinkett
Department of Neurology and the Isaac Albert Research
Institute of the Kingsbrook Jewish Medical Center
Rutland Road and East 49th Street, Brooklyn, N.Y. 11203

INTRODUCTION

Tay-Sachs disease (TSD) is a fatal, genetically determined disorder of sphingoglycolipid metabolism, associated with the absence of the lysosomal enzyme B-D-N-acetylhexosaminidase A (Hex A) (1). There is a massive accumulation of GM_2 ganglioside, and its asialo derivative GA_2 in cells of the central nervous system. A cell culture which reproduces these biochemical parameters would permit one to measure the effect of enzyme replacement therapy under controlled conditions that are not easily attainable in vivo. Although skin fibroblasts cultured from TSD patients lack Hex A, these cultured cells do not accumulate GM_2 ganglioside (2). Since TSD is a neuronal lipid storage disease, and since fetal TSD brain has the characteristic glycolipid patterns found in infant TSD brain, a cell strain from fetal TSD cerebellum was established and the glycolipid patterns were evaluated by TLC and GLC (3). The cells were labelled with ^{14}C-glucosamine in order to compare the metabolic activity of the gangliosides over an extended time period. The cells were also transformed with the oncogenic DNA SV-40 virus (4) since we wished to establish a permanent cell line for the study of this disease.

MATERIALS AND METHODS

Cell cultures were established as serially passaged diploid strains from the cerebellum and lung of an 18 and a 20 week old TSD fetus and an age matched control. Large quantities of cells were obtained from multiple roller cultures seeded from T60 flasks (5). Cultures derived from lung displayed typical fibro-

495

blastic morphology whereas cells established from brain were glial-
like. When confluent monolayers were established, each roller was
labelled for 2 hours in 5 ml. of serum free MEM with 8.5 uCi per
roller of D-glucosamine-1-C^{14} hydrochloride (specific activity
56.5 mCi/mM). After 2 hours the roller cultures were washed with
Hanks balanced salt solution to remove the unincorporated label
and were refed with complete MEM containing 10% heat inactivated
(57°C for 1 hr.) fetal calf serum. All cultures were refed bi-
weekly and at each selected time interval 4 rollers were washed
a total of 7 times and collected for analysis. Cultures were
transformed with the DNA tumorogenic SV-40 virus. Normal and TSD
transformed cultures were characterized by epithelioid morphology,
loss of contact inhibition, aneuploid chromosome number, reduced
cell size, and high density of cell growth. The hexosaminidase
activities were the same in the pretransformed and the transformed lines. Both lines were nontumorgenic in hamster cheek
pouches. The transformed TSD culture has undergone 67 subcultures
to date.

The total lipid extract obtained from the lyophilized cell
powder was partitioned according to the Suzuki (6) modification
of the method of Folch (7). The ganglioside fraction was subjected to alkaline methanolysis and separated from salt on a Sephadex
G-25 column. The lower phase from the partition was fractionated
on Unisil silicic acid columns. The individual gangliosides and
hexosylceramides in the sample were identified and quantitated by
thin layer and gas-liquid chromatography (3). The percent radioactivity in the individual ganglioside and hexosylceramide bands
was quantitated by liquid scintillation counting with appropriate
corrections being made for quenching.

RESULTS AND DISCUSSION

The thin layer chromatograms of gangliosides found in cell
cultures and in fetal and infant brain are shown in Fig. 1. These
patterns indicate that GM_2 is present in cultured cells derived
from fetal TSD cerebellum but not in the cells cultured from fetal
TSD lung. The thin layer patterns also show two other major
ganglioside bands: one having an Rf value corresponding to GM_3;
the other with an Rf value corresponding to GD_3. In contrast to
the ganglioside patterns found in the cerebellar cells, fetal
brain shows a greater percent of the more complex gangliosides,
GM_1, GD_{1a}, GD_{1b} and GT. The nature of these bands was confirmed
by GLC. N-glycolylneuraminic acid was not seen in the gangliosides. Table I indicates that the increased magnitude of GM_2
ganglioside in the TSD cultured cells is similar to that found in
fetal TSD cerebellum.

The thin layer patterns of hexosylceramides found in the cell
cultures and in fetal cerebellum are shown in Fig. 2. Whereas

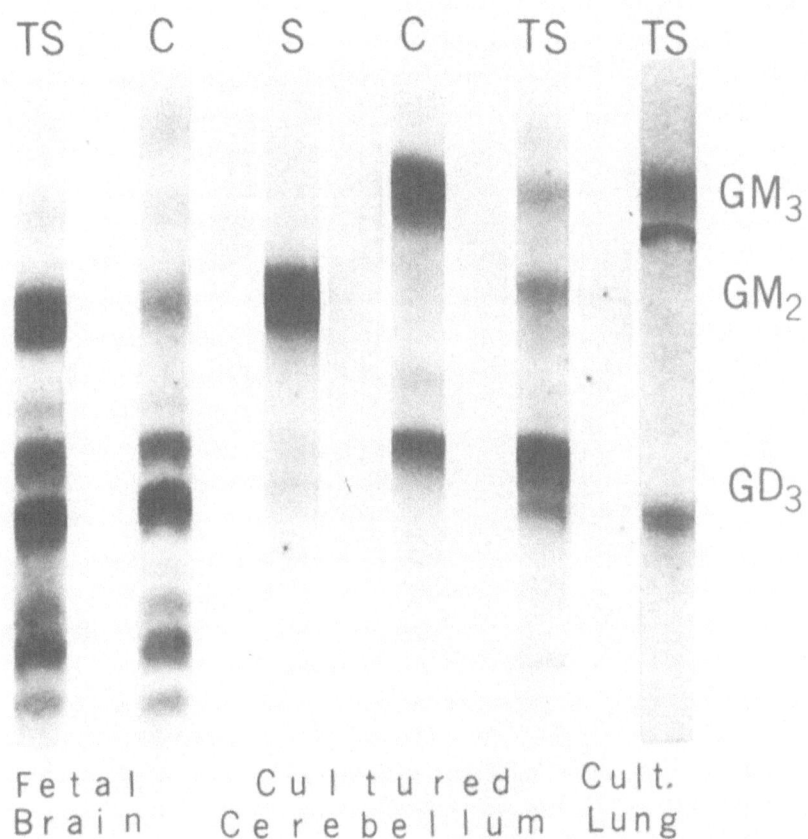

Fig. 1.　TLC of gangliosides from Tay-Sachs (TS) and normal (C) fetal brain and cultured cerebellum and lung.

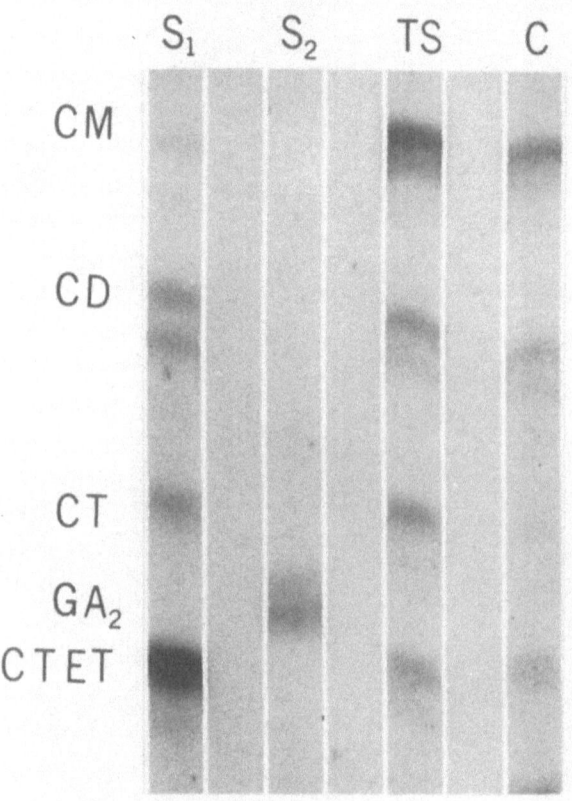

Fig. 2.   TLC of hexosylceramides from cultured TSD (TS) and
           normal (C) cells.

TABLE I. Gangliosides (mol %) in Fetal Cerebellum and Cultured
Fetal Cerebellar Cells[a]

	Cells			Cerebellum	
	TSD	Normal		TSD	Normal
GM_3	29.8	31.1	GM_3	2.2	5.7
GM_2	33.3	6.6	GM_2	32.7	13.9
GM_1	9.2	4.6	GM_1	25.5	21.5
GD_3	15.0	43.5	GD_{1a}	17.7	24.9
GD_{1a}	8.8	10.5	GD_{1b}	8.5	9.9
GD_{1b}	3.3	3.1	GT	10.3	13.9
GT	Trace	Trace	G_o	3.1	10.2

a   Quantitated by densitometry

fetal and infant TSD brain contain the asialotrihexosylceramide
(GA_2) (8) the brain cells contain a trihexosyl ceramide which is
not GA_2. In addition a tetrahexosyl ceramide, globoside, is
found in the cultured cells but not in fetal or infant brain. As
can be seen in Table II there are no essential differences between the ceramide patterns in the TSD and normal cultured cells.

TABLE II. Hexosylceramides (mol %) in Fetal Cerebellum and
Cultured Fetal Cerebellar Cells[a]

	Cells			Cerebellum	
	TSD	Normal		TSD	Normal
CM	63.3	64.1	CM	71.0	68.9
CD	11.9	11.6	CD	3.2	24.3
CT	12.4	2.9	GA_2	25.8	6.8
CTET	12.4	21.4	CTET	b	b

a   Determined by densitometry
b   not detected

The cerebroside from the cultured cerebellar cells is exclusively glucosylceramide, whereas in fetal TSD brain both glucosyl- and galactosylceramides are present with a preponderance of glucosyl-ceramide. TSD infant brain cerebroside consists mainly of galactosylceramide. The dihexosylceramides were identified as lactosylceramide in both the cultured cells and fetal brains. Table III summarizes the ganglioside and hexosylceramide patterns of the glycosphingolipids in fetal TSD and normal cells from the cerebellum and the lung.

TABLE III. Glycosphingolipids (nmoles/mg. protein) in Cultured Cells from Cerebellum and Lung

	Cerebellum		Lung	
	TSD	Normal	TSD	Normal
Gangliosides:				
GM_3	1.2	1.1	1.2	0.4
GM_2	1.3	0.3	---	---
GD_3	1.2	1.4	0.9	0.3
Hexosylceramides:				
CM	1.6	1.3	1.7	0.3
CD	0.6	0.5	0.7	0.4
CT	0.6	0.4	2.0	1.3
CTET	0.4	0.3	1.3	1.1

In the cerebellar cells $C_{24:0}$ and $C_{24:1}$ are the predominant fatty acids of the gangliosides and trihexosylceramides. In contrast, $C_{18:0}$ and $C_{18:1}$ are the predominant fatty acids of gangliosides and hexosylceramides from fetal and infant brain. The gangliosides from fetal brain have a higher percentage of $C_{18:1}$ unsaturated fatty acids when compared to infant brain. Furthermore, while long chain hydroxy fatty acids are observed in infant brain cerebroside, no hydroxy fatty acids are seen in cerebroside from fetal brain or fetal cerebellar cells. The fatty acid composition of GA_2 is similar to the ganglioside fatty acid patterns in both fetal and infant brain.

TABLE IV. Distribution of C_{18} and C_{24} Fatty Acids in the GM_2 and
GA_2 or Trihexosylceramides of TSD Infant, Fetal,
Cerebellum and Cultured Cerebellar Cells

	18:0	18:1	24:0	24:1	18:0	18:1	24:0	24:1
Infant	79.4	2.9	a	a	66.2	10.3	a	a
Fetal	63.2	16.4	a	a	75.0	9.0	a	a
Cells	4.0	4.0	36.2	29.4	1.4	2.7	38.1	38.8

a less than 0.5%

TABLE V. Sphingolipids in TSD

	Cultured Cells	Fetal	Infant
GM_2	increased	increased	increased
GD_3	present	absent	absent
GA_2	absent	present	present
Globoside	present	absent	absent
Major Fatty Acids			
GM_2	24:0, 24:1	18:0, 18:1	18:0
GA_2	--- ---	18:0, 18:1	18:0
CM[a]	24:0, 24:1	18:0, 18:1	24:0[b], 24:1[b]

a In cultured and fetal brain - mainly glucosylceramide; in
   infant brain - mainly galactosylceramide
b Non-hydroxy and hydroxy fatty acids

Table V summarizes the similarities and differences in the
glycosphingolipids between cultured cells, fetal, and infant TSD
brain.

Relative degradation rates of gangliosides were studied in
cultured cells utilizing ^{14}C-glucosamine, a ganglioside precursor.

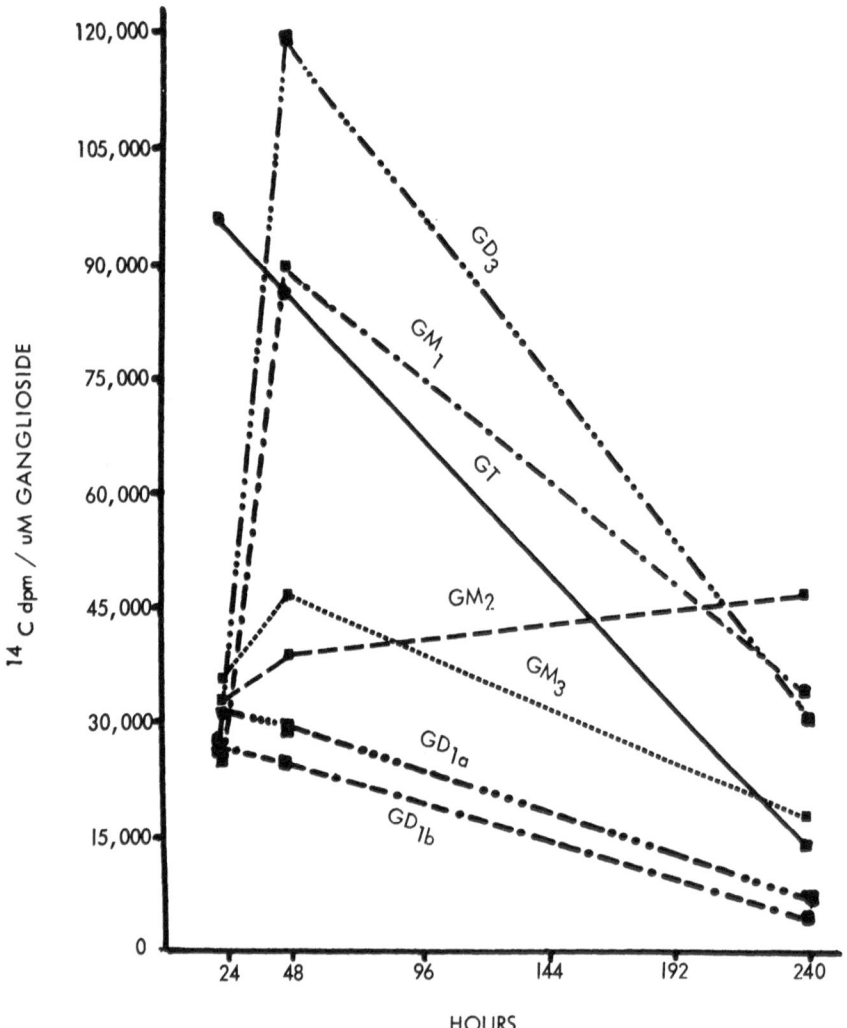

Fig. 3.   Radioactivity of TSD cerebellar cell gangliosides, over
          a 10 day period.

Ninety percent of the incorporated radioactivity was found in the non-lipid residue. Of the remaining 10 percent which was found in the chloroform:methanol extract, 90 percent was in the ganglioside fraction. By 240 hours, there was a decrease in the radioactivity of all the ganglioside bands except for GM_2 which then had the highest percent of radioactivity (Fig. 3). These results are consistent with decreased degradation of GM_2 ganglioside. In the hexosylceramide fraction, 93 percent of the radioactivity was associated with the globoside area. The remaining 7% of the radioactivity was found in the trihexosylceramide area. Since D-glucosamine is a precursor for glycolipids which contain amino sugars, it is presumed that the trihexosylceramide band contains a small amount of GA_2 which cochromatographed with the trihexosylceramide. The relative percent distribution of the gangliosides remained the same over the 10 day trial course.

TABLE VI. Distribution of Gangliosides (nmole/mg. dry weight) in TSD Cultured Cerebellar Cells over a Ten Day Time Period.[a]

	24 hrs	48 hrs	10 days
GM_3	.31	.47	.63
GM_2	.30	.44	.60
GM_1	.15	.22	.30
GD_3	.27	.40	.54
GD_{1a}	.15	.22	.30
GD_{1b}	.09	.14	.19
GT	.04	.05	.07
NANA (% dry wt)	.06	.10	.12

a   Quantitated by densitometry

Figure 4 shows that there is a simplification of the ganglioside patterns in both TSD and normal SV-40 transformed cell lines. Although the normal transformed line did not exhibit reduced Hex A activity there appears to be an increased concentration of the band with a mobility similar to GM_2. The hexosylceramide patterns

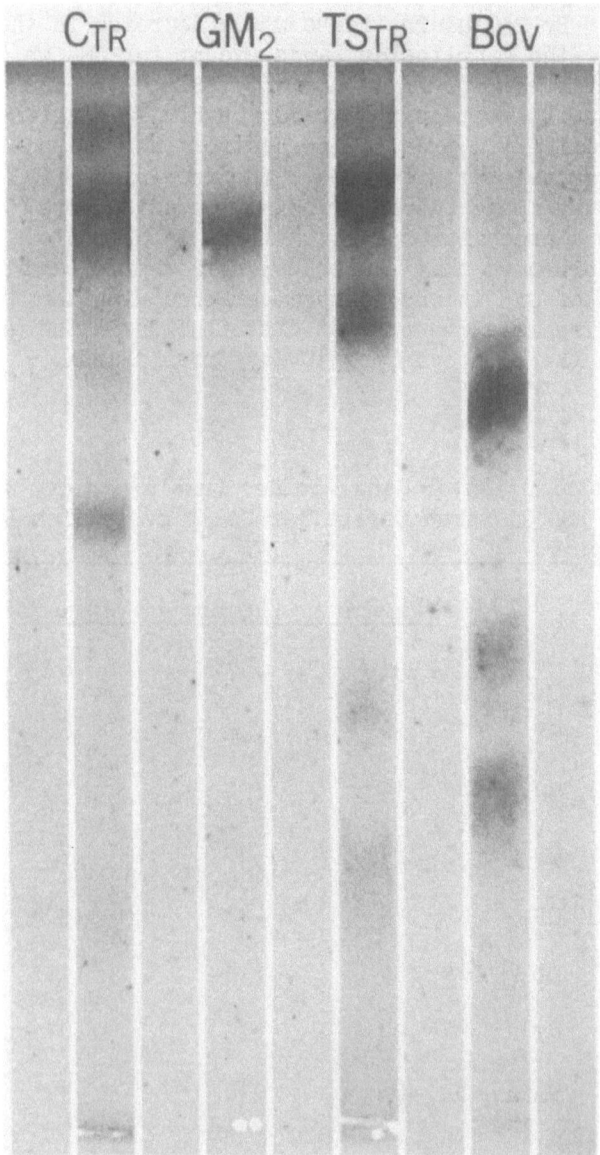

Fig. 4.   TLC of gangliosides from transformed (TR) normal (C)
           and Tay-Sachs (TS) cultured cerebellar cells. Bovine
           (Bov) brain ganglioside pattern for comparison.

in the pretransformed and transformed lines are similar. The nature of these bands require more definite identification.

Biochemically, the TSD cerebellar line is similar to TSD brain tissue in that there is an increased concentration of GM_2. This increase is caused by impaired degradation as shown by the labeled GM_2. However, there are major differences between these cells and fetal and infant brain. While there is a significant increase of GA_2 in fetal and infant TSD brain (8), no GA_2 was identified in the TSD cultured cells. Since Hex B is capable of hydrolyzing GA_2 in vitro (9), there is no obvious explanation for the increased concentration of this asialo trihexosylceramide in fetal and infant TSD brain. It has been suggested that increased concentrations of GM_2 inhibit the activity of Hex B against GA_2 (10). However, no GA_2 was found in a Niemann-Pick disease brain that had an increased concentration of GM_2 similar in magnitude to that found in fetal TSD brain (11). In juvenile GM_2 gangliosidosis (AB variant) even though Hex A and B are present, there is an accumulation of both GM_2 and GA_2 (12). Conversely, there are reports of asymptomatic cases with complete absence of Hex A activity (13). Thus, a nonenzymatic protein, subtle structural alterations in the enzyme, or relationships between substrate and enzyme may play a role in the pathogenesis of TSD.

In addition to the absence of GA_2 in the cells, there are two other major differences between these cultured brain cells and brain. One is the large percent of $C_{24:0}$ and $C_{24:1}$ fatty acids in the gangliosides and hexosylceramides from the cultured cells. Since the fetal calf serum used was found not to contain free C24 fatty acids, uptake from the culture medium is improbable. The other major difference between the cells and brain is the substantial amounts of GM_3 and GD_3 in the cultured cell line. One could argue that these cells are not of neuroglial origin. However, cultured fibroblasts from TSD skin and lung do not contain GM_2. Electron microscopically, glial filaments were seen in the cultured brain cells. Furthermore, smaller quantities of these long chain fatty acids in GM_3 and GD_3 gangliosides have been isolated from infant white matter (14). Finally, Robert et al found that a primary culture of rat embryonal glial cells contained only GM_3 and GD_3 (15). Thus, in spite of the differences noted, this brain-derived cell culture line can be considered a workable in vitro model for Tay-Sachs disease.

REFERENCES

1. Okada, S., and O'Brien, J. S., Tay-Sachs disease: Generalized absence of a Beta-D-N-Acetylhexosaminidase component, Science 165 (1969) 698-700.

2. Dawson, G., Matalon, R., and Dorfman, A., Glycosphingolipids
    in cultured human fibroblasts. II. Characterization and
    metabolism in fibroblasts from patients with errors of glyco-
    sphingolipid and mucopolysaccharide metabolism. J. Biol.
    Chem., 247 (1972) 5951-5958.

3. Hoffman, L. M., Amsterdam, D., and Schneck, L., GM_2 ganglio-
    side in fetal Tay-Sachs disease brain cell culture: A model
    system for the disease. Brain Res. (1975) In press.

4. Shein, H. M., Transformation of astrocytes and destruction of
    spongioblasts induced by Simian tumor virus (SV40) in cul-
    tures of human fetal neuroglia, J. Neuropath. & Exp. Neurol.
    26 (1967) 60-76.

5. Amsterdam, D., and Brooks, S. E., Methodology: Cell culture.
    In B. W. Volk and L. Schneck (Eds.), The Gangliosidoses,
    Plenum Press, New York, 1975, pp. 265-270.

6. Suzuki, K., The pattern of mammalian brain gangliosides.
    II. Evaluation of the extraction procedures, post-mortem
    changes and the effect of formalin preservation, J. Neurochem.
    12 (1965) 629-638.

7. Folch, J., Lees, M., and Sloane-Stanley, G. H., A simple
    method for the isolation and purification of total lipides
    from animal tissues, J. Biol. Chem., 226 (1957) 497-509.

8. Schneck, L., Pinkett, B., and Volk, B. W., Asialo GM2-gan-
    glioside in fetal Tay-Sachs disease brain, J. Neurochem. 24
    (1975) 183-184.

9. Sandhoff, K., The hydrolysis of Tay-Sachs ganglioside (TSG)
    by human N-acetyl-B-D-hexosaminidase A, FEBS Lett. 11 (1970)
    342-344.

10. Wenger, D. A., Okada, S., and O'Brien, J. S., Studies on the
    substrate specificity of hexosaminidase A and B from liver,
    Arch. Biochem. Biophys. 153 (1972) 116-129.

11. Greenbaum, M., Hoffman, L. M., and Schneck, L., Unpublished
    observations.

12. Sandhoff, K., Harzer, K., Wassle, W., and Jatzkewitz, H.,
    Enzyme alterations and lipid storage in three variants of
    Tay-Sachs disease, J. Neurochem. 18 (1971) 2469-2489.

13. Navon, R., Padeh, B. and Adam, A., Apparent deficiency of hexosaminidase A in healthy members of a family with Tay-Sachs disease, Am. J. Hum. Genet. 25 (1973) 287-293.

14. Vanier, M. T., Holm, M., Mansson, J. E., and Svennerholm, L., Gangliosides of infant brain, J. Neurochem. 21 (1973) 1375-1384.

15. Robert, J., Freysz, L., Sensenbrenner, M., Mandel, P., and Rebel, G., Gangliosides of glial cells: A comparative study of normal astroblasts in tissue culture and glial cells isolated on sucrose-ficoll gradients, FEBS Lett. 50 (1975) 144-146.

THE CORRECTION, IN VITRO, OF LYSOSOMAL ENZYME DEFICIENCIES BY
MEANS OF IMMUNOGLOBULIN-COATED LIPOSOMES

Gerald Weissmann, Charles Cohen, Sylvia Hoffstein

New York University Medical Center, Division of
Rheumatology, Department of Medicine, 550 First Avenue
New York, New York 10016

Introduction: Lysozyme In Liposomes

In 1965, we described, with A. D. Bangham (1) the formation
of artificial lipid structures which could serve as models for the
membranes of cells and/or organelles. By 1968 (2), we had coined
the term "liposome" to describe these artificial, multilamellar
structures, which, in their response to steroids, lytic proteins,
polyene antibiotics, etc. closely resembled natural biomembranes.
(The term "liposome" has now been generally accepted). Yet it was
not until 1970 (3) that it became possible to encapsulate an enzyme, rather than low molecular weight solutes such as ions, glucose or dyes, into the aqueous interstices between the multilamellar lipid bilayers of liposomes. We utilized the enzyme lysozyme
and established its mode of trapping in the following fashion:

Gel filtration resolved liposomes formed in the absence of
enzyme from free enzyme when both were chromatographed immediately
after mixing. In contrast, if liposomes were permitted to form in
the presence of lysozyme, subsequent chromatography disclosed two
peaks of enzyme activity: one associated with liposomes, the other
emerging as free lysozyme. The activity of lysozyme associated
with liposomes was "latent"; i.e. there was little or no activity
on substrate unless the liposomes were disrupted by Triton X-100,
amphotericin B, or nystatin. Lysozyme unassociated with lipid was
as available to substrate in the absence of detergent or polyenes
as in their presence. Charge-induced associations were not crucial
for enzyme capture since both positively and negatively charged
liposomes captured lysozyme in latent form. As a measure of their
integrity, liposomes could also be shown to capture the marker

509

molecule, glucose, the bulk of which was released together with
lysozyme from liposomes by detergent or polyenes. As the aqueous
interspaces of positively charged liposomes were increased by in-
cremental incorporation of stearylamine, capture of both glucose
and lysozyme was increased proportionally. For these and other
reasons, it was considered likely that the liposomes had captured
lysozyme in the water spaces between the lipid lamellae of liposomes (3).

*Entrapment Of Enzymes And Other Substances In Liposomes And Their
In Vivo Distribution*

        Since these descriptions of the trapping of lysozyme in
liposomes (3), over thirty reports have appeared in which various
substances have been trapped in liposomes. In many instances these
liposome-entrapped materials have been injected into living animals and their fate has been followed by biochemical and ultrastructural methods. Thus liposomes have been used to capture
drugs such as actinomycin D, methotrexate, EDTA (4, 5, 6); enzymes
such as invertase, amyloglucosidase, alpha-mannosidase (reviews in
7, 8), dextranase; proteins such as ^{131}I-albumin, diptheria tox-
oid (8, 9, 10), and other materials such as poly I:C (10) and per-
technetate (11). The results have been summarized in review art-
icles by Gregoriadis (7) and by Ryman (8), and can be outlined as
follows:
        1. Substances, especially enzymes, entrapped in uncoated
liposomes remain in the circulation longer than when injected in
untrapped form.
        2. Liposomes retain their membrane integrity whilst in the
circulation and do not release their trapped substances into plasma.
        3. Liposomes are rapidly taken up in Kupffer cells of the
liver and, to a smaller extent, spleen.
        4. Liposomes are rapidly destroyed in Kupffer cell lyso-
somes ultrastructure and biochemistry).
        5. Antigens presented in liposomes do not lead to fatal
anaphylaxis on repeat injection, in contrast to free antigen.

        Many of the reported experiments (e.g. ref. 12), seem, how-
ever, to be lacking in rigid controls, both with respect to the
adequacy of liposomal trapping (e.g. lack of controls for surface
adherence to liposomes vs. true aqueous phase solution) and with
respect to controls for simple adherence to surfaces of cells in
injected hosts. In the experiments of Gregoriadis and Ryman (8,
9), for example, it cannot be determined whether the injected material was truly interiorized or whether the liposomes did not
simply adhere to the cell surface, subsequently to sediment with
subcellular fractions. Since enzyme-laden liposomes were injected
as long as a week after their preparation, it is possible that

lipid-enzyme debris (formed in response to surface adsorption or fusion) may have become adherent to the surface of organelles during homogenization. Studies of cellular or lysosomal integrity were not reported. It is therefore not possible to exclude the real possibility that the enzyme-lipid complex produced injury to the reticuloendothelial cells which participated in their clearance. Indeed most *in vivo* studies with uncoated liposomes are thrown open to question by the very careful studies of Pagano et al (13) who presented strong evidence for *fusion* of uncoated liposomes with plasma membranes of target cells (*in vitro*). This mechanism, rather than selective uptake by lysosomes, may provide a partial explanation for results of double-label studies which have shown discrepancies between labels of liposomal lipids and their contents (13, 8).

Immunoglobulins And The Coating Of Liposomes

Consequently, we were not impressed with the possibilities of using simple, uncoated, enzyme-filled liposomes for trials of lysosomal enzyme replacement therapy, although we had tentatively suggested this approach (14). The reasons for our lack of confidence are that when liposomes encounter the membranes of cells or organelles, they tend to resist uptake (15), provoke fusion of cells or organelles (16), or remain adsorbed to the cell surface where their contents are poorly available to the cell interior(13).

The difficulties are due to the fact that the bare phospholipid surfaces of liposomes do not constitute a strong stimulus for endocytosis, but this problem might be overcome if liposomes were coated with substances capable of engaging cell surface receptors. Lattices of aggregated human IgG adhere to various phagocytes by attaching to the cells' surface Fc receptors (17), a process which triggers uptake either of the aggregated protein itself, or any particle coated with such aggregates. We had previously studied in detail the interaction of immunoglobulins with liposomes (18) utilizing enhanced diffusion of small (but not large!) molecules as one index of membrane insertion. Heat-aggregated human immunoglobulins (Ig) exceeded native immunoglobulins in their capacity to release anions and glucose from either anionic or cationic liposomes; this interaction was not dependent upon the presence of cholesterol in the membrane. Heat-aggregation (10 min at 62°C) increased the membrane-perturbing activity of certain Ig. Activity varied among classes and subclasses: IgG_1 > pooled IgG> IgG_4 > IgA_1 > IgG_3. IgG_2, IgA_2, and IgM were inert. Fc fragments of IgG were as active as IgG_1, whereas Fab fragments were inactive. Prolonging aggregation to 60 min destroyed the activity of Ig. Membrane-activity could not be induced in non-Ig molecules such as bovine serum albumin by 10 or 60 min heat aggregation. Density gradient centrifugation of IgG_1 molecules indicated that membrane perturbing activity was associated with 15-20s aggregates. Sepharose 4B chromatography demonstrated preferential interaction between cationic membranes and aggregated Ig, whereas anionic membranes interacted nonselectively with both native and aggregated Ig via salt-like interactions. One explanation for these data is that heat aggregation induces a conformational change in the Fc regions of certain Ig, permitting them to interact with liposomes, presumably by enhancing their hydrophobic associations with membrane phospholipids (18).

Introduction Of Peroxidase Into Phagocytes With Ig-Coated Liposomes

Since aggregated Ig form lattices in which the key Fc regions are disposed both towards the interior of the outermost lamellae of the liposomes, and *also* towards the surrounding medium, it would be expected that these would act as ligands for the Fc receptors of phagocytes in order to provoke endocytosis (17). These considerations led us to consider coating liposomes with aggregated immunoglobulins which would serve as surface ligands to engage the Fc receptors on lysosome-containing cells.

In the summer of 1974, at the Marine Biological Laboratory, we were able to test our hypothesis that Ig coating engendered significantly greater uptake of liposome-entrapped enzyme than of free enzyme (19). Phagocytes of the smooth dogfish (*Mustelus canis*) contain no endogenous peroxidase within their lysosomes and constitute models for cells genetically deficient in lysosomal enzymes such as myeloperoxidase. (Peroxidase deficiency in man results in impaired killing of intracellular fungi such as *candida* (20). We have obtained uptake of over 50% of exogenous horseradish peroxidase provided that the enzyme is exhibited to cells after incorporation into liposomes coated with heat-aggregated, isologous IgM. Elasmobranchs possess only IgM's of both the 19 and 7s variety: these resemble mammalian Ig's in membrane-perturbing capacity (19). Trapping of horseradish peroxidase was established by chromatographic resolution (Sephadex G-200; Sepharose 2B and 4B) of free enzyme from that associated with liposomes; liposome-associated horseradish peroxidase, together with trapped markers of the aqueous compartment (glucose, CrO_4^-) were excluded, whereas free enzyme and markers were retained. Enzyme and marker trapping was not electrostatic, varied with the molar ratio of charged membrane components, and was reversed by detergent lysis (Triton X-100) of liposomes. Uptake at 30° of aggregated IgM-coated liposomes containing trapped horseradish peroxidase exceeded that of free enzyme by 100-fold, and was more efficient than uptake of horseradish peroxidase presented in uncoated liposomes or in liposomes coated with native IgM. After phagocytosis, peroxidase-rich liposomes were localized exclusively in lysosomes of the phagocytes by ultrastructural histochemistry; the enzyme displayed over 50% latency to osmotic lysis. Activity could be demonstrated to remain intact at 4° for at least 60 hours, and at 70% of maximum at 18° (elasmobranch maximum temperature).

Introduction Of Purified Hexosaminidase A Into Leukocytes Of Patients With Tay-Sachs Disease

However useful for the restitution of the enzymic equipment of dogfish, our technique was next applied (21) to a human lyso-somal storage disease: Tay-Sachs. Aggregated human IgG was used to coat liposomes which had previously trapped purified hexosamin-idase A (hex A). By a new, high-yield procedure, hex A was puri-fied 7000-fold from human placenta: the homogeneous protein had a pI of 5.4, permitting non-electrostatic trapping in the aqueous interstices of anionic multilamellar liposomes (phosphatidylcho-line 7:dicetylphosphate 2:cholesterol 1, molar ratios). Trapped hex A was separated from free enzymes by means of Sephadex G-200 chromatography: 1.3 ± 0.3 mUnits of hex A/μmole phospholipid be-came associated with liposomes using glucose as a marker of the aqueous compartment. Once sequestered, the enzyme remained latent until lamellae were disrupted by Triton X-100. Presence of enzyme in aqueous compartments was proved by the demonstration of in-creased trapping (0.02 to 1.33 mUnits/μmoles of phospholipid) with increments in like-sign repulsion of the bilayers produced by in-creasing molar ratios of anionic dicetylphosphate (5-20%). To provide for ligand-receptor interaction with surface Fc receptors of human polymorphonuclear leukocytes (PMN's), liposomes were coated by heat-aggregated (62°, 10') human IgG. PMN's from Tay-Sachs patients genetically deficient in hex A activity readily in-corporated exogenous hex A provided in this fashion. PMN's ex-posed to enzyme laden liposomes coated with aggregated IgG incor-porated significantly more hex A than when the enzyme was presented in uncoated liposomes or in liposomes coated with native IgG, which engages Fc receptors with less avidity. Free enzyme was *not* endo-cytized. Acquisition of specific hex A isozyme activity by cells (determined by DEAE-cellulose chromatography) was not due to sur-face adsorption since cytochalasin B, which prevents phagocytosis but not surface adherence, blocked uptake. Incorporation of the isozyme by deficient cells was also demonstrated by starch gel electrophoresis, and ultrastructural studies showed that the im-munoglobulin-coated, hex A-containing liposomes were taken up into PMN lysosomes after membrane fusion.

The successful application of the coating technique to human cells *in vitro* leaves one with the following problems:
    1. Finding a method of introducing the enzyme into circu-lating phagocytes *in vivo*.
    2. Persuading the phagocytes *in vivo* to enter parenchymal organs such as liver, spleen, and perhaps, brain.

3. Causing the phagocytes which have liposome-entrapped enzyme to selectively discharge this material within parenchymal organs which contain the offending, stored substrate (e.g. GM_2 ganglioside).

Selective Non-Cytotoxic Release Of Lysosomal Constituents From Phagocytes

A series of experiments in our laboratory exploring the mechanisms of enzyme release (22-25) have suggested means for inducing phagocytes to release their vacuolar contents into surrounding media.

Since 1970 it has been evident that polymorphonuclear leukocytes, macrophages, and monocytes of man and other species selectively release lysosomal, but not cytoplasmic constituents when they are exposed to particulate challenges (24-26). Originally demonstrated after the uptake of zymosan particles (23, 24), this phenomenon also includes the release of lysosomal constituents when white cells are exposed to immune complexes either in the bulk phase or dispersed upon surfaces (24, 25). The former process, release of lysosomal hydrolases during the process of phagocytosis of discrete particles by white cells, has been termed "regurgitation during feeding", whereas the latter, extrusion of lysosomal enzymes after the exposure of white cells to immune complexes on a supporting surface has been termed, "reverse endocytosis" or "frustrated phagocytosis" (25). In these two circumstances the white cells release such enzymes as beta-glucuronidase, acid phosphatase, aryl sulphatase, and myeloperoxidase (constituents of azurophil granules) as well as lysozyme and alkaline phosphatase (constituents of specific granules). Viability is maintained during release and it has become appreciated that the stimuli to release of lysosomal hydrolases act via 1) Fc receptors on the polymorphonuclear leukocyte which recognize altered immunoglobulins such as those present in the form of immune complexes and 2) C3 receptors which recognize C3b fragments present upon such particles as serum-treated zymosan (25).

Release of lysosomal hydrolases in response to these two forms of stimulation appears, however, to depend upon a defined sequence of continuous, but separable, steps. These include the capacity of white cells to respond to appropriate stimuli in the bulk phase or upon a surface, upon their capacity to move towards the particle, upon their adherence to or deformation in response to particulates, upon the internalization of material present in the bulk phase, and finally, upon the merger of the two types of lysosomal granules with the phagocytic vacuole (formed in response to materials present in the fluid phase) or merger directly with the plasma membrane (when immune reactants are present on a solid surface).

We have previously shown that cyclic nucleotides, and colchicine, influence the release of lysosomal hydrolases in the "regurgitation during feeding" and in the "reverse endocytosis" model
systems (23-25). It was impossible however to be certain whether
the inhibitory effects of cyclic AMP and theophylline, for example,
on enzyme release were due to direct effects of these agents upon
translocation of the granules to the phagocytic vacuole (or the
plasma membrane) or upon the earliest events in this sequence.
In "regurgitation during feeding" enzyme extrusion is accidental
to the incomplete closure of the external stoma of the secondary
lysosome. Were a pharmacologic agent to influence lysosomal enzyme release in this model (which closely mimicks events of immune-
mediated tissue injury or of the inflammation following ingestion
of particles) it would be impossible to determine at which of the
several steps antecedent to this final regurgitation such agents
were to act. Indeed, publications by numerous authors have confirmed our original observations that agents which elevate the
levels within cells of cyclic AMP (or exogenous cyclic AMP itself)
have the effect of inhibiting enzyme release in this model (22-
25). Moreover, agents which cause the disassembly of microtubules,
such as colchicine or vinblastine, also inhibit enzyme release
(22-25). In contrary fashion, agents which elevate the levels
within cells of cyclic GMP enhance the release of lysosomal hydrolases when cells are stimulated to regurgitate during feeding of
zymosan particles coated with immune complexes. And likewise,
agents such as D_2O, which induce assembly of cytoplasmic microtubules also enhance release. However, the difficulty with the
interpretation of such experiments is that it has been demonstrated
by a number of investigators that cyclic nucleotides influence
1) chemotaxis; 2) adherence of polymorphonuclear leukocytes to
surfaces and, 3) phagocytosis *per se*. Consequently, since and
analysis of the response of polymorphonuclear leukocytes to the
ingestion of particles requires that each of these steps be
distinguished from the others in order to determine the site at
which cyclic nucleotides might exert these effects, it became
necessary to devise systems in which these aspects of leukocyte
function could be eliminated from experimental consideration.

To this end we have employed the drug cytochalasin B which
inhibits the phagocytosis of particles by polymorphonuclear leukocytes but does not inhibit many of their subsequent responses to
the particles. Indeed, cytochalasin B transforms the "regurgitation during feeding" mechanism into the "reverse endocytosis"
mechanism of enzyme release (24-26). Lysosomes merge with the
outer plasma membrane, perturbed as a consequence of the cell's
interaction with or contact by, particulates, as if this portion
of the plasma membrane were internalized as in the form of a
phagocytic vacuole. Cytochalasin B, may however, have other effects upon phagocytic cells in addition to that mediated by its in-

terference with the function of cytoplasmic microfilaments. Thus, cytochalasin B reversibly inhibits glucose transport in mammalian cells and may have other metabolic effects. However, it has been clearly demonstrated that cytochalasin B in the human polymorphonuclear leukocyte: 1) inhibits phagocytosis; 2) that in the presence of cytochalasin B, C-1 oxidation of glucose proceeds in response to contact with zymosan particles (providing the C 1-labeled glucose is given to the cells before cytochalasin B is administered); 3) that cytochalasin B has no effect upon the passive flux of potassium nor upon the ouabain-inhibitable sodium/potassium pump; 4) that no effect is observed of the drug upon amino acid translocation; 5) that cells respond with appropriate elevations of cyclic AMP or cyclic GMP following stimulation with adrenergic and cholinergic agents respectively; 6) that cytochalasin B does not interfere with the appropriate assembly or disassembly of cytoplasmic microtubules following administration of colchicine or exposure to deuterium oxide; 7) that superoxide production and nitroblue tetrazolium reduction are unimpaired; and 8) that cytologic viability is maintained as manifest by failure of lactate dehydrogenase to appear in supernatants of these cells or by dye exclusion studies (24-27).

In such cytochalasin B-treated cells (in which pharmacologic agents can now exert no effects upon any of the stages other than a) attachment or b) fusion of lysosomes with the plasma membrane, it becomes possible to study the effect of added cyclic nucleotides. When guinea pig peritoneal polymorphonuclear leukocytes are studied in this fashion it is again observed that cyclic GMP enhances the release of lysosomal enzymes, whereas cyclic AMP and theophylline inhibit the release of lysosomal enzymes from polymorphonuclear leukocytes provided they have been stimulated by zymosan in the presence of fresh guinea pig serum. This effect, as in human cells, seems to be associated with the assembly of cytoplasmic microtubules, and is sensitive to colchicine.

Nevertheless, the effects of particles such as zymosan (in the presence of fresh serum) upon enzyme release from polymorphonuclear leukocytes could still be influenced by the attachment to the surface of the phagocyte by the particle to be ingested. This step was the last remaining variable to be excluded before it was possible to be certain that the agents we were adding affected the critical step of fusion of granules with the phagocytic vacuole or the plasma membrane. It was therefore important to identify, if possible, humoral mediators of enzyme release in order to eliminate the possibility of drug effects upon the early step of particle/membrane attachment and contact. We have previously shown that the interaction of zymosan with fresh serum causes the generation of a lysosomal enzyme releasing factor (LRF) which was shown to be identical with the complement component C5a (25, 26). Purified human C5a has therefore been used as a stimulus for lysosomal enzyme release in order to determine whether a simple humoral mediator can cause lysosomal enzyme release, microtubule assembly, and whether these processes are again responsive, in reciprocal fashion, to the Yin/Yang control of the cyclic nucleotides: cyclic GMP and cyclic AMP. C5a causes selective lysosomal enzyme release from cytochalasin B-treated human or guinea-pig leukocytes, the transient assembly of cytoplasmic microtubules, and other metabolic consequences of phagocytosis such as C-1 oxidation, superoxide production, and reduction of nitroblue tetrazolium. This small protein (M.W. approx. 17,000) can therefore be considered hormone-like, in that its exhibition is followed by secretion of stored material from a secretory cell (25).

Each of the foregoing experiments have made it clear that constituents of lysosomes *can*, at least *in vitro*, be discharged from living phagocytes.

Introduction Of Ig-Coated Liposomes Into Phagocytes In Vivo

During the summer of 1975 at the Marine Biological Laboratory, we have been able to take advantage of such experiments to re-equip the phagocytes of *Mustelus canis* with peroxidase *in vivo*. We have injected Ig-coated liposomes containing horseradish peroxidase into the peritoneal cavity of *Mustelus canis*. As early as 30 min after injection, circulating phagocytes acquired lysosomally located peroxidase (in liposomes). These cells had obviously been chemotactically attracted to the Ig-coated liposomes in the peritoneal exudate, re-entered the circulation, and were now ready to migrate to organs and tissues of the deficient host. High levels of peroxidase were still found in phagocytes at 10-12 hrs after I-P injection, but *little* or *no* enzyme was present in plasma (such as after I-V injection, or after I-P injection of free enzyme). We then attempted to obtain discharge of the sequestered enzyme. To this end we injected zymosan particles I-V, both to induce "regurgitation during feeding" and to generate C5a anaphylotoxin which would be expected to open up tight junctions in systemic and brain capillaries. Two hours after non-lethal injections of zymosan, we achieved entry of enzyme into brain and massive accumulation of enzyme in spleen, without significant elevations of plasma enzyme levels. These early (and rudimentary) experiments confirm the postulate that means can, indeed, be devised for the delivery of phagocyte-borne, liposome-entrapped, enzymes to organs or tissues.

Comparison With Direct Enzyme Replacement

This subject has been reviewed recently in great detail (28-32), and a useful volume has emerged (33). Since not only Tay-

Sachs disease, but other lysosomal deficiency diseases are caused
by a genetic deficiency of specific acid hydrolases in lysosomes,
reversal of this deficiency has been approached by means of direct
enzyme replacement. Because it is the affected system, the lysosomal apparatus of cells, which normally takes up extracellular
macromolecules such as enzymes by endocytosis (28), attempts have
been made to mobilize the stored GM_2 ganglioside present in Tay-
Sachs diseases by direct administration of purified enzyme. Unfortunately, the injected enzyme disappears rapidly from the circulation, and most of it becomes localized in the liver rather
than at other affected sites such as the central nervous system.
Similar results are obtained when glucocerebrosidase and ceramidetrihexosidase are infused (29-32). The problems associated with
the direct administration of enzyme include 1) the inability of
this method to direct the enzyme to parenchymal tissues containing
the stored material; 2) the potential antigenicity of the enzyme;
3) the presence of competing substrates in the circulation; 4) interaction with components of the circulation such as the complement or kinin system, and finally 5) the inability of free enzyme
to cross the blood brain barrier. These problems prompted Brady
et al (32) to suggest that: *"Enzyme replacement therapy by simple
intravenous infusion of the deficient enzyme seems unlikely to
benefit patients with central nervous system damage. Other procedures must be devised, such as temporarily opening the blood-
brain barrier, chemical modification of the enzyme so that it will
pass from the circulation into the brain, or linking the enzyme
to the patients' own leukocytes, before a beneficial effect can
be expected"*. The last point is the chief reason for the use of
immunoglobulin-coated liposomes.

Attempts have been made to apply ligand-receptor models to
influence the uptake of enzymes by cells or organs (7, 33-35).
In such experiments, the mechanism of endocytosis of lysosomal
enzymes appears to depend on the nature of the oligosaccharide
portion of the molecule, and uptake can be influenced by modification of this part of the glycoprotein (36, 37). N-acetyl-alpha-
glucosaminidase, purified from human urine, is taken up by selective endocytosis (i.e.: receptor-dependent) in San Fillipo B fibroblasts, whereas the same enzyme, purified from human placenta, is
taken up by non-selective (bulk phase) endocytosis (38, 39).
Since differences in electrophoretic mobility and antigenicity between lysosomal enzymes from various human tissues have been
attributed to differences in sialic acid residues (7), previous
studies have suggested the use of a desialylated glycoprotein as
a surface ligand for protein-containing liposomes (7). However,
inconclusive results have been obtained from *in vivo* experiments
which utilized ^{3}H-fetuin and its desialylated derivative to coat

^{125}I-albumin linked covalently to liposomes. (Desialylated fetuin has an affinity for parenchymal cells of liver.) After the animals were sacrificed, 80% of the injected ^{125}I was found to be concentrated in the liver when the fetuin-liposome was injected, whereas 84% was localized to liver after treatment with the desialylated derivative (7). This is the only other experiment reported in which the ligand-receptor model has been used to introduce liposomes into specific target organs.

References

1. Bangham, A.D., Standish, M.M. and Weissmann, G. (1965) J. Mol. Biol. 13:253-259.

2. Sessa, G. and Weissmann, G. (1968) J. Lipid Res. 9:310-318.

3. Sessa, G. and Weissmann, G. (1970) J. Biol. Chem. 245:325-3301.

4. Rahman, Y.E. (1974) Proc.Soc.Exp.Biol. & Med. 145:1173.

5. Colley, C.M. and Ryman, B.E. (1975) Biochem. Soc. Trans. 3:157.

6. Rahman, Y.E., Rosenthal, M.W. and Cerny, E.A. (1973) Science. 180:300.

7. Gregoriadis, G. in "Enzyme Therapy in Lysosomal Storage Diseases" (eds. J.M. Tager, G.J.M. Hoogwinkel and W. Th. Daems) North-Holland Publishing, Amsterdam, p. 131, 1974.

8. Ryman, B.E. in "Enzyme Therapy in Lysosomal Storage Diseases" (eds. J.M. Tager, G.J.M. Hoogwinkel and W. Th. Daems) North-Holland Publishing, Amsterdam, p. 149, 1974.

9. Gregoriadis, G. and Allison, A.C. (1974) FEBS Letters 45:71.

10. Straub, S.X., Garry, R.F. and Magee, W.E. (1974) Infect. Immun. 10:783.

11. McDougall, I.R., Dunnick, J.K., McNamee, M.G. and Kriss, J.P. (1974) Proc. Natl. Acad. Sci. (U.S.) 71:3487.

12. Segal, A.W., Wills, E.J., Richmond, J.E., Slavin, G., Black, C.D.V. and Gregoriadis, G. (1974) Brit. J. Exp. Path. 55:320.

13. Pagano, R.E., Huang, L. and Wey, C. (1974) <u>Nature</u> 242:166-167.

14. Sessa, G. and Weissmann, G. (1969) <u>J. Clin. Invest</u>. 48:77a.

15. Magee, W.E. and Miller, O. (1972) <u>Nature</u> 235:339-341.

16. Papahadjopoulos, D., Poste, G. and Schaeffer, B.E. (1973) <u>Biochim. Biophys. Acta</u> 323:23-42.

17. Henson, P.M., Johnson, H.B. and Spiegelberg, H.L. (1972) <u>J. Immun</u>. 109:1182-1191.

18. Weissmann, G., Brand, A. and Franklin, E.C. (1974) <u>J. Clin. Invest</u>. 53:536-543.

19. Weissmann, G., Bloomgarden, D., Kaplan, R., Cohen, C., Hoffstein, S., Collins, T., Gottlieb, A. and Nagle, D. (1975) <u>Proc. Nat. Acad. Sci</u>. 72:88-92.

20. Lehrer, R.I. and Cline, M.J. (1969) <u>J. Clin. Invest</u>. 48:1487-1496.

21. Cohen, C.M., Weissmann, G., Hoffstein, S., Awasthi, Y.C. and Srivastava, S.K. (submitted to Biochemistry).

22. Zurier, R.B., Hoffstein, S. and Weissmann, G. (1973) <u>J. Cell Biol</u>. 58:27-41.

23. Zurier, R.B., Weissmann, G., Hoffstein, S., Kammerman, S. and Tai, H.-H. (1974) <u>J. Clin. Invest</u>. 53:297-309.

24. Zurier, R.B., Hoffstein, S. and Weissmann, G. (1973) <u>Proc. Nat. Acad. Sci</u>. 70:844-848.

25. Goldstein, I., Hoffstein, S., Gallin, J. and Weissmann, G. (1973) <u>Proc. Nat. Acad. Sci</u>. USA. 70:2916-2920.

26. Dunham, P.G., Goldstein, I.M. and Weissmann, G. (1974) <u>J. Cell Biol</u>. 63:215-226.

27. Goldstein, I.M., Roos, D., Weissmann, G., Kaplan, H. (1975) <u>J. Clin. Invest</u>. (in press).

28. deDuve, C.D., deBarsy, T., Poole, B., Trouet, A., Tulkens, Pa. and vanHoof, F. (1974) <u>Biochem. Pharm</u>. 23:2495.

29. Johnson, W.G., Desnick, R.J., Long, D.M., Sharp, H.L., Krivit, W., Brady, B. and Brady, R.O. (1973) in "Enzyme Therapy in Genetic Disease" (Bergsma, D. ed.) Vol. 9, William and Wilkins Co., Baltimore, p. 120-124.

30. Brady, R., Pentchev, P., Gal, A., Hibbert, S. and Dekaban, A. (1974) N. Engl. J. Med. 291:989-993.

31. Brady, R.O., Tallman, J.F. and Johnson, W.G. (1973) N. Engl. J. Med. 289:9-14.

32. Brady, R.O., Pentchev, P.G. and Gal, A.E. (1975) Fed. Proc. 34:1310.

33. Weissmann, U.N. (1974) in "Enzyme Therapy in Lysosomal Storage Diseases" (J.M. Tager, G. Hoogwinkel and W. Th. Daems, eds.) North-Holland Co. Amsterdam, p. 85.

34. Weissmann, U.N., Rossi, E. and Herschkowitz, N. (1971) N. Engl. J. Med. 284:672.

35. Porter, M.T., Fluharty, A.L. and Kihara, H. (1971) Science 172:1263.

36. Morell, A.G., Irvine, R.A., Sternlieb, I., Scheinberg, I. and Ashwell, G. (1968) J. Biol. Chem. 243:155-159.

37. Hickman, S., Shapiro, L.J. and Neufeld, E. (1974) Biochem. Biophys. Res. Comm. 57:55-61.

38. VonFigura, K. and Kresse, H. (1974) J. Clin. Invest. 53: 85-90.

39. O'Brien, J.S., Miller, A.L., Loverde, A.W. and Veath, M.L. (1973) Science 181:753-755.

Acknowledgments

     Aided by grants from the National Institutes of Health (AM-11949 and HL-15140), The National Foundation and The Whitehall Foundation.

ENZYME REPLACEMENT THERAPY FOR THE SPHINGOLIPIDOSES

R. O. Brady, P. G. Pentchev, A. E. Gal, S. R. Hibbert,

J. M. Quirk, G. E. Mook, J. W. Kusiak, J. F. Tallman

and A. S. Dekaban

Developmental and Metabolic Neurology Branch, NINCDS
National Institutes of Health, Bethesda, Md. 20014

The greatest progress in the field of inheritable disorders during the past decade was made in the understanding and control of lipid storage diseases. Since original demonstrations in 1965 and 1966 of the metabolic defects in Gaucher's disease (6,7) Niemann-Pick disease (8), Fabry's disease (9), and metachromatic leukodystrophy (17), specific enzyme deficiencies were demonstrated in ten heritable disorders of lipid metabolism. These discoveries paved the way for the development of facile procedures for the diagnosis of homozygotes, the detection of heterozygous carriers, and the monitoring of pregnancies at risk for any of these diseases (1-4). These applications of basic research endeavors have provided much relief from human anguish and suffering and they are in wide use at this time. However, there still remains much to be done for affected patients and compassionate physicians continue to seek further help in the treatment of hundreds of patients with these diseases. In particular, the therapy of patients with Type I (adult) Gaucher's disease in whom skeletal involvement causes severe bone and joint pains, and patients with Fabry's disease with intractable pains in arms and legs and progressive renal impairment deserves intensive attention. During the past three years much of our research efforts have been devoted to these two disorders. The results have been generally encouraging and we present here the pertinent observations.

ENZYME REPLACEMENT IN TAY-SACHS DISEASE

Our initial investigation in enzyme replacement was an
examination of the effect of the intravenous injection of purified hexosaminidase A in a patient with the "O" variant (Sandhoff-
Jatzkewitz) form of Tay-Sachs disease. This study was carried out
in collaboration with investigators at the University of Minnesota
Medical School (16). Hexosaminidase A was purified from human
urine by a procedure later employed to obtain the enzyme from
human placental tissue (15). Injections of 70 µg of hexosaminidase
A were given on two successive days. The level of hexosaminidase
activity in the blood rose from 35 nanomoles per ml per hour to
940 nmoles/ml/hr immediately following infusion of the enzyme.
The latter value is well within the normal range for this enzyme
(1). Hexosaminidase was rapidly cleared from the circulation with
a half-life of about 7.5 minutes. Much of the injected enzyme
appeared to have been taken up by the liver. There was no increase
in hexosaminidase activity in the brain, spinal fluid, or urine.
The exogenous enzyme appeared to have catalyzed the catabolism
of globoside since there was a 40% reduction in the level of this
glycolipid in the blood four hours after the administration of
hexosaminidase A. Note that this fall in globoside was detected
long after the hexosaminidase had been cleared from the circulation
suggesting that the enzyme may have acted extracirculatorily.

One bit of information obtained in the course of these initial
investigations was quite unexpected. When the amount of hexosaminidase A activity in the liver was compared in a preinfusion biopsy
specimen with that in a sample of liver tissue obtained 45 minutes
after the enzyme was injected, it was found that there was an
increase of approximately 2.4×10^6 units of hexosaminidase
activity over the preinfusion level. The actual quantity of
hexosaminidase A injected was only 980×10^3 units. Thus, it
appears as if there was 2.4 times more hexosaminidase activity
in the liver than was actually infused into the patient (12). The
significance of this observation was not fully appreciated until a
similar augmentation of endogenous enzyme activity was observed in
replacement trials in Fabry's disease.

Since the exogenous hexosaminidase A did not appear to cross
the blood-brain barrier and there was no demonstrable improvement
in the clinical status of the patient, it seems reasonable to
conclude that simple replacement of hexosaminidase by intravenous
injection of enzyme is unlikely to benefit patients with Tay-Sachs
disease. Much additonal work needs to be done. First, it will
be necessary to determine whether the blood-brain barrier could be
opened temporarily without harm, then to establish if the enzyme
is taken up by the nerve cells, and once there, if it will catalyze
the metabolism of the accumulating ganglioside.

ENZYME REPLACEMENT IN FABRY'S DISEASE

Despite the lace of a clinically beneficial effect of enzyme replacement in Tay-Sachs disease, we felt that investigations should be undertaken in patients with disorders such as Fabry's disease where the central nervous system does not appear to be involved although there is extensive accumulation of lipid in parenchymal organs, autonomic ganglia, and other tissues. Accordingly, a procedure was devised for the isolation of ceramidetrihexosidase, the enzyme lacking in patients with Fabry's disease (9), from human placental tissue (14). We have infused this enzyme intravenously into three patients with Fabry's disease. In each case there was no adverse reaction to the exogenous protein. Unfortunately, the plasma samples from one of the patients were inadvertently contaminated with extraneous materials leached from organic polymeric columns used for the elution of ceramidetrihexoside from thin-layer chromatograms. These samples could not be further analyzed. In the two cases analyzed, there was a decrease in the elevated level of ceramidetrihexoside in the plasma of the recipients (Table I). The clearance of ceramidetrihexoside from the plasma appeared to be proportional to the amount of enzyme administered. Since the accumulating ceramidetrihexoside appears to arise for the most part from globoside in the stroma of senescent erythrocytes, the transport of this lipid by the blood from sites of erythrocytorrhexis such as the spleen and liver to affected tissues such as the kidneys, peripheral ganglia and blood vessels appears to play an important role in the pathogenesis of Fabry's disease.

TABLE I

EFFECT OF INTRAVENOUS INJECTION OF PURIFIED CERAMIDETRIHEXOSIDASE ON

CERAMIDETRIHEXOSIDE IN THE PLASMA OF PATIENTS WITH FABRY'S DISEASE*

Case	Enzyme Injected	Ceramidetrihexoside		Δ
		Prior to Infusion	1 hour after Infusion	
	mg	nanomoles per ml of plasma		%
1	5.0	5.3	2.2	-58
2	3.0	6.7	4.5	-33

*Summary of data from Reference 10.

Therefore, it may be anticipated that the reduction of circulating ceramidetrihexoside brought about by the administration of ceramide-trihexosidase will have a salutary effect on the course of the disease. Studies are currently underway to evaluate this tenet.

Several other important findings were disclosed in the course of these investigations. It appears likely that the injected ceramidetrihexosidase exerted its catalytic effect after it was taken up by tissues such as the liver. This supposition is derived from an inspection of the kinetics of the disappearance of the enzyme from the circulation, which as in the Tay-Sachs patient, was very rapid, and the fall in plasma ceramidetrihexoside that occurred after the enzyme had been cleared. Secondly, the infused placental ceramidetrihexosidase is catalytically active at acid pH's, and it is virtually inactive at the pH of blood. Third, there was no evidence of an increase in circulating ceramidelacto-side, the immediate product of the reaction, at a time when cera-midetrihexoside had fallen to the normal range.

An additional potentially significant observation was the finding that the exogenous placental ceramidetrihexosidase may have caused an activation of the endogenous catalytically inactive α-galactosidase in the liver of one of the recipients from whom we obtained liver biopsy specimens prior to and one hour after infusion of ceramidetrihexosidase. It was calculated that 3.9 times more enzymatic activity was present in this organ than was actually injected (10,12). Because the difference in tissue α-galactosi-dase activity was small, caution must be exercised in the inter-pretation of these observations. However, this finding is consis-tent with the earlier observation of apparent activation of endo-genous hexosaminidase A activity in the patient with Tay-Sachs disease. If this augmentation of catalytic activity can be sub-stantiated, it will provide considerable encouragement for enzyme replacement in hereditary metabolic disorders.

Another significant observation was made with regard to the possibility of sensitizing recipients of exogenous enzymes to the injected proteins. It seems to us unlikely that this will happen with placental enzymes for a number of reasons which are summarized elsewhere (5,12). Furthermore, we have recently carried out skin tests on the first recipient of ceramidetrihexosidase and found no indication whatsoever that he had developed a sensitivity to the placental enzyme. This finding provides considerable encouragement to pursue the treatment of patients with lipid storage diseases through replacement of the missing enzymes.

ENZYME REPLACEMENT IN GAUCHER'S DISEASE

Emboldened by the findings in Fabry's disease, we undertook an investigation of the effect of infusion of glucocerebrosidase in patients with Gaucher's disease who have subnormal levels of this enzyme in their organs and tissues. A procedure was developed for the isolation of glucocerebrosidase in apparently homogenous form from human placenta (18). When this enzyme was infused into three patients with Gaucher's disease, there was a decrease in the quantity of glucocerebroside in the liver of each recipient (Table II). In addition, the elevated level of glucocerebroside associated with circulating erythrocytes fell to the normal level within a period of 72 hours following infusion in two of the three recipients. This effect persisted over a comparatively long period of time (Fig. 1). In the first patient who received glucocerebrosidase, the amount of red cell glucocerebroside was still 41% below the pre-infusion level one year after administration of the enzyme. In the second patient, erythrocyte glucocerebroside was 20% lower than the pre-infusion level 16 months after injection of the enzyme. We did not observe a decrease of red cell glucocerebroside in the third recipient. We believe the lack of change in this patient was due to the extremely high level of glucocerebroside in the liver where we saw only an 8% diminution after administration of enzyme. Glucocerebroside in the circulation appears to be a function of the amount of exchangeable glucocerebroside in tissues such as the liver (13).

TABLE II

EFFECT OF INTRAVENOUS INJECTION OF PURIFIED
GLUCOCEREBROSIDASE ON GLUCOCEREBROSIDE IN THE
LIVER OF PATIENTS WITH GAUCHER'S DISEASE

Case No.	Total Enzymatic Activity Infused	Glucocerebroside			
		Before Infusion	24 Hours After Infusion	Change	
	nanomoles/hr.	micrograms/gram of liver		Δ	%
1*	1.5×10^6	702	519	183	-26
2*	3.3×10^6	1630	1210	420	-26
3	9.3×10^6	17900	16500	1400	- 8

*Summary of data from Reference 11.

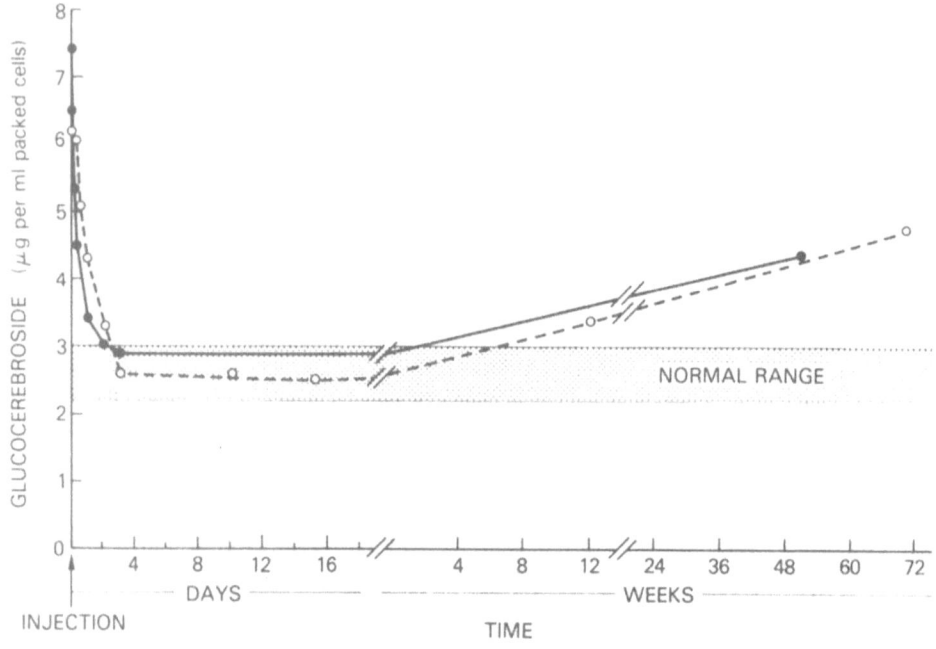

Fig. 1. Level of glucocerebroside in erythrocytes in two patients with Gaucher's disease who were infused with purified placental glucocerebrosidase.

Several other observations made in the course of these investigations deserve comment. 1. None of the patients had any fever or
other untoward reaction to the injected enzyme. 2. The amount
of glucocerebroside cleared from the liver of the recipients has
been calculated to be equivalent to the quantity of lipid that
accumulated over a considerable period of time (Table III). 3. Although the percentage of glucocerebroside calculated to have been
cleared from the liver of the third patient was considerably less
than that in the first and second recipients, it should be pointed
out that this patient had an extremely high level of hepatic glucocerebroside before infusion of the enzyme. In fact, the value of
17.9 mg of glucocerebroside per gram of liver is the highest value
yet recorded. This patient had a severe case of infectious hepa-
titis two years prior to infusion. It is not known whether this
antecedent illness contributed to the accumulation of this unusually
large amount of hepatic glucocerebroside. The clinical manifestations of Gaucher's disease in this patient were consistent with

TABLE III

ESTIMATION OF THE DURATION OF THE PHYSIOLOGICAL EFFECT OF
EXOGENOUS GLUCOCEREBROSIDASE ON LIVER GLUCOCEREBROSIDE

Case No.	Age of Patient	Enzyme Infused	Glucocerebroside cleared from the liver	Period of time over which lipid accumulated
	years	units x 10^{-6}	mg†	years
1*	15	1.5	396	4.0
2*	51	3.3	924	13.
3	22	9.3	3080	1.7

*Summary of data from Reference 19.

†Based on an estimated liver weight of 2200 grams.

a partial deficit of glucocerebrosidase which was 22 percent of
normal in her leukocytes. Liver function tests were normal at the
time of infusion. Nevertheless, even in this case, the amount of
glucocerebroside cleared from the liver seems to have been proportional to the amount of enzyme infused. The data obtained from
the three recipients are remarkably consistent in this regard
(Table IV). 4. The level of acid phosphatase activity was
measured in serum samples obtained from the third recipient. Prior
to infusion, the activity of this enzyme was 7.3 units. By one
month following infusion, it had fallen to 5.9 units. The normal
range is from 0.01 to 0.56 units. Although it is clearly impossible
to state from these few determinations that such an observation
carries any significance, if this finding can be confirmed, it may
indicate a potentially beneficial effect of enzyme replacement on
the bone lesions in these patients.

CONCLUDING REMARKS

We have now entered the era of enzyme replacement therapy.
This treatment appears to hold considerable promise for patients
with Fabry's disease and Gaucher's disease. Many additional
important aspects of enzyme replacement must now be intensively
examined. For example, we need to know what effect exogenous
ceramidetrihexocidase has on the frequent episodes of pain
in the extremities and whether it will reverse or prevent
further renal damage in Fabry patients. In addition, we

TABLE IV

ESTIMATION OF PROPORTIONALITY OF GLUCOCEREBROSIDASE
EFFECTIVENESS IN VIVO

Case No.	Amount of enzyme injected	Glucocerebroside cleared from the liver	
	units x 10^{-6*}	nmoles x $10^{-6\dagger}$	nmole/unit of enzyme
1	1.5	0.52	0.35
2	3.3	1.2	0.36
3	9.3	4.0	0.43

* Nanomoles of glucocerebroside hydrolyzed per hour.

† Based on an estimated liver weight of 2200 grams and an
  average molecular weight of 770 for glucocerebroside (20).

must determine whether the administration of glucocerebrosidase
will ameliorate the pain and skeletal system damage in patients
with Gaucher's disease. These long term investigations are
just beginning. Finally, we must undertake the development of
effective procedures to supply the missing enzymes to the central
nervous system in a form that can be utilized by neuronal cells
so that patients with brain damage may be benefited by enzyme
replacement.

REFERENCES

1. Brady, R. O. Enzyme defects in the sphingolipidoses and their
    application to diagnosis. Ann. Clin. Lab. Sci. 2, 285 (1972).

2. Brady, R. O. The chemistry and control of hereditary lipid
    diseases. Chem. Phys. Lipids 13, 271 (1974).

3. Brady, R. O. The lipid storage diseases: new concepts and
    control. Ann. Int. Med. 82, 257 (1975).

4. Brady, R. O. Sphingolipidoses and other metabolic disorders.
    In Basic Neurochemistry, 2nd Edition, Siegel, G. J., Albers,
    R. W., Katzman, R., and Agranoff, B. W. (Eds). Boston, Little,
    Brown and Co., 1976, in press.

5. Brady, R. O. Glucosyl ceramide lipidoses: Gaucher's disease.
    In The Metabolic Basis of Inherited Disease, Stanbury, J. B.,
    Wyngaarden, J. B., and Fredrickson, D. S., (Eds). New York,
    McGraw-Hill, Fourth Edition, in press, 1976.

6. Brady, R. O., Kanfer, J. N., and Shapiro, D. The metabolism
    of glucocerebrosides. II. Evidence of an enzymatic deficiency
    in Gaucher's disease. Biochem. Biophys. Res. Commun. 18, 221
    (1965).

7. Brady, R. O., Kanfer, J. N., Bradley, R. M., and Shapiro, D.
    Demonstration of a deficiency of glucocerebroside-cleaving
    enzyme in Gaucher's disease. J. Clin. Invest. 45, 1112 (1966).

8. Brady, R. O., Kanfer, J. N., Mock, M. B., and Fredrickson, D. S.
    The metabolism of sphingomyelin. II. Evidence of an enzymatic
    deficiency in Niemann-Pick disease. Proc. Natl. Acad. Sci.
    USA 55, 366 (1966).

9. Brady, R. O., Gal, A. E., Bradley, R. M., Martensson, E.,
    Warshaw, A. L., and Laster, L. Enzymatic defect in Fabry's
    disease: ceramidetrihexosidase deficiency. New Engl. J. Med.
    276, 1163 (1967).

10. Brady, R. O., Tallman, J. F., Johnson, W. G., Gal, A. E.,
    Leahy, W. R., Quirk, M. M., and Dekaban, A. S. Replacement
    therapy for inherited enzyme deficiency: use of purified
    ceramidetrihexosidase in Fabry's disease. New Engl. J. Med.
    289, 9 (1973).

11. Brady, R. O., Pentchev, P. G., Gal, A. E., Hibbert, S. R.,
    and Dekaban, A. S. Replacement therapy for inherited enzyme
    deficiency: use of purified glucocerebrosidase in Gaucher's
    disease. New Engl. J. Med.291, 989 (1974).

12. Brady, R. O., Pentchev, P. G., and Gal, A. E. Investigations in
    enzyme replacement therapy in lipid storage diseases. Fed.
    Proc. 34, 1310 (1975).

13. Dawson, G., and Sweeley, C. C. In vivo studies on glyco-
    sphingolipid metabolism in procine blood. J. Biol. Chem. 245
    410 (1970).

14. Johnson, W. G., and Brady, R. O. Ceramide trihexosidase from
    human placenta. Methods Enzymol. XXVIII, 849 (1972).

15. Johnson, W. G., Mook, G., and Brady, R. O. β-Hexosaminidase A
    from human placenta. Methods Enzymol. XXVIII, 857 (1972).

16. Johnson, W. G., Desnick, R. J., Long, D. M., Sharp, H. L., Krivit, W., Brady, B., and Brady, R. O. Intravenous injection of purified hexosaminidase A into a patient with Tay-Sachs disease. Birth Defects Orig. Art. Series IX, 120 (1973).

17. Mehl, E., and Jatzkewitz, H. Evidence for a genetic block in metachromatic leukodystrophy (ML). Biochem. Biophys. Res. Commun. 19, 407 (1965).

18. Pentchev, P. G., Brady, R. O., Hibbert, S. R., Gal, A. E., and Shapiro, D. Isolation and characterization of glucocere-brosidase from human placenta. J. Biol. Chem. 248, 5256 (1973).

19. Pentchev, P. G., Brady, R. O., Gal, A. E., and Hibbert, S. R. Replacement therapy for inherited enzyme deficiency. Sustained clearance of accumulated glucocerebroside in Gaucher's disease following infusion of purified glucocere-brosidase. J. Mol. Med. 1, 73 (1975).

20. Suomi, W. D. and Agranoff, B. W. Lipids of the spleen in Gaucher's disease. J. Lipid Res. 6, 211 (1965).

HIGH-PERFORMANCE LIQUID CHROMATOGRAPHIC ANALYSIS

OF GLYCOSPHINGOLIPIDS AND PHOSPHOLIPIDS

Robert H. McCluer and Firoze B. Jungalwala

Department of Biochemistry
Eunice Kennedy Shriver Center at
Walter E. Fernald State School
Waltham, Mass. 02154

INTRODUCTION

The modern form of liquid chromatography commonly referred to as high-speed or high-performance liquid chromatography (HPLC) has developed very rapidly in the past few years. HPLC implies the use of reusable columns, injection port sample application, the use of pumps for uniform solvent flow at high-pressure if necessary and automatic sample detection. Since 1969-1970 a better understanding of the factors which improve the speed and resolution in liquid chromatography has evolved. New column packing materials, column packing techniques, high pressure - low volume equipment and highly sensitive detectors have been developed. A large variety of such columns and equipment are now available commercially. The modern HPLC techniques have led to the development of sensitive, quantitative methods, analogous to that available for volatile materials by gas-chromatography, for a very large variety of relatively high molecular weight substances of biological interest.

The application of these HPLC techniques for the analysis of lipids and particularly of those of biochemical interest has lagged behind probably because most HPLC equipment was originally designed for pharmaceuticals and synthetic organic compounds. The major problems concern the facts that no totally satisfactory detectors for lipids have been available, that gradient elution analysis is generally desired, and groups or class separations have been predominant in the past whereas in most applications of HPLC individual substance separation and detection has been the goal.

We have been involved in an effort to exploit the techniques
and tools of modern HPLC for the analysis of compounds of interest
to the neurochemist and neurologist, particularly glycosphingolipids and phospholipids. Our initial approach involved the
preparation of derivatives which could exploit the highly sensitive
and stable minimum volume flow-through ultraviolet detectors that
were available. Perbenzoyl derivatives of glycosphingolipids have
been prepared and utilized for quantitative HPLC. Biphenylcarbonyl
derivatives of amino phospholipids have been prepared and similarly
used. 3-ketosphingolipids have also been prepared and utilized
for HPLC analysis. Sphingosine and other amine lipids chromatographed as their fluorsecamine derivatives with fluorescence
flow-through detection was shown to provide extreme sensitivity.
More recently we have exploited the fact that a large variety of
functional groups absorb ultraviolet light in the region of 200 nm
so that many compounds of interest can be chromatographed and
detected without derivatization. In the following pages these
methods will be reviewed with emphasis on some of the recent work
on the analysis of gangliosides and use of direct detection for
HPLC of phospholipids.

HPLC ANALYSIS OF GLYCOSPHINGOLIPIDS AS THEIR PERBENZOYL DERIVATIVES

A. Structure of Perbenzoyl Derivatives

The analysis of glycosphingolipids by HPLC becomes practical
if derivatives are prepared that allow the use of a sensitive UV
detector. For this reason, we have studied the reaction conditions
for the benzoylation of cerebrosides (1). The benzoylation of
cerebrosides, which contain non-hydroxy fatty acids (NFA),with
benzoylchloride in pyridine (60°C for 1 hr) results in amide
acylation in addition to normal O-acylation. Cerebrosides,which
contain α-hydroxy fatty acids (HFA), form only O-acyl derivatives
under these conditions. Cerebrosides and other sphingolipids
which contain non-hydroxy fatty acids cannot be recovered completely
after benzoylation because alkaline hydrolysis of the perbenzoyl
derivatives results in the formation of N-benzoyl compounds as
well as the parent N-acyl sphingolipid. Benzoylation of cerebrosides
with benzoic anhydride in pyridine forms only O-acyl derivatives
and the parent cerebrosides can be recovered after alkaline
methanolysis; however, the reaction is sluggish (110°C for 18 hrs.)
and sulfatides are completely converted to benzoylated cerebrosides
during the anhydride reaction. Furthermore, in our hands the
complete benzoylation of more complex glycosphingolipids is difficult
with benzoic anhydride even in the presence of triethylamine and/or
other bases and catalysts. Therefore, we have chosen the chloride
benzoylation for analytical purposes because the reaction times

are shorter, sulfatides do not desulfate under conditions required
for cerebroside derivatization and the more complex glycolipids
can be fully benzoylated. Ceramides, however, have been
conveniently derivatized with benzoic anhydride to yield products
that have proved highly useful for the HPLC analysis of normal
and Farber's disease tissues (2).

B. Analysis of Cerebrosides

An isocratic (single solvent elution) HPLC method for the
quantitative analysis of brain cerebrosides has been devised (3).
Samples containing 10 to 150 nmoles of monohexosylceramides are
benzoylated with benzoyl chloride in pyridine and the products are
purified by solvent distribution and analyzed by HPLC. The
benzoylated cerebrosides with nonhydroxy fatty acids are separated
from those with hydroxy fatty acids on a Zipax column with 7%
ethylacetate in hexane as a solvent and UV absorption at 280 nm
is recorded. This isocratic procedure can be applied directly to
chloroform-methanol extracts of adult brain, as well as to more
purified samples. Sulfatides do not interfere in the assay and
can be measured as cerebrosides after desulfation. This isocratic
procedure has the advantages of short analysis time, good sensitivity,
nondestructive measurement and requires a relatively inexpensive
monitor which operates at 280 nm. The isocratic elution can also
be conducted with a pneumatic pump because the Zipax column employed
can be operated at relatively low pressures with adequate flow
rates. Although total lipid extracts of adult brain can be analyzed
directly for cerebrosides without interference from other lipids,
tissue or tissue fractions which contain lower concentrations of
cerebrosides require the use of larger aliquots of total lipids
and inadequate chromatographic separations are obtained.

We have therefore, investigated the use of gradient elution
procedures for the analysis of samples which contain smaller amounts
of cerebrosides and the use of detection at 230 nm, the λmax of
the benzoyl derivatives, in order to provide increased sensitivity
(4). A microbenzoylation procedure was devised in which 0.4 to
10 nmoles of cerebrosides are benzoylated in "reactivials" with
50 μl of 10% benzoyl chloride in pyridine. The samples are heated
at 60°C for 1 hr and products are extracted into hexane. The
hexane phases are washed four times with alkaline 80% methanol
and products dissolved in a small volume of CCl_4 and suitable
portions are injected onto a Zipax column. Elution is with a
3 minute linear gradient of 3.8 to 5.5% dioxane in hexane generated
with a Water's Model 660 gradient programmer and pumps. The
solvents are pumped at a rate of 4 ml/min and detection is at 230 nm
with a Schoeffel Model SF 770 Spectroflow monitor. After completion
of an analysis the column is regenerated to its initial polarity

by reversing the gradient and pumping with the initial solvent
for 1 min so that the system is ready for the next injection in
3-4 minutes. Fig. 1. shows the cerebroside analysis of adult
rat and calf brain lipid extracts. The detector response is the
same for NFA and HFA cerebroside derivatives and as little as 10
picomoles of injected cerebroside can be quantitated. The procedure
gives a linear response in the range of 0.5 to 10 nmoles of reacted

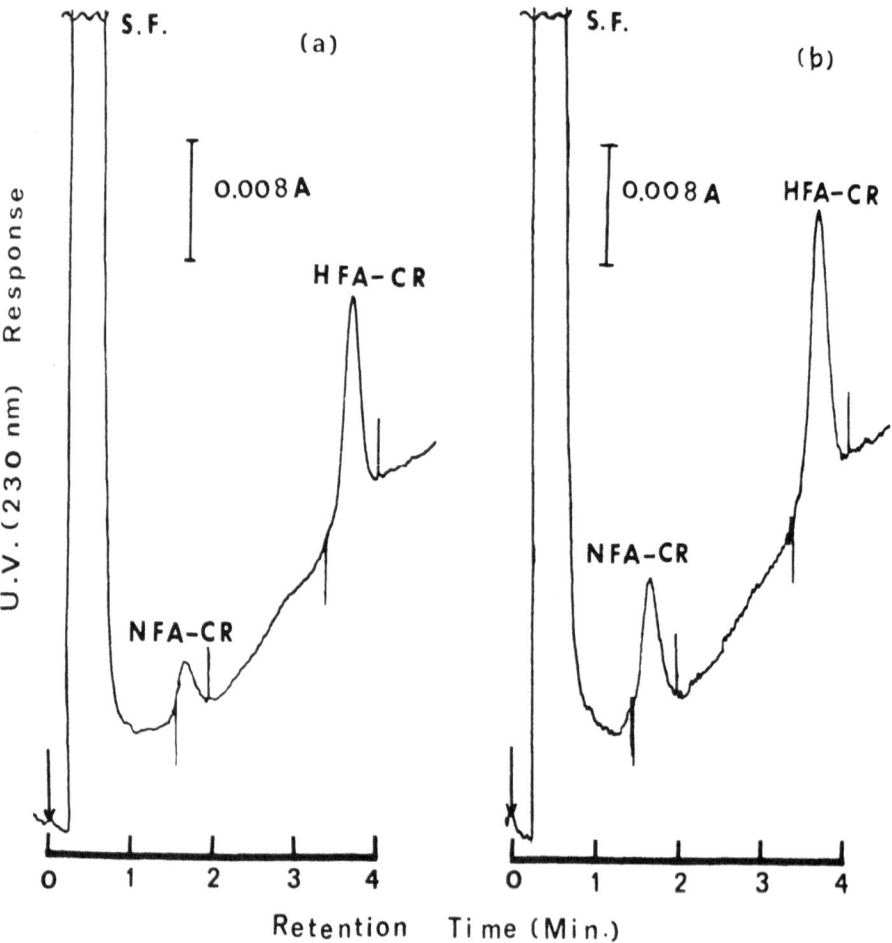

Fig. 1. Gradient-elution high-performance liquid chromatography
of the benzoylated cerebrosides in (a) adult rat brain lipid
extract (2 ug, dry wt) and (b) calf brain lipid extract (6 μg,
dry wt) on a Zipax column with detection at 230 nm. A 3 min
linear gradient of 2.8 to 5.% dioxane in hexane pumped at 4 ml
per min was used for elution,   represents point of injection.

cerebrosides as shown in Fig. 2. This procedure has been used to determine the ratio of NFA to HFA cerebrosides from rat brains of different ages. The ratios for 11 and 20 day old and adult brains were found to be 0.94, 0.71 and 0.48 respectively a result which is in general agreement with data obtained by gas chromatographic analysis of the fatty acids(4a).

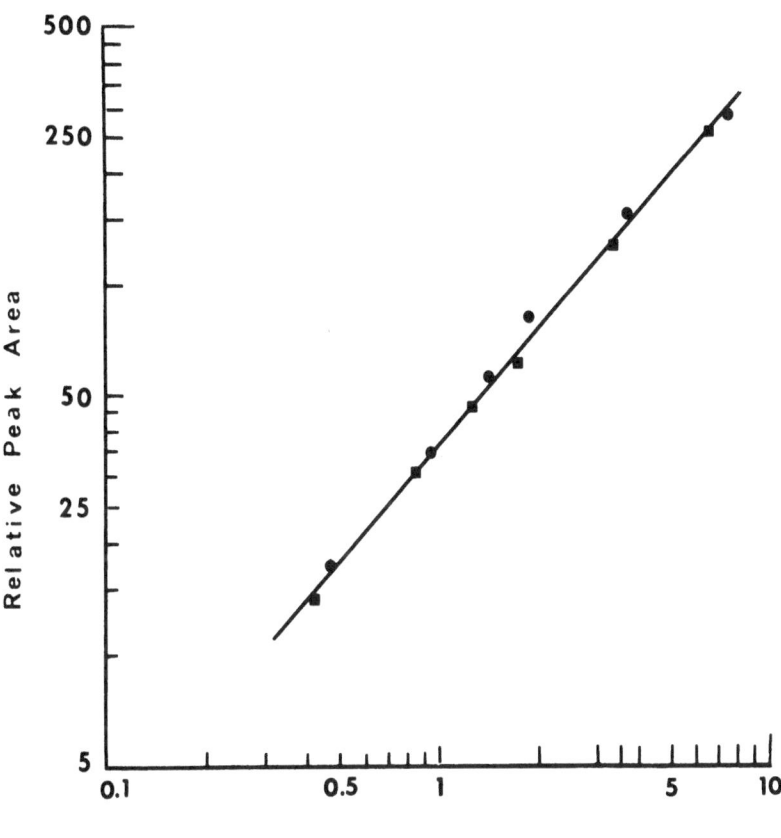

Cerebrosides Reacted, nmoles

Fig. 2. Quantitative analysis of individual benzoylated NFA (•) and HFA (■) cerebrosides by gradient-elution high-performance liquid chromatography. The amounts of individual cerebrosides indicated in the figure were benzoylated and suitable portions of the samples were injected. The response due to entire sample in terms of peak area is shown in the Figure. Gradient-elution was performed with dioxane in hexane and the derivatives were detected at 230 nm, as described in Fig. 1.

C. Analysis of Neutral Glycosphingolipids

Development of a quantitative HPLC method for the analysis of
neutral glycosphingolipids from human serum and erythrocyte
membranes has required the use of different benzoylation conditions
and gradient elution with modern HPLC equipment. Mono, di, tri
and tetraglycosyl ceramide are benzoylated in 20% benzoyl chloride
in pyridine at 90°C for 1 hr. (recent results have indicated that
more satisfactory results are obtained by benzoylation at 60°C for
5 hrs). Excess reagent is removed as described above for cerebrosides and the derivatives are dissolved in CCl$_4$ and appropriate
aliquots injected on a Zipax column. A chromatogram of benzoylated
neutral glycolipid standards obtained under conditions which provide
good quantitation is shown in Fig. 3.

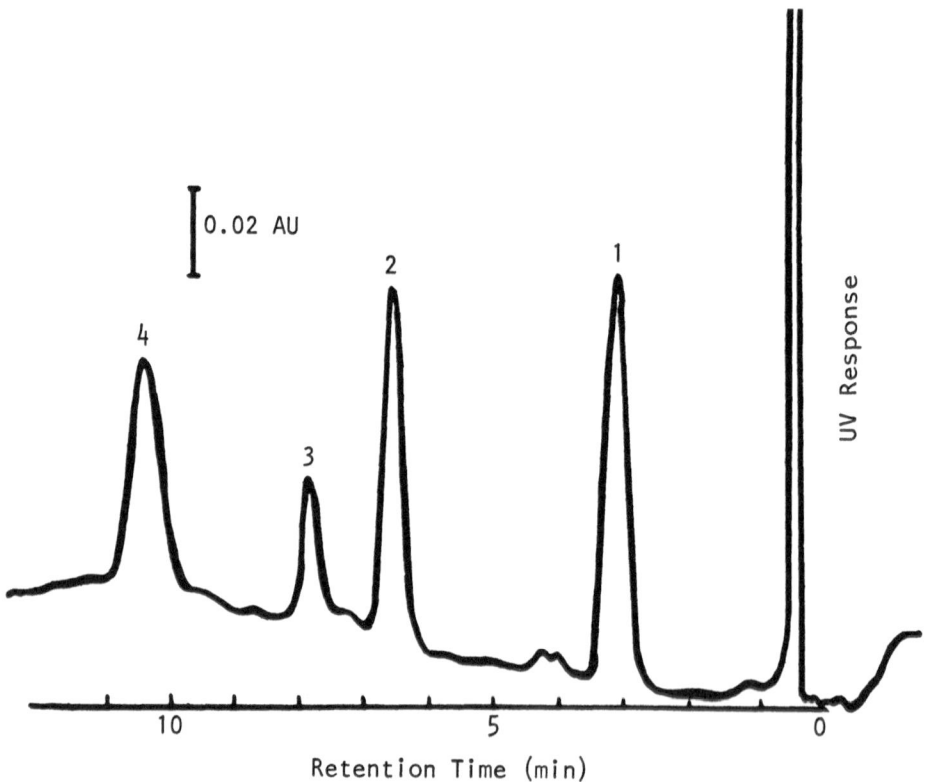

Fig. 3. Quantitative HPLC of benzoylated neutral glycolipids. A
2.1 x 50 cm Zipax column was employed with detection at 280 nm.
A 10 min linear gradient of 2% to 16% ethyl acetate (20% H$_2$O saturated) at a flow rate of 2.0 ml/min was used. Peaks are: 1, glucosyl
ceramide; 2, lactosyl ceramide; 3, galactosyl lactosylceramide and
4, globoside (N-acetylgalactosaminylgalactosyllactosylceramide)

D. Analysis of Gangliosides

Recently we attempted to develop an HPLC method for the analysis of gangliosides as their perbenzoyl derivatives. Although we are in the early stages of this work, this approach appears to be surprisingly successful. Pure ganglioside standards have been reacted with 10% benzoyl chloride in pyridine at 60°C for 5 hrs to yield single products as determined by TLC and HPLC. The chromatographic resolution of the major brain gangliosides was achieved with a Micro-Pak SI-10 (Varian) column and solvent gradient consisting of acetic acid in hexane (see Fig. 4).

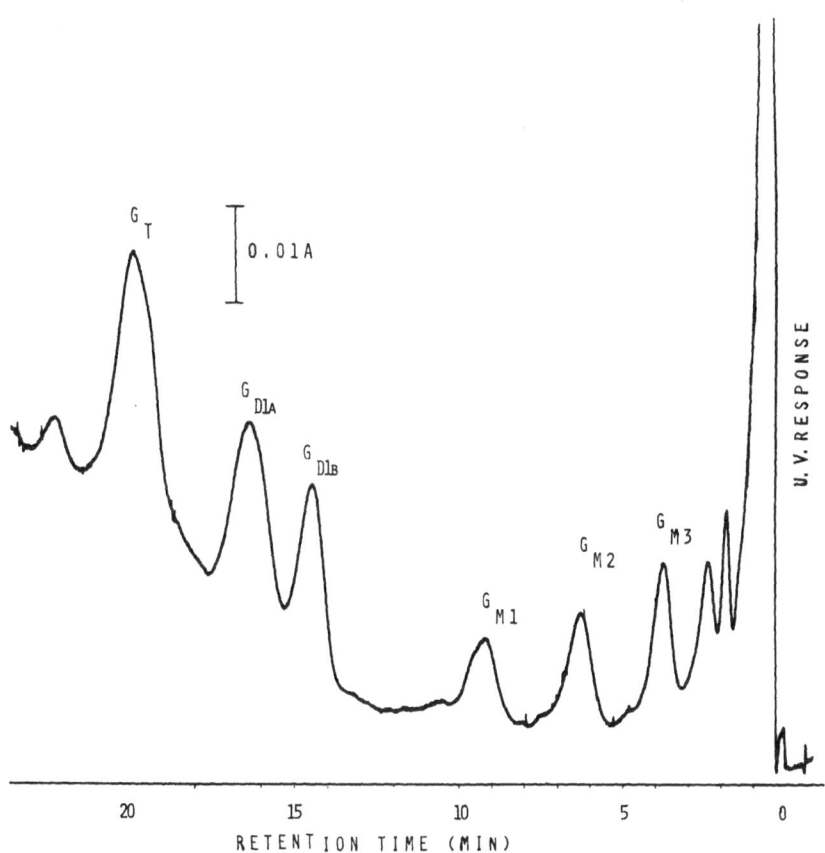

Fig. 4. Gradient-elution HPLC of benzoylated ganglioside standards on a 25 cm x 2.1 mm Micro Pak SI-10 (Varian) column with detection at 262 nm. A 45 min concave (#7 with Water's 660 programmer) gradient of 1% to 30% acetic acid in hexane pumped at 1.5 ml/min was used for elution.

Approximately 20 to 30 μg of each ganglioside was injected.
The positive slope of the baseline results from absorption of the
acetic acid and is the limiting factor in sensitivity at the
present time. Each ganglioside standard injected separately
produced a single peak except G_{M_3} and G_T. We believe the extra
peaks seen with these samples are due to impurities rather than
incompletely benzoylated material. The ganglioside derivatives
did not chromatograph adequately in neutral or basic solvent systems.

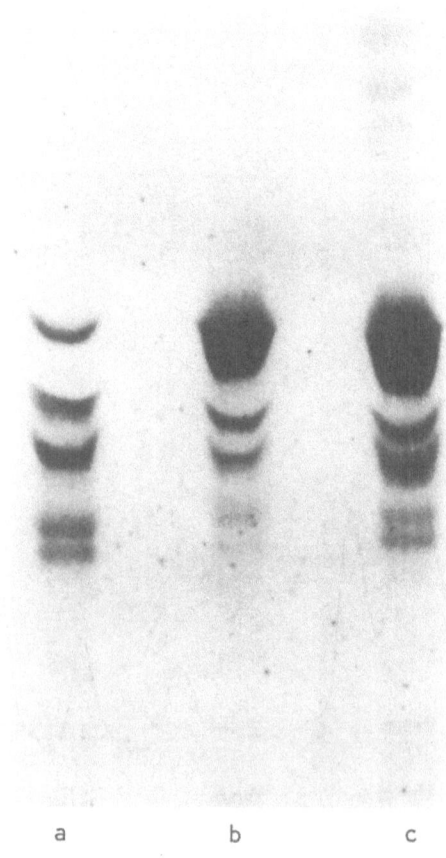

a   b   c

Fig. 5. TLC of ganglioside fractions prepared from the grey matter
of brains of individuals affected with adrenoleucodystrophy (a),
the classical form of G_{M2} gangliosidosis (b), Sandhoff-Jatzkewitz
variant of G_{M2} gangliosidosis (c). The plate was developed with
chloroform-methanol-2.5 N NH_3 (60:35:8) and the spots were visualized with resorcinol reagent.

In order to demonstrate the applicability of this procedure to biological samples, ganglioside fractions obtained from the grey matter of pathological brain tissue were analyzed. The TLC patterns of these samples are shown in Fig. 5.

The HPLC analysis of these ganglioside fractions are shown in Figures 6,7, and 8. Although the quantitative aspects of the ganglioside analysis by HPLC of their benzoates have not been completely examined as yet, we believe that these data show that the HPLC procedure can become a useful and quantitative method for the analysis of tissue gangliosides.

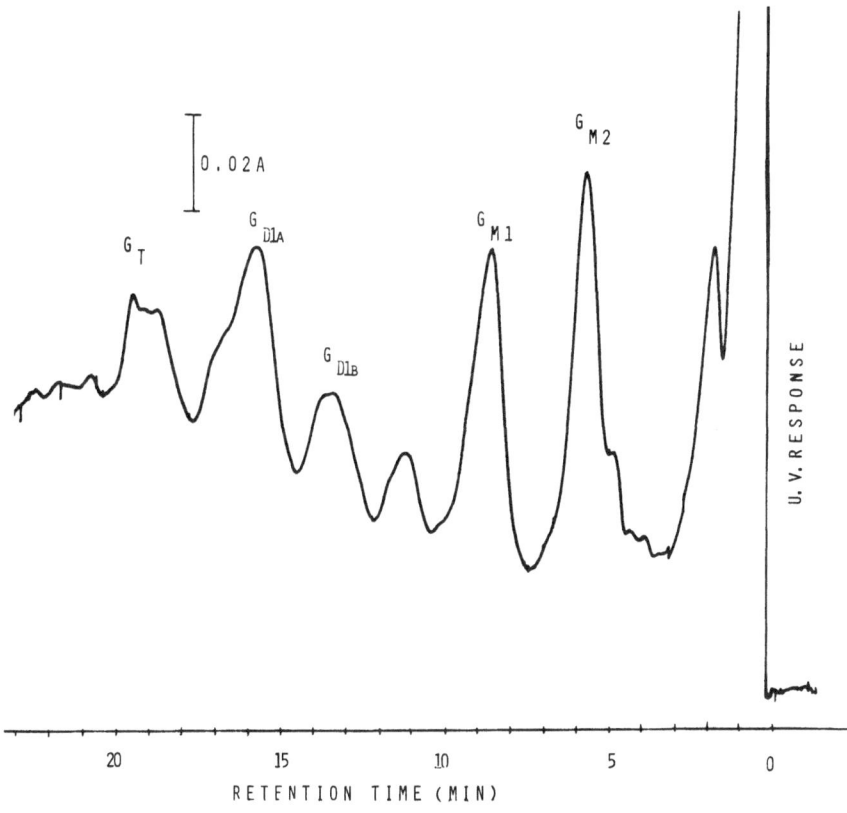

Fig. 6. Gradient elution HPLC of the benzoylated ganglioside fraction from the brain of a case of adrenoleucodystrophy . Chromatographic conditions as described in Fig. 4.

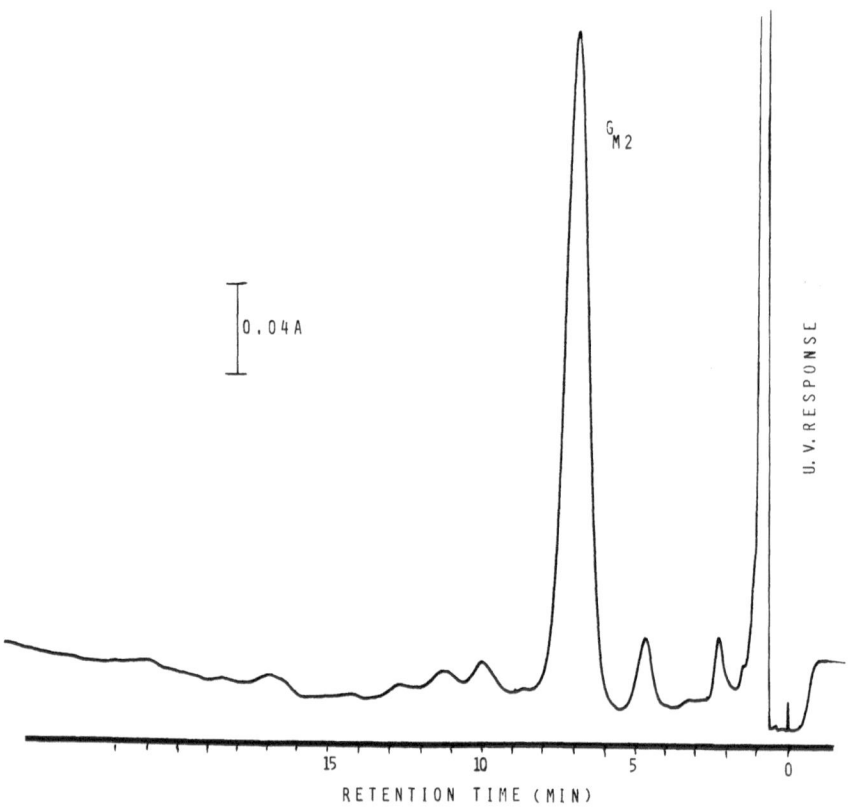

Fig. 7. Gradient elution HPLC of the ganglioside fraction from
the grey matter of the brain of a case of the classical form of
G_{M2} gangliosidosis. Chromatographic conditions as in Fig. 4.

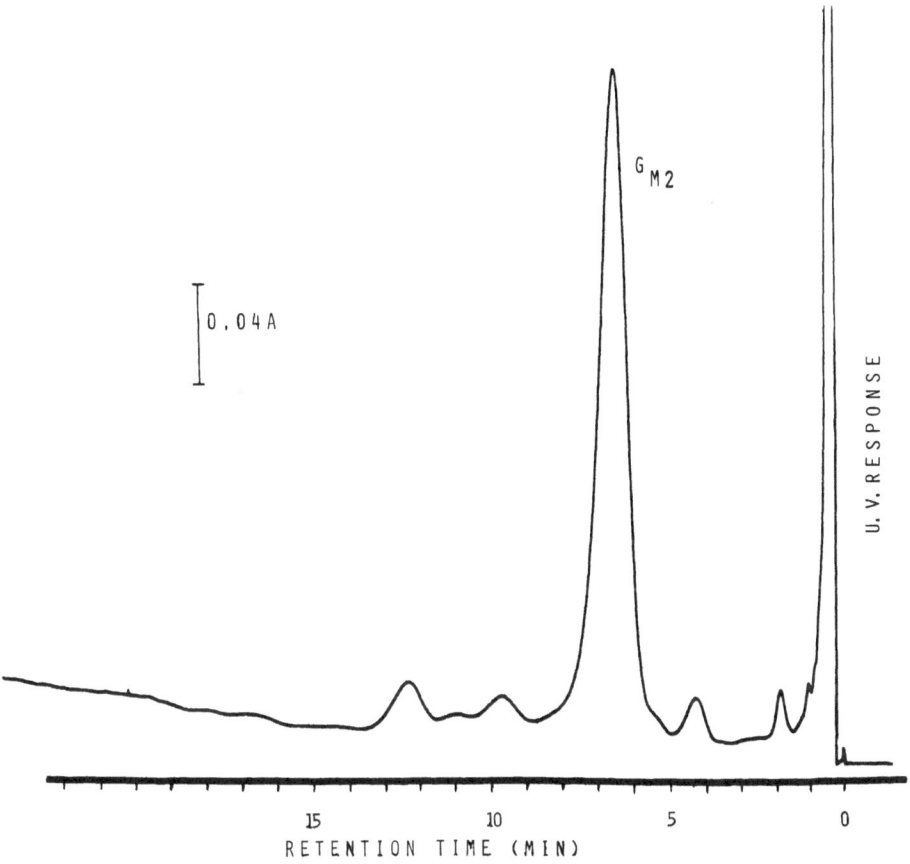

Fig. 8. Gradient elution HPLC of the ganglioside fraction from the grey matter of the brain of a case of Sandhoff-Jatzkewitz variant of G_{M2} gangliosidosis.

THE USE OF 3 KETOSPHINGOLIPIDS

Kishimoto and Mitry (5) reported that 2,3 dichloro-5,6-dicyano-
benzoquinone converts the allylic hydroxyl of sphingolipid long
chain base to the ketone. The allylic carbonyl group has strong
absorption at 230 nm. Based on this property of 3-ketosphingolipids,
high-performance liquid chromatographic methods for the analysis
of ceramides, cerebrosides and sulfatides with the use of UV detection
at 254 nm developed by Iwamori et al (6).

ANALYSIS OF AMINOPHOSPHOLIPIDS AS THEIR BIPHENYLCARBONYL DERIVATIVES

The phospholipids which contain primary amino groups, such as
ethanolamine and serine containing phosphoglycerides, have been
easily and quantitatively converted into their UV absorbing
N-biphenylcarbonyl derivatives (7). These have molar extinction
coefficients of about 20,000 at 280 nm. The phospholipid derivatives
were then separated and non-destructively determined by HPLC on a
prepacked MicroPak SI-10 column with dichloromethane-methanol -
15M NH_3 as solvent. Earlier, we have described isocratic elution
methods for the analysis of the biphenylcarbonyl derivative of
phosphatidylethanolamines with dichloromethanemethanol 15M NH_3,
92:8:1, by volume and for the lysophosphatidylethanolamine and
phosphatidylserine derivatives with the same solvents in the
proportions of 80:15:3, by volume (7). However, recently with
the use of gradient elution analysis, it has been possible to
separate and quantitate biphenylcarbonyl derivatives of phosphatidylethanolamine, phosphatidylserine and lysophosphatidylethanolamine, simultaneously (Fig. 9).

The adsorbent was re-equilibrated to its original activity
within five minutes by pumping the starting solvent. For the
analysis of ethanolamine-plasmalogens present in the phosphatidylethanolamine fraction of tissue extracts, a portion of the
derived extract was dried under N_2 and was exposed to conc. HCl
fumes for 10 min. The amount of the ethanolamine plasmalogens
was determined from the diminution of the phosphatidylethanolamine
derivative peak and increase in the lysophosphatidylethanolamine
derivative peak (7). The lower limit of detection by HPLC analysis
of the phospholipid derivatives was about 10-13 pmoles or 0.3-0.4 ng
of phospholipid phosphorus. The quantitative range of derivative
formation and analysis by HPLC of the phospholipids was shown to
be 10-500 nmole (7). Since the method is non-destructive we have
successfully employed the method for determining the specific-
radioactivity of ethanolamine- and serine-containing phosphoglycerides in various subcellular fractions of brain. The method
was also shown to be applicable to the analysis of these phospho-

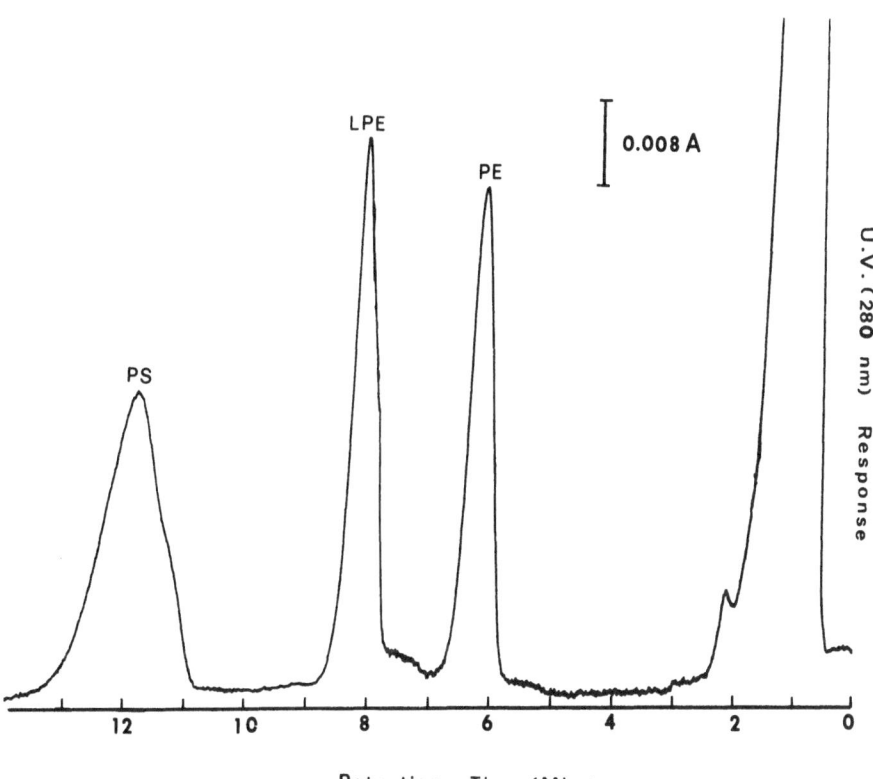

Fig. 9. Gradient-elution high-performance liquid chromatography
of biphenylcarbonyl derivatives of phosphatidylethanolamine, PE,
0.2 μg P; lysophosphatidylethanolamine, LPE, 0.211 ug P; and
phosphatidylserine, PS, 0.3 ug P, on a Li-Chrosorb SI 60, (20 μ
particle size) 2.5 mm, i.d x 50 cm column. The elution was with
a 10 min linear gradient of dichloromethane:methanol: 15M NH₃
94:7:0.75 (by volume) to the same solvents in proportions of
80:15:3 (by volume). The solvents were pumped at 2 ml per minute.
The detection was with a Laboratory Data Control Spectromonitor
set at 280 nm.

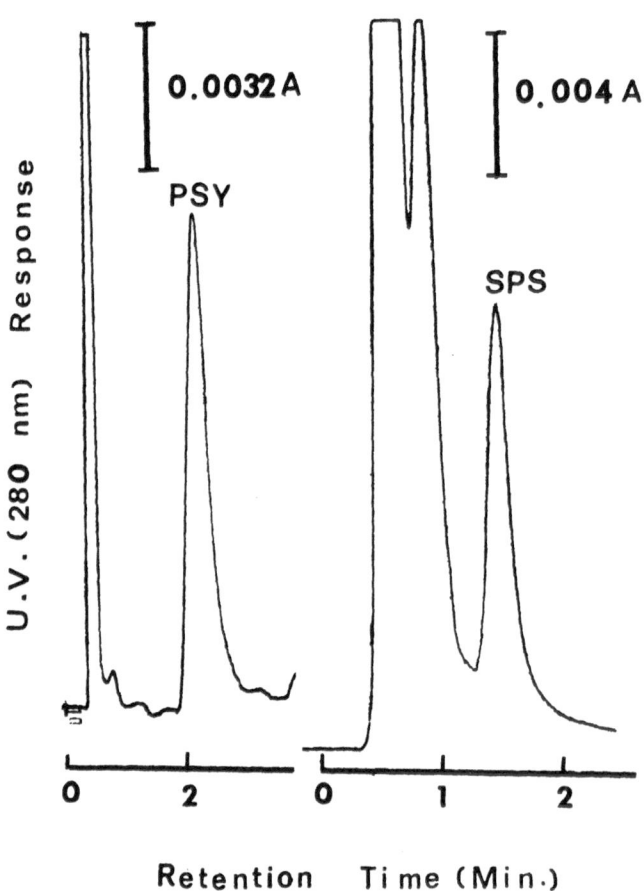

Fig. 10. High-performance liquid chromatography of biphenylcarbonyl
derivatives of psychosine (PSY) and sphingosine (SPS) on a MicroPak
SI-10 (50 cm x 2.1 mm, i.c.) column. For psychosine the solvent was
dichloromethane:methanol, 9:1, v/v flowing at 2 ml/min.
For sphingosine the solvent was acetonitrile:dichloromethane, 7.5:
2.5, v/v flowing at 0.5 ml/min. The amounts injected were equivalent
to 0.1 nmole of psychosine and 0.33 nmole of sphingosine. The
detection was with a Schoeffel spectromonitor set at 280 nm.

lipids in various other tissue samples (7). The derivatization method described here is also useful for the highly sensitive analysis of sphingolipids containing amino groups, such as sphingosine, psychosine and sphingosylphosphorylcholine, (Fig. 10).

DIRECT DETECTION IN THE REGION OF 200 nm

Until recently successful application of modern HPLC with ultraviolet detection has been primarily limited to materials that absorb ultraviolet light around 254 or 280 nm because commercially available minimum-volume flow-detectors operated only at these two fixed wavelengths. However, recent availability of the variable-wavelength ultraviolet flow-monitors prompted us to explore the possibility of direct detection of phospholipids and other complex-lipids in the low ultraviolet region where many different functional groups including isolated double bonds are known to absorb energy. We have employed HPLC method for the separation of lecithin, sphingomyelin and lysolecithin with direct detection at 205 nm, especially since these phospholipids do not have reactive functional groups and could not be easily subjected to derivative formation. The phospholipids were chromatographed on a MicroPak SI-10 column and eluted isocratically with acetonitrile methanol-water (75:21:14, by volume), Fig. 11.

We have shown, by employing synthetic phosphatidylcholines of known fatty acid composition and of varying degree of unsaturation, that the absorption at 203-205 nm was primarily due to isolated double bonds and the response measured was approximately proportional to the degree of unsaturation. Quantitation of lecithin and sphingomyelin by this method was obtained when the apparent extinction coefficient of the material analyzed was established. Alternatively, peaks were collected and quantitated by independent micromethods (8). The analysis of lecithin, sphingomyelin and lysolecithin present in the lipid extracts of animal tissues,blood and aminiotic fluids were performed without interference from other phospholipids or UV absorbing material. With the chromatographic system used for the analysis of these three phospholipids, phosphatidylethanolamine, phosphatidylserine, cerebrosides and sulfatides also gave response but they were eluted near the solvent front. Recently we have begun studies to analyze all the complex lipids present in the tissue lipid extracts, washed according to Folch procedure,with gradient elution HPLC analysis and detection at 203 nm. It has been possible so far to resolve the lipids of brain into four major fractions by this method (Fig. 12). Cholesterol, cerebrosides and sulfatides were eluted with the solvent front. Phosphotidylethanolamine was eluted next (peak 1) with small amounts of phosphatidylserine. Peak 2 was identified as mostly phosphatidylserine. Peak 3 and 4 were lecithin and sphingomyelin, respectively.

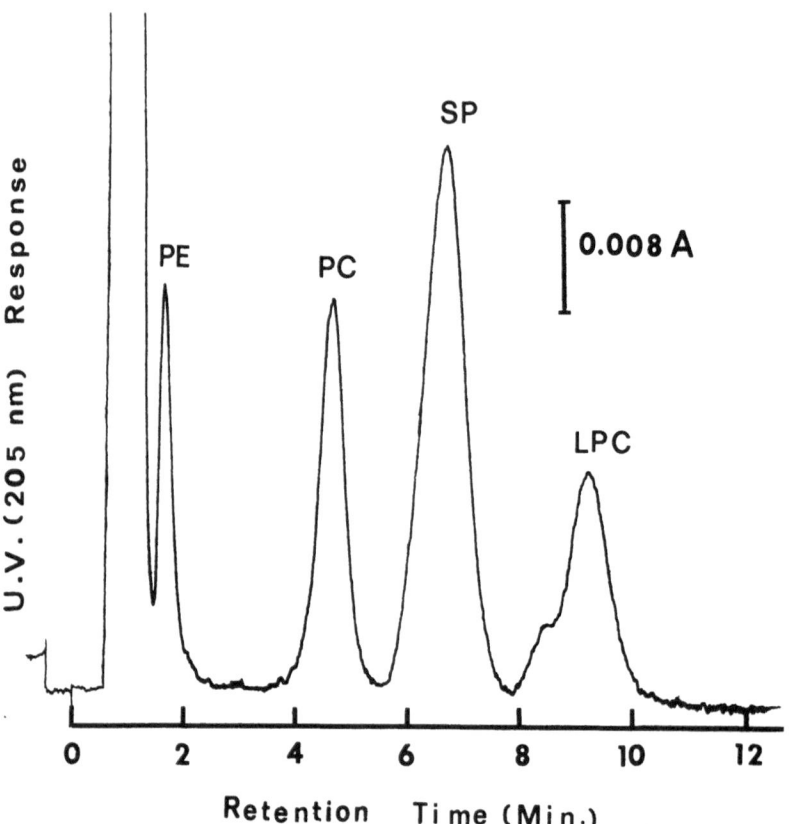

Fig. 11. High-performance liquid chromatography of phosphatidylethanolamine (dioleoyl form), PE; lecithin, (dioleoylform), PC;
sphingomyelin (bovine brain), SP; and lysolecithin (linolenoyl),LPC
on a MicroPak SI-10 column. The solvent was acetonitrile;methanol:
water 75:21:14, by volume, flowing at 1.5 ml/min. The amounts
injected were PE, 5 μg, PC, 10 ug; SP, 20 ug and LPC 5 μg. The
detection was with a Schoeffel spectromonitor set at 205 nm.

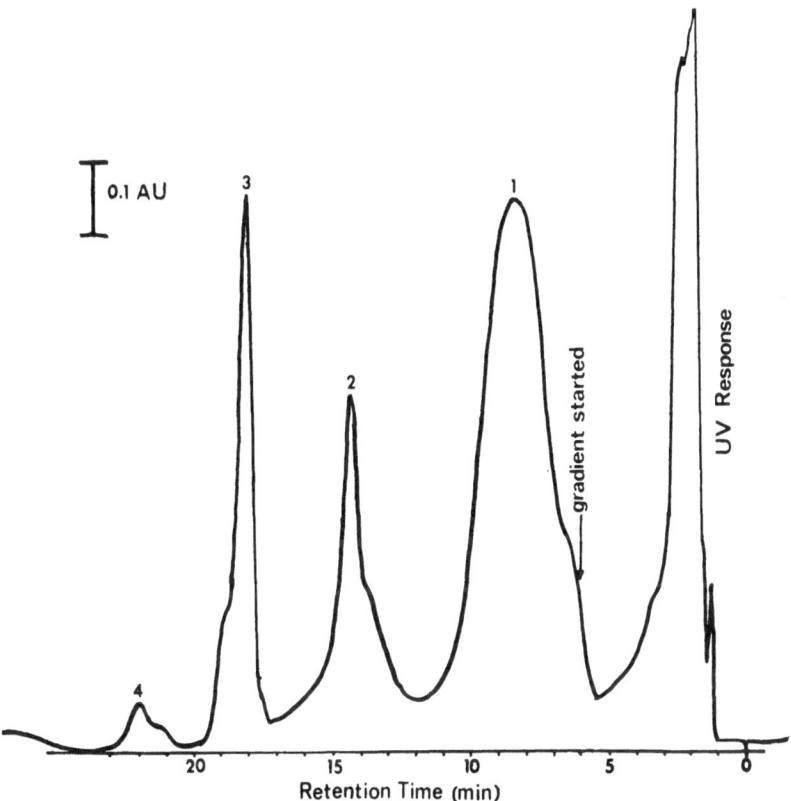

Fig. 12. Gradient-elution high-performance liquid chromatography of a lipid extract of rat brain (4 mg wet wt) on a MicroPak SI-10 column. The elution was with a 10 min linear gradient of 15% to 35% of methanol:water:ammonia, 15M (60:40:1, by vol.) in acetonitrile pumped at 1 ml/min. The detection was at 205 nm with a Schoeffel spectromonitor.

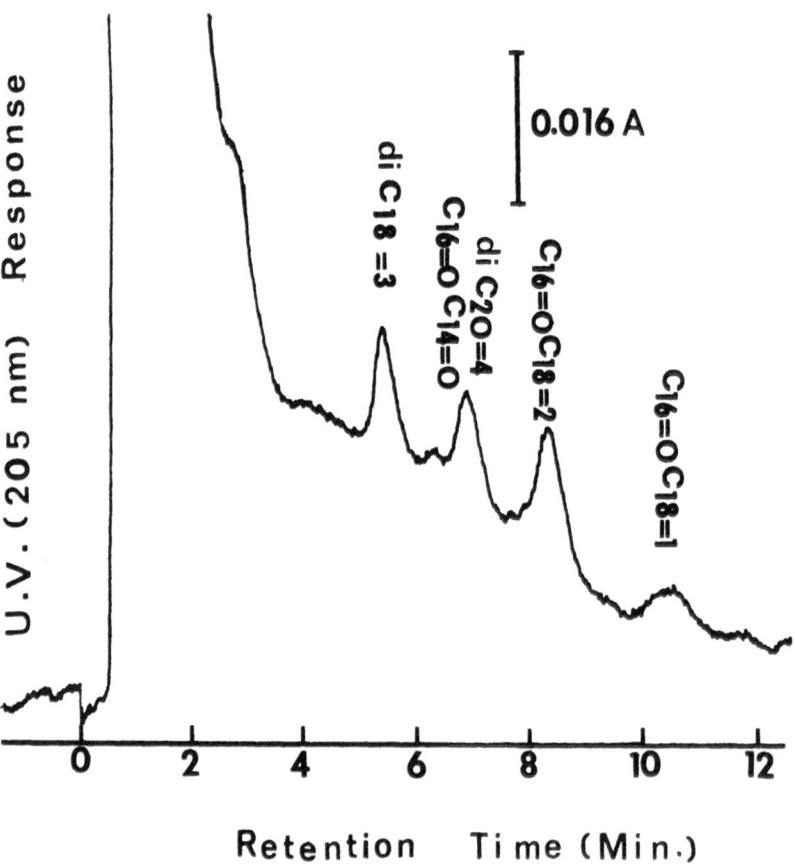

Fig. 13. Reversed-phase high-performance liquid-chromatography of dimethylphosphatidic acids on a μ-Bondapak C$_{18}$ column. The chromatography was performed at 60°C with methanol:phosphate buffer, 1mM, pH 8.0, 95:5 (v/v), with a flow rate of 2 ml/min. The detection was at 205 nm. The fatty acid chains of dimethyl-phosphatidic acids are shown over the corresponding peaks.

REVERSED-PHASE HPLC OF DIMETHYLPHOSPHATIDIC ACIDS

Recently a great interest has been generated in the analysis
of different molecular species of individual phospholipids. The
main molecular species of naturally occurring individual phospholipids, such as lecithin have been separated by counter-current
distribution or by rgentation (9) or reversed-phase partition
chromatography (10,11). However, these procedures are tedious
and the resolving power of such methods needs improvement.

We have initiated studies on the separation of the dimethylesters of phosphatidic acid which are obtainable in good yields
from several phospholipid classes by direct diazomethanolysis (12).
The dimethylesters of phosphatidic acid of known fatty acid
composition were prepared by diazomethanolysis reaction of
commercially available synthetic lecithins (12). The products of
the reaction were purified by silicic acid column chromatography.
The dimethyl esters of phosphatidic acids were eluted from the
silicic acid column with hexane:diethylether (1:1 by vol.).
Subsequent thin-layer chromatography with ether as solvent revealed
that dimethylphosphatidate had been formed in 75-80% yield. HPLC
of the dimethyl phosphatidic acids was performed on μ-Bondapak C_{18}
column (4.0 mm, i.d x 30 cm) at 60°C with methanol:phosphate
buffer, 1 mM, pH 8.0, 95:5 by vol. as the solvent at a flow rate
of 2 ml/min., Fig. 13. It is evident that the separation is based
on chain length as well as number of double bonds. However,
"critical pairs" could not be separated. A combination of
reversed-phase and silver-nitrate HPLC system should be able to
resolve the "critical pairs".

AN HPLC METHOD FOR SPHINGOMYELINASE

Niemann-Pick's disease is known to be due to deficiency of
sphingomyelinase (13). The current method for the measurement of
sphingomyelinase requires the use of radioactively labeled sphingomyelin which is difficult to obtain. Recently, however, Gal et al
(14) employed an artificial substrate, 2-hexadecanoylamino-4-
nitrophenylphosphorylcholine for this assay. We have used the
HPLC method for the measurement of sphingomyelin to follow the
action of sphingomyelinase from liver, brain or fibroblasts. The
tissues or the fibroblasts, 6-18 x 10^6 cells,were homogenized in
0.5 to 1 ml of Tris-HCl buffer, 0.05 M, pH 7.0 containing 1%
Triton X-100, by vol. The homogenate was centrifuged at 40,000 x
g for 1 hr. The supernatant was found to contain most of the
sphingomyelinase activity. The incubation mixtures contained
acetate buffer, 50 mM, pH 5.2; Triton X-100, 0.125%; bovine brain
sphingomyelin, 1.33 mM (0.266 μmoles) and enzyme protein (50 to

400 µg) in a final volume of 0.2 ml. The incubation was usually
for 4 hrs at 37°C with shaking. After the incubation 7.5 ml of
chloroform:methanol (2:1 v/v) was added and the mixture was washed
once with 0.2 vol. of 0.9% NaCl. The upper phase was removed and
the lower phase was washed three times with 0.2 vol. of methanol:
0.9% NaCl:chloroform (48:47"3 by vol.). The washed lower phase
was dried under N$_2$ and the residue was dissolved in 100 µl of
ethanol. Enzyme and substrate blanks were treated with the same
procedure. A suitable portion (usually 15 µl) of the sample was
injected, in triplicate, on a HPLC MicroPak column as described
in Fig. 11. The amount of sphingomyelin was determined from the
area of the peak as measured by cut and weigh method. The
sphingomyelinase activity was determined from the amount of
sphingomyelin that disappeared during the incubation. Initially,
it was shown that the activity in the supernatant of the fibroblast
homogenate was proportional to protein concentration up to 500 µg
of protein and the activity was linear up to 8 hours of incubation.
Table I shows the specific activity of sphingomyelinase in the
supernatant of human fibroblasts from normal individuals and from
a patient identified as having Niemann-Pick's Type A disease.
Attempts are being made to employ the HPLC method for the measurement of sphingomyelinase in human leuckocytes and for detection of
heterozygous carriers of Niemann-Pick's disease.

Table I: Sphingomyelinase activity in cultured human fibroblasts.
The enzyme activity was determined as described in the text.

Subject	Age	Sex	Specific Activity nmole/mg/hr
Normal	22 months	F	107.0
Normal	22 months	F	118.8
Normal	9.5 years	M	65.9
Normal	4 years	M	80.6
Niemann-Pick's (Type A)	6 months	F	27.3

We believe that the few applications of HPLC to the analysis of lipids, presented here, indicate that modern LC techniques will develop into a powerful tool for analytical work in neurochemistry.

Acknowledgements: The following individuals have participated in the work presented here:

> Dr. S. Gross, Dr. D. Ullman, J. Evans, Ms. B. Perelle,
> Ms. H. Heos, Dr. J. Pasquini, Dr. A. Milunsky and
> Dr. L. Hayes.

This work was supported in part by Grants HD-05515, HD-04147, NS-10613, CA 168533, NS 10437. Dr. Jungalwala is supported by a Research Career Development Award, CA 00144.

REFERENCES

1. McCluer, R.H. and Evans, J.E.: Preparation and analysis of benzoylated cerebrosides. J. Lipid Res., 14:611, 1973.

2. Sugita, M., Iwamori, M., Evans, J., McCluer, R.H., Moser, H.W. and Dulaney, J.T.: High-performance liquid chromatography of ceramides: application to analysis in human tissues and demonstration of ceramide excess in Farber's disease. J. Lipid Res., 15:223, 1974.

3. McCluer, R.H. and Evans, J.E.: Quantitative analysis of cerebroside by high-performance liquid chromatography of their perbenzoyl derivatives. J. Lipid Res., submitted.

4. Hayes, L., Jungalwala, F.B. and McCluer, R.H.: Determination of picomole quantities of cerebrosides by high-performance liquid chromatography with gradient elution analysis. In preparation.

4a. Hoshi, M., Williams, M. and Kishimoto, K.: Characterization of brain cerebrosides at early stages of development in the rat. J. Neurochem., 21:709, 1973.

5. Kishimoto, Y. and Mitry, M.I.T.: A new procedure for synthesis of 3-keto derivatives of sphingolipids and its application for study of fatty acid composition of brain ceramides and cerebrosides containing dihydro-sphingosine or sphingosine. Arch. Biochem. Biophys., 161:426, 1974.

6. Iwamori, M., Moser, H.W., McCluer, R.H. and Kishimoto, Y.: 2-ketosphingolipids: Application to the determination of sphingolipids which contain 4-sphingenine. Biochem. Biophys. Acta, 380:308, 1975.

7. Jungalwala, F.B., Turel, R.J., Evans, J.E. and McCluer, R.H.:
    Sensitive analysis of ethanolamine and serine containing
    phosphoglycerides by high performance liquid chromatography.
    Biochem. J., 145:517, 1975.

8. Dittmer, J.C. and Wells, M.A.: Quantitative and qualitative
    analysis of lipids and lipid components. Methods in Enzym.,
    14:482, 1969.

9. Arvidson, G.A.E.: Structural and metabolic heterogeneity of
    rat liver glycerophosphatides. European J. Biochem., 4:
    478, 1968.

10. Avidson, G.A.E.: Separation of naturally occurring lecithins
    according to fatty-acid chain-length and degree of unsaturation
    on a lipophilic derivative of Sephadex. J. of Chromatography,
    103:201, 1975.

11. Wurster, Jr., C.F. and Copenhaver, Jr., J.H.: Thin layer
    chromatographic separation of dimethylphosphatidates derived
    from lecithins. Lipids, 1:422, 1966.

12. Renkonen, O.: Mono-acid dimethyl phosphatidates from dif-
    ferent subtypes of choline and ethanolamine glycerophospha-
    tides. Biochim. Biophys. Acta, 152:114, 1968.

13. Kampine, J.P., Brady, R.O., and Kanfer, J.N.: Diagnosis of
    Gaucher's disease and Niemann-Pick disease with small samples
    of nervous blood. Science, N.Y., 155:86, 1967.

14. Gal, A.E., Brady, R.O., Hibbert, S.R. and Pentchev, P.G.:
    A practical chromatogenic procedure for the detection of
    homozygotes and heterozygous carriers of Niemann-Pick
    disease. New Engl. J. Med., 293, 632, 1975.

BRAIN GLYCOPROTEINS AND RECOGNITION FUNCTIONS:

RECOGNINS AND CANCER

Samuel Bogoch

Dreyfus Medical Foundation

New York, New York

INTRODUCTION AND SUMMARY

When the first determination of the structure of brain gangliosides (1) showed them to have a glucocerebroside basis, with
galactose, hexosamine and neuraminic acid residues attached, the
suitability of the structure for membrane, receptor and recognition functions was proposed (2). Because of the relationship of
gangliosides to Tay-Sachs disease, this conference has often been
the place where we have first reported the progress of our studies
over the past years on the structure and function of the brain
gangliosides and brain glycoproteins, that is, the brain mucoids.

The pharmacological properties of brain gangliosides, both in
active and passive roles, reported by us in the late 1950's and
early 1960's are now becoming subjects of interest (4). For example, we demonstrated the first in vivo pharmacological therapeutic use of the gangliosides in the inhibition of the neurotoxic
effects of influenza virus in mouse brain (24), and proposed with
this demonstration the "decoy" principle of therapeutic action.
This decoy principle is now being applied to the therapeutic binding of cholera toxin, and may be useful for other infectious
agents which may use gangliosides as receptors (4,24-27).

In the search for the protein to which gangliosides might be
attached in situ, we uncovered the presence of the brain glycoproteins - literally hundreds of them (5). We reported this finding at this conference in 1965 (6) together with the following
observations: 1) the fractionation of these glycoproteins into 16
groups permitted the quantitative examination of the groups in

normal developmental periods and in Tay-Sachs disease, 2) developmental patterns were indicated, 3) in addition to the Tay-Sachs
increase in gangliosides, there were increases in the carbohydrate-
rich glycoproteins of brain. This finding has been recently confirmed by others (7), 4) the general 'sign-post' theory of the
recognition and communication functions of the brain gangliosides
and glycoproteins was then proposed (8,9). The study of both the
concentration of each glycoprotein group and of the exchange of
radioactive carbohydrate unite of the glycoproteins in the pigeon
brain at rest, during training, and with learning, provided ample
evidence that these substances were indeed involved in the neural
processes which take place during the establishment of brain cir-
cuitry (10-16). Many of these observations have now been confirmed
in several other laboratories (17-21). The Biochemistry of Memory
was a somewhat unusual notion for a paper in 1965 (8) and for a
book in 1968 (9). That there is a biochemistry of memory is more
generally held now although its details will take much effort to
elaborate (22).

One test of the notion that the glycoproteins are involved in
high information states is to examine them in low information
states. The cancer cell is a 'dumb' cell in the sense that cell
division proceeds regardless of the fact that the space available
has been used up, and proceeds to the death of the host and hence
of the cancer cells themselves. And so we examined cancer of
brain cells.

Ten years ago we found that glycoprotein fraction 10B was increased in gliomas compared to normals and other disorders (6).
The increase was in the protein components but the carbohydrate
components were reduced (14). There was an increase in 10B in
Tay-Sachs disease also, but here the increase was seen to be in
the carbohydrate components as well as the protein (6). Antisera
prepared to crude fraction 10B from Tay-Sachs brain, or immunofluorescent study of brain sections containing tumor cells, did
not stain the tumor glia cells, did not stain normal resting glia
(23). Now, in retrospect, in view of the data I shall present,
it is clear that this Tay-Sachs antibody was a recognition substance (Recognin) to a component of reactive glia which are present
in high concentrations in both Tay-Sachs disease and brain tumors.

However, I have now found that there is another recognition
substance in the tumor cell itself. The identification of this
recognition substance has led to the following:

1) The production of the first cancer antigen of known
structure, Astrocytin, from crude fraction 10B of brain tumors;
2) The synthesis of new compounds (TARGET reagents) which
contain the immunochemical specificity of the _in situ_ cancer antigen;

3) The use of these TARGET reagents has permitted the isolation of pure specific antibody-like materials (TARGET-attaching
globulins, TAG) from human and animal serum;

4) The quantitative measure of serum TAG has provided the
first quantitative serum diagnostic method for malignant brain
tumors;

5) The TAG compounds react with the cancer antigen-like compounds in quantitative precipitin, Ouchterlony double diffusion
reactions, and label in situ glial cancer cells specifically in
double layer immunofluorescence - hence a new tissue diagnostic
method for malignant glia as well.

6) The cancer antigen-like material has been produced by
glioma cancer cell culture fermentation. This product, Malignin,
is structurally unique from the Astrocytin, but shares its immunochemical properties. Its bulk production permits the mass use of
TARGET reagent in diagnostic testing.

7) The percentage of extractable cancer protein which is
Malignin increases as the malignancy of the cancer growth increases.

8) Computer search of the library of protein structures re-
veals that Astrocytin and Malignin have unique structures, and that
the only proteins even remotely related are four in number - each a
respiratory protein. This finding may be of great significance
since it might provide the first biochemical insight into the basis
of the respiratory activity of cancer cells, and their dominance.
It may also provide new therapeutic means for their destruction
because -

9) TAG compounds have been found to be highly cytotoxic to
malignant glia in vitro

10) The implications of these findings extend beyond cancer
diagnosis and treatment and into tissue and organ specificity,
transplantation rejection, specific pharmacological delivery systems, and developmental disorders; thus for example

11) The third recognition substance of this type has been
identified as Reeler disease in mouse brain, to be of abnormal
molecular weight.

12) With the recognition of this third product, the family
name for the recognition substance, RECOGNINS, is here proposed,
together with the name of CHEMORECIPROCALS for their antibody-
like counterparts.

THE STRUCTURE OF ASTROCYTIN AND MALIGNIN

The two unique small molecular weight protein fragments, named
Astrocytin and Malignin, are produced from in vivo brain glial
tumor and in vitro cancer cell fermentation, respectively. They
bear specific tissue antigen and other immunochemical properties
characteristic of the malignancy.

Astrocytin has a molecular weight of approximately 8000 and

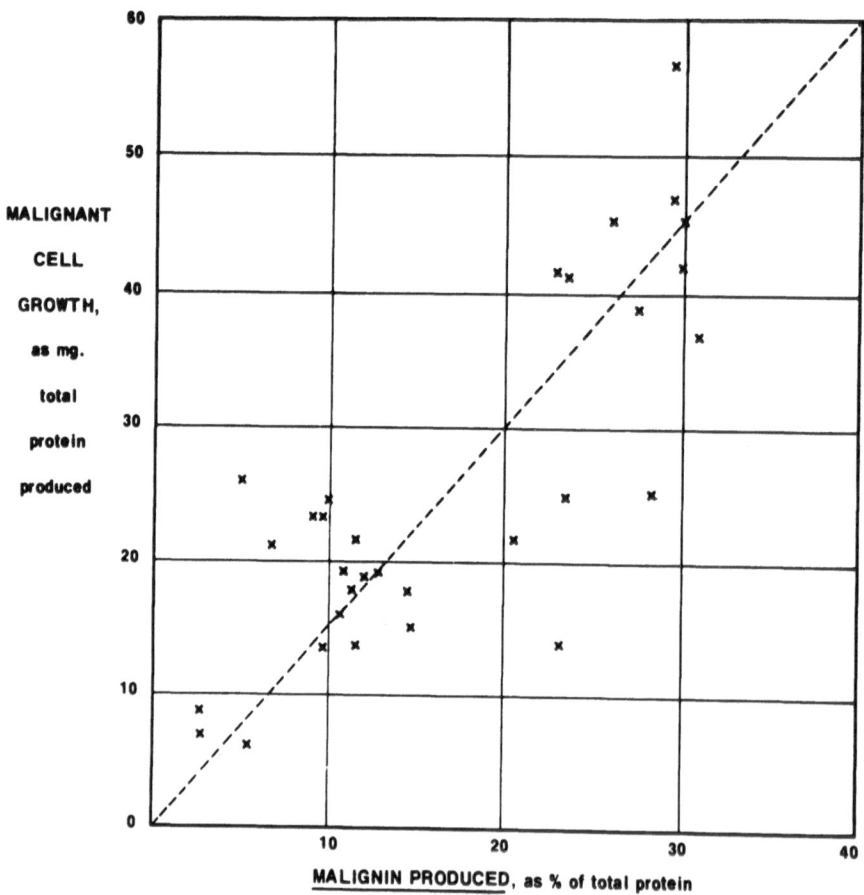

Figure 1

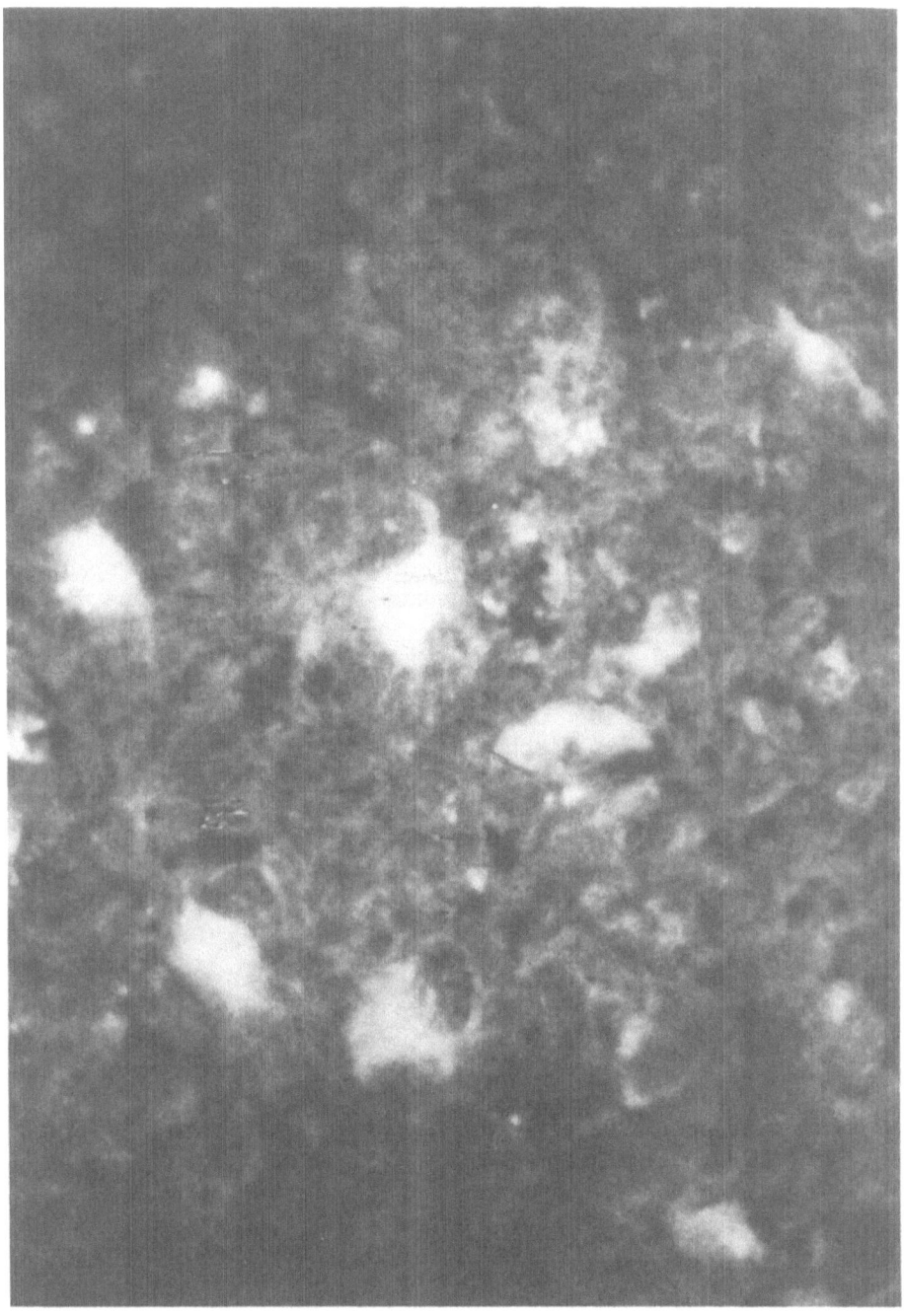

Figure 2

the following approximate composition: Asp 9, Threo 5, Ser 6, Glu 13, Pro 4, Gly 6, Ala 9, Val 4, 1/2 Cys 2, Meth 1, Isoleu 2, Leu 8, Tyr 2, Phe 3, Lys 8, His 2, Arg 4, Total 88.

Malignin, repeatedly produced over 60 generations from glioma cell culture fermentation, has a molecular weight of approximately 10,000, and the following approximate composition: Asp 9, Threo 5, Ser 5, Glu 13, Pro 4, Gly 6, Ala 7, Val 6, 1/2 Cys 1, Meth 2, Isoleu 4, Leu 8, Tyr 3, Phe 3, Lys 6, His 2, Arg 5, Total 89. The comparison of these two structures with that of structurally related proteins found by computer search is shown in Table II.

The percent of total extracted cancer cell protein which is malignin increases with the degree of malignancy of the growth (Figure 1).

ANTIBODIES TO ASTROCYTIN AND MALIGNIN

Antibodies prepared in rabbits are specific to these compounds, react with them in quantitative precipitin and Ouchterlony double diffusion reactions, and label in situ glial cancer cells specifically in double layer immunofluorescence (hence a new tissue diagnostic method).

Figure 2 shows a section of brain removed at surgery in the case of a malignant glial tumor. The section is stained with the new product TAG (TARGET-attaching globulin), an antibody-like protein fragment prepared from rabbits challenged with the Recognin, and with fluorescent goat anti-rabbit serum. In contrast to the results obtained with anti-Tay-Sachs antisera where only reactive (normal) glia, and no tumor glia stained, here we see the opposite, that is, only tumor glia stain.

This new tissue diagnostic test promises to be of use a) in identifying the presence of a malignant tumor (vs. a benign one) at surgery, and b) in defining whether there are still malignant glia present in the edges of the tissue removed at surgery, hence an indication of whether all of the tumor was removed.

Since TAG compounds also are highly cytotoxic to these cancer cells in vitro their therapeutic potential requires exploration in man.

SERUM TAG TEST FOR MALIGNANT BRAIN TUMORS

Synthesis of Astrocytin or Malignin complexes with carriers such as cellulose derivatives produces solid topographic antigen-like reagent templates (TARGET). These reagents react with antibody-like globulins in human serum and from the resulting complexes,

Table I

Normals*								Malignant Brain Tumors Primary		Malignant Other Tumors, Brain Secondaries	Malignant Other Tumors, No Brain Secondaries	Uncertain Cerebral Diagnosis
Serum TAG ug/ml		Serum TAG ug/ml		Serum TAG ug/ml		Serum TAG ug/ml		Serum TAG ug/ml		Serum TAG ug/ml	Serum TAG ug/ml	Serum TAG ug/ml
124	363[1]	19	99[6]	54	21	65	48	459	185	270	36[4]	165[8]
113	4	55	13[2]	27	0	113	20	397	253	257	31[5]	144[9]
105	31	51	270[3]	41	120	130	82	236	253	188	442[14]	13[9]
130	42	82	7	21	16	79	20	137	565	205	288[14]	209[10]
127	34	44	58	27	20	61	55	298	277	157[7]		75[10]
38	76	127	24	21	113	123	0	397	137[13]			184[11]
100	48	31	62	0	72	14		241	78[13]			27[11]
125	85	0	89	14		20		241	138			110[12]
30		125	89	62		41		217	650			192[15]
250[1]		118		38		34		147	160			
39		89		93		93		127	235			

*Includes normals, non-tumor medical and surgical disorders. 1-Very ill, undiagnosed; 2-Extra brain intracranial mass, undiagnosed; 3-Marked gliosis; 4-Malignant melanoma; 5-Osteosarcoma; 6-Brain cyst fluid; 7-Adenocarcinoma of colon; 8-Gastrectomy; 9-Headaches; 10-Emphysema; 11-Polymyalgia; 12-Colon cancer; 13-Convulsions; 14-Cancer of prostrate, secondaries to bone; 15-Clinically "normal" 18-Months earlier, when this abnormal serum TAG obtained: Now developed severe headaches, loss of smell and taste.

Table II

Comparison of the Structures of Astrocytin and Malignin to Nearest Structures* by Computer Search

	Astrocytin	Malignin	Cyto-chrome b5*	Ferre-doxin Leuc. Gl.*	Ferre-doxin Alfalfa*	Acyl Carrier E. Coli*	Neuro-physin Bovine	Neuro-physin Pig	Gonado-tropin Release
Aspartic acid	9	9	9	10	8	7	2	3	0
Threonine	5	5	6	4	6	6	2	2	0
Serine	6	5	5	7	8	3	6	7	1
Glutamic acid	13	13	14	13	13	14	9	9	0
Proline	4	4	3	5	3	1	8	7	1
Glycine	6	6	6	7	7	4	16	14	2
Alanine	9	7	4	6	9	7	6	7	0
Valine	4	6	4	6	9	7	4	2	0
1/2 Cysteine	2	1	0	5	5	0	14	14	0
Methionine	1	2	1	0	0	1	1	1	0
Isoleucine	2	4	4	4	4	7	2	2	0
Leucine	8	8	7	10	6	5	6	7	1
Tyrosine	2	3	3	3	4	1	1	1	1
Phenylalanine	3	3	3	3	2	2	3	3	0
Lysine	8	6	7	5	5	4	2	2	0
Histidine	2	2	7	1	2	1	0	0	1
Arginine	4	5	3	2	1	1	7	5	1
Asparagine	0	0	0	0	1	2	3	2	0
Tryptophane	0	0	1	1	1	0	0	0	1
Glutamine	0	0	0	4	3	4	5	4	0
Total No. Residues	88	89	87	96	97	77	97	92	10
Molecular Wt. **	8,000**	10,000**	10,035	10,588	10,483	8,509	10,065	9,488	1,201

*Only four close structures found; other three shown for comparison

** By thin-layer gel chromatog. Calculated mol. wt. above structures, Astrocytin 9,690, Malignin 10,067

TARGET-attaching globulins (TAG) can be isolated. Table I shows the quantity of serum TAG, in micrograms of protein per ml. for normals and tumors. TAG is 0 to 130 in 71, greater than 130 in 3 (mean 54.3) in normals and non-tumor medical and surgical disorders; 137 to 650 in 20, less than 130 in 2 (mean 246.4) in malignant brain tumors; 157 to 270 in 5 secondary malignant tumors in brain; 288 and 442 in 2 cancers of the prostate with no apparent brain secondaries, 31 and 36 in 2 sarcomas with no apparent secondaries to brain; and 9 with as yet uncertain clinical diagnoses. The above data represent two successive blind studies and a total of 114 serum specimens, and support the utility of the serum TAG determinations as a diagnostic procedure for malignant brain tumors.

REELER RECOGNIN

Because Reeler disease in mice represents a genetic nervous system disorder in which particular groups of nerve cells fail to migrate to their normal position (29), it was of interest to examine the recognins in this disorder.

Table III

Recognin Concentration in Mouse Brain, mg/g

	Normal	Reeler
Cerebellum (16-day old mouse)	2.50	0.71
Cortex (16-day old mouse)	0.60	0.96
Cortex (4-day old mouse)	0.29	0.53
Brainstem (16-day old mouse)	0.90	1.64
Whole Brain (17-day old mouse)	1.27	1.53
Whole Brain (1-day old mouse)	5.00	5.86

Table III shows the concentration of recognin in normal and reeler mouse brain. While there is a marked decrease in the concentration of recognin in cerebellum of Reeler mouse, there are the same or greater amounts of recognins in other areas of the brain. The recognin may not move from other areas of brain to the cerebellum, or the slight increase in other areas of Reeler brain may reflect some compensatory action.

The molecular weight of this Reeler Recognin was 3,600 to 5,000 in contrast to that of the recognins from all areas of normal mouse brain, which were 8,000.

This pathological recognin in Reeler brain is correlated with the inability for migrating brain cells to make the contacts they must in order to achieve proper placement, consistent with the role of the recognins in recognition and learning in cells.

STRUCTURAL RELATION TO RESPIRATORY PROTEINS

Computer search (29) shows Astrocytin and Malignin to be
unique in structure. The closest structures, surprisingly are
certain respiratory proteins: cytochrome b5 (human), ferredoxin of
leucaena glauca*, ferredoxin of alfalfa*, and the acyl carrier
protein of E. Coli. However, while Astrocytin and Malignin each
have only 2 histidines, cytochrome b5 for example, has 7 histidines,
and there are 6 to 13 other structural differences in each of the
structural neighbors. On the other hand, no proteins in the computer library are anywhere near as close as the above four, the
lack of even superficial similarity being chiefly due to the highly
unusual structural characteristics of Astrocytin and Malignin: the
fact that each has 13 residues of glutamic acid in an 88 and 89
residue total respectively. If the in situ equivalents of the
cancer Recognins in fact have respiratory functions in cancer cells,
since they account for such a large proportion of the extracted
cell protein, a biochemical mechanism may now be apparent for the
first time to account for the voracious respiratory activity* of
the cancer cell. This might also explain the absolute increase in
Malignin with increased malignancy (Figure 1), and why TAG is cytotoxic to cancer cells since it binds an essential respiratory protein.

DISCUSSION

The definition of recognition substances in mature brain cells
which operate during high information states of memory and learning
(1) has led to the observation that these substances are replaced
in cancer by in situ compounds which have the immunochemical specificities of Astrocytin and Malignin. These new compounds characterize
the low information (dumb) state of the cancer cell in that cell
division proceeds regardless of the fact that the space available
has been used up, and proceeds to the death of the host, and hence
of the cancer cells themselves. With the production of these first
two compounds of the group, the family name of Recognins is proposed. For the antibody-like compounds to the Recognins, the name
Chemoreciprocals is proposed.

The Recognins have immediate utility in the diagnosis of brain
malignancies, and possibly others, and represent a major advance in
our understanding of the structural basis of cancer antigens. The
same technology is being applied by us to other cancers. The
Recognins may simultaneously provide new insight into the respiratory
survival-efficacy of cancer cells, and new therapeutic means to
destroy them.

*- Note especially their anaerobic properties: neoplastic cells can
   survive for long periods of time in the absence of glucose and
   oxygen, even in the presence of cyanide (30).

These findings are also clearly relevant to other tissue and organ specificity studies, as in transplantation rejection, to disease specificity, and to means of specific delivery of pharmacological agents to particular subcellular and cellular addresses. There are also clear applications to defining and treating developmental disturbances, as those of cell positioning. Thus for example, we have now isolated a third Recognin - that in Reeler disease of mouse brain. In this genetic movement disorder in which particular groups of nerve cells fail to migrate to their normal position, Reeler Recognin is obviously abnormal, since it has a molecular weight of 3600 to 5000, compared to 8000 in normal mouse brain.

Acknowledgements

The technical assistance of G. Korsh, C. Gramm, and G. Kormby; the cooperation in the provision of serum samples by Dr. M.D. Walker, National Cancer Research Center, National Cancer Institute, Dr. Eli Goldensohn, Department of Neurology, Columbia-Presbyterian Medical Center, and Dr. Charles Fager, Department of Neurosurgery, Leahy Clinic, Boston; the cooperation in the provision of tumor and brain tissue specimens by Dr. William H. Sweet, Dr. Paul Kornblith, and Dr. R.G. DeLong, Departments of Neurosurgery and Neurology, Massachusetts General Hospital, and Dr. Charles Fager, Leahy Clinic; and the provision of immunofluorescent microscopic examination of tumor specimens by Dr. F.H. Hochberg, Department of Neuropathology, Massachusetts General Hospital, are all gratefully acknowledged. All of the studies reported here were supported entirely by Brain Research, Inc. The new products and processes in this communication are the subjects of filed patent applications.

REFERENCES

1. Bogoch, S., J. Am. Chem. Soc., 79:3286, 1957.
2. Bogoch, S., Virology, 4:458, 1957.
3. Bogoch, S., Biochem. J., 68:319, 1958.
4. Porcellati, G. (ed.) Biochemical and Pharmacological Implications of Ganglioside Function, International Society for Neurochemistry, Satellite Meeting, Cortona, Italy, August, 1975. Plenum Publishing Corp., (in press).
5. Bogoch, S., Rajam, P.C. and Belval, P.C., Nature, 204:73, 1964.
6. Bogoch, S. and Belval, P.C., in: Cerebral Sphingolipidoses. Aronson, S.M. and Volk, B.W. (eds.), Academic Press, New York, 1966, p. 273.
7. Berra, B., DePalma, S. and Brunngraber, E.G., Clin. Chim. Acta, 57:301, 1974.
8. Bogoch, S., Neurosci. Res. Prog. Bull., 3:38, 1965.
9. Bogoch, S., The Biochemistry of Memory: With an Inquiry into the Function of the Brain Mucoids. Oxford University Press,

10. Bogoch, S., Belval, P.C., Sweet, W.H., Sacks, W. and Korsh, G.,
     in: Protides of the Biological Fluids: Proceedings of the
     XVth Colloq. Bruge, Peters, H. (ed.), Elsevier, Amsterdam,
     1967, p. 131.

11. Bogoch, S., in: Handbook of Neurochemistry, Vo. I, Lajtha, A.
     (ed.), Plenum Publishing Corp., New York, 1969, p. 75.

12. Bogoch, S., in: Protein Metabolism of the Nervous System,
     Lajtha, A. (ed.), Plenum Publishing Corp., New York, 1970,
     p.555.

13. Quamina, A. and Bogoch, S., in: Protides of Biological Fluids,
     Proceedings of the XIIth Colloq. Bruges, Peters, H. (ed.),
     Elsevier, Amsterdam, 1966, p.211.

14. Bogoch, S., in: Functional and Structural Proteins of the
     Nervous System, Davison, A.N., Morgan, I.G. and Mandel, P.
     (eds.), Plenum Publishing Corp., New York, 1972, p.39.

15. Bogoch, S., in: Sphingolipids, Sphingolipidoses and Allied
     Disorders, Volk, B.W. and Aronson, S.M. (eds.), Plenum
     Publishing Corp., New York, 1972, p. 127.

16. Bogoch, S., in: Current Biochemical Approaches to Learning
     and Memory, Essman, W.B. and Nakajima, S. (eds.), Spectrum-
     Halstead-Wiley, 1973.

17. Routtenberg, A., George, D.R. and Davis, L.G., Behavioral
     Biology, 12:461, 1974.

18. Damstra-Entingh, T.D., Entingh, D.J., Wilson, J.E. and
     Glassman, E., Fed. Proc., 32:603, 1973.

19. Damstra-Entingh, T.D., Entingh, D.J., Wilson, J.E. and
     Glassman, E., Behavioral Biology, 13:121, 1975.

20. De Feudis, F.V., Biol. Psychiat., 4:239, 1972.

21. De Feudis, F.V., Biol. Psychiat., 7:3, 1973.

22. Bogoch, S., in: The Nervous System, Basic Sciences, 25th
     Anniversary Volume, National Institutes of Neurological
     and Communicative Disorders and Stroke, Brady, R. (ed.),
     in press.

23. Benda, P., Mori, T. and Sweet, W.H., J. Neurosurg., 33:281,
     1970.

24. Bogoch, S., Lynch, P. and Levine, A.S., Virology, 7:161, 1959.

25. Bogoch, S. and Bogoch, E.S., Nature, 183:53, 1959.

26. Bogoch, S., Paasonen, M.K. and Trendelenburg, U., Brit. J.
     Pharmacol., 18:325, 1962.

27. Bogoch, S., Nature, 185:392, 1960.

28. Sidman, R.L., in: The Cell Surface in Development, Moscona,
     A.A. (ed.), John Wiley and Sons, New York, 1974, p. 221.

29. Dayhoff, Margaret O. (ed.), Atlas of Protein Sequence and
     Structure, 1972. National Biomedical Research Foundation.
     P.O. Box 629, Silver Spring, Md. + Supplement 1, 1973.
     Computer search performed by Dr. Dayhoff and Associates.

30. Warburg, O., Gawehn, K., Geissler, A.W., Schroder, W.,
     Gewitz, H.S., and Volker, W., Arch. Biochem. Biophys.,
     78:573, 1958.

LIPIDS AND SLOW VIRUSES: COMPARISON OF MEASLES AND SSPE VIRIONS

R.W. Ledeen, C.A. Miller, J.E. Haley and
C.S. Raine

Departments of Neurology, Biochemistry,
Pathology and Neuroscience, Albert Einstein
College of Medicine, Bronx, N.Y. 10461

Slow virus diseases have attracted growing interest in recent years owing to recognition of their role in certain nervous system disorders and possible implication in multiple sclerosis. As with the sphingolipidoses, significant alterations in lipid composition occur in these conditions but the nature and origin of the changes are fundamentally different. Some are the direct consequence of demyelination while other changes, such as those involving gangliosides, have a less certain origin. Alterations among the glycosphingolipids might be anticipated in view of repeated findings (4,5,16,17) that virally transformed cells develop abnormal patterns of these constituents. A study of this phenomenon in slow virus conditions could be useful in elucidating the complex interactions between these atypical infectious agents and the host cell.

The lipids of the virions themselves are also important in the consideration of such interactions. The majority of viruses contain 20-35% lipid by weight and removal of this fraction generally results in loss of infectivity. Several viruses have already been subjected to detailed analysis (reviewed in ref. 3). We have recently begun a study of the lipid composition of two closely related paramyxoviruses, measles and

subacute sclerosing panencephalitis (SSPE) virus,
which have a well-established role in human neurological disorders. Our initial findings will be presented
along with a review of previous work on lipid changes
in SSPE-infected brain.

LIPID CHANGES IN SSPE

Significant ganglioside changes have been
described in brain tissue of patients with SSPE.
Wender (43) had earlier reported two cases which
showed an elevation of lipid hexosamine in cerebral
white matter, while Cumings (11) reported an increased
ganglioside level in cerebral cortex in one out of
three cases. The first detailed study, carried out by
Norton et al. (32), reported an abnormal pattern for
white matter in which the normally minor components
G_{M3}*, G_{M2}, G_{D3} and G_{D2} were significantly elevated. The
total ganglioside content of white matter was elevated
two-fold above normal but the level and pattern of gray
matter gangliosides were essentially normal.

Our own study of a different case (25) revealed
the same kind of pattern abnormality in white matter
gangliosides (Fig. 1), but in this instance gray matter
showed the same change. The above four gangliosides
were significantly elevated in both relative and
absolute terms, while G_{M1} was decreased due to

---

*The structures of these species are:

G_{M3}:   NeuNAc$(\alpha, 2-8)$Gal$(\beta, 1-4)$Glc$(\beta, 1-1)$Cer

G_{M2}:   NeuNAc$(\alpha, 2-3)$[GalNAc$(\beta, 1-4)$]Gal$(\beta, 1-4)$Glc$(\beta, 1-1)$Cer

G_{D3}:   NeuNAc$(\alpha, 2-8)$NeuNAc$(\alpha, 2-3)$Gal$(\beta, 1-4)$Glc$(\beta, 1-1)$Cer

G_{D2}:   NeuNAc$(\alpha, 2-8)$NeuNAc$(\alpha, 2-3)$[GalNAc$(\beta, 1-4)$]Gal$(\beta, 1-4)-$
        Glc$(\beta, 1-1)$Cer

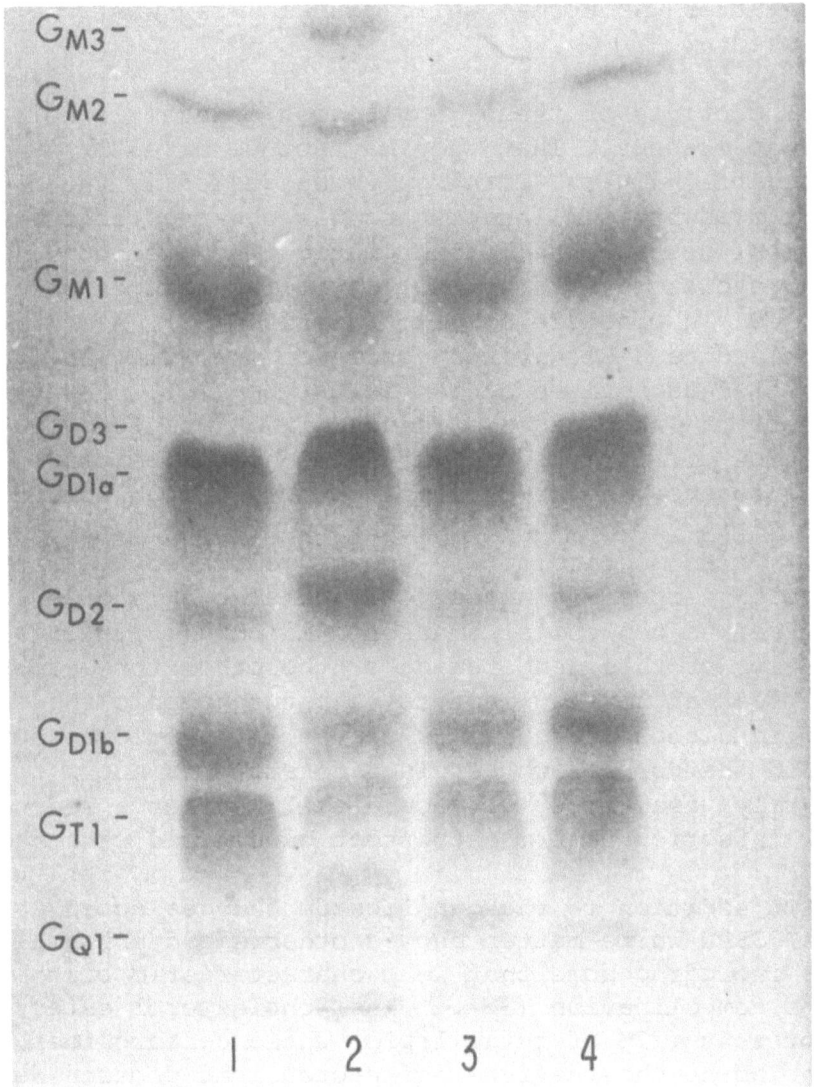

G_{M3}^-
G_{M2}^-

G_{M1}^-

G_{D3}^-
G_{D1a}^-

G_{D2}^-

G_{D1b}^-

G_{T1}^-

G_{Q1}^-

1   2   3   4

Fig. 1. TLC of gangliosides from SSPE brain (channel 2).
Channels 1,3,4 are gangliosides of normal human brain.
TLC plate, 20 cm x 40 cm, coated with 250 μ silica gel G.
Developing solvent: $CHCl_3$–CH_3OH–2.5N NH_4OH (60:40:9),
two ascending runs. Resorcinol-HCl spray.

demyelination. The total ganglioside concentration of
white matter was normal while that in gray was slightly
depressed.

The origin of these ganglioside changes is not
clear at present. That they may not be directly
related to the viral etiology is suggested by the fact
that a somewhat similar pattern was observed in such
non-viral diseases as metachromatic leucodystrophy (38)
and adrenoleucodystrophy (20). Similar changes were
also seen in Creutzfeldt-Jakob disease (39), now
recognized as a slow virus condition involving an agent
not yet characterized as to viral type (13). However,
Creutzfeldt-Jakob disease induced in chimpanzees by
injection of extracts from affected human brains
failed to show the abnormal pattern, although kuru did
so partially in having an elevation of ganglioside G_{D3}
(47). This ganglioside was greatly elevated in
multiple sclerosis plaques (46) and also in a case
diagnosed as congenital amaurotic idiocy (15). Thus,
elevation of this ganglioside or the other three does
not appear at first glance to be pathognomonic for any
specific disease category. However, it should be borne
in mind that brains whose diseased state is not
primarily viral in origin could still suffer a secondary
viral infection that might affect glycolipid patterns.

In addition to the ganglioside changes noted
above, SSPE white matter showed other lipid abnormalities including some that were characteristic of
severe demyelination (32). Thus, cholesterol ester
was present (27% of total lipid) while cerebrosides,
ethanolamine phosphatides and proteolipid protein were
significantly decreased below normal levels. Other
lipids showed smaller decreases. The myelin itself,
though having a normal lipid-protein ratio and normal
morphology, had a cholesterol content 50% above normal
with a concomitant decrease of cerebrosides, sulfatides
and proteolipid protein.

VIRUS ISOLATION AND CHARACTERIZATION

Virions were isolated in high purity by the procedure of Miller et al. (28,30). Doubly-clo..ed, early passage wild-type Edmonston strain measles virus and Hallé strain of SSPE virus were grown at 37° in CV-1 (monkey kidney) cells in Eagle's medium containing 10% fetal calf serum. The multiplicity of infection was 0.05 pfu/cell. At 42-48 hrs after infection, when the cytopathic effect involved over 80% of the cells, the supernatant fluids containing the released particles were collected and clarified by centrifugation at 1000 x g for five minutes. The virions were agglutinated and precipitated from the supernatant fluid with concanavalin A. After centrifugation at 10,000 x g for ten minutes, the complex was resuspended in NET buffer (pH 7.3) and the lectin eluted with 0.4M alpha methylmannoside. The virus was further purified by two successive equilibrium centrifugations through linear 15-60% sucrose gradients in NET buffer (pH 7.3). As observed previously (28), two major populations of infectious particles were produced which banded at 1.21 g/cc and 1.18 g/cc. A third minor population of virions was also present at a density of 1.15 g/cc but this was available in quantities insufficient for analysis. All three peaks contained infectious particles. Pooled samples of the two major fractions were used for lipid analysis.

A pelleted sample of each density population was fixed in phosphate-buffered 2.5% glutaraldehyde, post-fixed in 1% osmium tetroxide and processed for electron microscopy. Ultrastructural examination revealed close morphological similarities between the viruses. The predominant measles fraction, banding at 1.18 g/cc, appeared (Fig. 2B) identical to infectious particles noted in primary neural cultures and in vivo studies with hamster brain (2,35). These "standard particles" consisted of roughly circular structures, approximately 0.5 μ in diameter, enclosed by a unit membrane which is the lipid-containing envelope. The latter was seen to be coated with electron-dense external spike material. Within the virion could be seen fuzzy-coated

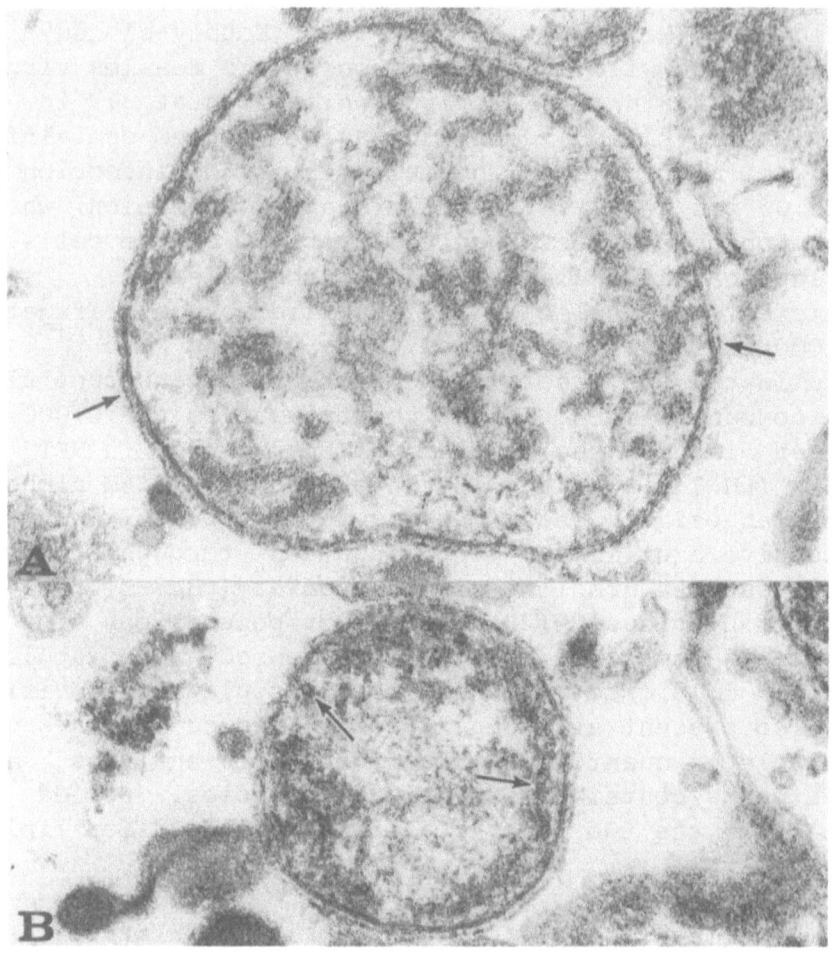

<u>Fig. 2.</u> Electron micrograph of typical measles virions.
<u>A</u> Large particle (high density, banding at 1.21 g/ml).
Note that the membrane is covered by an outer fuzzy
coating of spike material (arrows) while within the
particle, randomly scattered 16-18 nm granular nucleocapsids are seen. X 100,000.
<u>B</u> Standard particle (banding at 1.18 g/ml). The viral
envelope is covered with spike material (as above) but
in this smaller virion the nucleocapsid is aligned
beneath the membrane (arrows). X 100,000.

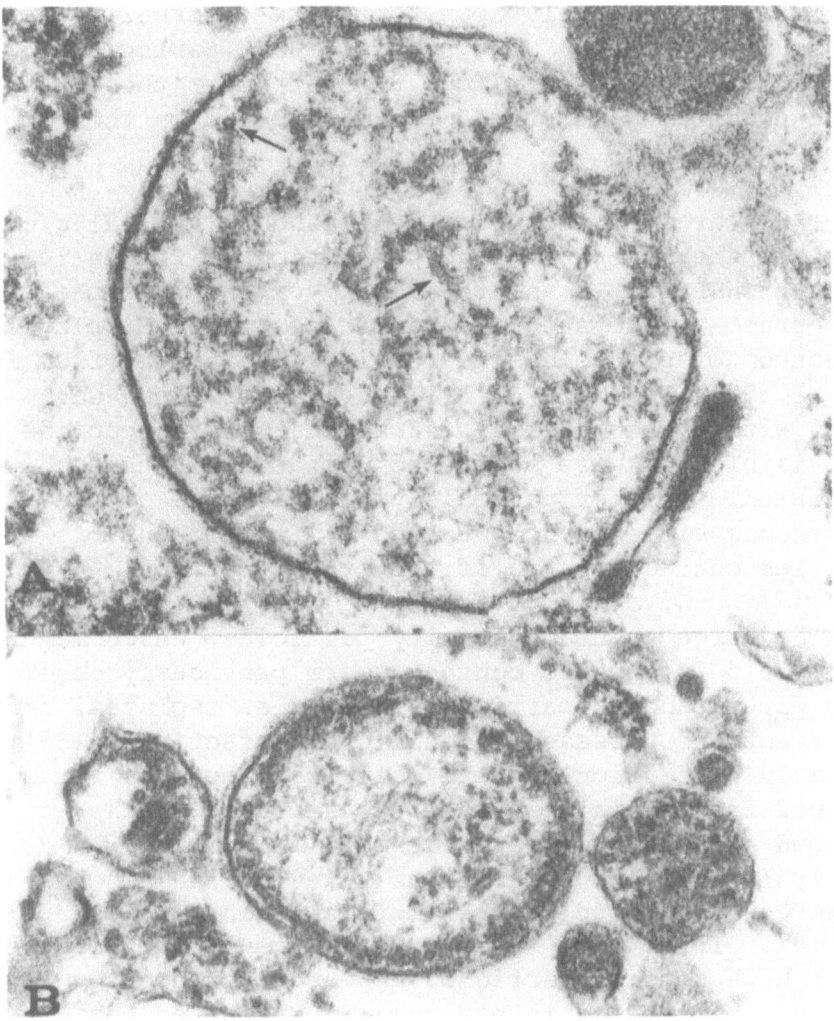

Fig. 3. Electron micrograph of typical SSPE virions.
A Large particle (high density, banding at 1.21 g/ml).
The virion envelope is covered with fuzzy spike material
and nucleocapsids (arrows) are randomly scattered
throughout the matrix of the particle. X 100,000.
B Standard particle (banding at 1.18 g/ml). Note
alignment of nucleocapsid beneath the envelope. The
latter is covered with spike material (as above). A
smaller virion is also seen to the left. X 100,000.

nucleocapsids (16-18 nm diameter), each a helically
coiled filament closely apposed to the internal surface
of the unit membrane. The standard SSPE particle had
an identical appearance (Fig. 3B) but under these
growth conditions comprised the minor band on the
sucrose gradient.

The "large" virion fraction, banding at 1.21 g/cc,
comprised the major particle population of the Hallé
strain of SSPE virus and the minor component of measles.
In contrast to the standard particles, these displayed
a spectrum of particle size ranging in diameter from
0.7 - 1.25 μ (Figs. 2A, 3A). The viral envelope was
coated with spike material and abundant nucleocapsids
were visible and were scattered haphazzardly throughout
the virion. Neither particle population was completely
homogeneous since each contained a minor amount of
particles characteristic of the other fraction.

The large or heavy density particles, which may be
heteroploid in genetic content, were previously observed
along with standard particles in measles isolates, and
both fractions possessed significant infectivity (33).
Similarly, infection of HeLa cells with measles virus
obtained from serial passages of undiluted stocks
produced at least two particle populations (7).
Negatively stained preparations revealed the denser
and larger virion to contain more abundant nucleocapsid
material. In both of these studies, generation of the
larger high density particles appeared enhanced by a
high multiplicity of infection. It was noted that the
decrease in cytopathic effect accompanying the use of
undiluted stocks could be correlated with inhibited
syncytial formation as well as decreasing yields of
infectious particles.

LIPID ISOLATION AND ANALYSIS

An aliquot of the virus suspension in sucrose was
taken for protein determination (27) and the remainder,
amounting to a few mg of virus, was pelleted by
centrifugation and washed to remove sucrose. Lipids

were extracted with chloroform-methanol (1:1)[*], an
aliquot taken for phosphorus determination, and the
remainder fractionated into acidic and non-acidic
lipids with a DEAE-Sephadex column (26). The F-1
fraction, eluted from the column with methanol-
chloroform-water (60:30:8), contained cholesterol and
the major phospholipids: lecithin, ethanolamine
phosphoglyceride and sphingomyelin. Cholesterol was
analyzed by GLC, using an OV-1 column (250°C) and
cholestane as internal standard. The three phospholipids were separated by TLC [silica gel H, chloroform-
methanol-15M NH_4OH (70:30:5)], and the zones after
iodine detection were scraped from the plate and
analyzed for phosphorus. Summation of the individual
phospholipids agreed well with the phosphorus value for
the entire F-1 fraction.

The F-2 fraction, eluted from DEAE-Sephadex with
methanol-chloroform-0.8M sodium acetate (60:30:8) and
containing acidic lipids, was reduced to a small volume
and adjusted to pH 3 with 1N HCl. It was lyophilized
to dryness and the lipids extracted from the sodium
chloride with chloroform-methanol (1:1). This solution
was applied to a 1 g Unisil column and the lipids were
eluted with 100 ml of the same solvent. For most
samples the entire F-2 fraction was utilized for GLC
assay of gangliosides (45) but one of the more abundant
samples was also analyzed for acidic phospholipids (see
below). The analytical results are summarized in Table 1,
all values being normalized to 1000 μg of viral protein.

In addition to the three major phospholipids in F-1
of DEAE-Sephadex,phosphorus-containing substances of
unknown structure were detected by analysis of zones
outside the major visible TLC bands; they amounted to
4-16% of total phospholipid. The quantities of acidic
phospholipid eluted in DEAE-Sephadex fraction F-2 were
too small for accurate determination in most samples
and they were accordingly estimated on the basis of
determinations made with the more abundant SSPE large

---

[*]All solvent ratios are by volume.

TABLE 1

LIPID COMPOSITION OF MEASLES AND SSPE VIRIONS

	MEASLES		SSPE	
	Standard	Large	Standard	Large
Protein	1000	1000	1000	1000
Cholesterol	102	75	59	49
Phospholipid, Total*	289	200	247	184
Phospholipid, F-1	245	164	174	131
Ethanolamine Phosphoglyceride	66 (26%)	54 (32%)	49 (27%)	40 (29%)
Lecithin	105 (42%)	70 (42%)	68 (37%)	53 (38%)
Sphingomyelin	50 (20%)	38 (23%)	36 (20%)	38 (27%)
Unidentified	30 (12%)	6 (4%)	30 (16%)	8 (6%)
Phospholipid, F-2 (Acidic)**	18	15	30	22
Gangliosides***	4.8	3.7	3.9	9.6
Total lipid	370	258	270	212
Phospholipid (F-1)/Cholesterol	2.17	2.16	2.60	2.68

Values are expressed on the basis of 1000 μg of viral protein; values in ( ) are % of F-1 phospholipid.

*Calculated by multiplying phosphorus content of the total C-M extract by 25. This includes an estimated 7-15% of non-lipid phosphorus, of unknown identity.

**Calculated as 42% of the difference between total and F-1 phospholipid.

***Calculated by multiplying sialic acid by 4.

particles. In this case it was found that only 42% of
phosphorus initially present in the fraction was eluted
from the final Unisil column. The remainder was
presumably non-lipid phosphorus that was retained by
the silica gel. The acidic phospholipids have not yet
been identified.

The ganglioside isolation procedure was based on
that previously described for tissues (26), with a
modification that eliminated dialysis and resultant
possible loss of gangliosides. In assaying by GLC,
sialic acid identification was affirmed by the use of
both OV-1 and OV-225 columns (45). N-acetylneuraminic
acid was the only type of sialic acid detected.

DISCUSSION

Measles virus is classified among the paramyxoviruses even though differing from the majority of these in
lacking neuraminidase. An important biological property
of virtually all members of this group is their ability
to cause persistent, noncytocidal infection of cultured
cells (42). SSPE virus is generally regarded as an
example of a persistent infection of the human central
nervous system by a measles virus, the evidence being
high antibody titers to measles in the sera, CSF and
brain extracts of SSPE patients (10,41) and the fact
that measles-like viruses have been isolated from SSPE
brain tissue by cocultivation with non-neural cell lines
(19,34,40). Suckling mice have also proved useful for
isolating virus from brain biopsy specimens of SSPE
patients (14).

The precise relationship between measles and SSPE
viruses is not yet clear. The possibility that SSPE
virus might be a genetically modified measles virus was
suggested by the need for specialized cultivation
techniques for virus isolation from infected cells (12)
and also by apparent differences between the virions of
certain strains in cell culture (36). Other considerations have led to speculation that they are actually
the same virus but behave differently in different

hosts due to defects in the plasma membrane (31).
Evidence for regions of non-homology between complement-
ary RNA from measles SSPE virions was provided by RNA-
RNA hybridization studies (44) while differences in
growth pattern and host range have also been reported
(40). In one comparison of structural polypeptides
(37) five of the proteins showed identical mobilities
on polyacrylamide gel electrophoresus but the sixth,
representing the smallest protein and the one associated
with the membrane, showed a slight difference in
molecular weights between measles and SSPE. Another
such study (29) found no differences in migration rates
between corresponding bands but more subtle differences
were not ruled out.

The first series of lipid analyses presented here
indicate envelope composition that would be expected
for two closely related viruses grown in identical
cultures. The same three major phospholipids were
present in approximately the same proportions in all
four isolates. Cholesterol, however, showed somewhat
greater variation than expected. The standard particles
had proportionately more total lipid than the corresponding heavy particles, in keeping with their relative
banding densities. The indication that both measles
particles had somewhat higher lipid content than the
corresponding SSPE fractions cannot yet be evaluated.

A large body of evidence suggests that the lipids
of the paramyxovirus virion are largely determined by
the host cell, in particular the plasma membrane from
which virus budding occurs (reviewed in ref. 8). A
different point of view holds that the viral envelope
proteins determine the lipid composition of the virion
by selective association with lipids (reviewed in ref. 3),
although the evidence for this theory is limited. Studies
employing spin-label electron spin resonance suggest
that the envelope lipids of paramyxovirus virions are
present in a bilayer (24). In addition to providing the
structural matrix for the viral membrane, lipids are
likely to have other functions as suggested by the
finding (18) that ethanolamine phosphoglyceride under-
went reaggregation with the glycoproteins of measles
virus to reconstitute active hemolytic activity. There

are also intriguing reports (1,6,14) of a non-specific phospholipid inhibitor against measles virus that prevents infection of certain cells in culture.

Ganglioside presence in the viral membrane was consistent with the absence of neuraminidase in these virions. They amounted to slightly over 1% of total lipid in three of the samples and about 4.5% in the SSPE large particles. Vesicular stomatitis virus, another virion lacking the enzyme, was found to contain the same ganglioside present in the plasma membrane of the host cell (23). The ganglioside concentration in that virus (4.4 µg/mg protein) was quite similar to that of the measles virus in this study. It has been suggested (9,21,22) that cells with relatively high ganglioside and low ethanolamine phosphoglyceride content are relatively more susceptible to cell fusion but the significance of this apparent correlation has not yet been determined.

ACKNOWLEDGEMENTS

This investigation was supported by research grants from the U.S. Public Health Service (NS-03356, NS-04834, NS-08952, NS-10931 and NS-70265), and a grant from the National Multiple Sclerosis Foundation (RG 1006-A-1). Fig. 1 is reproduced with permission of the Journal of Lipid Research. The skillful technical assistance of Mrs. Patricia Olenen is gratefully acknowledged.

REFERENCES

1.   Albrecht, P., and Schumacher, H.P., Markers for measles virus. I. Physical properties, Arch. ges. Virusforsch. 36, 23 (1972).

2.   Baringer, J.R. and Griffith, J.S., Experimental measles virus encephalitis. A light, phase, fluorescence and electron microscopic study, Lab. Invest. 23, 335 (1970).

3.   Blough, H.A., and Tiffany, J.M., Lipids in viruses,
      Adv. Lipid Res. 11, 267 (1973).

4.   Brady, R.O., Fishman, P.H., Biosynthesis of
      glycolipids in virus-transformed cells, Biochim.
      Biophys. Acta 355, 121 (1974).

5.   Brady, R.O., and Mora, P.T., Alterations in
      ganglioside pattern and synthesis in SV40- and
      polyoma virus-transformed mouse cell lines,
      Biochim. Biophys. Acta 218, 308 (1970).

6.   Burnstein, T., Swango, L.J., and Byington, D.P.,
      Non-specific brain inhibitor against measles
      virus, Arch. ges. Virusforsch. 34, 396 (1971).

7.   Chiarina, A., and Norrby, E., Separation and
      characterization of products of two measles
      variants, Arch. Res. Virusforsch. 29, 205 (1970).

8.   Choppin, P.W., and Compans, R.W., Reproduction of
      Paramyxovirus, in Comprehensive Virology, Vol. 4,
      (H. Fraenkel-Conrat and R.R. Wagner, eds.) New
      York and London, Plenum Press (1975) pp. 95-178.

9.   Choppin, P.W., Klenk, H.-D., Compans, R.W., and
      Caliguiri, L.A., The parainfluenza virus SV5 and
      its relationship to the cell membrane in
      "Perspectives in Virology", Vol. VII (M. Pollard,
      ed.) New York, Academic Press (1971) pp. 127-158.

10.   Connolly, J.H., Allen, I.V., Hurwitz, L.J., and
      Millar, J.H.D., Measles-virus antibody and antigen
      in subacute sclerosing panencephalitis, Lancet I,
      542 (1967).

11.   Cumings, J.N., Some biochemical considerations
      regarding different forms of demyelination, in
      "Mechanisms of Demyelination", (A.S. Rose and C.M.
      Pearson, eds.) New York, McGraw Hill, Inc. (1963)
      pp. 58-71.

12. Gajdusek, C.J., Slow virus diseases of the central nervous system, Amer. J. clin. Path. 56, 320 (1971).

13. Gajdusek, D.C., and Gibbs, C.J., Subacute and chronic disease caused by atypical infections with unconventional viruses in aberrant hosts, Perspectives in Virol., 8 279 (1973).

14. Greenham, L., Ferguson, M. and Peacock, D., SSPE measles virus: non-productive and productive infection in Vero cells and suckling mice, Med. Microbiol. & Immunol. 160, 201 (1974).

15. Hagberg, B., Hultquist, G., Ohman, R., and Svennerholm, L., Congenital amaurotic idiocy, Acta Paed. Scand. 54, 116 (1965).

16. Hakomori, S., and Murakami, W.T., Glycolipids of hamster fibroblasts and derived malignant-transformed cell lines, Proc. Natl. Acad. Sci. 59, 254 (1968).

17. Hakomori, S., Teather, C., and Andrews, H., Organization difference of cell surface "hematoside" in normal and virally transformed cells, Biochem. Biophys. Res. Comm. 33, 563 (1968).

18. Hall, W.W., and Martin, S.J., Structure and function relationships of the envelope of measles virus, Med. Microbiol. & Immunol. 160, 143 (1974).

19. Horta-Barbosa, L., Fuccillo, D.A., Sever, J.L., and Zeman, W., Subacute sclerosing panencephalitis: Isolation of measles virus from a brain biopsy, Nature 221, 974 (1969).

20. Igarashi, M., Schaumburg, H.H., Powers, J., Kishimoto, Y., Kolodny, E., and Suzuki, K., Fatty acid abnormality in adrenoleukodystrophy, J. Neurochem. in press.

21.   Klenk, H.-D., and Choppin, P.W., Lipids of plasma
      membranes of monkey and hamster kidney cells and
      of parainfluenza virions grown in these cells,
      Virology 38, 255 (1969).

22.   Klenk, H.-D., and Choppin, P.W., Plasma membrane
      lipids and parainfluenza virus assembly, Virology
      40, 939 (1970).

23.   Klenk, H.-D., and Choppin, P.W., Glycolipid content
      of vesicular stomatitis virus grown in baby hamster
      kidney cells, J. Virol. 7, 416 (1971).

24.   Landsberger, F.R., Compans, R.W., Choppin, P.W.,
      and Lenard, J., Organization of the lipid phase in
      viral membranes. Effects of independent variation
      of the lipid and the protein composition, Biochem.
      12, 4498 (1973).

25.   Ledeen, R., Salsman, K., and Cabrera, M.,
      Gangliosides in subacute sclerosing leukoencephali-
      tis: isolation and fatty acid composition of nine
      fractions, J. Lipid Res. 9, 129 (1968).

26.   Ledeen, R.W., Yu, R.K., and Eng, L.F., Gangliosides
      of human myelin: sialosylgalactosylceramide (G_7)
      as a major component, J. Neurochem. 21, 829 (1973).

27.   Lowry, O.H., Rosebrough, N.J., Farr, A.L., and
      Randall, R.J., Protein measurement with the Folin
      phenol reagent, J. Biol. Chem. 193, 269 (1951).

28.   Miller, C.A., and Fields, B.N., Biochemical
      analysis of measles and SSPE viruses (abst.)
      J. Neuropath. Exp. Neurol. in press.

29.   Miller, C.A., Raine, C.S., and Fields, B.N.,
      Comparative biochemical analysis of measles and
      SSPE viruses. In preparation.

30.   Miller, C.A., Raine, C.S., and Fields, B.N.,
      Biochemical characterization of measles virus
      after Concanavalin A purification, In preparation.

31. Norrby, E., Subacute sclerosing panencephalitis
     and measles virus, Ann. clin. Res. 5, 288 (1973).

32. Norton, W.T., Poduslo, S.E., and Suzuki, K.,
     Subacute sclerosing leukoencephalitis, J. Neuro-
     path. and Exptl. Neurol. 25, 582 (1966).

33. Numazaki, J., and Karzon, D., Density separable
     fractions during growth of measles virus, J. Immun.
     97, 458 (1966).

34. Payne, F.E., and Baublis, J.V., Measles virus
     strains isolated from SSPE patients, Internat.
     Virol. (Proc. 2nd Internat. Cong. for Virol.,
     Budapest), Vol. 2, p. 202, Basel:Karger (1972).

35. Raine, C.S., Feldman, L.A., Sheppard, R.D.,
     Bornstein, M.B., Ultrastructure of measles virus
     in cultures of hamster cerebellum, J. Virol. 4,
     169 (1969).

36. Raine, C.S., Feldman, L.A., Sheppard, R.D., and
     Bornstein, M.B., Subacute sclerosing panencephali-
     tis virus in cultures of organized central
     nervous tissue, Lab. Invest. 28, 627 (1973).

37. Schluederberg, A., Chavanick, S., Lipman, M.B.,
     and Carter, C., Comparative molecular weight
     estimates of measles and subacute sclerosing
     panencephalitis virus structural polypeptides by
     simultaneous electrophoresis in acrylamide gel
     slabs, Biochem. Biophys. Res. Comm. 58, 647 (1974).

38. Suzuki, K., Ganglioside patterns of normal and
     pathological brains, in "Inborn Disorders of
     Sphingolipid Metabolism" (S.M. Aronson and B.W.
     Volk, eds.), Oxford and New York, Pergamon Press,
     Inc., (1967) pp. 215-230.

39. Suzuki, K., and Chen, G., Chemical studies on
     Jakob-Creutzfeldt disease, J. Neuropathol. &
     Exptl. Neurol. 25, 396 (1966).

40. ter Meulen, V., Katz, M., and Müller, D., Subacute
     sclerosing panencephalitis: a review, Curr. Top.
     Microbiol. Immun. 57, 1 (1972).

41. Tourtellotte, W.W., Packer, J.A., Herndon, R.M.,
     and Cuadros, C.V., subacute sclerosing panencepha-
     litis: brain immunoglobulin-G, measles antibody
     and albumin, Neurol. 18, 117 (1968).

42. Walker, D.L., Persistent viral infection in cell
     cultures, in "Medical and Applied Virology" (M.
     Sanders, and E.H. Lennette, eds.) St. Louis,
     Warren H. Green, Inc. (1968) pp. 99-110.

43. Wender, M., Psychiat. Neurol. 141, 381 (1961).

44. Yeh, J., Characterization of virus-specific RNAs
     from subacute sclerosing panencephalitis virus-
     infected CV-1 cells, J. Virol. 12, 962 (1973).

45. Yu, R.K., and Ledeen, R.W., Gas-liquid chromato-
     graphic assay of lipid-bound sialic acids:
     measurement of gangliosides in brain of several
     species, J. Lipid Res. 11, 506 (1970).

46. Yu, R.K., Ledeen, R.W., and Eng, L.F., Ganglioside
     abnormalities in multiple sclerosis, J. Neurochem.
     23, 169 (1974).

47. Yu, R.K., Ledeen, R.W., Gajdusek, D.C., and Gibbs,
     C.J., Ganglioside changes in slow virus diseases:
     analyses of chimpanzee brains infected with kuru
     and Creutzfeldt-Jakob agents, Brain Res. 70, 103
     (1974).

Allen C. Crocker

Children's Hospital Medical Center and
Harvard Medical School
Boston, Massachusetts

The present (1975) Symposium on the Sphingolipidoses has
a secure and audacious tone--a reasonable reflection of
the state of the art in basic studies of the inborn errors
of metabolism in lipids, mucopolysaccharides, and saccharides. The prototypic lipidoses (Tay-Sachs, Gaucher,
Niemann-Pick diseases) no longer dominated the agenda.
More recently-described syndromes, such as fucosidosis
and mannosidosis, captured major attention, and there was
a comfortable acknowledgement that common features of
enzymology and tissue effects in the mucopolysaccharidoses and saccharidoses fully justified their joint consideration with the lipidoses. Of the 16 syndromes re-
ceiving primary consideration in the Symposium reports,
all but three (adrenoleukodystrophy, neuronal ceroid
lipofuscinosis, and polyunsaturated fatty acid lipidosis)
had an identified enzymopathy of relevance. Heterozygote
and prenatal homozygote diagnosis has now usually been
achieved or is thought technically possible in the
majority of these conditions. This more stable situation
allowed Symposium authors to devote their energies to an
advanced technology which, on occasion, leaves the
historic worker in the field of the lipidoses somewhat
breathless (to be an "historic worker" one must have been
active in this area before the time of the first Symposium,
in 1958!) It can assuredly be claimed that scientific
study of the inborn error syndromes related to large or
membrane-related molecules has come of age. The papers
in this Symposium constitute a progress report, part of
of a continuum of related works for these authors. In

the sum they are a documentation of handsome and substantial contributions in a difficult and heretofore
often obscure area of biologic inquiry. In the opinion
of this reviewer, the principal subjects of significance
can be gathered into the headings listed below.

IMPROVED UNDERSTANDING OF THE RELEVANT ENZYMOPATHY

Complexities of the enzyme situation for various reactions were discussed, including the soluble and
particulate forms of beta-glucosidase in Gaucher's
disease (Kanfer et al), the acid and alkaline components of ceramidase in Farber's disease (Dulaney et al),
the polymorphism of alpha-L-fucosidase in fucosidosis
(Hirschhorn et al)(Patel & Zeman), the isoenzymes of
mannosidase, with various cation effects, in mannosidosis (Desnick et al)(Lundblad et al), the various species
of sphingomyelinase in Niemann-Pick disease (Callahan &
Khalil), and the enzyme system components for hexosaminidase (Lowden et al).

Improved technology was presented for some assay systems,
such as iduronate sulfatase for carrier detection in
Hunter syndrome (Neufeld et al), a new substrate for
measurement of aryl sulfatase in fibroblasts and leukocytes in metachromatic leukodystrophy and Maroteaux-Lamy
syndrome (Kolodny & Mumford), and hexosaminidase A assay
in urine and tears in Tay-Sachs disease (Saifer et al).

Progress was reported in studies of the sulfatases of
Morquio and Maroteaux-Lamy syndromes (Dorfman et al),
difficulties were described in assessing peroxidase results in neuronal ceroid lipofuscinosis (Haust et al),
and the special features were mentioned of "an enzyme in
search of a disease," alpha-N-acetylgalactosaminidase
(Sung & Sweeley).

DOCUMENTATION OF BROADER TISSUE EFFECTS
FROM THE ENZYMOPATHY

It is now apparent that description of the biochemical
aberrations resulting from a single enzymatic deficiency
must per force be more extensive than was formerly considered. These effects can be due to the pertinence of
multiple potential substrates, such as for a beta- or
alpha-hexosidase enzyme, or, as Brunngraber et al point
out, turnover of membrane materials may involve sequential degradation of a variety of macro-molecular components and failure to degrade one may inhibit catabolism

of the entire complex. Many authors in this Symposium
provided information on tissue accumulation of somewhat
analogous catabolic products from glycoproteins in
seemingly dissimilar syndromes--such as oligosaccharides
and glycopeptides in G$_{M1}$-gangliosidosis, type I, and
Sandhoff disease (Wolfe & Ng Ying Kin), mannosidosis
(Lundblad et al), and fucosidosis (Dawson & Tsay).
Brunngraber et al mentioned as well the accumulation of
glycopeptides in Niemann-Pick and Gaucher's diseases and
in metachromatic leukodystrophy--but these are not found
in Tay-Sachs, Krabbe's, or neuronal ceroid lipofuscinosis
diseases. Unusual "fucolipids" are found in fucosidosis
(Hirschhorn et al)(Dawson and Tsay). Also of pertinence
is the identification of an increased psychosine level in
the brain of Krabbe's disease, plus several higher hexosylceramides (Vanier & Svennerholm), and various complex
sphingolipids in Farber's disease (Dulaney et al).

MORE COMPLETE DESCRIPTION OF NEWER SYNDROMES

This Symposium served as an occasion for recording considerably extended perimeters for the clinical definition
of certain syndromes, particularly fucosidosis (Landing
et al)(Hirschhorn et al)(Patel & Zeman) and adrenoleukodystrophy (Schaumburg et al), the latter suggesting an
abandonment of usage of the old term, Schilder's disease.
Mannosidosis was also well summarized (Desnick et al).
And the syndrome of "polyunsaturated fatty acid lipidosis," with its disturbance especially of arachidonic
acid metabolism, was presented in detail by Svennerholm.

EXPERIMENTAL MODELS OF INBORN ERROR SYNDROMES

Natural animal occurrences of analogous syndromes were
described for mannosidosis in Angus cattle (Lundblad et
al) and globoid leukodystrophy in dogs (Costantino-
Ceccarini et al). Attempts at induction of disease
pictures of relevance in animals included injection of
chlorphentermine in rats, with production of membranous
cytoplasmic bodies (Adachi et al), induction of globoid
cells in rat brain by injection of lactosylceramide
(Suzuki et al), and injection of mice with a beta-
glucosidase inhibitor, conduritol-B-epoxide to produce
a Gaucher-disease-like model (Kanfer et al). Schneck
et al established cultures of fetal Tay-Sachs disease
cerebellar cells, which showed similarities and differences chemically to fetal and infant Tay-Sachs disease
brain. Philippart & Kamensky pursued elaborate experiments in the chemical induction of lysosomal inclusions,

using retinol, chloroquine, AC 3579 (a diazafluoranthen
derivative), sphingomyelin, and n-acetyl-neuraminic acid;
their report contains a provocative inventory of possible
mechanisms for natural and experimental production of
lysosomal storage phenomena.

IMPROVED TECHNOLOGY FOR TISSUE STUDIES

Many of the papers from this Symposium have significant
new suggestions regarding analytical methods for the
study of enzymes and metabolites in tissues and body
fluids. Of particular note, however, are the reports of
McCluer & Jungalwala on the use of "high performance
liquid chromatography" for the analysis of glyco- and
phospholipids, and of Ellis & Patrick on procurement of
subcellular granules of white blood cells for enzyme
assay.

RELATED TISSUE STUDIES IN SPECIAL SITUATIONS

Bogoch has described interesting biologic aspects of
glycoproteins derived from brain tumors (with relation
to similar elements in Tay-Sachs disease brain), and
Ledeen reports on tissue ganglioside modification in
slow virus infection.

THERAPEUTIC IMPLICATIONS

It is a tribute to the level of resolve of many of the
contributors to this Symposium that the biochemical
modification for the described metabolic handicaps was
indeed considered approachable. The nihilism which has
dominated this field for years was no longer present, and
an atmosphere of high potential existed suggesting that
durable efforts in this area are within grasp. Intracellular incorporation of purified enzymes by fibroblasts
in tissue culture, a critically significant observation,
was again described, in this instance for fucosidase
(Hirschhorn et al). Possible modification of mannosidase
activity levels, per activation by zinc or cobalt cations
was also noted (Desnick et al). Radin speculated on the
use of enzyme inhibitors to slow accumulation of deleter-
ious metabolites, with particular reference to trials with
hexyl glucosyl sphingosine. Elaborate experiments were
reported by Weissmann et al on the intracellular transfer
of enzyme entrapped in liposomes coated with aggregated
immunoglobulin, including movement of hexosaminidase A
into Tay-Sachs disease neutrophils. The area of direct
replacement enzyme therapy by intravenous provision of

<u>purified materials</u> was summarized by Brady et al, repre-
senting the most advanced efforts of this sort--particu-
larly including work with Fabry and Gaucher diseases.
The technical concerns are listed, as well as the
significant evidences of important preliminary achieve-
ments.

FINAL COMMENTS

As has been noted, clinical concerns for the individuals
involved in the syndromes under discussion have indeed
been analyzed, particularly as they present specific
morbidity. It is also of relevance that in the majority,
the patients also have very commanding needs for developmental and educational supports. It is encouraging that
in current times a more favorable situation prevails for
the procurement of effective programs in this regard.
It is urged that workers who have responsibility for the
care and guidance of young people with inborn errors of
metabolism seek active consultation with child development, psychology, and special education resources.
Developmental assessment on a continuing basis, with
design of appropriate treatment and educational plans
(including stimulation programs, preschools, developmental day care programs, etc.) can provide critical
assistance for those children in whom developmental
handicap is a significant component.

CONTRIBUTORS AND PARTICIPANTS

MASAZUMI ADACHI, Department of Neuropathology, Isaac
    Albert Research Institute of the Kingsbrook Jewish
    Medical Center and Department of Pathology, State
    University of New York, Downstate Medical Center,
    Brooklyn, New York.

OMAR S. ALFI, Department of Pediatrics, Childrens
    Hospital of Los Angeles and University of Southern
    California School of Medicine, Los Angeles,
    California.

JUNE AMOROSO, Department of Biochemistry, Isaac Albert
    Research Institute of the Kingsbrook Jewish Medical
    Center, Brooklyn, New York.

DANIEL AMSTERDAM, Department of Microbiology, Isaac
    Albert Research Institute of the Kingsbrook Jewish
    Medical Center, Brooklyn, New York and Department
    of Microbiology, Mt. Sinai School of Medicine of
    The City University of New York, New York, New York.

PETER M. ANDERSON, Department of Genetics and Cell
    Biology and the Dight Institute for Human Genetics,
    University of Minnesota, Minneapolis, Minnesota.

BRADLEY ARBOGAST, Departments of Pediatrics and Biochem-
    istry, Joseph P. Kennedy, Jr. Mental Retardation
    Research Center and Pritzker School of Medicine,
    University of Chicago, Chicago, Illinois.

JAMES AUSTIN, Department of Neurology, University of
    Colorado Medical Center, Denver, Colorado.

NICOLE BAUMANN, Laboratoire de Neurochimie, Hôpital de
    la Salpêtrière, Paris, France.

NICOLAS G. BERATIS, Department of Pediatrics, Mt. Sinai
    School of Medicine of the City University of New
    York, New York, New York.

WILLIAM B. BERGREN, Department of Pathology, Childrens
    Hospital of Los Angeles and University of Southern
    California School of Medicine, Los Angeles,
    California.

591

BRUNO BERRA, Istituto Di Chimica Biologica Dell'Univer-
     sita Di Milano, Facolta di Medicina, Milano, Italy.

SAMUEL BOGOCH, Dreyfus Medical Foundation, New York,
     New York.

ROSCOE O. BRADY, Developmental and Metabolic Neurology
     Branch, National Institute of Neurological and
     Communicative Disorders and Stroke, National
     Institutes of Health, Bethesda, Maryland.

STEVEN BROOKS, Department of Microbiology, Isaac Albert
     Research Institute of the Kingsbrook Jewish Medical
     Center, Brooklyn, New York.

JOHN D. BROOME, Department of Pathology, State University
     of New York, Downstate Medical Center, Brooklyn,
     New York.

ERIC G. BRUNNGRABER, Missouri Institute of Psychiatry
     School of Medicine, University of Missouri-Columbia,
     St. Louis, Missouri, Illinois State Psychiatric
     Institute, Chicago, Illinois.

ROBERT M. BURTON, The Edward Mallinckrodt Department of
     Pharmacology, Washington University School of
     Medicine, St. Louis, Missouri.

JOHN W. CALLAHAN, Research Institute, The Hospital for
     Sick Children, Ontario, Canada.

CHARLES COHEN, Department of Medicine, Division of
     Rheumatology, New York University Medical Center,
     New York, New York.

JANET COLLINS, Department of Neurology, University of
     Colorado Medical Center, Denver, Colorado.

ELVIRA COSTANTINO-CECCARINI, The Saul R. Korey Depart-
     ment of Neurology and Rose F. Kennedy Center for
     Research in Mental Retardation and Human Development,
     Albert Einstein College of Medicine of Yeshiva
     University, Bronx, New York.

ALLEN C. CROCKER, Developmental Evaluation Clinic, Child-
     ren's Hospital Medical Center, Boston, Massachusetts.

LEONARD G. DAVIS, Illinois State Psychiatric Institute,
     Chicago, Illinois.

GLYN DAWSON, Departments of Pediatrics and Biochemistry, Joseph P. Kennedy Jr. Mental Retardation Research Center, University of Chicago, Chicago, Illinois.

ANATOLE S. DEKABAN, Developmental and Metabolic Neurology Branch, National Institute of Neurological and Communicative Disorders and Stroke, National Institute of Health, Bethesda, Maryland.

ROBERT DESNICK, Departments of Pediatrics, Genetics and Cell Biology and the Dight Institute for Human Genetics, University of Minnesota, Minneapolis, Minnesota.

GEORGE N. DONNELL, Department of Pediatrics, Childrens Hospital of Los Angeles and University of Southern California School of Medicine, Los Angeles, California.

ALBERT DORFMAN, Departments of Pediatrics and Biochemistry, Joseph P. Kennedy, Jr. Mental Retardation Research Center, Pritzker School of Medicine, University of Chicago, Chicago, Illinois.

GISÈLE DUBOIS, Laboratoire de Neurochimie, Hôpital de la Salpêtrière, Paris, France.

JOHN DULANEY, Department of Biochemistry, Eunice Kennedy Shriver Center for Mental Retardation, Waltham, Massachusetts and Massachusetts General Hospital, Boston, Massachusetts.

ROLAND B. ELLIS, MRC Clinical Genetics Unit and Department of Chemical Pathology, Institute of Child Health, London, England.

THOMAS F. FLETCHER, Department of Veterinary Biology, College of Veterinary Medicine, University of Minnesota, St. Paul, Minnesota.

JORDI FOLCH-PI, Department of Biological Chemistry, Harvard Medical School, Boston, Massachusetts.

ANDREW E. GAL, Developmental and Metabolic Neurology Branch, National Institute of Neurological and Communicative Disorders and Stroke, National Institutes of Health, Bethesda, Maryland.

BRUCE A. GORDON, Departments of Pathology, Biochemistry and Pediatrics, CPRI and the University of Western Ontario, Ontario, Canada.

MARK GREENBAUM, Department of Neurology, Isaac Albert
    Research Institute of the Kingsbrook Jewish Medical
    Center, Brooklyn, New York.

JAMES E. HALEY, Departments of Neurology, Biochemistry,
    Pathology and Neuroscience, Albert Einstein College
    of Medicine of Yeshiva University, Bronx, New York.

M. DARIA HAUST, Departments of Pathology, Biochemistry
    and Pediatrics, CPRI and the University of Western
    Ontario, Ontario, Canada.

SUE R. HIBBERT, Developmental and Metabolic Neurology
    Branch, National Institute of Neurological and
    Communicative Disorders and Stroke, National
    Institutes of Health, Bethesda, Maryland.

GEORGE G. HINTON, Departments of Pathology, Biochemi-
    stry and Pediatrics, CPRI and the University of
    Western Ontario, Ontario, Canada.

KURT HIRSCHHORN, Department of Pediatrics, Mt. Sinai
    School of Medicine of The City University of New
    York, New York, New York.

LINDA HOFFMAN, Department of Neurochemistry, Isaac
    Albert Research Institute of the Kingsbrook
    Jewish Medical Center, Brooklyn, New York.

SYLVIA HOFFSTEIN, New York University Medical Center,
    Division of Rheumatology, Department of Medicine,
    New York, New York.

PETER HÖSLI, Department of Molecular Biology, Institut
    Pasteur, Paris, France.

FELICITY N. HOWARD, Research Institute, The Hospital
    for Sick Children, Ontario, Canada.

MASAHIRO IGARASHI, The Saul R. Korey Department of
    Neurology and the Rose F. Kennedy Center for
    Research in Mental Retardation and Human Develop-
    ment, Albert Einstein College of Medicine of
    Yeshiva University, Bronx, New York.

JUSTUS C. IKONNE, Departments of Pediatrics, Genetics
    and Cell Biology and the Dight Institute for Human
    Genetics, University of Minnesota, Minneapolis,
    Minnesota.

JAVAID I. JAVAID, Illinois State Psychiatric Institute, Chicago, Illinois.

ANNE B. JOHNSON, The Saul R. Korey Department of Neurology and the Rose F. Kennedy Center for Research in Mental Retardation and Human Development, Albert Einstein College of Medicine of Yeshiva University, Bronx, New York.

FIROZE B. JUNGALWALA, Department of Biochemistry, Eunice Kennedy Shriver Center at the Walter E. Fernald State School, Waltham, Massachusetts.

ELSA KAMENSKY, Mental Retardation Center, University of California, Los Angeles, California.

SHIGEHIKO KAMOSHITA, Department of Pediatrics, Jichi Medical School, Tochigi-ken, Tokyo, Japan.

JULIAN N. KANFER, Eunice Kennedy Shriver Center at the Walter E. Fernald State School, Waltham, Massachusetts.

MARY KHALIL, Research Institute, The Hospital for Sick Children, Ontario, Canada.

N.M.K. NG YING KIN, The Donner Laboratory of Experimental Neurochemistry, Montreal Neurological Institute, McGill University, Montreal, Canada.

Y. KISHIMOTO, Eunice Kennedy Shriver Center at the Walter E. Fernald State School, Waltham, Massachusetts.

TERUO KITAGAWA, Department of Pediatrics, Nihon University School of Medicine, Tokyo, Japan.

EDWIN H. KOLODNY, Department of Neurology, Harvard Medical School, Boston, Massachusetts, and Department of Biochemistry, Eunice Kennedy Shriver Center at the Walter E. Fernald State School, Waltham, Massachusetts.

J.W. KUSIAK, Developmental and Metabolic Neurology Branch, National Institute of Neurological and Communicative Disorders and Stroke, National Institutes of Health, Bethesda, Maryland.

R.S. LABOW, Department of Biochemistry, University of Ottawa, Ontario, Canada.

BENJAMIN H. LANDING, Departments of Pathology and Pedia-
    trics, Childrens Hospital of Los Angeles and Univer-
    sity of Southern California School of Medicine,
    Los Angeles, California.

D.S. LAYNE, Department of Biochemistry, University of
    Ottawa, Ontario, Canada.

ROBERT W. LEDEEN, Departments of Neurology, Biochemistry,
    Pathology and Neuroscience, Albert Einstein College
    of Medicine of Yeshiva University, Bronx, New York.

FRED A. LEE, Department of Radiology, Childrens Hospital
    of Los Angeles and University of Southern California
    School of Medicine, Los Angeles, California.

G. LEGLER, Institut für Biochemie der Universitat Köln,
    Köln, Germany.

INGEBORG LIEBAERS, Section on Human Biochemical Genetics,
    National Institute of Arthritis, Metabolism and
    Digestive Diseases, National Institutes of Health,
    Bethesda, Maryland.

TIMPLE W. LIM, Section on Human Biochemical Genetics,
    National Institute of Arthritis, Metabolism and
    Digestive Diseases, National Institutes of Health,
    Bethesda, Maryland.

J. ALEXANDER LOWDEN, Research Institute, The Hospital
    for Sick Children, Ontario, Canada.

JACK LUBOWSKY, Scientific Computer Center, State Uni-
    versity of New York, Downstate Medical Center,
    Brooklyn, New York.

ARNE LUNDBLAD, Department of Clinical Chemistry,
    University Hospital, Lund, Sweden.

BARBARA MASK, Department of Neuropathology, Isaac Albert
    Research Institute of the Kingsbrook Jewish Medical
    Center, Brooklyn, New York.

PARVESH MASSON, Department of Clinical Chemistry,
    University Hospital, Lund, Sweden.

REUBEN MATALON, Departments of Pediatrics and Biochem-
    istry, Joseph P. Kennedy, Jr. Mental Retardation
    Research Center, Pritzker School of Medicine,
    University of Chicago, Chicago, Illinois

ROBERT H. McCLUER, Department of Biochemistry, Eunice Kennedy Shriver Center at the Walter E. Fernald State School, Waltham, Massachusetts.

CAROL A. MILLER, Departments of Neurology, Biochemistry, Pathology and Neuroscience, Albert Einstein College of Medicine of Yeshiva University, Bronx, New York.

AUBREY MILUNSKY, Eunice Kennedy Shriver Center at the Walter E. Fernald State School, Waltham, Massachusetts and Massachusetts General Hospital, Boston, Massachusetts.

GEORGE E. MOOK, Developmental and Metabolic Neurology Branch, National Institute of Neurological and Communicative Disorders and Stroke, National Institutes of Health, Bethesda, Maryland.

HUGO W. MOSER, Eunice Kennedy Shriver Center at the Walter E. Fernald State School, Waltham, Massachusetts and Massachusetts General Hospital, Boston, Massachusetts.

RICHARD A. MUMFORD, Eunice Kennedy Shriver Center at the Walter E. Fernald State School, Waltham, Massachusetts.

ELIZABETH F. NEUFELD, Section on Human Biochemical Genetics, National Institute of Arthritis, Metabolism and Digestive Diseases, National Institutes of Health, Bethesda, Maryland.

HARRY B. NEUSTEIN, Department of Pathology, Childrens Hospital of Los Angeles and University of Southern California School of Medicine, Los Angeles, California.

WON G. NG, Department of Pathology, Childrens Hospital of Los Angeles and University of Southern California School of Medicine, Los Angeles, California.

NILS E. NORDÉN, Department of Clinical Chemistry, University Hospital, Lund, Sweden.

PER-ARNE ÖCKERMAN, Department of Clinical Chemistry, University Hospital, Lund, Sweden.

MARIKO ODAWARA, Department of Pediatrics, Jichi Medical
     School, Tochigi-ken, Tokyo, Japan.

MISAO OWADA, Department of Pediatrics, Nihon University
     School of Medicine, Tokyo, Japan.

VIMALKUMAR PATEL, Division of Neuropathology, Indiana
     University Medical Center, Indianapolis, Indiana.

A.D. PATRICK, MCR Clinical Genetics Unit and Department
     of Chemical Pathology, Institute of Child Health,
     London, England.

PETER G. PENTCHEV, Developmental and Metabolic Neurology
     Branch, National Institute of Neurological and
     Communicative Disorders and Stroke, National
     Institutes of Health, Bethesda, Maryland.

GUTA PERLE, Genetic Laboratory, Isaac Albert Research
     Institute of the Kingsbrook Jewish Medical Center,
     Brooklyn, New York.

MICHEL PHILIPPART, Mental Retardation Center, University
     of California, Los Angeles, California.

BETTY PINKETT, Department of Neurology, Isaac Albert
     Research Institute of the Kingsbrook Jewish Medical
     Center, Brooklyn, New York.

CALVIN H. PLIMPTON, President, State University of New
     York, Downstate Medical Center, Brooklyn, New York.

JAMES M. POWERS, Department of Pathology, Medical
     University of South Carolina, Charleston, South
     Carolina.

JANE M. QUIRK, Development and Metabolic Neurology
     Branch, National Institute of Neurological and
     Communicative Disorders and Stroke, National
     Institutes of Health, Bethesda, Maryland.

NORMAN S. RADIN, Mental Health Research Institute and
     Department of Biological Chemistry, University of
     Michigan, Ann Arbor, Michigan.

SRINI S. RAGHAVEN, Eunice Kennedy Shriver Center at the
   Walter E. Fernald State School, Waltham, Massachusetts.

CEDRIC S. RAINE, The Saul R. Korey Department of Neurology
   and the Rose F. Kennedy Center for Research in Mental
   Retardation and Human Development, Albert Einstein
   College of Medicine of Yeshiva University, Bronx,
   New York.

MOHANRREDDY K. RAMAN, Departments of Pediatrics, Genetics
   and Cell Biology and the Dight Institute for Human
   Genetics, University of Minnesota, Minneapolis,
   Minnesota.

ABRAHAM SAIFER, Department of Biochemistry, Isaac Albert
   Research Institute of the Kingsbrook Jewish Medical
   Center, Brooklyn, New York.

HERBERT H. SCHAUMBURG, The Saul R. Korey Department of
   Neurology and the Rose F. Kennedy Center for Re-
   search in Mental Retardation and Human Development,
   Albert Einstein College of Medicine of Yeshiva
   University, Bronx, New York.

LARRY SCHNECK, Department of Neurology, Isaac Albert
   Research Institute of the Kingsbrook Jewish Medical
   Center, Brooklyn, New York.

HARVEY L. SHARP, Departments of Pediatrics, Genetics and
   Cell Biology, University of Minnesota, Minneapolis,
   Minnesota.

JAMES SIDBURY, National Institute of Child Health and
   Human Development, National Institutes of Health,
   Bethesda, Maryland.

C. SPIELVOGEL, Eunice Kennedy Shriver Center at the
   Walter E. Fernald State School, Waltham, Massachusetts.

PHILIP STURGEON, Brentwood Laboratories, Los Angeles,
   California.

J. SULLIVAN, Eunice Kennedy Shriver Center at the
   Walter E. Fernald State School, Waltham, Massachusetts.

SUN-SANG J. SUNG, Department of Biochemistry, Michigan
    State University, East Lansing, Michigan.

KINUKO SUZUKI, The Saul S. Korey Department of Neurology,
    and Rose F. Kennedy Center for Research in Mental
    Retardation and Human Development, Albert Einstein
    College of Medicine of Yeshiva University, Bronx,
    New York.

KUNIHIKO SUZUKI, The Saul S. Korey Department of Neurol-
    ogy and Rose F. Kennedy Center for Research in
    Mental Retardation and Human Development, Albert
    Einstein College of Medicine of Yeshiva University,
    Bronx, New York.

LARS SVENNERHOLM, Department of Neurochemistry, Psychi-
    atric Research Center, University of Göteborg,
    Göteborg, Sweden.

SIGFRID SVENSSON, Department of Clinical Chemistry,
    University Hospital, Lund, Sweden.

CHARLES C. SWEELEY, Department of Biochemistry, Michigan
    State University, East Lansing, Michigan.

JOHN F. TALLMAN, Developmental and Metabolic Neurology
    Branch, National Institute of Neurological and
    Communicative Disorders and Stroke, National
    Institutes of Health, Bethesda, Maryland.

HARUMI TANAKA, The Saul S. Korey Department of Neurology
    and Rose F. Kennedy Center for Research in Mental
    Retardation and Human Development, Albert Einstein
    College of Medicine of Yeshiva University, Bronx,
    New York.

CHHIN-YANG TSAI, Department of Pathology, Isaac Albert
    Research Institute of the Kingsbrook Jewish Medical
    Center, Brooklyn, New York.

GRACE CHEN TSAY, Departments of Pediatrics and Biochem-
    istry, Joseph P. Kennedy Jr. Mental Retardation
    Research Center, University of Chicago, Chicago,
    Illinois.

BRYAN M. TURNER, Department of Pediatrics, Mt. Sinai
    School of Medicine of The City University of New
    York, New York, New York.

JEAN-CLAUDE TURPIN, Laboratoire de Neurochimie, Hôpital
    de la Salpêtrière, Paris, France.

CARLO VALENTI, Department of Obstetrics and Gynecology, State University of New York, Downstate Medical Center, Brooklyn, New York.

MARIE-THÉRÈSE VANIER, Hôpital Sainte-Eugénie, Lyon, France.

BRUNO W. VOLK, Isaac Albert Research Institute of the Kingsbrook Jewish Medical Center, Department of Pathology, State University of New York, Downstate Medical Center, Brooklyn, New York.

LINDA L. WALLING, Departments of Pediatrics, Genetics and Cell Biology and the Dight Institute for Human Genetics, University of Minnesota, Minneapolis, Minnesota.

GERALD WEISSMANN, Department of Medicine, Division of Rheumatology, New York University Medical Center, New York, New York.

D.G. WILLIAMSON, Department of Biochemistry, University of Ottawa, Ontario, Canada.

LEONHARD S. WOLFE, The Donner Laboratory of Experimental Neurochemistry, Montreal Neurological Institute, McGill University, Montreal, Canada.

WILLIAM WORTH, Department of Neurology, University of Colorado Medical Center, Denver, Colorado.

WARREN YAMADA, Department of Neurology, University of Colorado Medical Center, Denver, Colorado.

MARIKO YOSHIDA, Department of Biochemistry, University of Tokyo School of Medicine, Tokyo, Japan.

WOLFGANG ZEMAN, Division of Neuropathology, Indiana University Medical Center, Indianapolis, Indiana.